Clinical Studies, Big Data, and Artificial Intelligence in Nephrology and Transplantation

Clinical Studies, Big Data, and Artificial Intelligence in Nephrology and Transplantation

Editors

Wisit Cheungpasitporn
Charat Thongprayoon
Wisit Kaewput

MDPI • Basel • Beijing • Wuhan • Barcelona • Belgrade • Manchester • Tokyo • Cluj • Tianjin

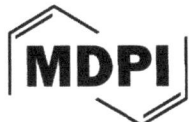

Editors
Wisit Cheungpasitporn
Division of Nephrology and
Hypertension, Department of
Medicine, Mayo Clinic
USA

Charat Thongprayoon
Division of Nephrology and
Hypertension, Department of
Medicine, Mayo Clinic
USA

Wisit Kaewput
Department of Medicine,
Phramongkutklao
College of Medicine
Thailand

Editorial Office
MDPI
St. Alban-Anlage 66
4052 Basel, Switzerland

This is a reprint of articles from the Special Issue published online in the open access journal *Journal of Clinical Medicine* (ISSN 2077-0383) (available at: https://www.mdpi.com/journal/jcm/special_issues/CS_BD_AI_NT).

For citation purposes, cite each article independently as indicated on the article page online and as indicated below:

LastName, A.A.; LastName, B.B.; LastName, C.C. Article Title. *Journal Name* **Year**, *Volume Number*, Page Range.

ISBN 978-3-0365-1134-4 (Hbk)
ISBN 978-3-0365-1135-1 (PDF)

© 2021 by the authors. Articles in this book are Open Access and distributed under the Creative Commons Attribution (CC BY) license, which allows users to download, copy and build upon published articles, as long as the author and publisher are properly credited, which ensures maximum dissemination and a wider impact of our publications.

The book as a whole is distributed by MDPI under the terms and conditions of the Creative Commons license CC BY-NC-ND.

Contents

About the Editors ix

Charat Thongprayoon, Wisit Kaewput, Karthik Kovvuru, Panupong Hansrivijit, Swetha R. Kanduri, Tarun Bathini, Api Chewcharat, Napat Leeaphorn, Maria L. Gonzalez-Suarez and Wisit Cheungpasitporn
Promises of Big Data and Artificial Intelligence in Nephrology and Transplantation
Reprinted from: *J. Clin. Med.* **2020**, *9*, 1107, doi:10.3390/jcm9041107 1

Luisa Averdunk, Jürgen Bernhagen, Karl Fehnle, Harald Surowy, Hermann-Josef Lüdecke, Sören Mucha, Patrick Meybohm, Dagmar Wieczorek, Lin Leng, Gernot Marx, David E. Leaf, Alexander Zarbock, Kai Zacharowski, on behalf of the RIPHeart Study Collaborators, Richard Bucala and Christian Stoppe
The *Macrophage Migration Inhibitory Factor* (MIF) Promoter Polymorphisms (rs3063368, rs755622) Predict Acute Kidney Injury and Death after Cardiac Surgery
Reprinted from: *J. Clin. Med.* **2020**, *9*, 2936, doi:10.3390/jcm9092936 15

Maria Irene Bellini, Aisling E Courtney and Jennifer A McCaughan
Living Donor Kidney Transplantation Improves Graft and Recipient Survival in Patients with Multiple Kidney Transplants
Reprinted from: *J. Clin. Med.* **2020**, *9*, 2118, doi:10.3390/jcm9072118 33

Wisit Cheungpasitporn, Charat Thongprayoon, Pradeep K Vaitla, Api Chewcharat, Panupong Hansrivijit, Felicitas L. Koller, Michael A Mao, Tarun Bathini, Sohail Abdul Salim, Sreelatha Katari, Lee S Cummings, Eddie Island, Jameson Forster and Napat Leeaphorn
Degree of Glomerulosclerosis in Procurement Kidney Biopsies from Marginal Donor Kidneys and Their Implications in Predicting Graft Outcomes
Reprinted from: *J. Clin. Med.* **2020**, *9*, 1469, doi:10.3390/jcm9051469 45

Michele F. Eisenga, Maarten A. De Jong, David E. Leaf, Ilja M. Nolte, Martin H. De Borst, Stephan J. L. Bakker and Carlo A. J. M. Gaillard
Erythropoietin, Fibroblast Growth Factor 23, and Death After Kidney Transplantation
Reprinted from: *J. Clin. Med.* **2020**, *9*, 1737, doi:10.3390/jcm9061737 59

Fabio Fabbian, Alfredo De Giorgi, Emanuele Di Simone, Rosaria Cappadona, Nicola Lamberti, Fabio Manfredini, Benedetta Boari, Alda Storari and Roberto Manfredini
Weekend Effect and in-Hospital Mortality in Elderly Patients with Acute Kidney Injury: A Retrospective Analysis of a National Hospital Database in Italy
Reprinted from: *J. Clin. Med.* **2020**, *9*, 1815, doi:10.3390/jcm9061815 73

Joana Gameiro, Tiago Branco and José António Lopes
Artificial Intelligence in Acute Kidney Injury Risk Prediction
Reprinted from: *J. Clin. Med.* **2020**, *9*, 678, doi:10.3390/jcm9030678 83

Edmund J. Gore, António W. Gomes-Neto, Lei Wang, Stephan J. L. Bakker, Hubert G. M. Niesters, Anoek A. E. de Joode, Erik A. M. Verschuuren, Johanna Westra and Coretta Van Leer-Buter
Torquetenovirus Serum Load and Long-Term Outcomes in Renal Transplant Recipients
Reprinted from: *J. Clin. Med.* **2020**, *9*, 440, doi:10.3390/jcm9020440 101

Caroline Jadlowiec, Maxwell Smith, Matthew Neville, Shennen Mao, Dina Abdelwahab, Kunam Reddy, Adyr Moss, Bashar Aqel and Timucin Taner
Acute Kidney Injury Patterns Following Transplantation of Steatotic Liver Allografts
Reprinted from: *J. Clin. Med.* **2020**, *9*, 954, doi:10.3390/jcm9040954 . . . . **115**

Wisit Kaewput, Charat Thongprayoon, Boonphiphop Boonpheng, Patompong Ungprasert, Tarun Bathini, Api Chewcharat, Narat Srivali, Saraschandra Vallabhajosyula and Wisit Cheungpasitporn
Inpatient Burden and Mortality of Goodpasture's Syndrome in the United States: Nationwide Inpatient Sample 2003–2014
Reprinted from: *J. Clin. Med.* **2020**, *9*, 455, doi:10.3390/jcm9020455 . . . . **125**

Aureliusz Kolonko, Joanna Musialik, Jerzy Chudek, Magdalena Bartmańska, Natalia Słabiak-Błaż, Agata Kujawa-Szewieczek, Piotr Kuczera, Katarzyna Kwiecień-Furmańczuk and Andrzej Więcek
Changes in Office Blood Pressure Control, Augmentation Index, and Liver Steatosis in Kidney Transplant Patients after Successful Hepatitis C Infection Treatment with Direct Antiviral Agents
Reprinted from: *J. Clin. Med.* **2020**, *9*, 948, doi:10.3390/jcm9040948 . . . . **135**

Andreas Kronbichler, Maria Effenberger, Jae Il Shin, Christian Koppelstätter, Sara Denicolò, Michael Rudnicki, Hannes Neuwirt, Maria José Soler, Kate Stevens, Annette Bruchfeld, Herbert Tilg, Gert Mayer and Paul Perco
Is There Decreasing Public Interest in Renal Transplantation? A Google Trends™ Analysis
Reprinted from: *J. Clin. Med.* **2020**, *9*, 1048, doi:10.3390/jcm9041048 . . . . **151**

Yukari Mae, Tomoaki Takata, Ayami Ida, Masaya Ogawa, Sosuke Taniguchi, Marie Yamamoto, Takuji Iyama, Satoko Fukuda and Hajime Isomoto
Prognostic Value of Neutrophil-To-Lymphocyte Ratio and Platelet-To-Lymphocyte Ratio for Renal Outcomes in Patients with Rapidly Progressive Glomerulonephritis
Reprinted from: *J. Clin. Med.* **2020**, *9*, 1128, doi:10.3390/jcm9041128 . . . . **163**

Kinga Musiał, Monika Augustynowicz, Izabella Miśkiewicz-Migoń, Krzysztof Kałwak, Marek Ussowicz and Danuta Zwolińska
Clusterin as a New Marker of Kidney Injury in Children Undergoing Allogeneic Hematopoietic Stem Cell Transplantation—A Pilot Study [†]
Reprinted from: *J. Clin. Med.* **2020**, *9*, 2599, doi:10.3390/jcm9082599 . . . . **175**

Eun Seop Seo, Se In Sung, So Yoon Ahn, Yun Sil Chang and Won Soon Park
Changes in Serum Creatinine Levels and Natural Evolution of Acute Kidney Injury with Conservative Management of Hemodynamically Significant Patent Ductus Arteriosus in Extremely Preterm Infants at 23–26 Weeks of Gestation
Reprinted from: *J. Clin. Med.* **2020**, *9*, 699, doi:10.3390/jcm9030699 . . . . **187**

Tara K. Sigdel, Andrew W. Schroeder, Joshua Y. C. Yang, Reuben D. Sarwal, Juliane M. Liberto and Minnie M. Sarwal
Targeted Urine Metabolomics for Monitoring Renal Allograft Injury and Immunosuppression in Pediatric Patients
Reprinted from: *J. Clin. Med.* **2020**, *9*, 2341, doi:10.3390/jcm9082341 . . . . **197**

Camilo G. Sotomayor, Charlotte A. te Velde-Keyzer, Martin H. de Borst, Gerjan J. Navis and Stephan J.L. Bakker
Lifestyle, Inflammation, and Vascular Calcification in Kidney Transplant Recipients: Perspectives on Long-Term Outcomes
Reprinted from: *J. Clin. Med.* **2020**, *9*, 1911, doi:10.3390/jcm9061911 211

J. Casper Swarte, Rianne M. Douwes, Shixian Hu, Arnau Vich Vila, Michele F. Eisenga, Marco van Londen, António W. Gomes-Neto, Rinse K. Weersma, Hermie J.M. Harmsen and Stephan J.L. Bakker
Characteristics and Dysbiosis of the Gut Microbiome in Renal Transplant Recipients
Reprinted from: *J. Clin. Med.* **2020**, *9*, 386, doi:10.3390/jcm9020386 231

Gerold Thölking, Nils Hendrik Gillhaus, Katharina Schütte-Nütgen, Hermann Pavenstädt, Raphael Koch, Barbara Suwelack and Stefan Reuter
Conversion to Everolimus was Beneficial and Safe for Fast and Slow Tacrolimus Metabolizers after Renal Transplantation
Reprinted from: *J. Clin. Med.* **2020**, *9*, 328, doi:10.3390/jcm9020328 243

Charat Thongprayoon, Javier A. Neyra, Panupong Hansrivijit, Juan Medaura, Napat Leeaphorn, Paul W. Davis, Wisit Kaewput, Tarun Bathini, Sohail Abdul Salim, Api Chewcharat, Narothama Reddy Aeddula, Saraschandra Vallabhajosyula, Michael A. Mao and Wisit Cheungpasitporn
Serum Klotho in Living Kidney Donors and Kidney Transplant Recipients: A Meta-Analysis
Reprinted from: *J. Clin. Med.* **2020**, *9*, 1834, doi:10.3390/jcm9061834 255

Johannes von Einsiedel, Gerold Thölking, Christian Wilms, Elena Vorona, Arne Bokemeyer, Hartmut H. Schmidt, Iyad Kabar and Anna Hüsing-Kabar
Conversion from Standard-Release Tacrolimus to MeltDose® Tacrolimus (LCPT) Improves Renal Function after Liver Transplantation
Reprinted from: *J. Clin. Med.* **2020**, *9*, 1654, doi:10.3390/jcm9061654 273

Christoph Weber, Lena Röschke, Luise Modersohn, Christina Lohr, Tobias Kolditz, Udo Hahn, Danny Ammon, Boris Betz and Michael Kiehntopf
Optimized Identification of Advanced Chronic Kidney Disease and Absence of Kidney Disease by Combining Different Electronic Health Data Resources and by Applying Machine Learning Strategies
Reprinted from: *J. Clin. Med.* **2020**, *9*, 2955, doi:10.3390/jcm9092955 289

Katie Wong, Amanda Owen-Smith, Fergus Caskey, Stephanie MacNeill, Charles RV Tomson, Frank JMF Dor, Yoav Ben-Shlomo, Soumeya Bouacida, Dela Idowu and Pippa Bailey
Investigating Ethnic Disparity in Living-Donor Kidney Transplantation in the UK: Patient-Identified Reasons for Non-Donation among Family Members
Reprinted from: *J. Clin. Med.* **2020**, *9*, 3751, doi:10.3390/jcm9113751 309

Manuela Yepes-Calderón, Camilo G. Sotomayor, Daniel Guldager Kring Rasmussen, Ryanne S. Hijmans, Charlotte A. te Velde-Keyzer, Marco van Londen, Marja van Dijk, Arjan Diepstra, Stefan P. Berger, Morten Asser Karsdal, Frederike J. Bemelman, Johan W. de Fijter, Jesper Kers, Sandrine Florquin, Federica Genovese, Stephan J. L. Bakker, Jan-Stephan Sanders and Jacob Van Den Born
Biopsy-Controlled Non-Invasive Quantification of Collagen Type VI in Kidney Transplant Recipients: A Post-Hoc Analysis of the MECANO Trial
Reprinted from: *J. Clin. Med.* **2020**, *9*, 3216, doi:10.3390/jcm9103216 325

Philip Zeuschner, Linda Hennig, Robert Peters, Matthias Saar, Johannes Linxweiler, Stefan Siemer, Ahmed Magheli, Jürgen Kramer, Lutz Liefeldt, Klemens Budde, Thorsten Schlomm, Michael Stöckle and Frank Friedersdorff
Robot-Assisted versus Laparoscopic Donor Nephrectomy: A Comparison of 250 Cases
Reprinted from: *J. Clin. Med.* **2020**, *9*, 1610, doi:10.3390/jcm9061610 . . . . **337**

Philip Zeuschner, Urban Sester, Michael Stöckle, Matthias Saar, Ilias Zompolas, Nasrin El-Bandar, Lutz Liefeldt, Klemens Budde, Robert Öllinger, Paul Ritschl, Thorsten Schlomm, Janine Mihm and Frank Friedersdorff
Should We Perform Old-For-Old Kidney Transplantation during the COVID-19 Pandemic? The Risk for Post-Operative Intensive Stay
Reprinted from: *J. Clin. Med.* **2020**, *9*, 1835, doi:10.3390/jcm9061835 . . . . **349**

About the Editors

Wisit Cheungpasitporn is American board certified in Nephrology and Internal Medicine. He completed his nephrology fellowship training at Mayo Clinic, Rochester, Minnesota. Here, Dr. Cheungpasitporn also completed additional training and has become an expert on kidney transplantation. He also completed a postdoctoral appointment as part of the clinical and translational science (CCaTS) program in 2015. Dr. Cheungpasitporn received the 2016 Donald C. Balfour Research Award, given in recognition of outstanding research as a junior scientist whose primary training is in a clinical field at Mayo Clinic, Rochester, Minnesota, as well as the 2016 William H.J. Summerskill Award, given in recognition of outstanding achievement in research for a clinical fellow at Mayo Clinic, Rochester, Minnesota. Dr. Cheungpasitporn joined the Division of Nephrology and Hypertension at Mayo Clinic, where he has served since August 2020.

Charat Thongprayoon MD; Division of Nephrology and Hypertension, Department of Medicine, Mayo Clinic, Rochester, MN, USA. Email: charat.thongprayoon@gmail.com. Dr. Charat Thongprayoon, MD is affiliated with Mayo Clinic Hospital, Rochester. Interests: nephrology; electrolytes; acute kidney injury; renal replacement therapy; epidemiology; outcome study.

Wisit Kaewput MD; Department of Medicine, Phramongkutklao College of Medicine, Bangkok, Thailand. Email: wisitnephro@gmail.com. Dr. Wisit Kaewput is affiliated with Phramongkutklao College of Medicine, Bangkok, Thailand. Interests: acute kidney injury; observational studies; statistical analysis; epidemiology.

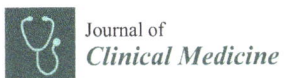 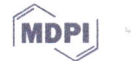

Editorial

Promises of Big Data and Artificial Intelligence in Nephrology and Transplantation

Charat Thongprayoon [1], Wisit Kaewput [2], Karthik Kovvuru [3], Panupong Hansrivijit [4], Swetha R. Kanduri [3], Tarun Bathini [5], Api Chewcharat [1], Napat Leeaphorn [6], Maria L. Gonzalez-Suarez [3] and Wisit Cheungpasitporn [3,*]

[1] Division of Nephrology, Department of Medicine, Mayo Clinic, Rochester, MN 55905, USA; charat.thongprayoon@gmail.com (C.T.); api.che@hotmail.com (A.C.)
[2] Department of Military and Community Medicine, Phramongkutklao College of Medicine, Bangkok 10400, Thailand; wisitnephro@gmail.com
[3] Division of Nephrology, Department of Medicine, University of Mississippi Medical Center, Jackson, MS 39216, USA; kkovvuru@umc.edu (K.K.); skanduri@umc.edu (S.R.K.); mgonzalezsuarez@umc.edu (M.L.G.-S.)
[4] Department of Internal Medicine, University of Pittsburgh Medical Center Pinnacle, Harrisburg, PA 17105, USA; hansrivijitp@upmc.edu
[5] Department of Internal Medicine, University of Arizona, Tucson, AZ 85721, USA; tarunjacobb@gmail.com
[6] Department of Nephrology, Department of Medicine, Saint Luke's Health System, Kansas City, MO 64111, USA; napat.leeaphorn@gmail.com
* Correspondence: wcheungpasitporn@gmail.com; Tel.: +1-601-984-5670; Fax: +1-601-984-5765

Received: 1 April 2020; Accepted: 9 April 2020; Published: 13 April 2020

Abstract: Kidney diseases form part of the major health burdens experienced all over the world. Kidney diseases are linked to high economic burden, deaths, and morbidity rates. The great importance of collecting a large quantity of health-related data among human cohorts, what scholars refer to as "big data", has increasingly been identified, with the establishment of a large group of cohorts and the usage of electronic health records (EHRs) in nephrology and transplantation. These data are valuable, and can potentially be utilized by researchers to advance knowledge in the field. Furthermore, progress in big data is stimulating the flourishing of artificial intelligence (AI), which is an excellent tool for handling, and subsequently processing, a great amount of data and may be applied to highlight more information on the effectiveness of medicine in kidney-related complications for the purpose of more precise phenotype and outcome prediction. In this article, we discuss the advances and challenges in big data, the use of EHRs and AI, with great emphasis on the usage of nephrology and transplantation.

Keywords: artificial intelligence; machine learning; big data; nephrology; transplantation; kidney transplantation; acute kidney injury; chronic kidney disease

1. Introduction

Kidney diseases, such as acute kidney injury (AKI) and chronic kidney disease (CKD) are major medical and public health issues worldwide, associated with high death and morbidity rates, together with great economic loss [1–6]. CKD is linked with a higher danger of argumentative outcomes, like cardiovascular complications, death, decreased quality of life, and substantial healthcare resource utilization [7–11], and it has been assessed that around 850 million individuals suffer different types of kidney diseases globally [12,13]. If left untreated, CKD may evolve into end-stage kidney disease (ESKD), which is associated with high mortality [14–16]. It is well-known that kidney diseases are very much multifactorial, with overlapping and complex clinical phenotypes, as well as morphologies [17].

The global distribution of nephrologists usually differs from one country to another, with bigger differences in its overall capacity [18]. Various nations across the world have established surveillance systems for kidney-related infections. Despite such attempts, the literature highlights that surveillance systems within third world countries are still not very strong [19]. In certain areas of some countries, basic records offices for transplantation and dialysis, as well as expert pathologists, are not even available [18,20]. Given how major gaps are always found in the main workforce in nephrology, the current eminence of kidney health management and research evidence in nephrology needs to be strengthened globally [21].

Traditionally, the randomized controlled trial (RCT) has always been used as the point of reference for offering evidence-based treatment. The numerical formulae applied in analyzing randomized control data have equally offered essential insights from numerous observational data. In the past few years, great emphasis has been placed on the pragmatic RCT, an essential component of real global research, which is applied when evaluating the great interventions within the actual clinical setting based on a great amount of samples so as to stimulate their individual practical value. A great amount of differences have been reported within nephrology, as well as some other relevant specialties. For instance, the literature indicates that nephrology trials were very limited in number and possessed minimally optimal features of high-quality designs [22]. Despite the fact that the already existing studies, as well as implemented works, have made major additions to a highly reliable prognostication, as well as an extensive understanding of the general histologic pathology, there is still a great amount of work which needs to be undertaken, as well as specific problems to be solved. The general capacity for undertaking cohort studies that involve a large sample size or Rapid Control trial is very much present across various parts of the globe, and has thereby resulted in the absence of research evidence within nephrology. In addition, limited activity in kidney research has impacted the evidence base for the treatment of kidney diseases, resulting in a lack of useful surrogate end-points for progression from the early stages of kidney disease-hindered trials [14,15]. On the same note, a great amount of cohort data could also be applied in generating relevant hypotheses and provide major insights into the etiology, pathogenesis, and prognosis of kidney diseases [23,24].

Those needs that are classified as unmet require provision of some ample spaces for the purpose of imagination in relation to leveraging the strength associated with big data, as well as relevant artificial intelligence (AI) to improve the overall status of patients with kidney diseases [25]. In this article, we discuss the big data concepts in nephrology, describe the potential use of AI in nephrology and transplantation, and also encourage researchers and clinicians to submit their invaluable research, including original clinical research studies [26–30], database studies from registries [31–33], meta-analyses [34–44], and artificial intelligence research [25,45–48] in nephrology and transplantation.

2. Big Data in Nephrology and Transplantation: Registries and Administrative Claims

Table 1 demonstrates known and commonly used databases that have provided big data in nephrology and transplantation [49–51]. For example, the United States Renal Data System (USRDS) is recognized as a state reconnaissance system that has the responsibility of collecting, analyzing, and subsequently distributing information regarding CKD and ESKD, all based on numerous big datasets. By delivering the yearly data report, the USRDS continuously tracks both the epidemiologic and economic burden linked to kidney diseases [52]. An important database in transplantation in the United States is the United Network for Organ Sharing (UNOS). The Organ Procurement and Transplantation Network (OPTN) data are linked by UNOS to the Social Security Death Master File for the purpose of augmenting ascertainment of different groups of candidates, as well as relevant deaths. The final data are attainable by different groups of researchers, and have always been applied in various studies regarding transplantation [50]. In addition to these databases in the United States, other countries worldwide also have big data within nephrology for researchers, such as the National Kidney Disease Surveillance Program in Ireland [53], the surveillance project on CKD management in

Canada [54], and the China Kidney Disease Network (CK-NET), a comprehensive CKD surveillance system for China [55].

Table 1. Nephrology and transplant databases and organizations.

Renal and Transplant Databases	Organizations
<ul><li>United States Renal Data System (USRDS) (https://www.usrds.org)</li><li>Organ Procurement and Transplantation Network (OPTN) (https://optn.transplant.hrsa.gov)</li><li>United Network for Organ Sharing (UNOS) (https://unos.org)</li><li>Scientific Registry of Transplant Recipients (SRTR) (https://www.srtr.org)</li><li>National Health and Nutrition Examination Survey Database (NHANES) (https://www.cdc.gov/nchs/nhanes/index.htm)</li><li>Chronic kidney disease database (CKDd) (http://www.padb.org/ckddb/)</li><li>National Death Index (NDI) (https://www.cdc.gov/nchs/ndi/index.htm)</li><li>Nephrotic Syndrome Study Network (NEPTUNE) (https://nephcure.org/2015/12/nephrotic-syndrome-study-network-neptune/)</li><li>National Inpatient sample (NIS) (https://www.hcup-us.ahrq.gov/news/exhibit_booth/nis_brochure.jsp)</li><li>Polycystic Kidney Disease Consortium Data Base (PKD) (https://pkdcure.org/research-medical-professionals/pkdoc/)</li><li>Kidney Early Evaluation Program Data base (KEEP) (https://www.kidney.org/news/keep)</li><li>Diabetes mellitus Treatment for Renal Insufficiency Consortium Database (DIAMETRIC) (https://www.diametric.nl/diametric-database/)</li><li>Center for Medicare And Medicaid Services (CMS) (https://www.cms.gov)</li><li>Jackson Heart Study (JHS) (https://www.jacksonheartstudy.org)</li></ul>**Gene Based Databases:**<ul><li>CKD- Gen Consortium Database (https://ckdgen.imbi.uni-freiburg.de)</li><li>Genome Wide Association Studies (GWAS) (https://dceg.cancer.gov/research/how-we-study/genomic-studies/gwas-overview)</li><li>Nephro Seq (https://www.nephroseq.org/resource/login.html)</li><li>Renal gene Expression Database (http://rged.wall-eva.net)</li><li>Humana Kidney and Urine Proteome Project (HKUPP) (http://www.hkupp.org)</li><li>Urine protein Biomarker Database (http://122.70.220.102/biomarker)</li><li>Urinary Peptidomics and Peak- maps (http://www.padb.org/updb/)</li><li>Kidney and Urinary Pathway Knowledge Database (KUPKB) (http://www.kupkb.org)</li></ul>	<ul><li>ESRD Networks (https://esrdnetworks.org)</li><li>American Society of Nephrology (ASN) (https://www.asn-online.org)</li><li>National Kidney Foundation (NKF) (https://www.kidney.org)</li><li>International Society of Nephrology (ISN) (https://www.theisn.org)</li><li>American Transplant Congress (ATC) (https://atcmeeting.org)</li><li>Renal Physician Association (RPA) (https://www.renalmd.org)</li><li>International Society of Peritoneal Dialysis (ISPD) (https://ispd.org)</li><li>National Renal Administrators Association (NRAA) (https://www.nraa.org/home)</li><li>Kidney and Urology Foundation of America (http://www.kidneyurology.org)</li><li>American Kidney Fund (https://www.kidneyfund.org/about-us/)</li><li>American Society of Artificial Internal Organs (https://asaio.org/about/)</li><li>Organ Procurement Organization (OPO) (https://unos.org/transplant/opos-increasing-organ-donation)</li><li>Acute Dialysis Quality Initiative (ADQI) (http://www.adqi.net/)</li><li>National Institute of Health (NIH) (https://www.nih.gov)</li><li>National Institute of Diabetes and Digestive and Kidney Diseases (https://www.niddk.nih.gov)</li><li>National Center for Health Statistics (NCHS) (https://www.cdc.gov/nchs/about/index.htm)</li></ul>

Numerous networks of international collaboration, like the International Network of CKD cohorts [56], the Therapeutic Evaluation of Steroids in IgA Nephropathy Global study [57], and the Chronic Kidney Disease Prognosis Consortium [58] have grown immensely within the last few years. There are possible advantages of introducing a traditional data element that are linked to kidney infections, like escalating the overall power of the groups which are under-represented [59]. There is, however, great need to address numerous challenges, like standardization of data, identification of the patient, plus some other additional infrastructure-related challenges. Additionally, the cadre of genomics is developing at a very rapid rate towards realizing an analysis of single cells, and subsequent great advances within metabolomics and proteomics have been developed within the past few years.

A great amount of progress has equally been realized within technological developments within the areas of large-scale molecular data generation in various databases that are gene-based (Table 1). The most recent advancements in technology have made it possible for us to produce larger amounts of data, more specifically regarding the omics data. Further development of somehow less expensive genotype arrays and the subsequent presence of samples within biobanks made it possible to undertake genome-wide association studies among numerous groups of patients, offering highly essential insights into the great risk factors and the pathogenesis of multiple kidney diseases [60–63].

Within nephrology, numerous consortia-collecting biopsy biobanks of kidney tissue have been started to undertake such forms of collaborative study. Several initiatives that are aimed at extensive characterization of the relevant kidney biopsies for various groups of kidney diseases subtypes have subsequently been launched, comprising of the NEPTUNE (Nephrotic Syndrome STudy Network), ERCB (European Renal cDNA Bank), EURenOmics, C-PROBE (Clinical Phenotyping and Resource Biobank), PKU-IgAN, and more recently, TRIDENT (for diabetic nephropathy), CureGN (for glomerulopathies), and the NIDDK (National Institute of Diabetes and Digestive and Kidney Diseases) Kidney Precision Medicine Project (KPMP) [64].

Big data within the medicine field might offer the opportunity to envision patients suffering from kidney diseases in a more holistic manner, using numerous lenses, each of which adequately presents the great opportunity of studying various scientific queries. Such data within the big databases might subsequently comprise of the general administrative health-related data, biometric data, biomarker data, as well as imaging, and might subsequently come from various sources, comprising of electronic health records, biobanks, reports in the internet, and various clinical registries [65]. These data from the large databases are collected and updated overtime. These data are valuable and can be used by researchers to answer numerous research questions and advance knowledge in nephrology and transplantation [66–68].

3. Using Electronic Health Record Data in Nephrology

Two major events have been reported within the last 10 years that seem to have changed the whole situation. To begin with is making it possible to digitalize all relevant medical information—more specifically, the initiation of EHRs that have the medical histories of the patients—and facilitate the processing of medical information using computers. This helps to make information-processing become automated by the use of given specialized software. EHRs have been greatly utilized with major regularity, clinical informatics strategies have subsequently been refined, and subsequently, the EHR field enabled [69,70].

The wide application of EHRs, when put together with the relevant novel of big data, tends to create some forms of unique opportunities for the purpose of nephrology research, as well as improvement in care for individual patients who might be suffering from kidney complications and transplantation. The data which is there within the EHR is considered big insofar as its volume is concerned. Such interventions have resulted in a new era of big data which has subsequently fueled precision medicine. These types of approach have already indicated an improved level of diagnosis, risk assessment, as well as treatment and management of numerous health conditions. With medicine getting digitalized, a great amount of data has since been developed from all aspects of health care, comprising the laboratory tests, EHR, together with medical imaging.

For instance, in the instance of electronic AKI, the automated diagnostic strategy tends to create a great opportunity to initiate predictive strategies, optimize the relevant AKI alerts, and subsequently trace AKI events across various institutions, as well as administrative datasets. The growth in the adoption of EHR and subsequent maturation of the relevant clinical informatics techniques might provide some sort of unique opportunity to advance the general predictive capabilities. Immediately, AKI has been properly diagnosed within real time, and several EHR-enabled interventions have become so viable. One of such great prospects is actually the prediction of detecting events prior to their occurrence [71]. AKI events might temporarily get anchored within the EHR, which develops a pre-disease phase of care, having the information which had accumulated before the development of

AKI. With a greater amount of content, high-throughput strategies can be applied to such a group of data so as to help in identifying a form of pre-AKI signal, which can subsequently assist in discriminating between patients who are of high risk and low risk for the AKI. The capability to predict AKI risk in this manner might subsequently have some forms of dramatic impact, as presently there is no scientifically proven treatment for AKI once one develops such conditions [72]. As patients who are considered to be of high risk get identified, the extent of care can get modified, and further strategies for harm prevention implemented. In the long run, such groups of patients, institutions, and population-based techniques will result in better long- and short-term outcomes for the respective hospitals, patients, and the whole of the healthcare system. Despite the fact that potential barriers are always there, and several nuanced groups need to be taken into consideration, such approaches that are EHR-enabled have the ability to greatly improve AKI-associated knowledge and care.

Patients suffering from kidney complications are reported to have the highest level of heterogeneity in manifestation of the disease, treatment response, and overall progression. The growth in big data actually tends to stimulate the general boom of artificial intelligence that is a perfect tool that helps in handling, and also processing the big data. AI can assist in shedding light on the specific accuracy of medicines used to treat kidney diseases, for outcome prediction, and also to gain a more precise phenotype.

4. Artificial Intelligence in Nephrology and Transplantation

AI presently shows a very important function in nearly all areas of the day-to-day lives of human beings, as well as within different academic disciplines. Based on the fact that there has been growth in the power of computers, developments in techniques and methods, and the overall blast of the quantity of medicine, data has never been an exemption. Literature clarifies that artificial intelligence can be used in disease risk assessment. Actually, disease risk assessment has a very important influence on the general prognosis, as well as clinical intervention strategies. Accurate and rapid assessment can assist clinicians in determining the conditions of the patient, out of which optimal treatment strategies can be implemented. Links between prognosis and risk factors of the diseases are very complex. The same risk factors can be experienced within different groups of diseases, and a single disease can actually be composed of several risk factors. In such case, the links between the known risk factors and the disease has very strong correlativity, instead of simple causality. Artificial intelligence can hence be applied in doing disease risk assessment in order to understand the main factors linked to disease prognosis so as to offer effective treatment for tertiary prevention of the disease. One of the important sections of AI is machine learning, which is characterized as the study of algorithms and statistical models that computer systems utilize to learn from sample data and previous experience without being explicitly programmed to achieve particular assignments. With the ability to identify obscure patterns in the data, we can use machine learning to solve many problems, including assessing relationships of two variables, creating predictions based on baseline characteristics, identifying objects with comparable patterns, and incorporating subjects by specific criteria. Machine learning techniques have the capacities of managing complex datasets and tremendous numbers of variables that are exceeding the capability of classical statistical methods [17]—see Figure 1A. Machine learning algorithms are usually utilized without initiating as many presumptions of the underlying data. In addition, a machine-learning method can determine complex patterns of health trajectories of immense numbers of characteristics and patients, which has exhibited high predictive certainty, and been confirmed and replicated with various validation investigations [73]. Well-known machine-learning algorithms include the artificial neural network (ANN), random forest, gradient boosting trees, and support vector machine [17].

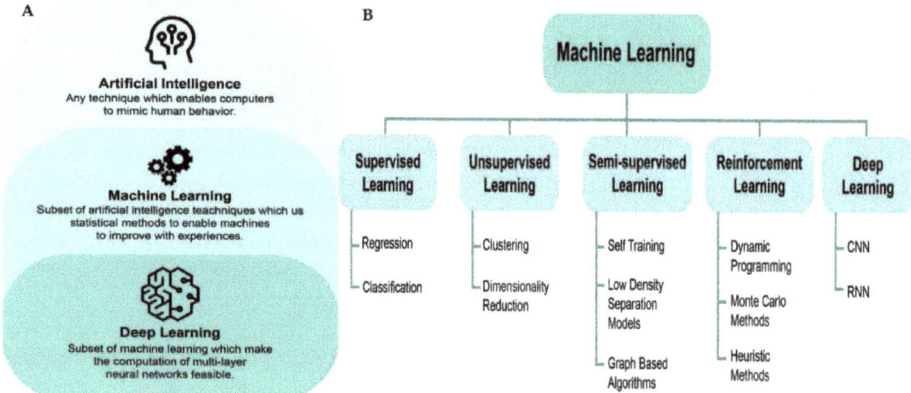

Figure 1. (a) Relationships between artificial intelligence, machine learning, and deep learning. (b) Types of machine learning. CNN, convolutional neural network; RNN, recurrent neural network.

Inspired by the idea of mimicking the biological structure of human brains, deep learning is a subfield of machine learning based on ANN [74]. Deep-learning models can learn many levels of data design with a multiple-processing-layers model structure, attaining more powerful model performance. This cutting-edge technology has significantly changed the paradigm of visual object recognition, speech recognition, and many other domains, such as genomics and drug discovery. Deep learning techniques are increasingly being applied to biomedical data, from image processing to genomic data analysis [75]. Such methods might outperform pathologists' fibrosis scores from histological renal biopsy images [76]. Well-known techniques include the convolutional neural network (CNN), fully connected neural network, generative adversarial network (GAN), deep reinforcement learning, and recurrent neural network (RNN) [17,77], shown in Figure 1B. AI-based clinical decision support systems (CDSS) can be implemented employing the expert system strategy, data-driven approach, or an ensemble approach by coupling both. An expert system consolidates a knowledge base containing a set of rules for specific clinical scenarios, and the initial rule set may be acquired from domain experts or learned from data through machine learning algorithms [72,78–80].

AI has recently been adopted for the prediction, diagnosis, and treatment of kidney diseases [76,81–85], as shown in Table 2. For example, a prediction model based on the combination of a machine learning algorithm and survival analysis has recently developed and can stratify risk for kidney disease progression among patients with IgA Nephropathy [86]. For AKI research, Tomasev et al. [83] recently used deep-learning methods to make a continuous prediction of AKI by developing a RNN model on the sequential health record data of >700,000 veterans, allowing physicians to practise with adequate data and sufficient time. In addition, regarding utilization of ANN and CNN methods, Kolachalama et al. [76] recently provided a perspicacity into the association of pathological fibrosis identified from histologic images with clinical phenotypes for patients with CKD, helping the diagnostics and prognostics of these phenotypes. Subsequently, there has been an increasing number of AI studies, with great emphasis on the usage of nephrology and transplantation [85,87–89].

Table 2. Selected articles reporting the utilization of artificial intelligence, machine learning, or deep learning in the field of nephrology and kidney transplantation.

Study	Country	Study Type	N	Subjects	Intervention
Zhou, 2020 [90]	China	R	212	Prediction of ARF and paraplegia after TAAAR	Machine learning classification models
Xu, 2020 [91]	USA	R	37,486	Identification the sub-phenotypes of AKI	Memory network-based deep learning approach
Song, 2020 [92]	USA	R	14,039	Longitudinal Risk Prediction of CKD in Diabetic Patients	Temporal-enhanced gradient boosting machine
Rashidi, 2020 [93]	USA	P, R	101	Early recognition of burn- and trauma-related AKI	Artificial intelligence/machine learning algorithms
Morid, 2020 [94]	USA	R	22,542	Prediction of adverse events in critical patients with AKI	Temporal pattern detection
Luo, 2020 [95]	China	R	519	Prediction of severe pneumonia during post-transplant hospitalization in recipients of a deceased-donor kidney transplant	Machine learning
Li, 2020 [96]	China	P	1952	Accuracy improvement of GFR estimation	Artificial neural network
Lei, 2020 [97]	China	R	1173	Prediction of AKI after liver cancer resection	Machine learning algorithms
Kate, 2020 [98]	USA	R	44,691	Prediction of AKI in hospitalized patients	Machine learning predictive models
Kang, 2020 [99]	South Korea	R	1571	Prediction of mortality in CRRT patients	Machine learning algorithms
Zimmerman, 2019 [100]	USA	R	23,950	Prediction of AKI following ICU admission	Machine learning models
Zhang, 2019 [101]	China	R	2456	Prediction of volume responsiveness in oliguric AKI	Machine learning models
Xu, 2019 [102]	USA	R	58,976	Prediction of mortality in patients with AKI in the ICU	Machine learning models
Xiao, 2019 [103]	China	R	551	Prediction of CKD progression	Machine learning tools
Mark, 2019 [104]	USA	R	100,000	Prediction of survival of kidney transplant recipients from UNOS	Machine learning models
Bae, 2019 [105]	USA	R	120,818	Prediction of survival after deceased donor kidney transplant from OPTN database	Machine learning methods

AKI, acute kidney injury; ARF, acute renal failure; AUC, area under curve; CKD, chronic kidney disease; CRRT, continuous renal replacement therapy; GFR, glomerular filtration rate; ICU, intensive care unit; OPTN, Organ Procurement and Transplantation Network; P, prospective; R, retrospective; TAAAR, thoracoabdominal aortic aneurysm repair; UNOS, United Network for Organ Sharing.

5. Potential Directions and Future Scope

In order to reinforce the usage and subsequent transformation of AI as well as data–based CDSSs in nephrology, AI, as well as big data, offers the chance to actually source knowledge from expert knowledge and big data and subsequently transform it into some form of intelligent system, which can be applied in risk classification, disease diagnosis, drug discovery, and prognostic evaluation, among some other things. AI might be useful in establishing the type of kidney disease and subsequently help in solving problems related to survival analysis of the patients who have gone through kidney transplants [106–114]. Renal biopsy images may be a good data base for application of machine learning algorithms.

Despite having numerous imperfections, big data, as well as artificial intelligence have been applied in the field of medication from numerous parts [115,116]. There are numerous possible guidelines of using big data and artificial intelligence in nephrology that requires greater attention, as well as further consideration [74,78,117–125].

6. Conclusions

In summary, the present status of kidney health care, and subsequently, research evidence in nephrology requires strengthening. Big data research that is problem-driven in nephrology is very much essential in promoting the interdisciplinary incorporation and subsequent improvements in kidney disease, and it may subsequently offer some greater insights to further studies in the future. Within the present era of using big data, it is strongly believed that big data and artificial intelligence will greatly reshape research done on kidney disease and consequently improve the general clinical practice of nephrology in the near future.

Funding: This research received no external funding.

Conflicts of Interest: We do not have any financial or non-financial potential conflicts of interest.

References

1. Sutherland, S.M.; Goldstein, S.L.; Bagshaw, S.M. Leveraging Big Data and Electronic Health Records to Enhance Novel Approaches to Acute Kidney Injury Research and Care. *Blood Purif.* **2017**, *44*, 68–76. [CrossRef] [PubMed]
2. Kashani, K.; Cheungpasitporn, W.; Ronco, C. Biomarkers of acute kidney injury: The pathway from discovery to clinical adoption. *Clin. Chem. Lab. Med.* **2017**, *55*, 1074–1089. [CrossRef] [PubMed]
3. Srivali, N.; Thongprayoon, C.; Cheungpasitporn, W.; Ungprasert, P.; Caples, S.M. Unusual cause of pleural effusion: Ovarian hyperstimulation syndrome. *QJM* **2016**, *109*, 197–198. [CrossRef] [PubMed]
4. Sanguankeo, A.; Upala, S.; Cheungpasitporn, W.; Ungprasert, P.; Knight, E.L. Effects of Statins on Renal Outcome in Chronic Kidney Disease Patients: A Systematic Review and Meta-Analysis. *PLoS ONE* **2015**, *10*, e0132970. [CrossRef] [PubMed]
5. Cheungpasitporn, W.; Thongprayoon, C.; Kittanamongkolchai, W.; Sakhuja, A.; Mao, M.A.; Erickson, S.B. Impact of admission serum potassium on mortality in patients with chronic kidney disease and cardiovascular disease. *QJM* **2017**, *110*, 713–739. [CrossRef]
6. Jadlowiec, C.; Smith, M.; Neville, M.; Mao, S.; Abdelwahab, D.; Reddy, K.; Moss, A.; Aqel, B.; Taner, T. Acute Kidney Injury Patterns Following Transplantation of Steatotic Liver Allografts. *J. Clin. Med.* **2020**, *9*, 954. [CrossRef]
7. Cheungpasitporn, W.; Thongprayoon, C.; O'Corragain, O.A.; Edmonds, P.J.; Kittanamongkolchai, W.; Erickson, S.B. Associations of sugar-sweetened and artificially sweetened soda with chronic kidney disease: A systematic review and meta-analysis. *Nephrology* **2014**, *19*, 791–797. [CrossRef]
8. Wijarnpreecha, K.; Thongprayoon, C.; Chesdachai, S.; Panjawatanana, P.; Ungprasert, P.; Cheungpasitporn, W. Associations of Proton-Pump Inhibitors and H2 Receptor Antagonists with Chronic Kidney Disease: A Meta-Analysis. *Dig. Dis. Sci.* **2017**, *62*, 2821–2827. [CrossRef]

9. Wijarnpreecha, K.; Thongprayoon, C.; Thamcharoen, N.; Panjawatanan, P.; Cheungpasitporn, W. Association of coffee consumption and chronic kidney disease: A meta-analysis. *Int. J. Clin. Pr.* **2017**, *71*. [CrossRef]
10. Wijarnpreecha, K.; Thongprayoon, C.; Nissaisorakarn, P.; Jaruvongvanich, V.; Nakkala, K.; Rajapakse, R.; Cheungpasitporn, W. Association of Helicobacter pylori with Chronic Kidney Diseases: A Meta-Analysis. *Dig. Dis. Sci.* **2017**, *62*, 2045–2052. [CrossRef]
11. Wijarnpreecha, K.; Thongprayoon, C.; Scribani, M.; Ungprasert, P.; Cheungpasitporn, W. Noninvasive fibrosis markers and chronic kidney disease among adults with nonalcoholic fatty liver in USA. *Eur. J. Gastroenterol Hepatol.* **2018**, *30*, 404–410. [CrossRef]
12. Glassock, R.J.; Warnock, D.G.; Delanaye, P. The global burden of chronic kidney disease: Estimates, variability and pitfalls. *Nat. Rev. Nephrol.* **2017**, *13*, 104–114. [CrossRef]
13. Jha, V.; Garcia-Garcia, G.; Iseki, K.; Li, Z.; Naicker, S.; Plattner, B.; Saran, R.; Wang, A.Y.; Yang, C.W. Chronic kidney disease: global dimension and perspectives. Chronic kidney disease: Global dimension and perspectives. *Lancet* **2013**, *382*, 260–272. [CrossRef]
14. Kaewput, W.; Thongprayoon, C.; Rangsin, R.; Ruangkanchanasetr, P.; Bathini, T.; Mao, M.A.; Cheungpasitporn, W. Association between serum uric acid and chronic kidney disease in patients with hypertension: A multicenter nationwide cross-sectional study. *J. Evid. Based Med.* **2019**, *12*, 235–242. [CrossRef]
15. Piccoli, G.B.; Breuer, C.; Cabiddu, G.; Testa, A.; Jadeau, C.; Brunori, G. Where Are You Going, Nephrology? Considerations on Models of Care in an Evolving Discipline. *J. Clin. Med.* **2018**, *7*, 199. [CrossRef] [PubMed]
16. Kaewput, W.; Thongprayoon, C.; Chewcharat, A.; Rangsin, R.; Satirapoj, B.; Kaewput, C.; Suwannahitatorn, P.; Bathini, T.; Mao, M.A.; Cato, L.D.; et al. Rate of kidney function decline and factors predicting progression of kidney disease in type 2 diabetes mellitus patients with reduced kidney function: A nationwide retrospective cohort study. *Ther. Apher. Dial.* **2020**. [CrossRef] [PubMed]
17. Xie, G.; Chen, T.; Li, Y.; Chen, T.; Li, X.; Liu, Z. Artificial Intelligence in Nephrology: How Can Artificial Intelligence Augment Nephrologists' Intelligence? *Kidney Dis.* **2020**, *6*, 1–6. [CrossRef] [PubMed]
18. Levin, A. Global challenges in kidney diseases. *Nephrol Dial. Transpl.* **2018**, *33*, 371–372. [CrossRef]
19. Yang, C.; Kong, G.; Wang, L.; Zhang, L.; Zhao, M.-H. Big data in nephrology: Are we ready for the change? *Nephrology* **2019**, *24*, 1097–1102. [CrossRef]
20. Kolachalama, V.B.; Singh, P.; Lin, C.Q.; Mun, D.; Belghasem, M.E.; Henderson, J.M.; Francis, J.M.; Salant, D.J.; Chitalia, V.C. Association of Pathological Fibrosis With Renal Survival Using Deep Neural Networks. *Kidney Int. Rep.* **2018**, *3*, 464–475. [CrossRef]
21. Bello, A.K.; Levin, A.; Tonelli, M.; Okpechi, I.G.; Feehally, J.; Harris, D.; Jindal, K.; Salako, B.L.; Rateb, A.; Osman, M.A.; et al. Assessment of Global Kidney Health Care Status. *JAMA* **2017**, *317*, 1864–1881. [CrossRef] [PubMed]
22. Inrig, J.K.; Califf, R.M.; Tasneem, A.; Vegunta, R.K.; Molina, C.; Stanifer, J.W.; Chiswell, K.; Patel, U.D. The landscape of clinical trials in nephrology: A systematic review of Clinicaltrials.gov. *Am. J. Kidney Dis.* **2014**, *63*, 771–780. [CrossRef] [PubMed]
23. Hulsen, T.; Jamuar, S.S.; Moody, A.R.; Karnes, J.H.; Varga, O.; Hedensted, S.; Spreafico, R.; Hafler, D.A.; McKinney, E.F. From Big Data to Precision Medicine. *Front. Med.* **2019**, *6*, 34. [CrossRef] [PubMed]
24. Shilo, S.; Rossman, H.; Segal, E. Axes of a revolution: Challenges and promises of big data in healthcare. *Nat. Med.* **2020**, *26*, 29–38. [CrossRef]
25. Gameiro, J.; Branco, T.; Lopes, J.A. Artificial Intelligence in Acute Kidney Injury Risk Prediction. *J. Clin. Med.* **2020**, *9*, 678.
26. Gore, E.J.; Gomes-Neto, A.W.; Wang, L.; Bakker, S.; Niesters, H.; de Joode, A.; Verschuuren, E.; Westra, J.; Leer-Buter, C.V. Torquetenovirus Serum Load and Long-Term Outcomes in Renal Transplant Recipients. *J. Clin. Med.* **2020**, *9*, 440. [CrossRef]
27. Swarte, J.C.; Douwes, R.M.; Hu, S.; Vich Vila, A.; Eisenga, M.F.; van Londen, M.; Gomes-Neto, A.W.; Weersma, R.K.; Harmsen, H.; Bakker, S. Characteristics and Dysbiosis of the Gut Microbiome in Renal Transplant Recipients. *J. Clin. Med.* **2020**, *9*, 386. [CrossRef]
28. Thölking, G.; Gillhaus, N.H.; Schütte-Nütgen, K.; Pavenstädt, H.; Koch, R.; Suwelack, B.; Reuter, S. Conversion to Everolimus was Beneficial and Safe for Fast and Slow Tacrolimus Metabolizers After Renal Transplantation. *J. Clin. Med.* **2020**, *9*, 328. [CrossRef]

29. Cheungpasitporn, W.; Kremers, W.K.; Lorenz, E.; Amer, H.; Cosio, F.G.; Stegall, M.D.; Gandhi, M.J.; Schinstock, C.A. De novo donor-specific antibody following BK nephropathy: The incidence and association with antibody-mediated rejection. *Clin. Transpl.* **2018**, *32*, e13194. [CrossRef]
30. Chewcharat, A.; Thongprayoon, C.; Cheungpasitporn, W.; Mao, M.A.; Thirunavukkarasu, S.; Kashani, K.B. Trajectories of Serum Sodium on In-Hospital and 1-Year Survival among Hospitalized Patients. *Clin. J. Am. Soc. Nephrol.* **2020**. [CrossRef]
31. Kaewput, W.; Thongprayoon, C.; Boonpheng, B.; Ungprasert, P.; Bathini, T.; Chewcharat, A.; Srivali, N.; Vallabhajosyula, S.; Cheungpasitporn, W. Inpatient Burden and Mortality of Goodpasture's Syndrome in the United States: Nationwide Inpatient Sample 2003–2014. *J. Clin. Med.* **2020**, *9*, 455. [CrossRef] [PubMed]
32. Cheungpasitporn, W.; Thongprayoon, C.; Ungprasert, P.; Wijarnpreecha, K.; Kaewput, W.; Leeaphorn, N.; Bathini, T.; Chebib, F.T.; Kröner, P.T. Subarachnoid Hemorrhage in Hospitalized Renal Transplant Recipients with Autosomal Dominant Polycystic Kidney Disease: A Nationwide Analysis. *J. Clin. Med.* **2019**, *8*, 524. [CrossRef] [PubMed]
33. Leeaphorn, N.; Thongprayoon, C.; Chon, W.J.; Cummings, L.S.; Mao, M.A.; Cheungpasitporn, W. Outcomes of kidney retransplantation after graft loss as a result of BK virus nephropathy in the era of newer immunosuppressant agents. *Am. J. Transpl.* **2019**. [CrossRef] [PubMed]
34. Lertjitbanjong, P.; Thongprayoon, C.; Cheungpasitporn, W.; O'Corragain, O.A.; Srivali, N.; Bathini, T.; Watthanasuntorn, K.; Aeddula, N.R.; Salim, S.A.; Ungprasert, P.; et al. Acute Kidney Injury after Lung Transplantation: A Systematic Review and Meta-Analysis. *J. Clin. Med.* **2019**, *8*, 1713. [CrossRef] [PubMed]
35. Thongprayoon, C.; Kaewput, W.; Thamcharoen, N.; Bathini, T.; Watthanasuntorn, K.; Lertjitbanjong, P.; Sharma, K.; Salim, S.A.; Ungprasert, P.; Wijarnpreecha, K.; et al. Incidence and Impact of Acute Kidney Injury after Liver Transplantation: A Meta-Analysis. *J. Clin. Med.* **2019**, *8*, 372. [CrossRef] [PubMed]
36. Wongboonsin, J.; Thongprayoon, C.; Bathini, T.; Ungprasert, P.; Aeddula, N.R.; Mao, M.A.; Cheungpasitporn, W. Acetazolamide Therapy in Patients with Heart Failure: A Meta-Analysis. *J. Clin. Med.* **2019**, *8*, 349. [CrossRef]
37. Gonzalez Suarez, M.L.; Thongprayoon, C.; Mao, M.A.; Leeaphorn, N.; Bathini, T.; Cheungpasitporn, W. Outcomes of Kidney Transplant Patients with Atypical Hemolytic Uremic Syndrome Treated with Eculizumab: A Systematic Review and Meta-Analysis. *J. Clin. Med.* **2019**, *8*, 919. [CrossRef]
38. Chewcharat, A.; Thongprayoon, C.; Bathini, T.; Aeddula, N.R.; Boonpheng, B.; Kaewput, W.; Watthanasuntorn, K.; Lertjitbanjong, P.; Sharma, K.; Torres-Ortiz, A.; et al. Incidence and Mortality of Renal Cell Carcinoma after Kidney Transplantation: A Meta-Analysis. *J. Clin. Med.* **2019**, *8*, 530. [CrossRef]
39. Cheungpasitporn, W.; Thongprayoon, C.; Craici, I.M.; Sharma, K.; Chesdachai, S.; Khoury, N.J.; Ettore, A.S. Reactivation of BK polyomavirus during pregnancy, vertical transmission, and clinical significance: A meta-analysis. *J. Clin. Virol.* **2018**, *102*, 56–62. [CrossRef]
40. Thongprayoon, C.; Cheungpasitporn, W.; Lertjitbanjong, P.; Aeddula, N.R.; Bathini, T.; Watthanasuntorn, K.; Srivali, N.; Mao, M.A.; Kashani, K. Incidence and Impact of Acute Kidney Injury in Patients Receiving Extracorporeal Membrane Oxygenation: A Meta-Analysis. *J. Clin. Med.* **2019**, *8*, 981. [CrossRef]
41. Thongprayoon, C.; Kaewput, W.; Thamcharoen, N.; Bathini, T.; Watthanasuntorn, K.; Salim, S.A.; Ungprasert, P.; Lertjitbanjong, P.; Aeddula, N.R.; Torres-Ortiz, A.; et al. Acute Kidney Injury in Patients Undergoing Total Hip Arthroplasty: A Systematic Review and Meta-Analysis. *J. Clin. Med.* **2019**, *8*, 66. [CrossRef]
42. Kanduri, S.R.; Cheungpasitporn, W.; Thongprayoon, C.; Bathini, T.; Kovvuru, K.; Garla, V.; Medaura, J.; Vaitla, P.; Kashani, K.B. Incidence and Mortality of Acute Kidney Injury in Patients Undergoing Hematopoietic Stem Cell Transplantation: A Systematic Review and Meta-analysis. *QJM* **2020**. [CrossRef] [PubMed]
43. Thongprayoon, C.; Cheungpasitporn, W.; Mao, M.A.; Sakhuja, A.; Erickson, S.B. Admission calcium levels and risk of acute kidney injury in hospitalised patients. *Int. J. Clin. Pr.* **2018**, *72*, e13057. [CrossRef] [PubMed]
44. Thongprayoon, C.; Khoury, N.J.; Bathini, T.; Aeddula, N.R.; Boonpheng, B.; Leeaphorn, N.; Ungprasert, P.; Bruminhent, J.; Lertjitbanjong, P.; Watthanasuntorn, K.; et al. BK polyomavirus genotypes in renal transplant recipients in the United States: A meta-analysis. *J. Evid. Based Med.* **2019**, *12*, 291–299. [CrossRef] [PubMed]
45. Lin, S.Y.; Hsieh, M.H.; Lin, C.L.; Hsieh, M.J.; Hsu, W.H.; Lin, C.C.; Hsu, C.Y.; Kao, C.H. Artificial Intelligence Prediction Model for the Cost and Mortality of Renal Replacement Therapy in Aged and Super-Aged Populations in Taiwan. *J. Clin. Med.* **2019**, *8*, 995. [CrossRef] [PubMed]

46. Díez-Sanmartín, C.; Sarasa Cabezuelo, A. Application of Artificial Intelligence Techniques to Predict Survival in Kidney Transplantation: A Review. *J. Clin. Med.* **2020**, *9*, 572. [CrossRef]
47. Azuaje, F.; Kim, S.Y.; Perez Hernandez, D.; Dittmar, G. Connecting Histopathology Imaging and Proteomics in Kidney Cancer through Machine Learning. *J. Clin. Med.* **2019**, *8*, 1535. [CrossRef]
48. Hsiao, C.C.; Tu, H.T.; Lin, C.H.; Chen, K.H.; Yeh, Y.H.; See, L.C. Temporal Trends of Severe Hypoglycemia and Subsequent Mortality in Patients with Advanced Diabetic Kidney Diseases Transitioning to Dialysis. *J. Clin. Med.* **2019**, *8*, 420. [CrossRef]
49. Gout, A.M.; Martin, N.C.; Brown, A.F.; Ravine, D. PKDB: Polycystic Kidney Disease Mutation Database—A gene variant database for autosomal dominant polycystic kidney disease. *Hum. Mutat.* **2007**, *28*, 654–659. [CrossRef]
50. Massie, A.B.; Kucirka, L.M.; Segev, D.L. Big data in organ transplantation: Registries and administrative claims. *Am. J. Transpl.* **2014**, *14*, 1723–1730. [CrossRef]
51. Papadopoulos, T.; Krochmal, M.; Cisek, K.; Fernandes, M.; Husi, H.; Stevens, R.; Bascands, J.L.; Schanstra, J.P.; Klein, J. Omics databases on kidney disease: Where they can be found and how to benefit from them. *Clin. Kidney J.* **2016**, *9*, 343–352. [CrossRef] [PubMed]
52. Port, F.K.; Held, P.J. The US Renal Data System at 30 Years: A Historical Perspective. *Am. J. Kidney Dis.* **2019**, *73*, 459–461. [CrossRef] [PubMed]
53. Stack, A.G.; Casserly, L.F.; Cronin, C.J.; Chernenko, T.; Cullen, W.; Hannigan, A.; Saran, R.; Johnson, H.; Browne, G.; Ferguson, J.P. Prevalence and variation of Chronic Kidney Disease in the Irish health system: Initial findings from the National Kidney Disease Surveillance Programme. *Bmc Nephrol.* **2014**, *15*, 185. [CrossRef] [PubMed]
54. Bello, A.K.; Ronksley, P.E.; Tangri, N.; Singer, A.; Grill, A.; Nitsch, D.; Queenan, J.A.; Lindeman, C.; Soos, B.; Freiheit, E.; et al. A national surveillance project on chronic kidney disease management in Canadian primary care: A study protocol. *BMJ Open* **2017**, *7*, e016267. [CrossRef] [PubMed]
55. Saran, R.; Steffick, D.; Bragg-Gresham, J. The China Kidney Disease Network (CK-NET): "Big Data-Big Dreams". *Am. J. Kidney Dis.* **2017**, *69*, 713–716. [CrossRef]
56. Dienemann, T.; Fujii, N.; Orlandi, P.; Nessel, L.; Furth, S.L.; Hoy, W.E.; Matsuo, S.; Mayer, G.; Methven, S.; Schaefer, F.; et al. International Network of Chronic Kidney Disease cohort studies (iNET-CKD): A global network of chronic kidney disease cohorts. *BMC Nephrol.* **2016**, *17*, 121. [CrossRef]
57. Lv, J.; Zhang, H.; Wong, M.G.; Jardine, M.J.; Hladunewich, M.; Jha, V.; Monaghan, H.; Zhao, M.; Barbour, S.; Reich, H.; et al. Effect of Oral Methylprednisolone on Clinical Outcomes in Patients With IgA Nephropathy: The TESTING Randomized Clinical Trial. *JAMA* **2017**, *318*, 432–442. [CrossRef]
58. Matsushita, K.; Ballew, S.H.; Astor, B.C.; Jong, P.E.d.; Gansevoort, R.T.; Hemmelgarn, B.R.; Levey, A.S.; Levin, A.; Wen, C.-P.; Woodward, M.; et al. Cohort profile: The chronic kidney disease prognosis consortium. *Int. J. Epidemiol.* **2013**, *42*, 1660–1668. [CrossRef]
59. Levin, A.; Tonelli, M.; Bonventre, J.; Coresh, J.; Donner, J.-A.; Fogo, A.B.; Fox, C.S.; Gansevoort, R.T.; Heerspink, H.J.L.; Jardine, M.; et al. Global kidney health 2017 and beyond: A roadmap for closing gaps in care, research, and policy. *Lancet* **2017**, *390*, 1888–1917. [CrossRef]
60. O'Seaghdha, C.M.; Fox, C.S. Genome-wide association studies of chronic kidney disease: What have we learned? *Nat. Rev. Nephrol.* **2011**, *8*, 89–99. [CrossRef]
61. Wuttke, M.; Köttgen, A. Insights into kidney diseases from genome-wide association studies. *Nat. Rev. Nephrol.* **2016**, *12*, 549–562. [CrossRef]
62. Ahlqvist, E.; van Zuydam, N.R.; Groop, L.C.; McCarthy, M.I. The genetics of diabetic complications. *Nat. Rev. Nephrol.* **2015**, *11*, 277–287. [CrossRef] [PubMed]
63. Mohan, C.; Putterman, C. Genetics and pathogenesis of systemic lupus erythematosus and lupus nephritis. *Nat. Rev. Nephrol.* **2015**, *11*, 329–341. [CrossRef] [PubMed]
64. Lindenmeyer, M.T.; Kretzler, M. Renal biopsy-driven molecular target identification in glomerular disease. *Pflug. Arch.* **2017**, *469*, 1021–1028. [CrossRef] [PubMed]
65. Rumsfeld, J.S.; Joynt, K.E.; Maddox, T.M. Big data analytics to improve cardiovascular care: Promise and challenges. *Nat. Rev. Cardiol.* **2016**, *13*, 350–359. [CrossRef]
66. Cheungpasitporn, W.; Thongprayoon, C.; Ungprasert, P.; Wijarnpreecha, K.; Raimondo, M.; Kroner, P.T. Acute pancreatitis in end-stage renal disease patients in the USA: A nationwide, propensity score-matched analysis. *Eur. J. Gastroenterol. Hepatol.* **2019**, *31*, 968–972. [CrossRef]

67. Thongprayoon, C.; Kaewput, W.; Boonpheng, B.; Ungprasert, P.; Bathini, T.; Srivali, N.; Vallabhajosyula, S.; Castaneda, J.L.; Monga, D.; Kanduri, S.R.; et al. Impact of ANCA-Associated Vasculitis on Outcomes of Hospitalizations for Goodpasture's Syndrome in the United States: Nationwide Inpatient Sample 2003-2014. *Medicina* **2020**, *56*, 103. [CrossRef]
68. Ungprasert, P.; Koster, M.J.; Cheungpasitporn, W.; Wijarnpreecha, K.; Thongprayoon, C.; Kroner, P.T. Inpatient epidemiology and economic burden of granulomatosis with polyangiitis: A 10-year study of the national inpatient sample. *Rheumatology* **2020**. [CrossRef]
69. Evans, R.S. Electronic Health Records: Then, Now, and in the Future. *Yearb. Med. Inform.* **2016**, *25* (Suppl. 1), S48–S61. [CrossRef]
70. Sutherland, S.M.; Goldstein, S.L.; Bagshaw, S.M. Acute Kidney Injury and Big Data. *Contrib. Nephrol.* **2018**, *193*, 55–67.
71. Sutherland, S.M. Electronic Health Record-Enabled Big-Data Approaches to Nephrotoxin-Associated Acute Kidney Injury Risk Prediction. *Pharmacotherapy* **2018**, *38*, 804–812. [CrossRef] [PubMed]
72. Sutherland, S.M. Big Data and Pediatric Acute Kidney Injury: The Promise of Electronic Health Record Systems. *Front. Pediatr.* **2019**, *7*, 536. [CrossRef] [PubMed]
73. Shipp, M.A.; Ross, K.N.; Tamayo, P.; Weng, A.P.; Kutok, J.L.; Aguiar, R.C.; Gaasenbeek, M.; Angelo, M.; Reich, M.; Pinkus, G.S.; et al. Diffuse large B-cell lymphoma outcome prediction by gene-expression profiling and supervised machine learning. *Nat. Med.* **2002**, *8*, 68–74. [CrossRef]
74. Saez-Rodriguez, J.; Rinschen, M.M.; Floege, J.; Kramann, R. Big science and big data in nephrology. *Kidney Int.* **2019**, *95*, 1326–1337. [CrossRef] [PubMed]
75. Angermueller, C.; Pärnamaa, T.; Parts, L.; Stegle, O. Deep learning for computational biology. *Mol. Syst Biol.* **2016**, *12*, 878. [CrossRef] [PubMed]
76. SGarcelon, N.; Burgun, A.; Salomon, R.; Neuraz, A. Electronic health records for the diagnosis of rare diseases. *Kidney Int.* **2020**, *97*, 676–686. [CrossRef]
77. Stead, W.W. Clinical Implications and Challenges of Artificial Intelligence and Deep Learning. *JAMA* **2018**, *320*, 1107–1108. [CrossRef]
78. Obermeyer, Z.; Emanuel, E.J. Predicting the Future—Big Data, Machine Learning, and Clinical Medicine. *N. Engl. J. Med.* **2016**, *375*, 1216–1219. [CrossRef]
79. Russakovsky, O.; Deng, J.; Su, H.; Krause, J.; Satheesh, S.; Ma, S.; Huang, Z.; Karpathy, A.; Khosla, A.; Bernstein, M. Imagenet large scale visual recognition challenge. *Int. J. Comput. Vis.* **2015**, *115*, 211–252. [CrossRef]
80. Pennington, J.; Socher, R.; Manning, C.D. (Eds.) Glove: Global vectors for word representation. In Proceedings of the 2014 Conference on Empirical Methods in Natural Language Processing (EMNLP), Doha, Qatar, 25–29 October 2014.
81. Hermsen, M.; de Bel, T.; den Boer, M.; Steenbergen, E.J.; Kers, J.; Florquin, S.; Roelofs, J.; Stegall, M.D.; Alexander, M.P.; Smith, B.H.; et al. Deep Learning-Based Histopathologic Assessment of Kidney Tissue. *J. Am. Soc. Nephrol.* **2019**, *30*, 1968–1979. [CrossRef]
82. Ginley, B.; Lutnick, B.; Jen, K.Y.; Fogo, A.B.; Jain, S.; Rosenberg, A.; Walavalkar, V.; Wilding, G.; Tomaszewski, J.E.; Yacoub, R.; et al. Computational Segmentation and Classification of Diabetic Glomerulosclerosis. *J. Am. Soc. Nephrol.* **2019**, *30*, 1953–1967. [CrossRef] [PubMed]
83. Tomašev, N.; Glorot, X.; Rae, J.W.; Zielinski, M.; Askham, H.; Saraiva, A.; et al. A clinically applicable approach to continuous prediction of future acute kidney injury. *Nature* **2019**, *572*, 116–119. [CrossRef] [PubMed]
84. Escandell-Montero, P.; Chermisi, M.; Martínez-Martínez, J.M.; Gómez-Sanchis, J.; Barbieri, C.; Soria-Olivas, E.; Mari, F.; Vila-Francés, J.; Stopper, A.; Gatti, E.; et al. Optimization of anemia treatment in hemodialysis patients via reinforcement learning. *Artif. Intell. Med.* **2014**, *62*, 47–60. [CrossRef] [PubMed]
85. Barbieri, C.; Molina, M.; Ponce, P.; Tothova, M.; Cattinelli, I.; Ion Titapiccolo, J.; Mari, F.; Amato, C.; Leipold, F.; Wehmeyer, W.; et al. An international observational study suggests that artificial intelligence for clinical decision support optimizes anemia management in hemodialysis patients. *Kidney Int.* **2016**, *90*, 422–429. [CrossRef] [PubMed]
86. Chen, T.; Li, X.; Li, Y.; Xia, E.; Qin, Y.; Liang, S.; Xu, F.; Liang, D.; Zeng, C.; Liu, Z. Prediction and Risk Stratification of Kidney Outcomes in IgA Nephropathy. *Am. J. Kidney Dis.* **2019**, *74*, 300–309. [CrossRef]

87. Samal, L.; D'Amore, J.D.; Bates, D.W.; Wright, A. Implementation of a scalable, web-based, automated clinical decision support risk-prediction tool for chronic kidney disease using C-CDA and application programming interfaces. *J. Am. Med. Inf. Assoc.* **2017**, *24*, 1111–1115. [CrossRef]
88. Tangri, N.; Stevens, L.A.; Griffith, J.; Tighiouart, H.; Djurdjev, O.; Naimark, D.; Levin, A.; Levey, A.S. A predictive model for progression of chronic kidney disease to kidney failure. *JAMA* **2011**, *305*, 1553–1559. [CrossRef]
89. Ravizza, S.; Huschto, T.; Adamov, A.; Böhm, L.; Büsser, A.; Flöther, F.F.; Hinzmann, R.; König, H.; McAhren, S.M.; Robertson, D.H.; et al. Predicting the early risk of chronic kidney disease in patients with diabetes using real-world data. *Nat. Med.* **2019**, *25*, 57–59. [CrossRef]
90. Zhou, C.; Wang, R.; Jiang, W.; Zhu, J.; Liu, Y.; Zheng, J.; et al. Machine learning for the prediction of acute kidney injury and paraplegia after thoracoabdominal aortic aneurysm repair. *J. Card. Surg.* **2020**, *35*, 89–99. [CrossRef]
91. Xu, Z.; Chou, J.; Zhang, X.S.; Luo, Y.; Isakova, T.; Adekkanattu, P.; Ancker, J.S.; Jiang, G.; Kiefer, R.C.; Pacheco, J.A.; et al. Identifying sub-phenotypes of acute kidney injury using structured and unstructured electronic health record data with memory networks. *J. Biomed. Inform.* **2020**, *102*, 103361. [CrossRef]
92. Song, X.; Waitman, L.R.; Yu, A.S.; Robbins, D.C.; Hu, Y.; Liu, M. Longitudinal Risk Prediction of Chronic Kidney Disease in Diabetic Patients Using a Temporal-Enhanced Gradient Boosting Machine: Retrospective Cohort Study. *JMIR Med. Inform.* **2020**, *8*, e15510. [CrossRef] [PubMed]
93. Rashidi, H.H.; Sen, S.; Palmieri, T.L.; Blackmon, T.; Wajda, J.; Tran, N.K. Early Recognition of Burn- and Trauma-Related Acute Kidney Injury: A Pilot Comparison of Machine Learning Techniques. *Sci. Rep.* **2020**, *10*, 205. [CrossRef] [PubMed]
94. Morid, M.A.; Sheng, O.R.L.; Del Fiol, G.; Facelli, J.C.; Bray, B.E.; Abdelrahman, S. Temporal Pattern Detection to Predict Adverse Events in Critical Care: Case Study With Acute Kidney Injury. *JMIR Med. Inform.* **2020**, *8*, e14272. [CrossRef] [PubMed]
95. Luo, Y.; Tang, Z.; Hu, X.; Lu, S.; Miao, B.; Hong, S.; Bai, H.; Sun, C.; Qiu, J.; Liang, H.; et al. Machine learning for the prediction of severe pneumonia during posttransplant hospitalization in recipients of a deceased-donor kidney transplant. *Ann. Transl. Med.* **2020**, *8*, 82. [CrossRef]
96. Li, N.; Huang, H.; Qian, H.-Z.; Liu, P.; Lu, H.; Liu, X. Improving accuracy of estimating glomerular filtration rate using artificial neural network: Model development and validation. *J. Transl. Med.* **2020**, *18*, 120. [CrossRef]
97. Lei, L.; Wang, Y.; Xue, Q.; Tong, J.; Zhou, C.-M.; Yang, J.-J. A comparative study of machine learning algorithms for predicting acute kidney injury after liver cancer resection. *PeerJ* **2020**, *8*, e8583. [CrossRef]
98. Kate, R.J.; Pearce, N.; Mazumdar, D.; Nilakantan, V. A continual prediction model for inpatient acute kidney injury. *Comput. Biol. Med.* **2020**, *116*, 103580. [CrossRef]
99. Kang, M.W.; Kim, J.; Kim, D.K.; Oh, K.-H.; Joo, K.W.; Kim, Y.S.; Han, S.S. Machine learning algorithm to predict mortality in patients undergoing continuous renal replacement therapy. *Crit. Care* **2020**, *24*, 42. [CrossRef]
100. Zimmerman, L.P.; Reyfman, P.A.; Smith, A.D.R.; Zeng, Z.; Kho, A.; Sanchez-Pinto, L.N.; Luo, Y. Early prediction of acute kidney injury following ICU admission using a multivariate panel of physiological measurements. *Bmc Med. Inform. Decis. Mak.* **2019**, *19* (Suppl. 1), 16. [CrossRef]
101. Zhang, Z.; Ho, K.M.; Hong, Y. Machine learning for the prediction of volume responsiveness in patients with oliguric acute kidney injury in critical care. *Crit. Care* **2019**, *23*, 112. [CrossRef]
102. Xu, Z.; Luo, Y.; Adekkanattu, P.; Ancker, J.S.; Jiang, G.; Kiefer, R.C.; Pacheco, J.A.; Rasmussen, L.V.; Pathak, J.; Wang, F. Stratified Mortality Prediction of Patients with Acute Kidney Injury in Critical Care. *Stud. Health Technol. Inform.* **2019**, *264*, 462–466. [PubMed]
103. Xiao, J.; Ding, R.; Xu, X.; Guan, H.; Feng, X.; Sun, T.; Zhu, S.; Ye, Z. Comparison and development of machine learning tools in the prediction of chronic kidney disease progression. *J. Transl. Med.* **2019**, *17*, 119. [CrossRef]
104. Mark, E.; Goldsman, D.; Gurbaxani, B.; Keskinocak, P.; Sokol, J. Using machine learning and an ensemble of methods to predict kidney transplant survival. *PLoS ONE* **2019**, *14*, e0209068. [CrossRef] [PubMed]
105. Bae, S.; Massie, A.B.; Thomas, A.G.; Bahn, G.; Luo, X.; Jackson, K.R.; Ottmann, S.E.; Brennan, D.C.; Desai, N.M.; Coresh, J.; et al. Who can tolerate a marginal kidney? Predicting survival after deceased donor kidney transplant by donor-recipient combination. *Am. J. Transpl.* **2019**, *19*, 425–433. [CrossRef] [PubMed]

106. Yoo, K.D.; Noh, J.; Lee, H.; Kim, D.K.; Lim, C.S.; Kim, Y.H.; Lee, J.P.; Kim, G.; Kim, Y.S. A Machine Learning Approach Using Survival Statistics to Predict Graft Survival in Kidney Transplant Recipients: A Multicenter Cohort Study. *Sci. Rep.* **2017**, *7*, 8904. [CrossRef] [PubMed]
107. Niel, O.; Bastard, P. Artificial Intelligence in Nephrology: Core Concepts, Clinical Applications, and Perspectives. *Am. J. Kidney Dis.* **2019**, *74*, 803–810. [CrossRef] [PubMed]
108. Improta, G.; Mazzella, V.; Vecchione, D.; Santini, S.; Triassi, M. Fuzzy logic-based clinical decision support system for the evaluation of renal function in post-Transplant Patients [published online ahead of print, 2019 Nov 12]. *J. Eval. Clin. Pract.* **2019**. [CrossRef]
109. Atallah, D.M.; Badawy, M.; El-Sayed, A.; Ghoneim, M.A. Predicting kidney transplantation outcome based on hybrid feature selection and KNN classifier. *Multimed. Tools Appl.* **2019**, *78*, 20383–20407. [CrossRef]
110. Nematollahi, M.; Akbari, R.; Nikeghbalian, S.; Salehnasab, C. Classification Models to Predict Survival of Kidney Transplant Recipients Using Two Intelligent Techniques of Data Mining and Logistic Regression. *Int. J. Organ. Transpl. Med.* **2017**, *8*, 119–122.
111. Tapak, L.; Hamidi, O.; Amini, P.; Poorolajal, J. Prediction of Kidney Graft Rejection Using Artificial Neural Network. *Healthc Inf. Res.* **2017**, *23*, 277–284. [CrossRef]
112. Shahmoradi, L.; Langarizadeh, M.; Pourmand, G.; Fard, Z.A.; Borhani, A. Comparing Three Data Mining Methods to Predict Kidney Transplant Survival. *Acta Inf. Med.* **2016**, *24*, 322–327. [CrossRef] [PubMed]
113. Luck, M.; Sylvain, T.; Cardinal, H.; Lodi, A.; Bengio, Y. Deep learning for patient-specific kidney graft survival analysis. *arXiv* **2017**, arXiv:170510245.
114. Topuz, K.; Zengul, F.D.; Dag, A.; Almehmi, A.; Yildirim, M.B. Predicting graft survival among kidney transplant recipients: A Bayesian decision support model. *Decis. Support. Syst.* **2018**, *106*, 97–109. [CrossRef]
115. Lyell, D.; Coiera, E. Automation bias and verification complexity: A systematic review. *J. Am. Med. Inf. Assoc.* **2017**, *24*, 423–431. [CrossRef] [PubMed]
116. Agarwal, R.; Sinha, A.D. Big data in nephrology-a time to rethink. *Nephrol. Dial. Transpl.* **2018**, *33*, 1–3. [CrossRef]
117. Lee, C.H.; Yoon, H.-J. Medical big data: Promise and challenges. *Kidney Res. Clin. Pr.* **2017**, *36*, 3–11. [CrossRef]
118. Calvert, J.; Saber, N.; Hoffman, J.; Das, R. Machine-Learning-Based Laboratory Developed Test for the Diagnosis of Sepsis in High-Risk Patients. *Diagnostics* **2019**, *9*, 20. [CrossRef]
119. Lim, E.-C.; Park, J.H.; Jeon, H.J.; Kim, H.-J.; Lee, H.-J.; Song, C.-G.; Hong, S.K. Developing a Diagnostic Decision Support System for Benign Paroxysmal Positional Vertigo Using a Deep-Learning Model. *J. Clin. Med.* **2019**, *8*, 633. [CrossRef]
120. Heo, S.-J.; Kim, Y.; Yun, S.; Lim, S.-S.; Kim, J.; Nam, C.-M.; Park, E.-C.; Jung, I.; Yoon, J.-H. Deep Learning Algorithms with Demographic Information Help to Detect Tuberculosis in Chest Radiographs in Annual Workers' Health Examination Data. *Int. J. Env. Res. Public Health* **2019**, *16*, 250. [CrossRef]
121. Kooman, J.P.; Wieringa, F.P.; Han, M.; Chaudhuri, S.; van der Sande, F.M.; Usvyat, L.A.; Kotanko, P. Wearable health devices and personal area networks: can they improve outcomes in haemodialysis patients? *Nephrol. Dial. Transplant.* **2020**, *35* (Suppl. 2), ii43–ii50. [CrossRef]
122. Shortliffe, E.H.; Sepúlveda, M.J. Clinical Decision Support in the Era of Artificial Intelligence. *JAMA* **2018**, *320*, 2199–2200. [CrossRef] [PubMed]
123. Santo, B.A.; Rosenberg, A.Z.; Sarder, P. Artificial intelligence driven next-generation renal histomorphometry. *Curr. Opin. Nephrol. Hypertens.* **2020**, *29*, 265–272. [CrossRef] [PubMed]
124. Na, L.; Yang, C.; Lo, C.C.; Zhao, F.; Fukuoka, Y.; Aswani, A. Feasibility of Reidentifying Individuals in Large National Physical Activity Data Sets From Which Protected Health Information Has Been Removed With Use of Machine Learning. *JAMA Netw. Open* **2018**, *1*, e186040. [CrossRef] [PubMed]
125. Obermeyer, Z.; Lee, T.H. Lost in Thought—The Limits of the Human Mind and the Future of Medicine. *N. Engl. J. Med.* **2017**, *377*, 1209–1211. [CrossRef]

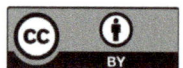

© 2020 by the authors. Licensee MDPI, Basel, Switzerland. This article is an open access article distributed under the terms and conditions of the Creative Commons Attribution (CC BY) license (http://creativecommons.org/licenses/by/4.0/).

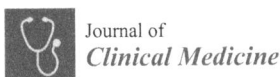

Article

The *Macrophage Migration Inhibitory Factor* (MIF) Promoter Polymorphisms (rs3063368, rs755622) Predict Acute Kidney Injury and Death after Cardiac Surgery

Luisa Averdunk [1,2], Jürgen Bernhagen [3,4,5], Karl Fehnle [6], Harald Surowy [2], Hermann-Josef Lüdecke [2], Sören Mucha [7,8], Patrick Meybohm [9], Dagmar Wieczorek [2], Lin Leng [10], Gernot Marx [1], David E. Leaf [11,12], Alexander Zarbock [13], Kai Zacharowski [9], on behalf of the RIPHeart Study Collaborators [†], Richard Bucala [10,*,‡] and Christian Stoppe [1,14,*,‡]

1. Department of Intensive Care Medicine, University Hospital Aachen, Rheinisch Westphälische Technische Hochschule Aachen, 52074 Aachen, Germany; luisa.aver@gmail.com (L.A.); gmarx@ukaachen.de (G.M.)
2. Institute of Human Genetics and Department of Pediatrics, Medical Faculty, Heinrich Heine University, 40225 Düsseldorf, Germany; harald.surowy@uni-duesseldorf.de (H.S.); Hermann-Josef.Luedecke@uni-duesseldorf.de (H.-J.L.); dagmar.wieczorek@hhu.de (D.W.)
3. Department of Vascular Biology, Institute for Stroke and Dementia Research, Klinikum der Universität München, Ludwig-Maximilians-University Munich, 80333 Munich, Germany; Juergen.Bernhagen@med.uni-muenchen.de
4. German Center for Cardiovascular Research (DZHK), Partner Site Munich Heart Alliance, 10785 Berlin, Germany
5. Munich Cluster for Systems Neurology (EXC 2145 SyNergy), 81377 Munich, Germany
6. Algora: Statistics and Clinical Research GmbH, 85540 Haar, Germany; karl.fehnle@algora.de
7. Institute of Clinical Molecular Biology, Christian Albrechts University of Kiel, 24118 Kiel, Germany; s.mucha@ikmb.uni-kiel.de
8. Institute for Cardiogenetics, University of Lübeck, Ratzeburger Allee 160, 23562 Lübeck, Germany
9. Department of Anesthesiology, Intensive Care Medicine & Pain Therapy, University Hospital Frankfurt, Goethe University, 60323 Frankfurt, Germany; meybohm_p@ukw.de (P.M.); kai.zacharowski@kgu.de (K.Z.)
10. Department of Internal Medicine, Yale University School of Medicine, New Haven, CT 06510, USA; lin.leng@yale.edu
11. Division of Renal Medicine, Brigham and Women's Hospital, Boston, MA 02115, USA; deleaf@bwh.harvard.edu
12. Harvard Medical School, Boston, MA 02115, USA
13. Intensive Care and Pain Medicine, Department of Anesthesiology, University of Münster, 48149 Münster, Germany; zarbock@uni-muenster.de
14. Department of Anesthesiology, Intensive Care Medicine and Pain Therapy, University Hospital Würzburg, 97080 Würzburg, Germany
* Correspondence: richard.bucala@yale.edu (R.B.); christian.stoppe@gmail.com (C.S.); Tel.: +49-241-8036575 (R.B. & C.S.); Fax: +49-241-8082406 (R.B. & C.S.)
† RIPHeart Study Collaborators are listed at the end of the manuscript. See Supplemental Acknowledgments for consortium details.
‡ Contributed equally as last authors.

Received: 3 August 2020; Accepted: 1 September 2020; Published: 11 September 2020

Abstract: Background: Macrophage Migration Inhibitory Factor (MIF) is highly elevated after cardiac surgery and impacts the postoperative inflammation. The aim of this study was to analyze whether the polymorphisms CATT$_{5-7}$ (rs5844572/rs3063368,"-794") and G>C single-nucleotide polymorphism (rs755622,-173) in the *MIF* gene promoter are related to postoperative outcome. Methods: In 1116 patients undergoing cardiac surgery, the *MIF* gene polymorphisms were analyzed and serum MIF was measured by ELISA in 100 patients. Results: Patients with at least one extended repeat allele (CATT$_7$) had a significantly higher risk of acute kidney injury (AKI) compared to others (23% vs. 13%; OR 2.01 (1.40–2.88), $p = 0.0001$). Carriers of CATT$_7$ were also at higher risk of death (1.8% vs. 0.4%; OR 5.12 (0.99–33.14), $p = 0.026$). The GC genotype was associated with

AKI (20% vs. GG/CC:13%, OR 1.71 (1.20–2.43), $p = 0.003$). Multivariate analyses identified CATT$_7$ predictive for AKI (OR 2.13 (1.46–3.09), $p < 0.001$) and death (OR 5.58 (1.29–24.04), $p = 0.021$). CATT$_7$ was associated with higher serum MIF before surgery (79.2 vs. 50.4 ng/mL, $p = 0.008$). Conclusion: The CATT$_7$ allele associates with a higher risk of AKI and death after cardiac surgery, which might be related to chronically elevated serum MIF. Polymorphisms in the *MIF* gene may constitute a predisposition for postoperative complications and the assessment may improve risk stratification and therapeutic guidance.

Keywords: acute kidney injury; genetic polymorphisms; risk prediction; (cardiac) surgery; inflammatory cytokines; clinical studies

1. Introduction

Conventional open-heart surgery is performed annually in more than one million patients worldwide, and the incidence of postoperative sequelae including acute organ dysfunction remains high [1,2]. A more precise identification of patients' risk for postoperative complications is desirable both for prognostic guidance and for the application of earlier and more effective interventions. While clinical scoring systems such as the well-established EuroSCORE were primarily developed for the preoperative risk stratification of mortality in cardiac surgery patients, only limited evidence exists about its value for postoperative organ dysfunction and other complications [3]. The identification of genomic risk alleles could be especially helpful to more accurately predict outcomes and to enable personalized medicine approaches.

Oxidative stress and a systemic inflammatory response contribution to the pathogenesis of postoperative organ dysfunctions following cardiac surgery [4]. Macrophage migration inhibitory factor (MIF) is a stress-regulating cytokine that increases in the circulation after cardiac surgery [5]. Within the *MIF* gene promoter, two polymorphisms, a G>C single nucleotide polymorphism 270 bases before *MIF* transcription start (−270) (originally described as −173; HGVS nomenclature: NM_002415.2 c.−270G>C, rs755622) and a CATT tetranucleotide repeat CATT$_{5-7}$ (rs3063368), have been associated with disease severity of multiple chronic inflammatory diseases, including osteoporosis, ankylosing spondylitis, and multiple sclerosis [6–8]. A higher number of CATT repeats has been reported to increase *MIF* promotor activity and to be associated with higher circulating MIF concentrations in different autoimmune and chronic inflammatory conditions [9–12]. The clinical significance of functional polymorphisms in *MIF* for postoperative outcome after cardiac surgery is unknown. In this study, we analyzed 1116 patients who underwent elective cardiac surgery with a cardiopulmonary bypass. We analyzed whether *MIF* promoter polymorphisms impact the risk of postoperative organ dysfunction and mortality in patients undergoing cardiac surgery. In a subset of patients, we also examined the correlation between *MIF* genotypes and circulating MIF levels.

2. Materials and Methods

2.1. Study Design and Patients

The present study is a predefined sub-study performed in cardiac surgery patients of the Remote Ischemic Preconditioning Heart (RIPHeart) study (January 2011–May 2014), which investigated whether upper limb remote ischemic conditioning reduced mortality and the incidence of myocardial infarction, stroke, and acute kidney injury (AKI) in adults scheduled for elective cardiac surgery requiring a cardiopulmonary bypass [13]. As the initial intervention study did not show group differences, this *MIF* polymorphism study includes all patients irrespective of the initial group assignment [13]. The trial was undertaken in compliance with International Conference on Harmonisation Good Clinical Practice guidelines, the Declaration of Helsinki (2008), and European Directive 2001/20/CE regarding the conduct of clinical trials (4 April 2001). The study was registered at ClinicalTrials.gov (NCT01067703). The study protocol was approved by the ethics committees of the University of Kiel, Aachen, and all participating centers of this prospective multicenter study.

Patients scheduled for elective cardiac surgery with use of cardiopulmonary bypass (e.g., coronary artery bypass graft (CABG), valve surgery, ascending aorta replacement) were eligible for this study. Of the 1403 patients screened for the study, blood samples were available from 1196 patients. Seven patients were excluded due to missing outcome data and 70 patients were excluded due to missing genotype information (Supplemental Figure S1). Thus, data from 1119 patients were included in the current study. The $CATT_8$ genotype was excluded from analysis because of its low frequency ($N = 3$), which is in accord with prior reports [14].

Blood samples were collected before surgery, at 45 min after cardiopulmonary bypass (CPB) initiation, at 2 min after opening of the cross-clamp (reperfusion), at 15 min after weaning from CPB, and at 1, 6, and 24 h after admission to ICU. Blood samples were processed no later than 2 h after collection and were stored at −70 °C or −20 °C until further transfer. The final study visit took place either before hospital discharge, or at the latest 30 days after ICU admission.

2.2. Outcome Measures

The primary exposure was the *MIF* genotype, which we analyzed according to the following groups: alleles (e.g., carriers of at least one C allele), genotypes (e.g., GC), and individual genotype combinations (e.g., $CATT_{5,7}$-GC). The endpoints were the association between the *MIF* genotype and the incidence of postoperative organ dysfunctions, including AKI, myocardial infarction, new onset of atrial fibrillation, stroke, delirium, and death. Each of these outcome parameters were analyzed as single events, and in the composite outcome "multiple organ dysfunction", when patients suffered from more than one organ dysfunction.

According to the KDIGO Clinical Practice Guideline 2012, AKI was defined as a $\geq$ 5-fold increase of serum creatinine from baseline, and a urine output of ≤0.5 mL/kg/h for more than 6 h, or the use of renal replacement therapy within 72 h [15]. However, a total creatinine increase of $\geq$ 0.3 mg/dL was not considered a diagnostic criterion for AKI, as this criterion had not yet been established in 2011 when the data collection started. Non-fatal myocardial infarction was defined by biomarker values more than five times higher than the 99th percentile of the normal reference range combined with new pathological Q-waves or new left bundle branch block within the first 72 h, standard clinical criteria for myocardial infarction from 72 h on, new ischemic finding by echocardiography or angiography, or myocardial infarction diagnosed at autopsy [16]. New onset of atrial fibrillation was defined as a new onset within the first four days after surgery [13]. The occurrence of postoperative delirium was assessed with the CAM-ICU score (preoperative, 24, 48, 72, and 96 h after surgery) [17]. Stroke was defined by any new, temporary or permanent, focal or global neurological deficit, or evidence of stroke on autopsy, and was evaluated according to the National Institutes of Health Stroke Scale ($\geq$4 points) [18].

Myocardial infarction, atrial fibrillation, and stroke were analyzed until hospital discharge with a maximum of 14 days after surgery.

2.3. ELISA

Serum was available from 100 patients in the RIPheart Study. Serum MIF levels were quantified by ELISA in duplicates as previously described and according to the manufacturer's instructions (R&D Systems, Minneapolis, MN, USA) ([5]). Samples were diluted 1:10 before analysis to obtain measures in the valid assay range.

2.4. Nomenclature and Genotyping of the Tetranucleotide Repeat Polymorphism $CATT_n$ (rs3063368)

In adherence to the U.S. National Library of Medicine dbSNP database (ncbi.nlm.nih.gov/snp/), the tetranucleotide repeat polymorphism formerly described as rs5844572, referring to the $CATT_6$

allele, will be referred to with the reference SNP number rs3063368, which comprises the multiallelic repeat polymorphism CATT$_n$ present at this site. The tetranucleotide repeat polymorphism is located at position chr22:23893566-23893569: (GRCh38.p12) (ncbi.nlm.nih.gov/snp/rs3063368), and based on older transcript annotations (NM_002415.2) -794 nucleotides, or based on more accurate transcript annotations (NM_002415.2) -909 nucleotides upstream of the start codon. The repeat polymorphism is a deletion, or respectively a duplication, of TTCA tetranucleotide repeats. In parallel with former publications, in this study this SNP will be referred to as a tetranucleotide 5-, 6-, 7-, or 8- fold repeat of CATT. The DNA sequence of this SNP is illustrated in Supplemental Figure S2 (UCSC Genome Browser, genome.ucsc.edu).

EDTA-anticoagulated whole blood was used for genotyping. DNA was extracted with the Autopure LS automated system according to the manufacturer's recommendations (Qiagen, Hilden, Germany).

For the analysis of the tetranucleotide repeat (rs3063368), as formerly described, a fragment length polymorphism PCR with fluorescently labeled primers and fragment length analysis via capillary electrophoresis was applied [10]. Of note, with this technique a phase analysis with the rs755622 single nucleotide polymorphism (SNP) is not possible. DNA was amplified in a Mastercycler gradient (Eppendorf AG, Germany). The PCR reaction mix contained 2.5 µL 10× PCR buffer, 3 µL (25 mM) MgCl2, 2 µL dNTP Mix, 0.8 µL of each primer, 0.15 µL (1 U) Taq polymerase, and 13.75 µL of purified DNA, in a total end volume of 25 µL. The PCR consisted of the following steps: an initial denaturation step (95 °C, 12 min), 35 amplification cycle (95 °C, 30 s; X (primer annealing temperature see Supplemental Table S1, 30 s; 72 °C, 30 s) and a final elongation step (72 °C, 10 min). The reverse primer was labeled with 6-Carboxyfluorescein (6-FAM) [19]. The PCR was performed in a SimpliAmp Thermal Cycler (Life Technologies, Carlsbad, CA, USA). The PCR products were subjected to capillary electrophoresis on an ABI 3730XL Genetic Analyzer (Applied Biosystems, Foster City, CA, USA). Data collection was performed with Data Collection v3.0 software (Applied Biosystems, Foster City, CA, USA) and the results were analyzed by GeneMapper ID v5 software (Applied Biosystems, Foster City, CA, USA).

2.5. Nomenclature and Genotyping of the SNP G>C Substitution (rs755622)

The SNP rs755622 is a substitution of G>C in the non-coding region at position chr22:23,894,205 (GRCh38.p12). Based on the older transcript annotations (NM_002415.1), this SNP has been formerly described with the position NM_002415.1:m.-173. According to the more accurate transcript annotation (NM_002415.2), the G>C substitution is located at position NM_002415.2:m.-178 and NM_002415.2:c.-270 G>C. (The start codon is located at position chr22:23,894,475.)

DNA was extracted from EDTA-anticoagulated whole blood with Autopure (Qiagen, Hilden, Germany). Genotyping of the SNP rs755622 G>C was performed using an Assays-on-Demand® allelic discrimination on a TaqMan platform according to the manufacturer's instructions (ThermoFisher Scientific, Waltham, MA, USA). The polymerase chain reaction (PCR) contained 10 ng of genomic DNA, 10 µL TaqMan master mix, and 0.125 µL of 40× assay mix. PCR was performed using 96-well plates on an ABI 9700 thermal cycler (Applied Biosystems, Foster City, CA, USA) (reaction conditions 50 °C for 2 min, 95 °C for 10 min, followed by 40 cycles of 95 °C for 15 s and 60 °C for 1 min). The TaqMan 7700 platform was used to perform an end-plate reading using the allelic discrimination option.

Sample and marker quality control (QC) was performed with PLINK (v1.9; https://www.cog-genomics.org/plink/1.9)(PMID:25722852).

2.6. Statistics

Baseline characteristics were analyzed using of Wilcoxon Rank Sum test for continuous variables and Fisher's exact test for binary variables. Associations between *MIF* polymorphisms and outcome parameters were analyzed using univariate logistic regression and results are presented together with odds ratios and 95% confidence intervals.

Multivariable logistic regression analysis was performed to analyze the influence of relevant baseline variables. Model selection was based on the postoperative complication (dependent variable) and the genotype (independent variable). Further variables were selected on the basis of univariate analyses and significant differences. Model selection was accomplished by a backward elimination or a stepwise procedure.

Serum MIF levels at individual time points were compared using Wilcoxon Rank Sum test according to the *MIF* genotype. Analyses were calculated with SAS 9.4 (SAS Institute Inc., Cary, NC, USA) and SPSS (IBM SPSS, version 21.0, Armonk, NY, USA). All *p*-Values refer to two-sided tests, and $p < 0.05$ was considered statistically significant.

2.7. Study Approval

Each patient provided written informed consent prior to inclusion in the study.

3. Results

3.1. Patients, Baseline Characteristics, and Postoperative Complications

The median age was 68 years and 25.1% were females (Table 1). Postoperative AKI was associated with older age ($p < 0.001$), female gender ($p = 0.007$), the intake of aspirin ($p = 0.01$), lower baseline hemoglobin (<14 g/dL) ($p < 0.001$), peripheral artery disease ($p = 0.02$), hypertension ($p = 0.01$), insulin-dependent diabetes mellitus (IDDM) ($p = 0.01$), and a higher EuroSCORE ($p < 0.001$) (Table 1). Death was associated with older age ($p = 0.03$) and IDDM ($p = 0.03$) (Table 1).

Table 1. Baseline and operative characteristics by AKI and death.

	AKI					Death			
	Yes (N = 170)		No (N = 946)		*p*-Value	Yes (N = 8)		No (N = 1108)		*p*-Value
Demographics										
Age, years	72	(66–77)	67	(58–73)	<0.001	73	(70–80)	68	(59–73)	0.03
Sex (female)	57	(33.5)	223	(23.6)	0.007	3	(37.5)	277	(25.0)	0.42
Active smokers	32	(18.8)	198	(20.9)	0.61	1	(12.5)	229	(20.7)	1.00
Medication										
Beta blockers	109	(64.1)	587	(62.1)	0.67	6	(75.0)	690	(62.3)	0.72
ACE inhibitors	91	(53.5)	478	(50.5)	0.51	3	(37.5)	566	(51.1)	0.50
Cholesterol-lowering drug	110	(64.7)	624	(66.0)	0.79	6	(75.0)	728	(65.7)	0.72
Insulin	21	(12.4)	77	(8.1)	0.08	3	(37.5)	95	(8.6)	0.03
Aspirin	128	(75.3)	619	(65.4)	0.01	4	(50.0)	743	(67.1)	0.45
Clopidogrel	17	(10)	76	(8.0)	0.37	2	(25.0)	91	(8.2)	0.14
Comorbidities										
Hypertension	153	(90.0)	772	(81.6)	0.01	6	(75.0)	919	(82.9)	0.63
Ischemic heart disease	132	(77.6)	706	(74.6)	0.39	5	(62.5)	833	(75.2)	0.42
Previous MI						1	(12.5)	315	(28.4)	0.45
Congestive heart disease	43	(25.3)	193	(20.4)	0.15	2	(25.0)	234	(21.1)	0.68
PAD	20	(11.8)	62	(6.6)	0.02	2	(25.0)	80	(7.2)	0.68
COPD	15	(8.8)	80	(8.5)	0.88	0	0	95	(8.6)	1.00
Chronic kidney disease	24	(14.1)	107	(11.3)	0.30	1	(12.5)	130	(11.7)	1.00
IDDM	56	(32.9)	219	(23.2)	0.01	4	(50.0)	271	(24.5)	0.11
Laboratory, at baseline										
Serum creatinine mg/dL	0.92	(0.8–1.1)	0.91	(0.8–1.1)	0.66	0.99	(0.73–1.14)	0.91	(0.80–1.07)	0.82
Hemoglobin, g/dL	13.6	(12.5–14.6)	14.2	(13.4–14.9)	<0.001	13.6	(12.1–14.4)	14.1	(13.2–14.9)	0.31
EuroSCORE	5	(3–7)	4	(2–6)	<0.001	6	(5–8)	4	(2–6)	0.03
Type of surgery										
CABG (alone)	64	(37.6)	434	(45.9)		3	(37.5)	495	(44.7)	
Aortic valve *	37	(12.8)	190	(20.1)		2	(12.5)	225	(20.3)	
Mitral valve *	6	(3.5)	32	(3.4)	0.26	0	(37.5)	38	(3.4)	0.25
Aorta ascendens *	3	(1.8)	30	(3.2)		0	(25.0)	33	(3.0)	
Combined procedures	57	(33.5)	245	(25.9)		2	25.0	300	(27.1)	
Other type of surgery	3	(1.8)	15	(1.6)		1	12.5	17	(1.5)	

Data are expressed as the median and interquartile range (Q1–Q3) or absolute numbers and (percentage). The association of baseline characteristics with AKI and death was analyzed by Wilcoxon rank sum or Fisher's exact test. ACE, angiotensin converting enzyme; CABG, coronary artery bypass graft; COPD, chronic obstructive pulmonary disease; IDDM, insulin-dependent diabetes mellitus; MI, myocardial infarction; PAD, peripheral artery disease, *, replacement or reconstruction (alone). Bold fonts indicate *p*-values < 0.05.

3.2. Genotype Frequencies

The most common genotypes were CATT$_{6,6}$-GG (32.3%) and CATT$_{5,6}$-GG (30.9%) (Table 2); 24.8% of patients carried at least one CATT$_7$ allele; 29.6% of patients were heterozygous and 2.3% of patients were homozygous carriers of the G>C substitution. The allele frequencies in our study cohort were comparable to the frequencies published in the reference database gnomAD (Table 1) [20]. The frequency of the GC genotype and the $CATT_7$-repeat allele was higher than in patients with AKI compared to patients without AKI (X^2 test for trend, $p = 0.001$) (Figure 1).

Table 2. Frequencies of the *MIF* $CATT_{5-7}$ repeat allele (rs3063368) and the G>C single-nucleotide polymorphism (rs755622) in 1116 patients undergoing cardiac surgery.

$CATT_{5-7}$ Repeat Allele Carrier Frequencies (rs3063368)			
	N Carriers	%	Allele Frequency (Europe) % [1]
$CATT_5$	488	43.7	- *
$CATT_6$	957	85.8	84.3
$CATT_7$	277	24.8	24.9
G>C SNP Genotype Frequencies (rs755622)			
	N Genotypes	%	Allele Frequency (Europe) % [1]
GG (homozygous)	762	68.3	65.2
GC (heterozygous)	328	29.4	31.7
CC (homozygous)	26	2.3	3.1
Individual Genotype Combination Frequencies (rs3063368 & rs755622)			
	N	%	
$CATT_{5,5}$-GG	68	6.1	
$CATT_{5,6}$-GG	329	29.5	
$CATT_{6,6}$-GG	360	32.3	
$CATT_{5,7}$-GG	2	0.2	
$CATT_{6,7}$-GG	3	0.3	
$CATT_{5,5}$-CG	3	0.3	
$CATT_{5,6}$-CG	16	1.4	
$CATT_{6,6}$-CG	63	5.6	
$CATT_{5,7}$-CG	69	6.2	
$CATT_{6,7}$-CG	176	15.8	
$CATT_{7,7}$-CG	1	0.1	
$CATT_{5,7}$-CC	1	0.1	
$CATT_{6,7}$-CC	10	0.9	
$CATT_{7,7}$-CC	15	1.3	
All	1116	100.00	

The most frequent genotypes observed were $CATT_{5,6}$-GG (29.5%), $CATT_{6,6}$-GG (32.3%), and $CATT_{6,7}$-CG (15.8%). The frequency of the polymorphisms was comparable to the frequency in the general reference population (Europe) [1]; SNP, Single nucleotide polymorphism; $CATT_7$, patients carrying at least one $CATT_7$ allele. Data presented as absolute numbers and percentage. [1] calculated from reference gnomAD Database (including >7500 genomes from unrelated non-Finnish European individuals sequenced as part of various population genetic studies) [20]. * As $CATT_5$ is the wildtype allele, there is no information regarding $CATT_5$ in the gnomAD Database.

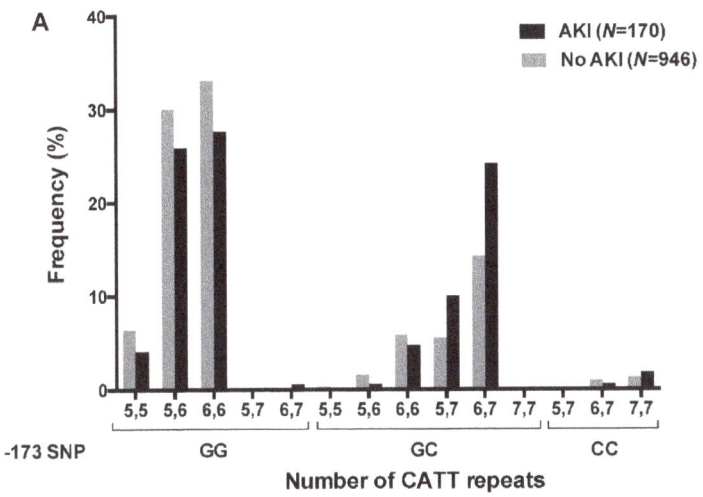
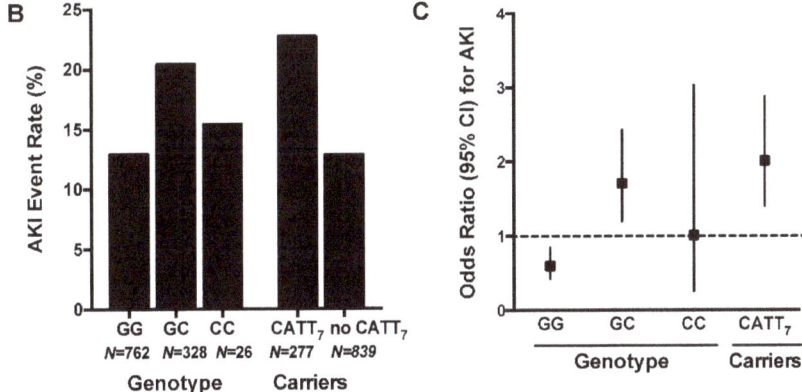

Figure 1. Frequency distribution of the CATT microsatellite repeat (rs3063368) and the G>C SNP (rs755622) in patients with AKI versus patients not affected by AKI after cardiac surgery. (**A**) In patients with AKI, the frequency of the GC genotype and the CATT$_7$ allele is higher than in patients without AKI (X^2 test for trend, $p = 0.001$). (**B**) The AKI event rate was higher in patients with the GC genotype (20%) versus patients with the CC or the GG genotype (13%), and higher in CATT$_7$ carriers (23%) compared to non-carriers. (**C**) Patients carrying the GC genotype or the CATT$_7$ allele had a significantly increased relative risk of AKI compared to all other patients.

3.3. Association of the Tetranucleotide Repeat CATT$_{5-7}$ (rs3063368) and the G>C Single-Nucleotide Polymorphism (rs755622) with Postoperative Outcome

All patients ($N = 1116$) were examined for the association between the two polymorphisms in the *MIF* promoter and risk of postoperative complications. The overall incidence of AKI after cardiac surgery was 15.2% ($N = 170$) (Table 3). Patients who were either homozygous or heterozygous carriers of the *MIF* CATT$_7$ allele had a significantly increased risk of AKI after cardiac surgery when compared to all other patients (22.7% vs. 12.8%, OR 2.01, 95% CI 1.40–2.88, $p = 0.0001$) (Table 4).

Table 3. Absolute and relative frequency of postoperative complications. * Patients affected by at least two of the predefined organ dysfunctions.

	Patients (N = 1116)	
	N	%
Death	8	0.7
Myocardial infarction (MI)	93	8.3
Stroke	24	2.2
Delirium	144	12.9
Acute kidney injury (AKI)	170	15.2
Stage 1	108	9.7
Stage 2	38	3.4
Stage 3	24	2.1
Atrial Fibrillation	245	21.9
Multiple Complications (≥) *	139	12.4

Table 4. Association of the MIF promoter polymorphisms with AKI.

MIF Polymorphism	AKI (N = 170)				OR	(95% CI)	p-Value
	Patients Carrying This Allele/Genotype		Patients NOT Carrying this Allele/Genotype				
	N	Incidence, %	N	Incidence, %			
CATT Repeat Allele Carriers (rs3063368)							
CATT$_5$	69	14.1	101	16.1	0.86	(0.61–1.21)	0.401
CATT$_6$	143	14.9	27	17.0	0.86	(0.54–1.40)	0.551
CATT$_7$	63	22.7	107	12.8	2.01	(1.40–2.88)	0.0001
Genotypes							
G>C (rs755622)							
GG	99	12.9	71	20.1	0.60	(0.42–0.85)	0.0031
GC	67	20.4	103	13.1	1.71	(1.20–2.43)	0.0025
CC	4	15.4	166	15.2	1.01	(0.25–3.03)	1.000
CATT repeat (rs3063368)							
CATT$_{5,5}$	7	9.9	163	15.6	0.59	(0.22–1.32)	0.233
CATT$_{5,6}$	45	13.0	125	16.2	0.78	(0.52–1.13)	0.178
CATT$_{5,7}$	17	23.6	153	14.7	1.80	(0.95–3.25)	0.060
CATT$_{6,6}$	55	13.0	115	16.6	0.75	(0.52–1.07)	0.122
CATT$_{6,7}$	43	22.8	127	13.7	1.86	(1.23–2.77)	0.003
CATT$_{7,7}$	3	18.8	167	15.2	1.29	(0.23–4.76)	0.723
Individual genotype combinations *							
CATT$_{5,5}$-GG (6.1%)	7	10.3	163	15.6	0.62	(0.24–1.40)	0.297
CATT$_{5,6}$-GG (29.5%)	44	13.4	126	16.0	0.81	(0.55–1.19)	0.275
CATT$_{6,6}$-GG (32.3%)	47	13.1	123	16.3	0.77	(0.53–1.12)	0.182
CATT$_{6,6}$-CG (5.6%)	8	12.7	162	15.4	0.80	(0.32–1.73)	0.718
CATT$_{5,7}$-CG (6.2%)	17	24.6	153	14.6	1.91	(1.01–3.46)	0.036
CATT$_{6,7}$-CG (15.8%)	41	23.3	129	13.7	1.91	(1.25–2.87)	0.002

The incidence of AKI was higher among patients carrying the CATT$_7$ allele, in patients with the GC or CATT$_{6,7}$ genotype, and in patients with the genotype combinations CATT$_{5,7}$-CG and CATT$_{6,7}$-CG. AKI, acute kidney injury; CI, confidence interval; OR, odds ratio; SNP, Single nucleotide polymorphism; CATT$_7$, patients carrying at least one CATT$_7$ allele. * genotype combinations with a frequency of >5%. Data presented as absolute numbers and percentage. p-value calculated by Fisher exact test; bold fonts indicate p-values < 0.05.

Patients carrying the G>C SNP were also at increased risk of AKI (20.4% vs. 13.1%, OR 1.71, 95% CI 1.20–2.43, $p = 0.0025$) (Table 4). The 26 homozygote carriers of the CC genotype did not show an increased risk of AKI when compared to others ($p = 1.000$).

Multiple complications, defined as at least two of the predefined organ dysfunctions, were observed in 12.4% of patients (N = 139) (Table 3). The CATT$_7$ repeat and the G>C SNP were significantly associated with the occurrence of multiple postoperative complications when compared to all other genotypes (CATT$_7$: 17.7% vs. 10.7%, OR 1.79, 95% CI 1.20–2.65, p = 0.003; GC: 16.8% vs. 10.7%, OR 1.69, 95% CI 1.15–2.47, p = 0.007) (Table 5).

Table 5. Association of the *MIF* promoter polymorphisms with multiple complications *.

MIF Polymorphism	Multiple Complications * (N = 139)						*p*-Value
	Patients Carrying this Allele/Genotype		Patients NOT Carrying this Allele/Genotype				
	N	Incidence, %	N	Incidence, %	OR	(95% CI)	
-CATT repeat allele carriers (rs3063368)							
CATT $_5$	50	10.3	89	14.2	0.69	(0.47–1.01)	0.055
CATT $_6$	120	12.5	19	12.0	1.06	(0.62–1.88)	0.898
CATT $_7$	49	17.7	90	10.7	1.79	(1.20–2.65)	**0.003**
Genotypes							
G>C (rs755622)							
GG	80	10.1	59	16.7	0.59	(0.40–0.86)	**0.005**
GC	55	16.8	84	10.7	1.69	(1.15–2.47)	**0.007**
CC	4	15.4	135	12.4	1.29	(0.32–3.87)	0.554
CATT repeat (rs3063368)							
CATT $_{5,5}$	4	5.6	135	12.9	0.40	(0.10–1.11)	0.092
CATT $_{5,6}$	33	9.6	106	13.8	0.66	(0.42–1.02)	0.050
CATT $_{5,7}$	13	18.1	126	12.1	1.61	(0.78–3.06)	0.140
CATT $_{6,6}$	53	12.5	86	12.4	1.01	(0.69–1.48)	1.000
CATT $_{6,7}$	34	18.0	105	11.3	1.72	(1.09–2.66)	**0.015**
CATT $_{7,7}$	2	12.5	137	12.5	1.00	(0.11–4.45)	1.000
Individual genotype combinations †							
CATT $_{5,5}$-GG (6.1%)	4	5.9	135	12.9	0.42	(0.11–1.16)	0.126
CATT $_{5,6}$-GG (29.5%)	32	9.7	107	13.6	0.68	(0.44–1.05)	0.091
CATT $_{6,6}$-GG (32.3%)	44	12.2	95	12.6	0.97	(0.65–1.44)	0.923
CATT $_{6,6}$-CG (5.6%)	9	14.3	130	12.4	1.18	(0.50–2.49)	0.693
CATT $_{5,7}$-CG (6.2%)	13	18.4	126	12.0	1.70	(0.83–3.25)	0.127
CATT $_{6,7}$-CG (15.8%)	32	18.2	107	11.4	1.73	(1.08–2.70)	**0.018**

The incidence of multiple complications was higher among patients carrying the CATT$_7$ allele, in patients with the GC or CATT $_{6,7}$ genotype, and in patients with the genotype combinations CATT $_{5,7}$-CG and CATT $_{6,7}$-CG. CI, confidence interval; OR, odds ratio; SNP, Single nucleotide polymorphism; CATT$_{7x}$, patients carrying at least one CATT$_7$ allele. † genotype combinations with a frequency of > 5%. * Patients affected by at least two of the predefined organ dysfunctions. † defined as at least two of the predefined organ dysfunctions. Data presented as absolute numbers and percentage. *p*-value calculated by Fisher's exact test; bold fonts indicate *p*-values < 0.05.

The incidence of death during the first 30 days after surgery was 0.7% (N = 8) (Table 3). The mortality of carriers of the *MIF* CATT$_7$ allele was significantly higher compared to patients not carrying the CATT$_7$ repeat (1.81% vs. 0.36%, p = 0.026, OR 5.12, 95% CI 0.99–33.14) (Table 6). Likewise, patients with the *MIF* CATT$_{6,7}$ repeat genotype also had an increased risk of death when compared to all other patients (2.1% vs. 0.4%, OR 4.99, 95% CI 0.92–26.98, p = 0.032). Mortality rates in carriers of the GC genotype were increased with borderline significance (1.5% vs. 0.4%, OR 4.05, 95% CI 0.78–26.20, p = 0.053).

There was no significant difference in the incidence of AKI or death in heterozygous or homozygous carriers of the C allele or the CATT7 repeat allele (AKI-C-allele: 20.4% vs. 15.4%, OR 1.41 (0.47–4.24), p = 0.537; AKI-CATT7: 21.7% vs. 18.8%, OR 1.11 (0.30–4.05), p = 0.879; death-C allele: 0% vs. 1.5%, OR 0.90 (0.05–16.75), p = 0.526; death-CATT7: 0% vs. 1.9%; OR 0.66 (0.03–12.54), p = 0.589). While *MIF* promoter polymorphisms were significantly associated with AKI, multiple complications, and death, no significant association was found with regards to the incidence of postoperative myocardial infarction, atrial fibrillation, stroke, or delirium (Supplemental Tables S2–S5).

Table 6. Association of the *MIF* promoter polymorphisms with death.

MIF Polymorphism	Death (N = 8)						p-Value
	Patients Carrying This Allele/Genotype		Patients NOT Carrying This Allele/Genotype				
	N	Incidence, %	N	Incidence, %	OR	(95% CI)	
CATT repeat allele carriers (rs3063368)							
$CATT_5$	2	0.4	6	1.0	0.43	(0.04–2.40)	0.478
$CATT_6$	7	0.7	1	0.6	1.16	(0.15–52.80)	1.000
$CATT_7$	5	1.8	3	0.4	5.12	(0.99–33.14)	0.026
Genotypes							
G>C (rs755622)							
GG	3	0.4	5	1.4	0.28	(0.04–1.43)	0.118
GC	5	1.5	3	0.4	4.05	(0.78–26.20)	0.053
CC	0	0	8	0.7	0.00	(0.00–19.77)	1.000
CATT repeat (rs3063368)							
$CATT_{5,5}$	0	0	8	0.8	0.00	(0.00–6.75)	1.000
$CATT_{5,6}$	1	0.3	7	0.9	0.32	(0.01–2.49)	0.447
$CATT_{5,7}$	1	1.4	7	0.7	2.09	(0.05–16.59)	0.415
$CATT_{6,6}$	2	0.5	6	0.9	0.54	(0.05–3.06)	0.717
$CATT_{6,7}$	4	2.1	4	0.4	4.99	(0.92–26.98)	0.032
$CATT_{7,7}$	0	0	8	0.7	0.00	(0.00–33.33)	1.000
Individual genotype combinations *							
$CATT_{5,5}$-GG (6.1%)	0	0	8	0.8	0.00	(0.00–7.07)	1.000
$CATT_{5,6}$-GG (29.5%)	1	0.3	7	0.9	0.34	(0.01–2.66)	0.449
$CATT_{6,6}$-GG (32.3%)	2	0.6	6	0.8	0.70	(0.07–3.93)	1.000
$CATT_{6,6}$-CG (5.6%)	0	0	8	0.8	0.00	(0.00–7.68)	1.000
$CATT_{5,7}$-CG (6.2%)	1	1.5	7	0.7	2.18	(0.05–17.39)	0.401
$CATT_{6,7}$-CG (15.8%)	4	2.3	4	0.4	5.44	(1.00–29.44)	0.025

The incidence of death was higher among patients carrying the $CATT_7$ allele, in patients with the $CATT_{6,7}$ genotype, and in patients with the genotype combination $CATT_{6,7}$-CG.; OR, odds ratio; SNP, Single nucleotide polymorphism; $CATT_7$, patients carrying at least one $CATT_7$ allele. * genotypes with a frequency of > 5%. Data presented as absolute numbers and percentage. p-value calculated by Fisher's exact test; bold fonts indicate p-values < 0.05.

3.4. MIF Genotypes as a Predictor of AKI in Multivariable Analyses

To assess if the *MIF* genotype improves preoperative risk prediction, a multivariable logistic regression was performed for AKI and death. For risk modeling, all baseline patients' characteristics (Table 1), including the well-established EuroSCORE, a preoperative risk stratification tool, were considered, and a logistic regression parameter selection procedure was performed. For the prediction of AKI, the variables EuroSCORE, hemoglobin, hypertension, and the presence of the *MIF* $CATT_7$ allele were selected. When adjusted for these variables, the *MIF* $CATT_7$ allele remained a significant predictor of AKI (OR 2.13, 95% CI, 1.46–3.1) (Table 7). The resulting model had an AUC of 0.71 (95% CI, 0.67–0.76).

For prediction of death, the statistical variable selection procedure resulted in a model containing the variables EuroSCORE, insulin-dependent diabetes, and the *MIF* $CATT_7$ allele. The presence of a *MIF* $CATT_7$ repeat allele significantly improved the prediction of postoperative mortality in this model (OR 5.58, 95% CI 1.29–24.04, $p = 0.021$). The resulting model had an AUC (receiver operating statistics—area under the curve) of 0.874 (95% CI, 0.786–0.962) (Table 7, Figure 2). In summary, the *MIF* $CATT_7$ allele is a significant predisposing risk factor for AKI and death after cardiac surgery.

The multivariable logistic regression model for AKI includes the variables *MIF* $CATT_7$ allele carriers and arterial hypertension as binary variables, and EuroSCORE and hemoglobin levels as continuous variables (according to Table 7). The model for death includes the variables *MIF* $CATT_7$ carrier status and insulin-dependent diabetes as binary variables and EuroSCORE as a continuous variable. AUC, area under the curve; CI, confidence interval.

Table 7. Predictors of Acute Kidney Injury (AKI) and death using multivariable logistic regression.

Variable	ß	OR	(95% CI)	p-Value
AKI (N = 170) *	−1.066			
CATT$_7$ carrier	0.755	2.13	(1.46–3.09)	**<0.001**
EuroSCORE	0.202	1.22	(1.38–1.32)	**<0.001**
Hemoglobin	−0.183	0.83	(0.74–0.94)	**0.004**
Hypertension	0.701	2.03	(1.11–3.72)	**0.022**
Death (N = 8) †	−6.709			
CATT$_7$ carrier	1.719	5.58	(1.29–24.04)	**0.021**
EuroSCORE	0.342	1.41	(1.05–1.88)	**0.021**
IDDM	1.923	6.84	(1.55–30.26)	**0.011**

In addition to the well-established EuroSCORE and other baseline characteristics, the *MIF* CATT$_7$ was identified as a significant predictor of AKI and death. AKI, acute kidney injury; OR, odds ratio; CI, confidence interval. IDDM, insulin-dependent diabetes mellitus. Bold fonts indicate p-values < 0.05. * Area under the curve (AUC), 0.71; 95% CI, 0.67 - 0.76; Hosmer und Lemeshow Goodness-of-Fit Test, 0.8432. † Area under the curve (AUC), 0.87; 95% CI, 0.79–0.96; Hosmer und Lemeshow Goodness-of-Fit Test, 0.9702.

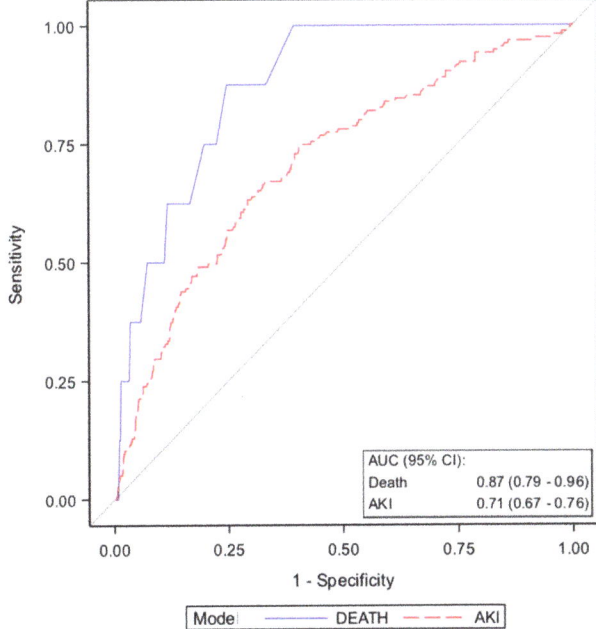

Figure 2. Receiver operating characteristics (ROC) curves for the prediction of AKI (red) and death (blue) after elective cardiac surgery. The grey line indicates the reference values of a diagnostic test that is no better than chance level.

3.5. MIF Serum Levels Before Surgery Are Increased in Patients Carrying the CATT$_7$ Allele

To assess the association of the *MIF* promoter polymorphisms and the circulating MIF levels in cardiac surgery patients, perioperative kinetics of serum MIF were analyzed in 100 patients in relation to the underlying *MIF* polymorphisms. In patients carrying at least one CATT$_7$ allele (CATT$_7$), serum MIF was significantly elevated before surgery (79.2 vs. 50.4 ng/mL, p = 0.008) and one hour after surgery (154.8 vs. 79.5 ng/mL, p = 0.02) (Figure 3). The comparison of all other alleles, genotypes, and individual genotype combinations did not show significant differences between groups.

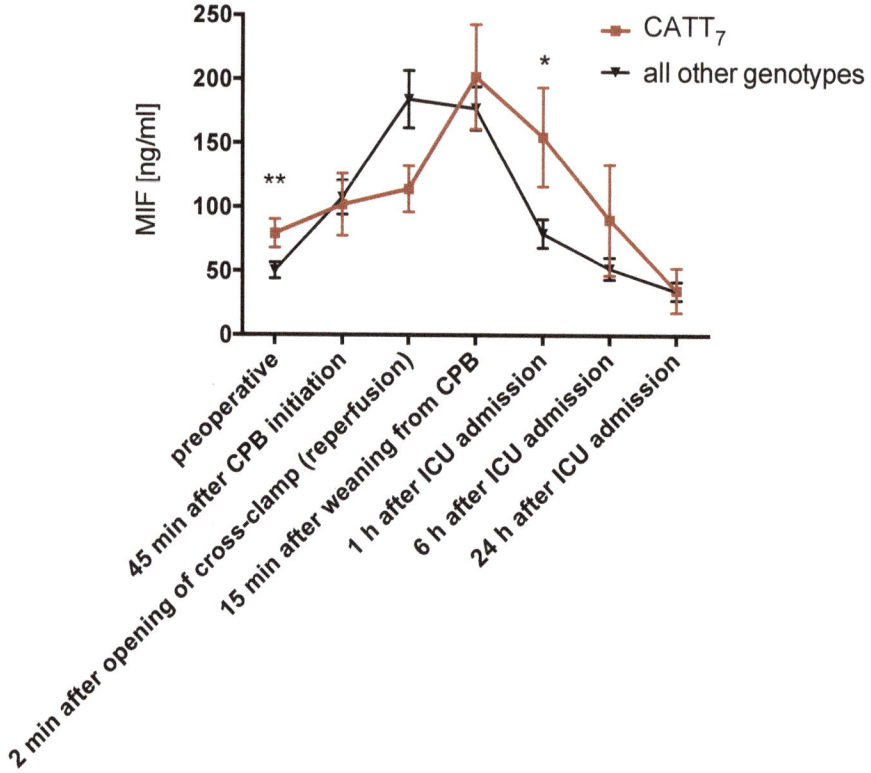

Figure 3. Perioperative kinetics of serum MIF in patients undergoing cardiac surgery. * $P < 0.05$, ** $P < 0.01$.

Serum MIF was quantified with ELISA in 100 patients. Patients heterozygous or homozygous for the *MIF* CATT$_7$ allele had significantly increased serum MIF before surgery (preoperative) and significantly lower serum MIF 1 h after surgery. Data are means ± SEM. ** $p < 0.01$, * $p < 0.05$ versus other groups at the corresponding time point (difference between groups) analyzed by Wilcoxon Rank Sum test.

4. Discussion

MIF is an inflammatory cytokine that is rapidly released from preformed intracellular pools in response to diverse cellular and systemic stressors, including ischemia-reperfusion, endotoxemia and surgery [21]. Previous studies demonstrated a significant peak of circulating MIF during cardiac surgery, as well as an association between circulating MIF and adverse postoperative outcomes [5,22–24]. Two polymorphisms in the *MIF* gene regulatory region, a CATT$_{5-7}$ microsatellite repeat (rs3063368) and a -270 (formerly described as -173) G>C single-nucleotide polymorphism (rs755622), which is in linkage disequilibrium with CATT$_7$, have been studied regarding their association with different pathologic conditions (e.g., pulmonary tuberculosis, acute coronary syndrome, carotid artery atherosclerosis, systemic lupus erythematosis, multiple sclerosis) [8,14,25–28]. However, the impact of the *MIF* gene polymorphisms on postoperative outcomes after cardiac surgery has not been analyzed.

The cardiac surgery patients in the present study displayed similar allele frequencies of the *MIF* CATT$_{5-7}$ microsatellite repeat (rs3063368) and G>C single nucleotide variant (rs755622) as in the general population [20]. Approximately 25% of patients carried at least one longer CATT repeat (CATT$_7$) (rs3063368) and 30% carried at least one C allele (rs755622). Demographic characteristics and procedural data revealed no significant differences between genotypes. Heterozygous or homozygous carriers of the $CATT_7$ allele had an almost 5-fold increased risk of death after cardiac surgery. Patients carrying either the $CATT_7$ or the C allele had an approximately 2-fold increased risk of suffering from AKI or multiple organ dysfunctions. While the risk for AKI was 12.8% in patients not carrying a $CATT_7$ allele, it was 22.7% for carriers of the $CATT_7$ allele. In addition to the well-established EuroSCORE, the *MIF* $CATT_7$ was identified as a significant predictor of death and development of AKI in a multivariable logistic regression model. The reason why we observed no significant association between homozygosity of the CC genotype might be attributed to the very low number of patients (N = 26, frequency 2.3%), but should be reevaluated in larger cohorts.

The *MIF* promoter microsatellite was suggested to influence MIF mRNA expression, as assessed by luciferase reporter assays in normal and patient cells [11,14]. The longer $CATT_7$ repeat further has been associated with higher serum MIF levels in various patient cohorts, including those with coronary artery disease [10,29,30]. In this study, we found that patients carrying the $CATT_7$ allele had higher serum MIF preoperatively and one hour after surgery, but serum MIF did not differ at the other intra- and postoperative timepoints.

In recent literature, MIF has already been associated with AKI in divergent clinical settings of septic shock, liver transplantation, glomerulonephritis, and renal allograft rejection [31–34].

However, there are indications that MIF can have a protective role against renal tubular injury in experimental models of ischemic AKI [23,35]. In one study, high MIF serum levels during cardiac surgery were associated with a reduced risk of postoperative AKI [23]. This contrasts with our observation of the $CATT_7$ and G>C, that are the proposed high expression alleles, being associated with AKI. An important risk factor for postoperative AKI is pre-existing chronic kidney disease (CKD), genetic studies support an association between the presence of at least one *MIF* G>C allele (rs755622) with chronic kidney and cardiovascular disease [36,37]. In a cross-sectional study MIF serum levels were significantly increased in patients with CKD [38]. It is well established that chronic kidney disease (CKD) predisposes to AKI [39]. Therefore, it can be speculated that the association between proposed high expression *MIF* genotypes with AKI is related to CKD that may inflate the risk for postoperative AKI. We suggest that preoperatively, chronically elevated MIF serum levels are associated with detrimental effects and may need to be discriminated from high intraoperative MIF serum levels, which might in fact mediate organ-protective effects during ischemia-reperfusion. This is in line with the notion that acute elevations of MIF serum levels may ameliorate ischemia-reperfusion injury after cardiac surgery, whereas long-term elevations in MIF may aggravate inflammatory pathways in atherosclerosis [40,41]. The observation of MIF correlating with markers of oxidative stress (8-hydroxy-2-deoxyguanosine) and endothelial activation (ICAM-1) in a cohort of CKD patients, supports the thesis that chronically elevated MIF levels might contribute to cardiovascular and associated CKD [38].

Mechanistically, MIF induces intracellular signal cascades via binding to its receptors including the cardioprotective CD74/AMPK kinase axis and the MIF CXC motif chemokine receptors, CXCR2, CXCR4, or CXCR7. Serum MIF may influence the expression of MIF receptors, and there are indications from mouse models that genetic *MIF* deficiency downregulates the expression of the MIF-signalling co-receptor CD44, which is required for signaling responses through CD74 [42,43]. Accordingly, chronically elevated levels of MIF might lead to an altered or injurious response to an acute, perioperative MIF increase, and potentially explain why MIF may be renoprotective in healthy mice but deleterious in multimorbid patients with chronic, underlying inflammation. The results of the present study nevertheless remain observational and cannot explain causative pathophysiology. Further studies investigating the mechanisms by which high expression of the *MIF* genotype may mediate the observed deleterious effects may help in the development of protective strategies for high risk cardiac surgery patients.

We acknowledge several limitations of our study, including the observational design. The event rate for death was very low, and therefore the analysis addressing the association of *MIF* genotypes with mortality should be interpreted cautiously and requires validation in larger cohorts. Although we measured serum MIF in a subcohort of patients and observed a relationship with increased CATT repeat length, this observation has not been consistently observed in prior studies, in part due to limitations of the serum compartment in reflecting systemic or regional tissue *MIF* expression levels [44,45]. Moreover, the study focused on Caucasian subjects and population stratification at the *MIF* locus exists [46]. While we did not study different geographic cohorts, our homogenous study population allows generalisability across predominantly European populations. Finally, the genotyping technique employed does not allow a concise phase analysis, and single haplotypes, e.g., the co-localization of a specific CATT allele (rs3063368) with the G or C allele (rs755622), cannot be explored.

In the same study cohort, one genome-wide association study (GWAS) has been undertaken and did not identify an association of the *MIF* gene polymorphisms with postoperative outcome [47]. Therefore, our findings underscore the necessity of candidate gene studies, including of common structural variants such as microsatellite repeats that are not detectable by SNP-based GWAS platforms [47–49]. As technological advances and declining costs in next-generation sequencing technologies pave the way for the broader availability of genomic testing, the implementation of genetic susceptibility data will help to improve risk stratification and to reduce the incidence and sequelae of cardiac surgery [50].

5. Conclusions

In the setting of cardiac surgery, we identified the *MIF* promotor polymorphisms $CATT_7$ (rs3063368) and -270 (formerly -173) G>C (rs755622), to be predictive of development of postoperative AKI and death. These *MIF* promoter alleles could improve current clinical risk prediction models and thus serve as a helpful decision-making tool for clinicians and patients in the near future.

Supplementary Materials: The following are available online at http://www.mdpi.com/2077-0383/9/9/2936/s1. Supplemental Figure S1. Flowchart of the patients screened and included in the study. Supplemental Figure S2. SNP rs5844572 region ($CATT_n$ tetranucleotide repeat) and rs755622 (G>C) with UCSC genome browser (Geb. 2009; GRCh37/hg19 Assembly). Supplemental Table S1. Primer sequences used for genotyping of the tetranucleotide repeat polymorphism $CATT_n$ (rs3063368). Supplemental Table S2. Association of *MIF* promoter polymorphisms with Myocardial Infarction. Supplemental Table S3. Association of *MIF* promoter polymorphisms with Stroke. Supplemental Table S4. Association of *MIF* promoter polymorphisms with delir. Supplemental Table S5. Association of MIF regulatory polymorphisms with atrial fibrillation.

Author Contributions: Conceptualization, L.A., C.S. and K.Z.; Methodology, L.A., C.S., K.F.; Software, K.F., C.S.; Validation, K.F., L.A., C.S.; Formal Analysis, K.F., L.A., C.S., J.B.; Investigation, L.A., K.F., S.M., C.S.; Resources, C.S., K.Z., R.B., J.B., G.M.; Data Curation, K.F., L.A.; Writing—Original Draft Preparation, L.A., C.S.; Writing—Review and Editing, J.B., R.B., H.S., H.-J.L., S.M., P.M., D.W., L.L., G.M., D.E.L., A.Z.; Project Administration, C.S.; Funding Acquisition, C.S., K.Z., J.B. All authors have read and agreed to the published version of the manuscript.

Funding: This study was partly supported by the Deutsche Forschungsgemeinschaft (DFG; STO 1099/8-1 to CS BE 1977/9-1; BE 1977/14-1 to JB; SFB1123/A3 to JB). The RIPHeart Study was funded by the German Research Foundation (ME 3559/1-1).

Acknowledgments: We are thankful for the technical support received from Christian Beckers. RIPHeart Study Collaborators: Ana Stevanovic, Rolf Rossaint, Marc Felzen, Andreas Goetzenich, Tobias Moormann, Katharina Chalk, Pascal Knuefermann, Thomas Recht, Andreas Hoeft, Michael Winterhalter, Sonja Iken, Carolin Wiedenbeck, Gerhard Schwarzmann, Simone Lindau, Andreas Zierer, Stephan Fichtlscherer, Gerold Goerlach, Matthias Wollbrueck, Ursula Boening, Markus Weigand, Julia Strauchmann, Kai U. Morsbach, Markus Paxian, Konrad Reinhard, Jens Scholz, Jochen Renner, Ole Broch, Helga Francksen, Bernd Kuhr, Hermann Heinze, Hauke Paarmann, Hans-Hinrich Sievers, Stefan Klotz, Thomas Hachenberg, Christian Werner, Susanne Mauff, Angela Alms, Stefan Bergt, and Norbert Roewer. Aachen (Department of Anesthesiology, Medical Faculty RWTH Aachen University, Aachen, Germany): Ana Stevanovic, Rolf Rossaint, Marc Felzen, (Department of Thoracic and Cardiovascular Surgery): Andreas Goetzenich; 195 patients; Berlin (Department of Anesthesiology and Intensive Care Medicine, Charité-Universitätsmedizin Berlin, Campus Charité Mitte, Berlin, Germany): Tobias Moormann, Katharina Chalk; 37 patients; Bonn (Department of Anesthesiology and Intensive Care Medicine, University Hospital Bonn, Bonn, Germany): Pascal Knuefermann, Thomas Recht, Andreas Hoeft; 73 patients; Duesseldorf (Department of Anesthesiology and Intensive Care Medicine, University Hospital Duesseldorf, Germany): Michael Winterhalter; 65 patients; Frankfurt am Main (Department of Anesthesiology, Intensive Care Medicine and Pain Therapy, University Hospital Frankfurt, Frankfurt am Main, Germany): Sonja Iken, Carolin Wiedenbeck, Gerhard Schwarzmann, Simone Lindau, (Department of Thoracic and Cardiovascular Surgery): Andreas Zierer, (Internal Medicine III: Cardiology, Angiology, Nephrology): Stephan Fichtlscherer; 117 patients; Giessen (Department of Cardiovascular Surgery, University of Giessen, Germany): Gerold Goerlach,

Matthias Wollbrueck, Ursula Boening; (Department of Anesthesiology): Markus Weigand; 148 patients; Goettingen (Department of Anesthesiology and Intensive Care Medicine, University Hospital Goettingen, Germany): Julia Strauchmann, Konrad August; 91 patients; Jena (Department of Anesthesiology and Intensive Care Medicine, Jena University Hospital, Jena, Germany): Kai U. Morsbach, Markus Paxian, Konrad Reinhard; 76 patients; Kiel (Department of Anesthesiology and Intensive Care Medicine, University Hospital Schleswig-Holstein, Campus Kiel, Germany): Jens Scholz, Jochen Renner, Ole Broch, Helga Francksen, Bernd Kuhr; 237 patients; Luebeck (Department of Anesthesiology, University Hospital Luebeck, Luebeck, Germany): Hermann Heinze, Hauke Paarmann; (Department of Cardiac and Thoracic Vascular Surgery): Hans-Hinrich Sievers, Stefan Klotz; 56 patients; Magdeburg (Department of Anesthesiology, University Hospital Magdeburg, Germany); Thomas Hachenberg; 14 patients; Mainz (Department of Anesthesiology, Medical Center of Johannes Gutenberg-University, Mainz, Germany): Christian Werner, Susanne Mauff; 116 patients; Rostock (Clinic of Anesthesiology and Intensive Care Medicine, University Hospital Rostock, Rostock, Germany): Angela Alms, Stefan Bergt; 146 patients; Wuerzburg (Department of Anesthesiology, University Hospital Wuerzburg, Wuerzburg, Germany): Norbert Roewer; 32 patients.

Conflicts of Interest: R.B. has significant financial interests. He is a co-inventor on patents related to therapeutic MIF modulation and MIF genotyping, and owns more than 5% of the voting shares in MIFCOR, Inc, a Yale University biotechnology start-up company. J.B. is a co-inventor on patents describing the therapeutic utility of MIF antagonists (modest interests). D.E.L. has received research grant support from BioPorto Diagnostics (modest interests). R.B., J.B., and D.E.L. did not shape or manipulate the design and execution of the study. They contributed by helping with interpretation of data and by reviewing the manuscript.

References

1. Brown, P.P.; Kugelmass, A.D.; Cohen, D.J.; Reynolds, M.R.; Culler, S.D.; Dee, A.D.; Simon, A.W. The Frequency and Cost of Complications Associated with Coronary Artery Bypass Grafting Surgery: Results from the United States Medicare Program. *Ann. Thorac. Surg.* **2008**, *85*, 1980–1986. [CrossRef]
2. Grover, A.; Gorman, K.; Dall, T.M.; Jonas, R.; Lytle, B.; Shemin, R.; Wood, D.; Kron, I. Shortage of Cardiothoracic Surgeons Is Likely by 2020. *Circulation* **2009**, *120*, 488–494. [CrossRef] [PubMed]
3. Roques, F.; Nashef, S.A.; Michel, P.; Gauducheau, E.; De Vincentiis, C.; Baudet, E.; Cortina, J.; David, M.; Faichney, A.; Gavrielle, F.; et al. Risk factors and outcome in European cardiac surgery: Analysis of the EuroSCORE multinational database of 19030 patients. *Eur. J. Cardio-Thorac. Surg.* **1999**, *15*, 816–823. [CrossRef]
4. Sureshbabu, A.; Ryter, S.W.; Choi, M.E. Oxidative stress and autophagy: Crucial modulators of kidney injury. *Redox Biol.* **2015**, *4*, 208–214. [CrossRef] [PubMed]
5. Stoppe, C.; Rex, S.; Goetzenich, A.; Kraemer, S.; Emontzpohl, C.; Soppert, J.; Averdunk, L.; Sun, Y.; Rossaint, R.; Lue, H.; et al. Interaction of MIF Family Proteins in Myocardial Ischemia/Reperfusion Damage and Their Influence on Clinical Outcome of Cardiac Surgery Patients. *Antioxid. Redox Signal.* **2015**, *23*, 865–879. [CrossRef] [PubMed]
6. Ozsoy, A.Z.; Karakus, N.; Tural, S.; Yigit, S.; Kara, N.; Alaylı, G.; Tumer, M.K.; Kuru, O. Influence of the MIF polymorphism −173G > C on Turkish postmenopausal women with osteoporosis. *Z. Rheumatol.* **2017**, *77*, 629–632. [CrossRef] [PubMed]
7. Vishwakarma, S.K.; Lakkireddy, C.; Sravani, G.; Sastry, B.V.S.; Raju, N.; Ahmed, S.I.; Owaisi, N.; Jaisawal, A.; Khan, M.A.; Khan, A.A. Association of CD14 and macrophage migration inhibitory factor gene polymorphisms with inflammatory microRNAs expression levels in ankylosing spondylitis and polyarthralgia. *Int. J. Immunogenet.* **2018**, *45*, 190–200. [CrossRef]
8. Benedek, G.; Meza-Romero, R.; Jordan, K.; Zhang, Y.; Nguyen, H.; Kent, G.; Li, J.; Siu, E.; Frazer, J.; Piecycha, M.; et al. MIF and D-DT are potential disease severity modifiers in male MS subjects. *Proc. Natl. Acad. Sci. USA* **2017**, *114*, E8421–E8429. [CrossRef]
9. Bae, S.-C.; Lee, Y.H. Circulating macrophage migration inhibitory factor levels and its polymorphisms in systemic lupus erythematosus: A meta-analysis. *Cell. Mol. Biol.* **2017**, *63*, 74–79. [CrossRef]
10. Baugh, J.A.; Chitnis, S.; Donnelly, S.C.; Monteiro, J.; Lin, X.; Plant, B.J.; Wolfe, F.; Gregersen, P.K.; Bucala, R. A functional promoter polymorphism in the macrophage migration inhibitory factor (MIF) gene associated with disease severity in rheumatoid arthritis. *Genes Immun.* **2002**, *3*, 170–176. [CrossRef]
11. Yao, J.; Leng, L.; Sauler, M.; Fu, W.-L.; Zheng, J.; Zhang, Y.; Du, X.; Yu, X.; Lee, P.; Bucala, R. Transcription factor ICBP90 regulates the MIF promoter and immune susceptibility locus. *J. Clin. Investig.* **2016**, *126*, 732–744. [CrossRef] [PubMed]

12. Guo, P.; Wang, J.; Liu, J.; Xia, M.; Li, W.; He, M. Macrophage immigration inhibitory factor promotes cell proliferation and inhibits apoptosis of cervical adenocarcinoma. *Tumor Biol.* **2015**, *36*, 5095–5102. [CrossRef] [PubMed]
13. Meybohm, P.; Bein, B.; Brosteanu, O.; Cremer, J.T.; Gruenewald, M.; Stoppe, C.; Coburn, M.; Schaelte, G.; Böning, A.; Niemann, B.; et al. A Multicenter Trial of Remote Ischemic Preconditioning for Heart Surgery. *N. Engl. J. Med.* **2015**, *373*, 1397–1407. [CrossRef] [PubMed]
14. Sreih, A.; Ezzeddine, R.; Leng, L.; Lachance, A.; Yu, G.; Mizuec, Y.; Subrahmanyan, L.; Pons-Estel, B.A.; Abelson, A.-K.; Gunnarsson, I.; et al. Dual effect of the macrophage migration inhibitory factor gene on the development and severity of human systemic lupus erythematosus. *Arthritis Rheum.* **2011**, *63*, 3942–3951. [CrossRef]
15. Palevsky, P.M.; Liu, K.D.; Brophy, P.D.; Chawla, L.S.; Parikh, C.R.; Thakar, C.V.; Tolwani, A.J.; Waikar, S.S.; Weisbord, S.D. KDOQI US Commentary on the 2012 KDIGO Clinical Practice Guideline for Acute Kidney Injury. *Am. J. Kidney Dis.* **2013**, *61*, 649–672. [CrossRef]
16. Thygesen, K.; Alpert, J.S.; White, H.D.; Jaffe, A.S.; Apple, F.S.; Galvani, M.; Katus, H.A.; Newby, L.K.; Jan, R.; Chaitman, B.; et al. Universal Definition of Myocardial Infarction. *Circulation* **2007**, *116*, 2634–2653. [CrossRef]
17. Ely, E.W.; Inouye, S.K.; Bernard, G.R.; Gordon, S.; Francis, J.; May, L.; Truman, B.; Speroff, T.; Gautam, S.; Margolin, R.; et al. Delirium in mechanically ventilated patients: Validity and reliability of the confusion assessment method for the intensive care unit (CAM-ICU). *JAMA* **2001**, *286*, 2703–2710. [CrossRef] [PubMed]
18. Wityk, R.J.; Pessin, M.S.; Kaplan, R.F.; Caplan, L.R. Serial assessment of acute stroke using the NIH Stroke Scale. *Stroke* **1994**, *25*, 362–365. [CrossRef]
19. Harris, J.; Morand, E.F. *Macrophage Migration Inhibitory Factor Methods and Protocols*; Methods in Molecular Biology; Springer: Berlin, Germany, 2020; Volume 2080.
20. Karczewski, K.J.; Francioli, L.C.; Tiao, G.; Cummings, B.B.; Alfoldi, J.; Wang, Q.; Collins, R.L.; Laricchia, K.M.; Ganna, A.; Birnbaum, D.P.; et al. The mutational constraint spectrum quantified from variation in 141,456 humans. *Nature* **2020**, *581*, 434–443. [CrossRef]
21. Bacher, M.; Meinhardt, A.; Lan, H.Y.; Mu, W.; Metz, C.N.; Chesney, J.A.; Calandra, T.; Gemsa, D.; Donnelly, T.; Atkins, R.C.; et al. Migration inhibitory factor expression in experimentally induced endotoxemia. *Am. J. Pathol.* **1997**, *150*, 235–246.
22. Gando, S.; Nishihira, J.; Kemmotsu, O.; Kobayashi, S.; Morimoto, Y.; Matsui, Y.; Yasuda, K. An increase in macrophage migration inhibitory factor release in patients with cardiopulmonary bypass surgery. *Surg. Today* **2000**, *30*, 689–694. [CrossRef] [PubMed]
23. Stoppe, C.; Averdunk, L.; Goetzenich, A.; Soppert, J.; Marlier, A.; Kraemer, S.; Vieten, J.; Coburn, M.; Kowark, A.; Kim, B.-S.; et al. The protective role of macrophage migration inhibitory factor in acute kidney injury after cardiac surgery. *Sci. Transl. Med.* **2018**, *10*, aan4886. [CrossRef]
24. Stoppe, C.; Grieb, G.; Rossaint, R.; Simons, D.; Coburn, M.; Götzenich, A.; Strüssmann, T.; Pallua, N.; Bernhagen, J.; Rex, S. High Postoperative Blood Levels of Macrophage Migration Inhibitory Factor Are Associated with Less Organ Dysfunction in Patients after Cardiac Surgery. *Mol. Med.* **2012**, *18*, 843–850. [CrossRef] [PubMed]
25. Liu, A.; Bao, F.; Voravuthikunchai, S.P. CATT polymorphism in MIF gene promoter is closely related to human pulmonary tuberculosis in a southwestern China population. *Int. J. Immunopathol. Pharmacol.* **2018**, *32*. [CrossRef] [PubMed]
26. Valdes-Alvarado, E.; Muñoz-Valle, J.F.; Valle, Y.; Sandoval-Pinto, E.; García-González, I.J.; Valdez-Haro, A.; De La Cruz-Mosso, U.; Flores-Salinas, H.E.; Padilla-Gutierrez, J.R. Association between the −794 (CATT)5-8 MIF Gene Polymorphism and Susceptibility to Acute Coronary Syndrome in a Western Mexican Population. *J. Immunol. Res.* **2014**, *2014*, 704854. [CrossRef] [PubMed]
27. Lan, M.-Y.; Chang, Y.-Y.; Chen, W.-H.; Tseng, Y.-L.; Lin, H.-S.; Lai, S.-L.; Liu, J.-S. Association between MIF gene polymorphisms and carotid artery atherosclerosis. *Biochem. Biophys. Res. Commun.* **2013**, *435*, 319–322. [CrossRef] [PubMed]
28. Sanchez, E.; Gómez, L.M.; Lopez-Nevot, M.A.; González-Gay, M.A.; Sabio, J.M.; Ortego-Centeno, N.; De Ramón, E.; Anaya, J.; González-Escribano, M.F.; Koeleman, B.P.; et al. Evidence of association of macrophage migration inhibitory factor gene polymorphisms with systemic lupus erythematosus. *Genes Immun.* **2006**, *7*, 433–436. [CrossRef]

29. Mitchell, R.A.; Liao, H.; Chesney, J.; Fingerle-Rowson, G.; Baugh, J.; David, J.; Bucala, R. Macrophage migration inhibitory factor (MIF) sustains macrophage proinflammatory function by inhibiting p53: Regulatory role in the innate immune response. *Proc. Natl. Acad. Sci. USA* **2001**, *99*, 345–350. [CrossRef]
30. Qian, L.; Wang, X.-Y.; Thapa, S.; Tao, L.-Y.; Wu, S.-Z.; Luo, G.-J.; Wang, L.-P.; Wang, J.-N.; Wang, J.; Li, J.; et al. Macrophage migration inhibitory factor promoter polymorphisms (-794 CATT5-8): Relationship with soluble MIF levels in coronary atherosclerotic disease subjects. *BMC Cardiovasc. Disord.* **2017**, *17*, 144. [CrossRef]
31. Payen, D.; Lukaszewicz, A.-C.; Legrand, M.; Gayat, E.; Faivre, V.; Mégarbane, B.; Azoulay, E.; Fieux, F.; Charron, D.; Loiseau, P.; et al. A Multicentre Study of Acute Kidney Injury in Severe Sepsis and Septic Shock: Association with Inflammatory Phenotype and HLA Genotype. *PLoS ONE* **2012**, *7*, e35838. [CrossRef]
32. Baron-Stefaniak, J.; Schiefer, J.; Miller, E.J.; Berlakovich, G.A.; Baron, D.M.; Faybik, P. Comparison of macrophage migration inhibitory factor and neutrophil gelatinase-associated lipocalin-2 to predict acute kidney injury after liver transplantation: An observational pilot study. *PLoS ONE* **2017**, *12*, e0183162. [CrossRef] [PubMed]
33. Brown, F.G.; Nikolic-Paterson, D.J.; Hill, P.A.; Isbel, N.M.; Dowling, J.; Metz, C.M.; Atkins, R.C. Urine macrophage migration inhibitory factor reflects the severity of renal injury in human glomerulonephritis. *J. Am. Soc. Nephrol.* **2002**, *13*, S7–S13. [PubMed]
34. Brown, F.G.; Nikolic-Paterson, D.J.; Chadban, S.J.; Dowling, J.; Jose, M.D.; Metz, C.N.; Bucala, R.; Atkins, R.C. Urine Macrophage Migration Inhibitory Factor Concentrations as a Diagnostic Tool in Human Renal Allograft Rejection. *Transplantion* **2001**, *71*, 1777–1783. [CrossRef] [PubMed]
35. Djudjaj, S.; Martin, I.V.; Buhl, E.M.; Nothofer, N.J.; Leng, L.; Piecychna, M.; Floege, J.; Bernhagen, J.; Bucala, R.; Boor, P. Macrophage Migration Inhibitory Factor Limits Renal Inflammation and Fibrosis by Counteracting Tubular Cell Cycle Arrest. *J. Am. Soc. Nephrol.* **2017**, *28*, 3590–3604. [CrossRef]
36. Herder, C.; Illig, T.; Baumert, J.; Müller-Nurasyid, M.; Klopp, N.; Khuseyinova, N.; Meisinger, C.; Martin, S.; Thorand, B.; Koenig, W. Macrophage migration inhibitory factor (MIF) and risk for coronary heart disease: Results from the MONICA/KORA Augsburg case-cohort study, 1984–2002. *Atherosclerosis* **2008**, *200*, 380–388. [CrossRef]
37. Tong, X.; He, J.; Liu, S.; Peng, S.; Yan, Z.; Zhang, Y.; Fan, H. Macrophage migration inhibitory factor -173G/C gene polymorphism increases the risk of renal disease: A meta-analysis. *Nephrology* **2015**, *20*, 68–76. [CrossRef]
38. Bruchfeld, A.; Carrero, J.J.; Qureshi, A.R.; Lindholm, B.; Bárány, P.; Heimburger, O.; Hu, M.; Lin, X.; Stenvinkel, P.; Miller, E.J. Elevated Serum Macrophage Migration Inhibitory Factor (MIF) Concentrations in Chronic Kidney Disease (CKD) Are Associated with Markers of Oxidative Stress and Endothelial Activation. *Mol. Med.* **2009**, *15*, 70–75. [CrossRef]
39. Chawla, L.S.; Kimmel, P.L. Acute kidney injury and chronic kidney disease: An integrated clinical syndrome. *Kidney Int.* **2012**, *82*, 516–524. [CrossRef]
40. Rassaf, T.; Weber, C.; Bernhagen, J. Macrophage migration inhibitory factor in myocardial ischaemia/reperfusion injury. *Cardiovasc. Res.* **2014**, *102*, 321–328. [CrossRef]
41. Tilstam, P.V.; Qi, D.; Leng, L.; Young, L.; Bucala, R. MIF family cytokines in cardiovascular diseases and prospects for precision-based therapeutics. *Expert Opin. Ther. Targets* **2017**, *21*, 671–683. [CrossRef]
42. Yoo, S.-A.; Leng, L.; Kim, B.-J.; Du, X.; Tilstam, P.V.; Kim, K.H.; Kong, J.-S.; Yoon, H.-J.; Liu, A.; Wang, T.; et al. MIF allele-dependent regulation of the MIF coreceptor CD44 and role in rheumatoid arthritis. *Proc. Natl. Acad. Sci. USA* **2016**, *113*, E7917–E7926. [CrossRef] [PubMed]
43. Ochi, A.; Chen, N.; Schulte, W.; Leng, L.; Moeckel, N.G.; Piecychna, M.; Averdunk, L.; Stoppe, C.; Bucala, R.; Moeckel, G.W. MIF-2/D-DT enhances proximal tubular cell regeneration through SLPI- and ATF4-dependent mechanisms. *Am. J. Physiol. Physiol.* **2017**, *313*, F767–F780. [CrossRef] [PubMed]
44. Herder, C.; Klopp, N.; Baumert, J.; Müller-Nurasyid, M.; Khuseyinova, N.; Meisinger, C.; Martin, S.; Illig, T.; Koenig, W.; Thorand, B. Effect of macrophage migration inhibitory factor (MIF) gene variants and MIF serum concentrations on the risk of type 2 diabetes: Results from the MONICA/KORA Augsburg Case–Cohort Study, 1984–2002. *Diabetologia* **2007**, *51*, 276–284. [CrossRef] [PubMed]
45. Matia-García, I.; Salgado-Goytia, L.; Muñoz-Valle, J.F.; García-Arellano, S.; Hernández-Bello, J.; Salgado-Bernabé, A.B.; Parra-Rojas, I. Macrophage Migration Inhibitory Factor Promoter Polymorphisms (−794 CATT5–8 and −173 G > C): Relationship with mRNA Expression and Soluble MIF Levels in Young Obese Subjects. *Dis. Markers* **2015**, *2015*, 461208. [CrossRef] [PubMed]

46. Zhong, X.-B.; Leng, L.; Beitin, A.; Chen, R.; McDonald, C.; Hsiao, B.; Jenison, R.D.; Kang, I.; Park, S.-H.; Lee, A.; et al. Simultaneous detection of microsatellite repeats and SNPs in the macrophage migration inhibitory factor (MIF) gene by thin-film biosensor chips and application to rural field studies. *Nucleic Acids Res.* **2005**, *33*, e121. [CrossRef]
47. Westphal, S.; Stoppe, C.; Gruenewald, M.; Bein, B.; Renner, J.; Cremer, J.; Coburn, M.; Schälte, G.; Boening, A.; Niemann, B.; et al. Genome-wide association study of myocardial infarction, atrial fibrillation, acute stroke, acute kidney injury and delirium after cardiac surgery—A sub-analysis of the RIPHeart-Study. *BMC Cardiovasc. Disord.* **2019**, *19*, 26. [CrossRef]
48. Saw, K.M.E.; Ng, R.G.R.; Chan, S.P.; Ang, Y.H.; Ti, L.K.; Chew, T.H.S. Association of genetic polymorphisms with acute kidney injury after cardiac surgery in a Southeast Asian population. *PLoS ONE* **2019**, *14*, e0213997. [CrossRef]
49. Leaf, D.E.; Body, S.C.; Muehlschlegel, J.D.; McMahon, G.M.; Lichtner, P.; Collard, C.D.; Shernan, S.K.; Fox, A.A.; Waikar, S.S. Length Polymorphisms in Heme Oxygenase-1 and AKI after Cardiac Surgery. *J. Am. Soc. Nephrol.* **2016**, *27*, 3291–3297. [CrossRef]
50. Suwinski, P.; Ong, C.; Ling, M.H.T.; Poh, Y.M.; Khan, A.M.; Ong, H.S. Advancing Personalized Medicine Through the Application of Whole Exome Sequencing and Big Data Analytics. *Front. Genet.* **2019**, *10*, 49. [CrossRef]

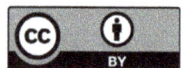

© 2020 by the authors. Licensee MDPI, Basel, Switzerland. This article is an open access article distributed under the terms and conditions of the Creative Commons Attribution (CC BY) license (http://creativecommons.org/licenses/by/4.0/).

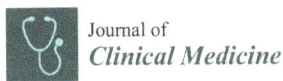

Article

Living Donor Kidney Transplantation Improves Graft and Recipient Survival in Patients with Multiple Kidney Transplants

Maria Irene Bellini *, Aisling E Courtney and Jennifer A McCaughan

Regional Nephrology and Transplant Unit, Belfast City Hospital, 51 Lisburn Road, Belfast BT9 7AB, UK; aisling.courtney@belfasttrust.hscni.net (A.E.C.); jennifer.mccaughan@belfasttrust.hscni.net (J.A.M.)
* Correspondence: mariairene.bellini@nhs.net; Tel.: +44-0-2896156671

Received: 3 June 2020; Accepted: 2 July 2020; Published: 5 July 2020

Abstract: Background: Failed kidney transplant recipients benefit from a new graft as the general incident dialysis population, although additional challenges in the management of these patients are often limiting the long-term outcomes. Previously failed grafts, a long history of comorbidities, side effects of long-term immunosuppression and previous surgical interventions are common characteristics in the repeated kidney transplantation population, leading to significant complex immunological and technical aspects and often compromising the short- and long-term results. Although recipients' factors are acknowledged to represent one of the main determinants for graft and patient survival, there is increasing interest in expanding the donor's pool safely, particularly for high-risk candidates. The role of living kidney donation in this peculiar context of repeated kidney transplantation has not been assessed thoroughly. The aim of the present study is to analyse the effects of a high-quality graft, such as the one retrieved from living kidney donors, in the repeated kidney transplant population context. Methods: Retrospective analysis of the outcomes of the repeated kidney transplant population at our institution from 1968 to 2019. Data were extracted from a prospectively maintained database and stratified according to the number of transplants: 1st, 2nd or 3rd+. The main outcomes were graft and patient survivals, recorded from time of transplant to graft failure (return to dialysis) and censored at patient death with a functioning graft. Duration of renal replacement therapy was expressed as cumulative time per month. A multivariate analysis considering death-censored graft survival, decade of transplantation, recipient age, donor age, living donor, transplant number, ischaemic time, time on renal replacement therapy prior to transplant and HLA mismatch at HLA-A, -B and -DR was conducted. In the multivariate analysis of recipient survival, diabetic nephropathy as primary renal disease was also included. Results: A total of 2395 kidney transplant recipients were analysed: 2062 (83.8%) with the 1st kidney transplant, 279 (11.3%) with the 2nd graft, 46 (2.2%) with the 3rd+. Mean age of 1st kidney transplant recipients was 43.6 ± 16.3 years, versus 39.9 ± 14.4 for 2nd and 41.4 ± 11.5 for 3rd+ ($p < 0.001$). Aside from being younger, repeated kidney transplant patients were also more often males ($p = 0.006$), with a longer time spent on renal replacement therapy ($p < 0.0001$) and a higher degree of sensitisation, expressed as calculated reaction frequency ($p < 0.001$). There was also an association between multiple kidney transplants and better HLA match at transplantation ($p < 0.0001$). A difference in death-censored graft survival by number of transplants was seen, with a median graft survival of 328 months for recipients of the 1st transplant, 209 months for the 2nd and 150 months for the 3rd+ ($p = 0.038$). The same difference was seen in deceased donor kidneys ($p = 0.048$), but not in grafts from living donors ($p = 0.2$). Patient survival was comparable between the three groups ($p = 0.59$). Conclusions: In the attempt to expand the organ donor pool, particular attention should be reserved to high complex recipients, such as the repeated kidney transplant population. In this peculiar context, the quality of the donor has been shown to represent a main determinant for graft survival—in fact, kidney retrieved from living donors provide comparable outcomes to those from single-graft recipients.

Keywords: living donation; repeated kidney transplantation; graft survival; prolonged ischaemic time; patient survival; pre-emptive transplantation

1. Introduction

The proportion of end-stage renal disease (ESRD) patients with a failed kidney transplant is increasing each year [1,2]; 25% of patients on the US kidney transplant waiting list have a failed transplant [3] and in the Eurotransplant area, the number of patients being re-waitlisted after returning to dialysis steadily ranges between 17.9% and 18.9% [4].

Morbidity and mortality for patients with a failed kidney transplant on dialysis is high; there is a two- to three-fold risk of death compared to patients with a functioning graft and a median recipient survival after graft failure of three years [3,5]. This increased mortality [6] relates to higher rates of cardiovascular, neoplastic and infective events, in which the burden of immunosuppressive therapy is no longer counterbalanced by the benefits of a working kidney transplant [7]. The single modifiable factor which has the greatest impact on recipient survival in this group is the time to re-transplantation [6]; however, the suboptimal outcome of repeated kidney re-transplantation has generated increasing debate regarding the overall management and resource allocation within this subgroup. Nevertheless, previous reports have shown that there is a significative survival benefit after repeat deceased donor kidney transplantation over remaining on the waiting list, due to significant improvement in better immunological screening, crossmatching, HLA matching, post-operative management and immunosuppression protocols [8], although the overall outcome remains impaired by an inferior survival compared to first kidney transplant recipients [9].

Yet, other fundamental outcome drivers, for example the impact of a high-quality living donor graft, have not been fully investigated in the peculiar context of repeated kidney transplantation.

One of the primary advantages in fact of receiving a kidney from a living donor is that the organ is generally healthier and more resistant to the occurrence and extension of the subsequent ischaemic reperfusion injury. To become eligible, living donors undergo full screening of their kidney function, tissue and immunological compatibility with the recipient and a comprehensive overall physical health check. This is in contrast with grafts retrieved from deceased donors, where already the stress and the damage related to the death of the individual determine a systemic storm summing up to the usual longer time in cold storage to allow retrieval and transfer between different teams and hospitals. All together, these factors can temporarily reduce and potentially compromise the organ function irreversibly [10].

The incidence of delayed graft function in kidneys from deceased donors varies, but is overall as high as 30%; it might also take weeks before the recipient is fully dialysis independent [11,12], thus the recipients are more exposed and vulnerable in the post-operative period. Conversely, kidneys from living donors tend to function immediately, reducing the risk of hospitalisation and renal replacement therapy after transplant to less than 4% [13] and setting in this way the recipient for the best short- and long-term outcome.

Why is it so important an immediate graft function? As stated above, the more complex the procedure, the higher the likelihood of the prolonged ischaemic insult and the resultant impact on challenging recipients. Previously failed grafts, a long history of comorbidities, side effects of long-term immunosuppression and previous surgical interventions are common characteristics in the repeated kidney transplant population, leading to significant immunological and technical challenges.

Intuitively, it might initially seem sensible to withdraw immunosuppression in patients after graft failure to reduce the risk of cardiovascular, neoplastic and infective complications. However, for those who are fit for a subsequent transplant, this commonly results in a high degree of sensitisation to HLA, namely the production of donor-specific HLA antibodies (DSA) and other panel-reactive antibodies (PRAs) [14]. This reduces access to compatible donors and may result in an extremely prolonged wait for transplantation, with the associated morbidity and mortality [15]. This increased waiting time might also have a worse synergistic effect with the often extended ischemic time, due to the technical challenges associated with re-transplantation, namely adhesions from previous surgery, difficulties accessing the iliac vasculature or earlier manipulation of the bladder to establish the ureterovesical anastomosis [16].

The aim of this study is to analyse the experience of repeated kidney transplantation in our institution over 50 years, with a focus on outcomes in recipients of first, second and third/fourth kidney transplants and factors which impact these outcomes.

2. Methods

All recipients of kidney transplants in Northern Ireland between 1968 and 2019 were included in the analysis. Recipients were identified using a prospectively maintained database which records data on all transplant recipients. Recipients were followed up until death or 1 September 2019. The clinical and research activities being reported are consistent with the principles of the Declaration of Helsinki and comply with the Declaration of Istanbul. Approval for this study was granted by the Regional Ethics Committee (12/NI/1078).

Death-censored graft survival was measured from time of transplant to graft failure (return to dialysis) and censored when a patient died with a functioning graft. Duration of renal replacement therapy was expressed as cumulative time per month. Recipient survival was measured from transplantation to death. Pre-transplant sensitisation levels were expressed as a calculated reaction frequency (cRF), which is calculated as the proportion of the last 10,000 UK, blood group-identical, deceased donors to which the patient has DSAs. Recipients were considered highly sensitized if they had a cRF greater than 85%.

Immunosuppression: No routine induction was used in any era. Maintenance regimen was on prednisolone and azathioprine before 1989; from 1989 to 1998, cyclosporine was introduced and patients commenced on triple therapy; in 1998, mycophenolate mofetil replaced azathioprine in the triple-therapy regimen; and from 2000, tacrolimus replaced cyclosporine. Overall, the majority of patients were maintained on two agents in the long term, with 25% on the calcineurin inhibitor-free regimen.

Living donors: Numbers of living donors performed varied according to the decade considered: 3.3% from 1968 to 1977; 9.8% from 1978 to 1987; 4% from 1988 to 1997; 10.6% from 1998 to 2007 and 55.3% from 2008 to 2017.

Statistical Analysis

Continuous variables are presented as the mean ± standard deviation. Analysis of variance and t test were used to compare continuous variables between groups. For nominal or non-parametric variables, the Pearson χ^2 test was performed. Kaplan–Meier and Cox regression analyses were applied for survival analysis. In a multivariate analysis for death-censored graft survival, factors previously associated in our population were included: decade of transplantation, recipient age, donor age, living donor, transplant number, ischaemic time, time on renal replacement therapy prior to transplant and HLA mismatch at HLA-A, -B and -DR. In the multivariate analysis of recipient survival, diabetic nephropathy as primary renal disease was also included. Confidence interval was set to 95%, and p was considered significant at less than 0.05. Analysis was performed using SPSS (IBM SPSS Statistics for Windows, Version 20.0; IBM Corp, Armonk, NY, USA).

3. Results

A total of 2395 kidney transplant recipients were included: 2062 (83.8%) received a 1st kidney transplant, 279 (11.3%) received a 2nd kidney transplant, 46 (1.9%) received a 3rd kidney transplant and 8 (0.3%) received a 4th kidney transplant. The outcomes of the 3rd and 4th kidney transplants were grouped together (3rd+).

Table 1 summarises donor and recipient characteristics. Recipients of 3rd+ kidney transplants were significantly more likely to receive a living donor kidney ($p < 0.0001$).

Table 1. Demographics of kidney transplants performed in Northern Ireland in the period 1968–2019.

	1st Transplant $n = 2062$	2nd Transplant $n = 279$	3rd+ Transplant $n = 54$	p Value
Recipient				
Recipient age (mean+SD, years)	43.6 ± 16.3	39.9 ± 14.4	41.4 ± 11.5	0.001
Recipient sex (male)	1244 (60%)	187 (67%)	38 (73%)	0.006
Renal replacement therapy duration (mean+SD, months)	22.5 ± 26.6	124.7 ± 95.8	207.3 ± 106.8	<0.0001
Calculated reaction frequency (cRF) (mean+SD, %)	15.3 ± 29.7	54.1 ± 40.3	75.7 ± 34.5	<0.0001
Donor				
Donor age (mean+SD, years)	49.7 ± 9	39.4 ± 16.1	43.5 ± 16	0.166
Donor sex (male)	1159 (56%)	152 (54%)	28 (54%)	0.171
Living donor	549 (26%)	82 (29%)	22 (42%)	<0.0001
Transplant				
Pre-emptive transplantation	308 (14.9%)	22 (7.9%)	3 (5.6%)	<0.0001
HLA-A, -B, -DR mismatch (mean+SD, number)	2.4 ± 1.3	2 ± 1.4	1.4 ± 1.4	<0.0001
Ischaemic time (mean+SD, hours)	17.5 + 18	16.6 + 16.5	13 + 9.9	0.197

Donor age, donor sex and cold ischaemic time did not statistically differ between the groups.

In total, 99% of recipients were White. Recipients of repeated kidney transplants were more likely to be male ($p = 0.006$) and were younger ($p < 0.001$): mean age of 1st KTRs was 43.6 ± 16.3 years, versus 39.9 ± 14.4 for 2nd and 41.4 ± 11.5 for 3rd+ KTRs. Furthermore, these patients were also significantly more sensitised, with an increasing cRF from 15% (1st transplant) to 54% (2nd transplant), to 76% (3rd+ transplant) ($p < 0.0001$). As a consequence, there was also an association between multiple kidney transplants and better HLA match at transplantation ($p < 0.0001$). The pre-emptive rate was significantly lower in recipients of multiple transplants ($p < 0.0001$).

3.1. Surgical Information

All kidney transplants were performed extraperitoneally and graft nephrectomy was only performed in four cases: one in relation to uncontrolled antibody mediated rejection with systemic involvement, one following a catastrophic bleed, one simultaneously to the implant and one to create space for a potential 4th graft. The final patient had had multiple gynaecology procedures and the peritoneal content would not have been easily mobilised to allow graft implantation.

Only one major bleeding event occurred that required graft nephrectomy (2nd implant), but the recipient underwent successful implantation of a 3rd graft three years later. Urological complications were not recorded.

3.2. Death-Censored Graft and Recipient Survival

Figure 1 shows death-censored graft survival, with a median of 328 months for 1st kidney transplant recipients (KTRs) in blue, 209 months for 2nd KTRs in green and 150 months for 3rd+ KTRs in red ($p = 0.04$).

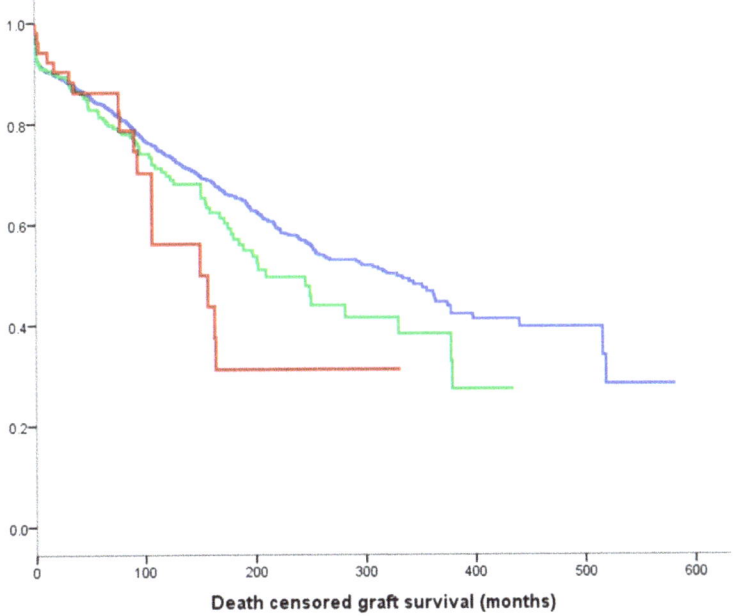

Figure 1. Median death-censored graft survival: 328 months for 1st graft (blue line), 209 months for 2nd (green line) and 150 months for 3rd+ (red line). ($p = 0.04$).

Death-censored graft survival remained significantly different between the three groups in the case of deceased donor transplants (Figure 2a), but there was no significant difference in death-censored graft survival between the groups in living donor transplantation (Figure 2b).

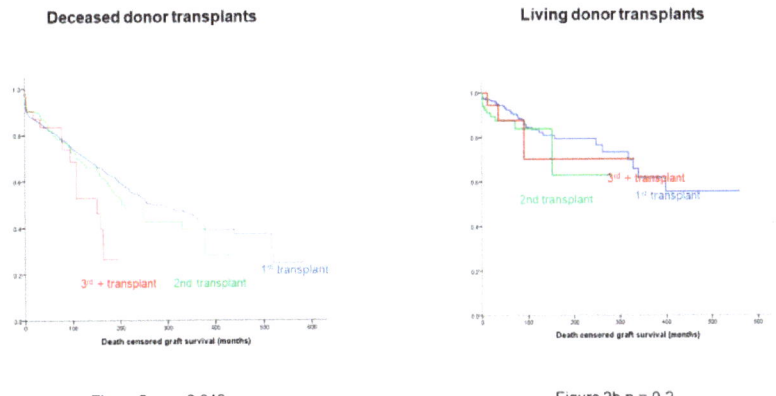

Figure 2. Difference in death-censored graft survival is seen in deceased donor transplants (**a**) but not in kidneys retrieved from living donors (**b**). Prolonged ischaemia is significantly detrimental to long-term survival in deceased donor grafts and 3rd and 4th transplants are associated with prolonged ischaemic times. These are marginal patients with difficult vasculature—marginal kidneys do less well in this context while good kidneys cope fine. Blue line: recipients of 1st kidney transplant; green line: recipients of 2nd kidney transplant; red line: recipients of 3rd kidney transplant.

Recipient survival was comparable between the three groups ($p = 0.59$), with a median of 234 months for 1st KTRs in blue, 256 months for 2nd KTRs in green and 298 months for 3rd+ KTRs in red (Figure 3). The 10 year recipient survival for all groups exceeded 70%.

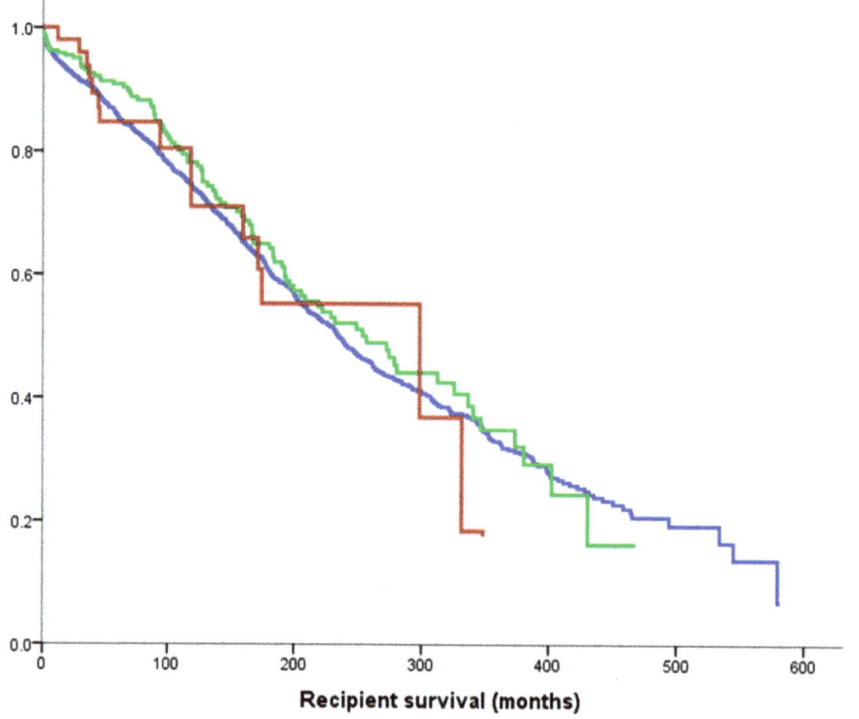

Figure 3. Median recipient survivals: 234 months for 1st graft (blue line); 256 months for 2nd (green line); 298 months for 3rd+ (red line) ($p = 0.59$).

In multivariate analysis, earlier decade of transplantation, older donor and recipient age, longer ischemic time, and transplant number were significantly associated with death-censored graft loss. Living donor transplantation was associated with improved death-censored graft survival (Table 2).

Table 2. Factors associated with death-censored graft survival in all recipients on a multivariate analysis.

Covariate	HR	95% CI	p Value
Decade of transplant	0.84	0.78–0.90	<0.001
Recipient age (per decade)	0.90	0.86–0.96	<0.001
Living donor	0.61	0.45–0.83	0.002
Donor age (per decade)	1.14	1.08–1.20	<0.001
Transplant number	1.23	1.03–1.48	0.02
Ischaemic time (per 6h)	1.09	1.01–1.17	0.02

Time on RRT and HLA mismatch at HLA-A, - B and -DR were not significant and dropped out of model.

For recipients of 3rd+ transplants, the association with a living donor is the only factor associated with death-censored graft survival (Table 3).

Table 3. Multivariate analysis for death-censored graft survival in 3rd+ recipients.

Covariate	HR	95% CI	p Value
Decade of transplant	0.98	0.49–1.96	0.9
Recipient age (per decade)	0.85	0.51–1.39	0.5
Living donor	0.10	0.01–0.89	0.04
Donor age (per decade)	0.76	0.63–1.40	0.8
Ischaemic time (per 6h)	0.57	0.30–1.10	0.08

Despite small numbers, a living donor transplant was associated with a 90% reduction in death-censored graft loss.

In multivariate analysis for recipient survival, significant factors were decade of transplant, recipient age, recipient primary disease of diabetic nephropathy, duration of RRT pre-transplant, living donor, donor age and ischaemic time (Table 4).

Table 4. Multivariate analysis for recipient survival in all transplants.

Covariate	HR	95% CI	p Value
Decade of transplant	0.60	0.56–0.65	<0.001
Recipient age (per decade)	1.7	1.6–1.8	<0.001
Recipient primary disease diabetic nephropathy	2.8	2.3–3.5	<0.001
RRT pre-transplant (per month)	1.002	1.00–1.004	0.02
Living donor	0.75	0.56–1.00	0.05
Donor age (per decade)	1.07	1.02–1.1	0.03
Ischaemic time (per 6h)	1.1	1.04–1.2	0.002

HLA mismatch at HLA-A, -B and -DR and transplant number were not significant and dropped out of model.

4. Discussion

This study investigated the outcomes of repeated kidney transplantation at our institution and demonstrated excellent graft and recipient outcomes (Figures 1 and 3), despite a significantly more sensitised population and a longer vintage of ESRD. There was also an association between multiple kidney transplants and better HLA match at transplantation ($p < 0.0001$); this is unsurprising, as more highly sensitised patients require better matched kidneys. Our results are in contrast to a recent European multicentre analysis reporting that mortality and graft loss after 3rd+ KTRs were higher as compared to 1st KTRs, despite receiving grafts with more favourable HLA matches [17]. More in detail, Assfalg et al. analysed the outcomes of 1464 patients from 42 centres in the Eurotransplant area who received a third or fourth kidney transplant in the period 1996–2010, confirming a younger age compared to first transplant recipients, a more frequently favourable HLA match, but a higher rate of graft loss, death with functioning graft and primary non-function. Their conclusion was, therefore, to set an upper limit for the number of sequential transplantations in order to consider also the prospect of success of transplantation. In our study, it was confirmed that there is a significant difference in death-censored graft survival by number of transplants, as shown in Figure 1, with a median graft survival of 328 months for 1st KTRs, 209 months for 2nd KTRs and 150 months for 3rd+ KTRs, but the death-censored graft survival remained significantly different in the case of deceased donor transplants (Figure 2a), but not after living donor transplantation (Figure 2b). This suggests that living donor transplantation confers a significant benefit in the context of repeated kidney transplantation and challenges the assumption that repeated transplant recipients as well as any other special group of patients should be a priori denied access to transplantation [18]. Important modifiable factors, such as the quality of the implanted graft or the time at which the operation is performed, could significantly affect the overall outcome and this should be taken into consideration when planning such a complex procedure and before fixing an arbitrary cut off number to waitlist transplant candidates.

In this regard, an extensive patient work up with multidisciplinary input is highly recommended to maximise the chances of successful waitlisting for the candidate, to be followed by a successful repeated kidney transplantation. Further, in our study, in fact, 3rd+ KTRs are overall better matched compared to 1st or 2nd KTRs ($p < 0.001$), reflecting the broad immunological work up. Yet, despite a similar finding to the study from Dabare et al. [19], where patient survival did not differ significantly by transplant number even considering third or fourth KTRs and, therefore, confirming the survival benefit for this population over remaining on dialysis, we disagree with the authors' conclusion. In our present analysis, we observed a significant decline in graft survival only in the case of deceased donor grafts, with a progressive worsening survival curve in parallel with the progressive increase in repeated kidney transplant number (Figure 2a). The conclusion that regardless of the donor type, there is an inferior graft survival for the repeated kidney transplant population is not confirmed instead for grafts retrieved from living donors (Figure 2b). Therefore, the authors' suggestion to use HLA-incompatible living donors and extended criteria deceased donors in the peculiar context of the repeated kidney transplant population is not justifiable from our experience.

Prolonged ischaemic time is significantly detrimental to long-term survival for deceased donor grafts [20], with preservation strategies being key for suboptimal and extended criteria deceased donor organs [12]. Often 3rd and 4th kidney transplants are associated with prolonged ischaemic times due to increasing technical complexity: KTRs of 3rd and 4th transplants may have difficult vasculature that often requires additional surgical time. The deceased donor kidney performs less well in this context, while better-quality living donor kidneys can tolerate the insult. In our centre, where there is a high rate of living donor transplantation, there is for this reason an even higher proportion of organs retrieved from living donors in the case of 3rd+ KTRs (Table 1). To overcome living donor shortage, broad educational campaigns aiming to educate and inform the general population [21] and particularly via social media, have demonstrated an increase in donation rates [22]. With the current organ donor shortage and more patients dying on the waiting list, living donor kidney donation seems, therefore, to satisfy and significantly contribute to expand the donor pool for the general population, and more specifically for those who might not survive a long waiting list time or a major operation, like in the case of the repeated kidney transplantation subgroup. In addition, every living donor transplant that occurs removes one person from the transplant waiting list, shortening the waiting list for a deceased donor transplant, too.

With increasing evidence of how the preservation time and modality significantly impact organs retrieved from marginal donors [10] and with an even increasing debate in how to safely implement the donor pool, without compromising recipient outcomes, until a general consensus on how to best treat and preserve deceased donor grafts [23], an effort to find alternative ways of influencing patient and graft survivals should be canvassed in the ethical attempt to provide the best renal replacement therapy to those who need it.

Another important advantage offered by living donation is that an elective operation allows diligent planning and the presence of additional surgical expertise for complex cases [24]. This might also contribute to better outcomes, independently from the quality of the donor [19], with a standardised elective procedure taking place at an optimal time and that, despite being a major operation, has a minor impact [25] on the recovery of the healthy donor, who usually can plan ahead for time off work, for family care for and for a full recovery.

With deceased donor transplantation, the surgery often takes place out of hours; additionally, emergency procedures usually carry out extra unanticipated risks [26], along with the impossibility to schedule the time and avoid the waitlist consequences and deterioration on the general health status of the candidate, who might even be transplanted after several years, because of the complex immunological status. Inevitably, the elderly and sickest candidates might, therefore, be more susceptible to the vicious cycle of repeated kidney transplantation, becoming not transplantable, with a significant drop out from the list, or a detrimental transplant outcome. In our opinion, this is, therefore, why living donor kidney donation is so fundamental to expand the donor pool: removing successfully a difficult transplant candidate from the transplant waiting list and ensuring that the next person on the list will not have to wait as long for a deceased donor transplant.

The preferred surgical approach in the case of repeated kidney transplantation at our centre is extraperitoneal to avoid ileus and expedite an enhanced recovery [27]. In the case of native polycystic kidney disease, further space for transplantation might become a challenge, and therefore the affected patients are more likely to undergo native nephrectomy before the planned transplant, as they are already vintage patients [28]. In our series, 13 patients (23.6% of the total population) underwent bilateral native nephrectomy.

Differently from native nephrectomy, kidney transplantectomy was rarely performed in the case of a failed graft. The British Transplant Society guidelines [29] suggest limited indications for graft nephrectomy: localised symptoms that are resistant to medical therapy, to create space for re-transplantation, to enable complete withdrawal of immunosuppression and where there is risk of graft rupture or graft malignancy. This caution with regard to graft nephrectomy is partly due to its immunological effect [30], as nephrectomy and the cessation of immunosuppression can precipitate the development of HLA antibodies (DSAs and PRAs), which limits access to re-transplantation. In our series, only four graft nephrectomies were recorded: because of antibody mediated rejection with systemic involvement, because of a bleeding catastrophe after the transplant and to create space for a potential further kidney transplant. The limited number of graft nephrectomy at our institution is in contrast with other centres' experiences, estimated at approximately 40% from a Turkish report [31] and up to 75% in a UK single-centre experience from 2009 [32]. We tend to avoid, as a general principle, an additional operation, unless not strictly required, in consideration of the controversy affecting the immunological recipient status and the likelihood of finding a suitable match, with antibody absorption from the graft itself. [30,32]. As previously stated, in fact the graft nephrectomy would imply the cessation of the immunosuppression, giving rise to antibody production due to the persistence of donor antigen-presenting cells after the transplantectomy. Furthermore, with the evidence that HLA matching plays a fundamental role in the context of repeated kidney transplantation, from the present study and another large registry analysis [17], we think that a synergistic approach to optimise the recipient condition and general immunological status would better satisfy increased complexity at the moment of transplantation in the eventuality that a prolonged surgical time would be required to find a suitable implantation site. Once again, we emphasize the importance of a high-quality graft, like the one retrieved from a living donor, to better resist a prolonged ischaemic insult.

Finally, given the increased morbidity in patients with failed kidney transplants, special attention should be paid to the attainment of cardiovascular and other infective or malignant events [33], the main cause of death in the long term and also in particular for the repeated KTRs. In our centre, we acknowledge this extra care and, notably, recipient survival did not differ between the groups.

5. Limitations

The main limitation of this study is the retrospective data assessment from a single institution, subjected to selection bias by the nature of the study itself, with a change in the immunosuppression and overall management of kidney transplant recipients over time. There is also an immortal bias due to younger age and higher fitness of the recipients of repeated kidney transplantation, possibly leading to comparable patient survival between the subgroups. Nevertheless, the comprehensive assessment from the same institution over a period of more than 50 years shed light on the context of the failing kidney transplant population, for which the best treatment and donor selection remains unclear in terms of long-term outcomes.

6. Conclusions

In conclusion, a living donor kidney has the greatest impact on improving graft and recipient survival in patients with multiple kidney transplants. We recommend early work up of recipients with failing grafts to achieve pre-emptive transplantation and minimise time on dialysis, and early pursuit of a living donor option for these individuals.

In our view, it is fundamental to consider that not only recipients' factors but also donors' characteristics are strongly related to short- and long-term results after kidney transplantation and that the higher the risk represented by the recipient, as in the case of the repeated kidney transplant population, the more likely stress and damage in the immediate and longer follow up will occur, therefore potentially irreversibly compromising the graft.

Living donor kidneys represent an undervalued resource significantly impacting the transplant outcome for higher-risk candidates, where a standard donor is instead more likely to be affected by the recipient status.

Author Contributions: M.I.B.: study conception; writing the original manuscript and revision; data analysis; A.E.C.: study conception; data collection; manuscript revision; J.A.M.: study conception, data collection and analysis; manuscript revision. All authors have read and agreed to the published version of the manuscript.

Funding: This research was supported by the Northern Ireland Kidney Research Fund (NIKRF).

Conflicts of Interest: The authors declare no conflict of interest with relevance to the present study.

Abbreviations

Abbr.	Original Word
DSA	Donor-specific antibody
ESRD	End-stage renal disease
KTR	Kidney transplant recipient
PRA	Panel-reactive antibody
RRT	Renal replacement therapy (cumulative time)

References

1. U.S. Renal Data System, USRDS 2009 Annual Data Report: Atlas of Chronic Kidney Disease and End-Stage Renal Disease in the United States; National Institutes of Health, National Institute of Diabetes and Digestive and Kidney Diseases: Bethesda, MD, USA, 2009.
2. U.S. Renal Data System, USRDS 2010 Annual Data Report: Atlas of Chronic Kidney Disease and End-Stage Renal Disease in the United States; National Institutes of Health, National Institute of Diabetes and Digestive and Kidney Diseases: Bethesda, MD, USA, 2010.
3. Kaplan, B.; Meier-Kriesche, H.U. Death after graft loss: An important late study endpoint in kidney transplantation. *Am. J. Transplant.* **2002**, *2*, 970–974. [CrossRef] [PubMed]
4. Mehrabi, S.; Sohn, S.; Li, D.; Pankratz, J.J.; Therneau, T.; Sauver, J.L.S.; Liu, H.; Palakal, M. Temporal pattern and association discovery of diagnosis codes using deep learning. In Proceedings of the 2015 International Conference on Healthcare Informatics, Richardson, TX, USA, 21–23 October 2015; pp. 408–416.
5. Fernandez Fresnedo, G.; Ruiz, J.C.; Gomez Alamillo, C.; de Francisco, A.L.; Arias, M. Survival after dialysis initiation: A comparison of transplant patients after graft loss versus nontransplant patients. *Transplant. Proc.* **2008**, *40*, 2889–2890. [CrossRef]
6. McCaughan, J.A.; Patterson, C.C.; Maxwell, A.P.; Courtney, A.E. Factors influencing survival after kidney transplant failure. *Transplant. Res.* **2014**, *3*, 18. [CrossRef] [PubMed]
7. Knoll, G.; Muirhead, N.; Trpeski, L.; Zhu, N.; Badovinac, K. Patient survival following renal transplant failure in Canada. *Am. J. Transplant.* **2005**, *5*, 1719–1724. [CrossRef] [PubMed]
8. Coupel, S.; Giral-Classe, M.; Karam, G.; Morcet, J.F.; Dantal, J.; Cantarovich, D.; Blancho, G.; Bignon, J.D.; Daguin, P.; Soulillou, J.P.; et al. Ten-year survival of second kidney transplants: Impact of immunologic factors and renal function at 12 months. *Kidney Int.* **2003**, *64*, 674–680. [CrossRef]

9. Redfield, R.R.; Gupta, M.; Rodriguez, E.; Wood, A.; Abt, P.L.; Levine, M.H. Graft and patient survival outcomes of a third kidney transplant. *Transplantation* **2015**, *99*, 416–423. [CrossRef]
10. Bellini, M.I.; Nozdrin, M.; Yiu, J.; Papalois, V. Machine perfusion for abdominal organ preservation: A systematic review of kidney and liver human grafts. *J. Clin. Med.* **2019**, *8*, 1221. [CrossRef]
11. Perico, N.; Cattaneo, D.; Sayegh, M.H.; Remuzzi, G. Delayed graft function in kidney transplantation. *Lancet* **2004**, *364*, 1814–1827. [CrossRef]
12. Bellini, M.I.; Charalampidis, S.; Herbert, P.E.; Bonatsos, V.; Crane, J.; Muthusamy, A.; Dor, F.; Papalois, V. Cold pulsatile machine perfusion versus static cold storage in kidney transplantation: A single centre experience. *BioMed. Res. Int.* **2019**, *2019*, 7435248. [CrossRef]
13. Redfield, R.R.; Scalea, J.R.; Zens, T.J.; Muth, B.; Kaufman, D.B.; Djamali, A.; Astor, B.C.; Mohamed, M. Predictors and outcomes of delayed graft function after living-donor kidney transplantation. *Transpl. Int.* **2016**, *29*, 81–87. [CrossRef]
14. Lucisano, G.; Brookes, P.; Santos-Nunez, E.; Firmin, N.; Gunby, N.; Hassan, S.; Gueret-Wardle, A.; Herbert, P.; Papalois, V.; Willicombe, M.; et al. Allosensitization after transplant failure: The role of graft nephrectomy and immunosuppression—A retrospective study. *Transpl. Int.* **2019**, *32*, 949–959. [CrossRef]
15. McCaughan, J.A.; Courtney, A.E. Successful kidney transplantation in highly sensitized, ultra-long-term dialysis patients. *Transpl. Int.* **2017**, *30*, 844–846. [CrossRef]
16. Ooms, L.S.; Roodnat, J.I.; Dor, F.J.; Tran, T.C.; Kimenai, H.J.; Ijzermans, J.N.; Terkivatan, T. Kidney retransplantation in the ipsilateral iliac fossa: A surgical challenge. *Am. J. Transplant.* **2015**, *15*, 2947–2954. [CrossRef]
17. Assfalg, V.; Selig, K.; Tolksdorf, J.; van Meel, M.; de Vries, E.; Ramsoebhag, A.M.; Rahmel, A.; Renders, L.; Novotny, A.; Matevossian, E.; et al. Repeated kidney re-transplantation-the Eurotransplant experience: A retrospective multicenter outcome analysis. *Transpl. Int.* **2020**. [CrossRef] [PubMed]
18. Morath, C.; Süsal, C. Three is not enough. *Transpl. Int.* **2020**, *33*, 612–614. [CrossRef] [PubMed]
19. Dabare, D.; Kassimatis, T.; Hodson, J.; Khurram, M.A.; Papadakis, G.; Rompianesi, G.; Shaw, O.; Karydis, N.; Callaghan, C.; Olsburgh, J.; et al. Outcomes in third and fourth kidney transplants based on the type of donor. *Transplantation* **2019**, *103*, 1494–1503. [CrossRef]
20. Aubert, O.; Kamar, N.; Vernerey, D.; Viglietti, D.; Martinez, F.; Duong-Van-Huyen, J.P.; Eladari, D.; Empana, J.P.; Rabant, M.; Verine, J.; et al. Long term outcomes of transplantation using kidneys from expanded criteria donors: Prospective, population based cohort study. *Br. Med. J.* **2015**, *351*, h3557. [CrossRef] [PubMed]
21. Bellini, M.I.; Charalampidis, S.; Stratigos, I.; Dor, F.; Papalois, V. The effect of Donors' demographic characteristics in renal function post-living kidney donation. Analysis of a UK single centre cohort. *J. Clin. Med.* **2019**, *8*, 883. [CrossRef]
22. Bellini, M.I.; Parisotto, C.; Dor, F.J.M.F.; Kessaris, N. Social Media Use Among Transplant Professionals in Europe: A Cross-Sectional Study From the European Society of Organ Transplantation. *Exp. Clin. Transpl.* **2020**, *18*, 169–176. [CrossRef]
23. Bellini, M.I.; D'Andrea, V. Organ preservation: Which temperature for which organ? *J. Int. Med. Res.* **2019**, *47*, 2323–2325. [CrossRef]
24. Chandak, P.; Byrne, N.; Coleman, A.; Karunanithy, N.; Carmichael, J.; Marks, S.D.; Stojanovic, J.; Kessaris, N.; Mamode, N. Patient-specific 3D printing: A novel technique for complex pediatric renal transplantation. *Ann. Surg.* **2019**, *269*, e18–e23. [CrossRef] [PubMed]
25. Bellini, M.; Wilson, R.S.; Veitch, P.; Brown, T.; Courtney, A.; Maxwell, A.P.; D'Andrea, V.; McDaid, J. Hyperamylasemia post living donor nephrectomy does not relate to pain. *Cureus* **2020**, *12*, e8217. [CrossRef] [PubMed]
26. The National Confidential Enquiry into Patient Outcome and Death. National Confidential Enquiry into Perioperative Outcome and Death. Who Operates when 1995/6? Available online: www.ncepod.org.uk/1995_6.html (accessed on 13 October 2019).
27. Mazzucchi, E.; Danilovic, A.; Antonopoulos, I.M.; Piovesan, A.C.; Nahas, W.C.; Lucon, A.M.; Srougi, M. Surgical aspects of third and subsequent renal transplants performed by the extraperitoneal access. *Transplantation* **2006**, *81*, 840–844. [CrossRef]
28. Bellini, M.I.; Charalmpidis, S.; Brookes, P.; Hill, P.; Dor, F.; Papalois, V. Bilateral nephrectomy for adult polycystic kidney disease does not affect the graft function of transplant patients and does not result in sensitisation. *BioMed. Res. Int.* **2019**, *2019*, 7423158. [CrossRef]

29. British Transplantation Society guidelines. Available online: https://bts.org.uk/wp-content/uploads/2016/09/13_BTS_Failing_Graft-1.pdf (accessed on 13 October 2019).
30. Lin, J.; Wang, R.; Xu, Y.; Chen, J. Impact of renal allograft nephrectomy on graft and patient survival following retransplantation: A systematic review and meta-analysis. *Nephrol. Dial. Transplant.* **2018**, *33*, 700–708. [CrossRef] [PubMed]
31. Yagmurdur, M.C.; Emiroğlu, R.; Ayvaz, I.; Sozen, H.; Karakayali, H.; Haberal, M. The effect of graft nephrectomy on long-term graft function and survival in kidney retransplantation. *Transplant. Proc.* **2005**, *37*, 2957–2961. [CrossRef] [PubMed]
32. Ahmad, N.; Ahmed, K.; Mamode, N. Does nephrectomy of failed allograft influence graft survival after re-transplantation? *Nephrol. Dial. Transplant.* **2009**, *24*, 639–642. [CrossRef]
33. McCaughan, J.A.; Courtney, A.E. The clinical course of kidney transplant recipients after 20 years of graft function. *Am. J. Transplant.* **2015**, *15*, 734–740. [CrossRef]

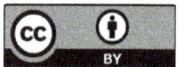

© 2020 by the authors. Licensee MDPI, Basel, Switzerland. This article is an open access article distributed under the terms and conditions of the Creative Commons Attribution (CC BY) license (http://creativecommons.org/licenses/by/4.0/).

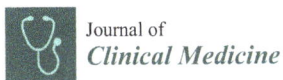

Article

Degree of Glomerulosclerosis in Procurement Kidney Biopsies from Marginal Donor Kidneys and Their Implications in Predicting Graft Outcomes

Wisit Cheungpasitporn [1,*], Charat Thongprayoon [2,*], Pradeep K Vaitla [1], Api Chewcharat [2], Panupong Hansrivijit [3], Felicitas L. Koller [4], Michael A Mao [5], Tarun Bathini [6], Sohail Abdul Salim [1], Sreelatha Katari [7], Lee S Cummings [7], Eddie Island [7], Jameson Forster [7] and Napat Leeaphorn [7,*]

[1] Division of Nephrology, Department of Medicine, University of Mississippi Medical Center, Jackson, MS 39216, USA; pvaitla@umc.edu (P.K.V.); sohail3553@gmail.com (S.A.S.)
[2] Division of Nephrology and Hypertension, Mayo Clinic, Rochester, MN 55905, USA; chewcharat.api@mayo.edu
[3] Department of Internal Medicine, University of Pittsburgh Medical Center Pinnacle, Harrisburg, PA 17105, USA; hansrivijitp@upmc.edu
[4] Department of Transplant and Hepatobiliary Surgery, University of Mississippi Medical Center, Jackson, MS 39216, USA; fkoller@umc.edu
[5] Division of Nephrology, Division of Nephrology and Hypertension, Mayo Clinic, Jacksonville, FL 32224, USA; mao.michael@mayo.edu
[6] Department of Internal Medicine, University of Arizona, Tucson, AZ 85721, USA; tarunjacobb@gmail.com
[7] Renal Transplant Program, School of Medicine/Saint Luke's Health System, University of Missouri-Kansas City, Kansas City, MO 64110, USA; skatari@saint-lukes.org (S.K.); lscummings@saint-lukes.org (L.S.C.); eisland@saint-lukes.org (E.I.); jforster@saint-lukes.org (J.F.)
* Correspondence: wcheungpasitporn@gmail.com (W.C.); charat.thongprayoon@gmail.com (C.T.); napat.leeaphorn@gmail.com (N.L.)

Received: 25 April 2020; Accepted: 9 May 2020; Published: 14 May 2020

Abstract: Background: This study aimed to assess the association between the percentage of glomerulosclerosis (GS) in procurement allograft biopsies from high-risk deceased donor and graft outcomes in kidney transplant recipients. **Methods:** The UNOS database was used to identify deceased-donor kidneys with a kidney donor profile index (KDPI) score > 85% from 2005 to 2014. Deceased donor kidneys were categorized based on the percentage of GS: 0–10%, 11–20%, >20% and no biopsy performed. The outcome included death-censored graft survival, patient survival, rate of delayed graft function, and 1-year acute rejection. **Results:** Of 22,006 kidneys, 91.2% were biopsied showing 0–10% GS (58.0%), 11–20% GS (13.5%), >20% GS (19.7%); 8.8% were not biopsied. The rate of kidney discard was 48.5%; 33.6% in 0–10% GS, 68.9% in 11–20% GS, and 77.4% in >20% GS. 49.8% of kidneys were discarded in those that were not biopsied. Death-censored graft survival at 5 years was 75.8% for 0–10% GS, 70.9% for >10% GS, and 74.8% for the no biopsy group. Among kidneys with >10% GS, there was no significant difference in death-censored graft survival between 11–20% GS and >20% GS. Recipients with >10% GS had an increased risk of graft failure (HR = 1.27, $p < 0.001$), compared with 0–10% GS. There was no significant difference in patient survival, acute rejection at 1-year, and delayed graft function between 0% and 10% GS and >10% GS. **Conclusion:** In >85% KDPI kidneys, our study suggested that discard rates increased with higher percentages of GS, and GS >10% is an independent prognostic factor for graft failure. Due to organ shortage, future studies are needed to identify strategies to use these marginal kidneys safely and improve outcomes.

Keywords: procurement kidney biopsy; glomerulosclerosis; kidney transplantation; transplantation; outcomes

1. Introduction

In the United States, more than 90,000 patients with end-stage kidney disease (ESKD) are currently waiting for a kidney transplant [1,2]. A significant gap between the number of kidney transplant candidates and donors remains an ongoing problem, resulting in a median wait time exceeding four years [3–6]. This delay has a dramatic impact on ESKD patients on the transplant waiting list, as their survival is, on average, below 40% after 5 years on dialysis [7]. Despite the severe organ shortage, a significant number of procured organs are discarded every year [8,9].

The shortage of deceased donor organs continues to be a problem in kidney transplantation despite the implementation of expanded criteria donor (ECD) programs in 2002 to increase the use of organs from donors with ≥60 years or comorbidities [10]. In 2013, the United Network of Organ Sharing (UNOS) Kidney Transplantation Committee approved a new allocation policy based on the kidney donor profile index (KDPI), a percentile score that compares an organ to previously recovered kidneys and signifies donor factors affecting transplant function [11]. KDPI >85% kidneys, previously designated as expanded criteria donor (ECD) kidneys, are offered to patients who have consented to accept a non-ideal renal allograft, thereby increasing access to earlier kidney transplantation [11]. Unfortunately, the discard rate for KDPI >85% kidneys continues to be high, close to 50% under the new kidney allocation system (KAS). The major determinants of discarded kidneys are donor comorbidities and procurement wedge biopsy findings, especially the percentage of glomerulosclerosis (GS) [8,12–16].

Despite conflicting evidence regarding the prognostic capability of histologic findings for differentiating donor kidneys at greater risk of inferior outcomes [17–19], the use of procurement biopsies has become an increasingly common practice, particularly in KDPI >85% kidneys in which 95% of recovered kidneys were biopsied [9,18,20]. The percentage of GS is commonly the primary biopsy information reviewed because it provides a convenient cutoff for offer turndowns [8,21,22]. This is in spite of studies noting that the percentage of GS has failed to consistently predict graft outcomes [18,21,23–29].

The aim of this study is to explore the association between the percentage of GS and graft outcomes in kidney transplant recipients who received KDPI >85% kidneys between 1 January 2005 to 2 December 2014 using the Organ Procurement and Transplantation Network (OPTN)/UNOS database.

2. Methods

2.1. Data Source and Study Population

We used the OPTN/UNOS database to identify deceased-donor kidneys recovered from January 1, 2005 to December 2, 2014 (before implementation of the kidney allocation system). The study was exempt from the institutional review board due to the publicly available nature of the de-identified database of the OPTN/UNOS database. All data used in the analysis were provided by UNOS through the Standard Transplant Analysis and Research (STAR) database. The database is a de-identified, patient-level data source that contains donor, waitlist, and transplant recipient variables derived from UNet forms for any transplant in the United States after October 1, 1987. KDPI (reference year of 2017) was calculated based on donor factors to summarize the likelihood of graft failure after deceased donor kidney transplant. Higher KDPI scores are associated with shorter estimated graft function. Although the KDPI was not formally introduced into allocation policy until implementation of the new kidney allocation system (KAS) on December 2014, the OPTN/UNOS database has KDPI values for 99% of all deceased donor recipients who underwent kidney transplantation during the study period. To assess the predictive value of procurement biopsy GS percentage in high-risk deceased donors, we only included deceased-donor kidneys with a KDPI score > 85%. We excluded recovered kidneys for dual-kidney transplant and kidneys from donors with body weight < 20 kg. Subsequently, we assess the post-transplant outcomes based on GS percentage in deceased-donor kidney transplant recipients who received kidney with KDPI > 85%. We excluded patients undergoing kidney re-transplants or multi-organ transplant from the analysis.

2.2. Outcomes

We categorized deceased donor kidneys into four groups based on the percentage of GS: 0–10%, 11–20%, >20% and no biopsy performed. We investigated the kidney discard rates and post-transplant deceased donor allograft outcomes based on GS groups. The primary outcome was death-censored graft survival. Death-censored graft survival began at kidney transplant, was followed until graft failure, defined as the requirement of renal replacement therapy and/or kidney re-transplant, and was censored at death or the end of study (6 September 2018), whichever was earlier. The secondary outcomes were patient survival, rate of delayed graft function, and 1-year acute rejection. Delayed graft function was defined as a requirement of dialysis within the first week of transplantation. As there was no statistical difference in any post-transplant outcomes between 11–20% and >20% GS (Table S1), we combined these two groups together (>10% GS) when assessing post-transplant outcomes.

2.3. Covariates

Donor-related factors included donor age, sex, race, diabetes mellitus, hypertension, body mass index, the last serum creatinine before kidney procurement, donation after cardiac death, hepatitis C virus (HCV) antibody status, cause of death, and machine perfusion. Recipient-related factors included recipient age, sex, race, body mass index, diabetes mellitus, preemptive transplant, dialysis duration, and panel reactive antibody. Transplant-related factors included HLA-DR mismatch, cold ischemic time, transplant period, and induction therapy.

2.4. Statistical Analysis

Baseline characteristics were described using mean ± standard deviation (SD) for continuous variables or frequencies with percentage for categorical variables. Continuous variables were compared between GS groups using the student's *t*-test or ANOVA, as appropriate. Categorical variables were compared between GS groups using the Chi-squared test. Patient survival and death-censored graft survival outcomes were estimated using the Kaplan–Meier method with significance tested using the log-rank test. The associations of the GS percentage group with death-censored graft failure and patient mortality was assessed using Cox proportional hazards analysis. The proportional hazards assumption was tested using Schoenfeld residuals ($p = 0.29$). Because the OPTN/UNOS database did not specify the date of occurrence, the associations of the GS percentage group with delayed graft function and 1-year acute rejection were assessed using logistic regression analysis. Multivariable analysis was performed to adjust for covariates associated with outcomes of interest with $p < 0.05$ in univariate analysis. All *p*-values were two-tailed, and *p*-values of <0.05 were considered significant. Stata version 13 (StataCorp, College Station, TX, USA) was used for all statistical analyses.

3. Results

3.1. Kidney Procurement Cohort and Rate of Kidney Discard

During the study period, 25,154 kidneys were recovered from deceased donors with KDPI > 85%. A total of 3014 kidneys recovered for dual-kidney transplant and 134 kidneys from donors with a body weight < 20 kg were excluded. A total of 22,006 kidneys with KDPI > 85% were included in the kidney procurement cohort. Of these kidneys, 58.0% had 0–10% GS, 13.5% had 11–20% GS, 19.7% had >20% GS, and 8.8% had no kidney biopsy performed (Figure S1). Overall, the rate of kidney discard was 48.5%; 33.6% in 0–10% GS, 68.9% in 11–20% GS, and 77.4% in >20% GS. 49.8% kidneys were discarded in the no kidney biopsy group.

3.2. Kidney Transplant Recipient Cohort

In this cohort of 22,006 deceased donor kidneys with KDPI > 85%, 10,662 kidneys were discarded. After excluding 1032 recipients with prior kidney transplants or undergoing multi-organ transplant, a total of 10,312 recipients with donor KDPI > 85% were included in the post-transplant outcome analysis. Of these patients, 75.6% had 0–10% GS, 11.9% had 11–20% GS, 4.9% had >20% GS, and 7.6% had no kidney biopsy performed (Figure S2). The median (IQR) number of glomeruli in each kidney biopsy was 47 (IQR: 28, 69). There was no association between KDPI and percent of GS ($p = 0.70$). The donor, recipient, and transplant-related characteristics stratified by percent of GS are shown in Table 1.

Table 1. Characteristics of donors, recipients, and transplant according to percent GS in transplanted allograft.

	Glomerulosclerosis				
	0–10%	11–20%	>20%	No-Biopsy	p-Value
N	7796	1230	500	786	
Donor					
Age (years)	60.7 ± 7.1	60.5 ± 6.9	60.6 ± 6.7	58.5 ± 7.4	<0.001
Male (%)	46.7	41.1	46.4	36.6	<0.001
Black (%)	28.8	29.5	25.2	30.0	0.26
Diabetes (%)	26.5	34.2	30.6	20.2	<0.001
Hypertension (%)	79.0	81.8	80.8	73.8	<0.001
BMI (kg/m^2)	28.8 ± 6.9	29.2 ± 7.5	29.2 ± 7.5	27.3 ± 6.5	<0.001
Creatinine (mg/dL) before kidney procurement	1.2 ± 1.0	1.2 ± 0.6	1.2 ± 0.5	1.2 ± 1.0	0.04
Donor after cardiac death (%)	10.0	7.1	6.8	4.6	<0.001
HCV antibody positive (%)	5.8	2.4	2.8	12.9	<0.001
Cause of death (%)					
Cerebrovascular accident	78.1	79.4	83.0	82.8	0.002
Machine perfusion (%)	49.9	51.2	47.8	19.5	<0.001
Expanded criteria donor (%)	85.4	87.7	86.4	75.5	<0.001
Recipient					
Age (years)	61.5 ± 9.8	62.4 ± 9.6	61.6 ± 9.8	59.9 ± 10.6	0.001
Male (%)	64.0	63.1	63.2	63.9	0.92
Black (%)	36.4	36.8	40.6	33.3	0.07
BMI	27.9 ± 5.3	28.4 ± 5.5	27.5 ± 5.0	27.6 ± 5.4	0.001
Diabetes (%)	47.2	46.8	48.8	47.1	0.90
Dialysis duration (%)					
Preemptive	9.8	8.9	9.8	9.0	0.70
<1 years	8.7	8.1	7.0	9.5	0.41
1–3 years	29.6	26.7	30.8	30.7	0.13
>3 years	49.4	54.0	48.4	46.8	0.006
PRA (%)					
<10	81.7	84.7	81.8	78.1	0.003
10–60	12.0	9.8	12.6	15.0	0.005
>60	5.9	4.6	4.4	5.7	0.21
Missing	0.5	0.9	1.2	1.2	0.01
Transplant					
HLA DR mismatch (%)					
0	8.2	7.2	7.8	8.9	0.42
1	39.0	36.3	38.4	36.9	0.27
2	52.8	56.5	53.8	54.2	0.12
Cold ischemic time (hours)	19.5 ± 9.4	20.5 ± 9.5	19.8 ± 9.1	15.7 ± 9.2	<0.001
Transplant period					
2005–2007	28.6	22.7	35.0	45.2	<0.001
2008–2010	33.8	31.6	35.6	27.4	0.001
2011–2014	37.6	45.7	29.4	27.5	<0.001
Induction therapy (%)					
Thymoglobulin	46.1	52.3	51.4	47.3	<0.001
Alemtuzumab	14.7	13.5	16.0	9.5	0.001
Basiliximab	18.9	19.2	17.2	24.7	0.001
Other induction	7.6	8.1	5.2	7.1	0.19
No induction	16.3	11.0	13.4	15.0	<0.001

GS, glomerulosclerosis; HCV, hepatitis C virus; BMI, body mass index; PRA, panel reactive antibody; HLA, human leukocyte antigen.

3.3. Baseline Characteristics Based on Percentages of Glomerulosclerosis

Table 2 summarizes and compares donor, recipient, and transplant-related characteristics between 0–10% and >10% GS allograft groups. Kidneys donors with >10% GS had a higher prevalence of female sex, diabetes and hypertension. Kidney donors with 0–10% GS had a higher prevalence of donation after cardiac death and positive hepatitis C antibody. Recipients of kidneys with GS > 10% were older and had longer dialysis vintage, whereas recipients of kidneys with 0–10% GS had higher panel reactive antibodies. Kidney transplants with >10% GS had more HLA DR mismatch, cold ischemic time, and thymoglobulin induction. Kidney transplants with 0–10% GS had more transplants without induction therapy.

Table 2. Comparison of donors, recipients, and transplant characteristics between GS 0–10% and GS > 10% transplanted allografts.

	Glomerulosclerosis		
	0–10%	>10%	p-Value
N	7796	1730	
Donor			
Age (years)	60.7 ± 7.1	60.5 ± 6.8	0.18
Male (%)	46.7	42.7	0.002
Black (%)	28.8	28.3	0.66
Diabetes (%)	26.5	33.1	<0.001
Hypertension (%)	79.0	81.5	0.02
BMI (kg/m^2)	28.8 ± 6.9	29.2 ± 7.5	0.04
Creatinine (mg/dL) before kidney procurement	1.2 ± 1.0	1.2 ± 0.6	0.85
Donor after cardiac death (%)	10.0	7.0	<0.001
HCV antibody positive (%)	5.8	2.5	<0.001
Cause of death (%)			
Cerebrovascular accident	78.1	80.4	0.04
Machine perfusion (%)	49.9	50.2	0.82
Expanded criteria donor (%)	85.4	87.3	0.04
Recipient			
Age (years)	61.5 ± 9.8	62.2 ± 9.6	0.003
Male (%)	64.0	63.1	0.48
Black (%)	36.4	37.9	0.26
BMI	27.9 ± 5.3	28.1 ± 5.4	0.35
Diabetes (%)	47.2	47.4	0.86
Dialysis duration (%)			
Preemptive	9.8	9.1	0.40
<1 years	8.7	7.8	0.25
1–3 years	29.6	27.9	0.16
>3 years	49.4	52.4	0.02
PRA (%)			
<10	81.7	83.9	0.03
10–60	12.0	10.6	0.10
>60	5.9	4.6	0.03
Missing	0.5	1.0	0.01
Transplant			
HLA DR mismatch (%)			
0	8.2	7.4	0.30
1	39.0	36.9	0.10
2	52.8	55.7	0.03
Cold ischemic time (hours)	19.5 ± 9.4	20.3 ± 9.4	<0.001
Transplant period			
2005–2007	28.6	26.2	0.05
2008–2010	33.8	32.8	0.40
2011–2014	37.6	41.0	0.008
Induction therapy (%)			
Thymoglobulin	46.1	52.0	<0.001
Alemtuzumab	14.7	14.2	0.59
Basiliximab	18.9	18.6	0.79
Other induction	7.6	7.3	0.67
No induction	16.3	11.7	<0.001

GS, glomerulosclerosis; HCV, hepatitis C virus; BMI, body mass index; PRA, panel reactive antibody; HLA, human leukocyte antigen.

3.4. Post-Transplant Outcomes Based on Percentages of Glomerulosclerosis

The median (IQR) follow-up was 4.87 (2.90, 7.02) years after kidney transplant. During follow-up, 3015 (29.2%) patients had allograft failure, and 4433 (43.0%) patients died. A total of 1443 (14.0%) patients had acute rejection within one year, and 3436 (33.3%) patients had delayed graft function. Figure 1 compares death-censored graft survival between 0–10% and >10% GS. Graft survival rate at 5 years was 75.8% for 0–10% GS and 70.9% for >10% GS ($p < 0.001$).

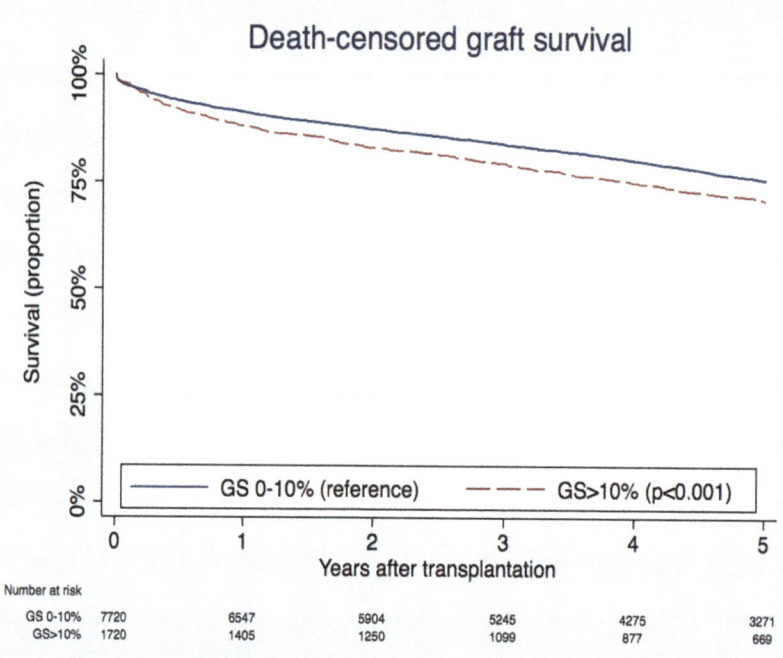

Figure 1. Kaplan–Meier death-censored graft survival curves between 0–10% and >10% allograft glomerulosclerosis (GS) groups.

In unadjusted analysis, kidneys with >10% GS were associated with a 24% higher risk of graft failure compared to kidneys with 0–10% GS (HR 1.24; 95% CI 1.13–1.36, $p < 0.001$). After adjusting for baseline donor, recipient, and transplant-related factors, kidneys with >10% GS remained significantly associated with a 27% higher risk of graft failure compared to kidneys with 0–10% GS (HR 1.27; 95% CI 1.15–1.40, $p < 0.001$) (Table S2). Of note, there was no difference in death-censored graft survival between 11–20% GS and >20% GS (Figure 2 and Table S1). There was no significant difference in patient survival (HR 1.03; 95% CI 0.96–1.12, $p = 0.40$), rate of acute rejection at 1-year (HR 1.13; 95% CI 0.97–1.31, $p = 0.11$), and rate of delayed graft function (HR 1.10; 95% CI 0.98–1.23, $p = 0.11$) between 0–10% GS and >10% GS (Table S2).

We examined the graft outcomes of >85% KDPI kidney with a low degree of GS, compared with 71–85% KDPI kidneys. The death-censored graft survival at 5 years in >85% KDPI kidneys with 0–10% GS was inferior to in 71–85% KPDI kidneys (75.8% vs. 81.2%; $p < 0.001$), as shown in Figure 3.

3.5. Characteristics and Outcomes of Kidneys with No Biopsy Performed

Kidneys donors with no biopsy performed were younger, more were female, and had a greater prevalence of positive hepatitis C antibody, but had a lower prevalence of diabetes, hypertension, body weight, donation after cardiac death, use of machine perfusion, and expanded criteria donation when compared with kidneys with 0–10% GS (Table 1). Graft survival rate at 5 years was comparable between 0% and 10% GS and the no biopsy group (75.8% vs. 74.8%; $p = 0.62$), as shown in Figure 2.

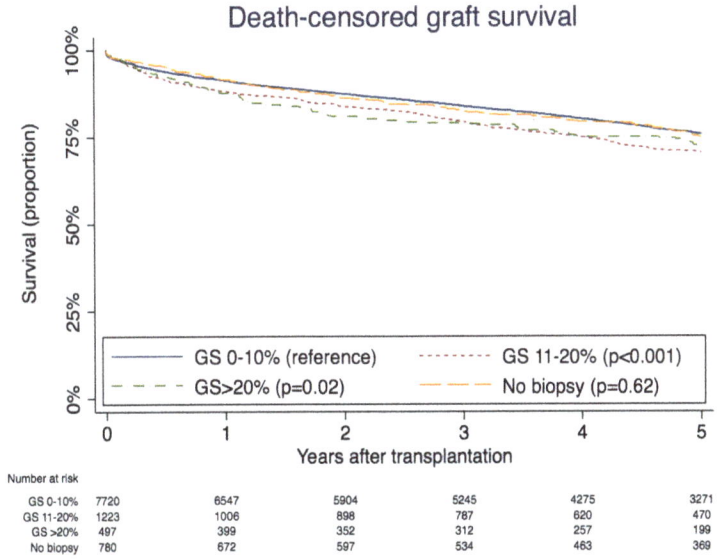

Figure 2. Kaplan–Meier death-censored graft survival curves according to percent glomerulosclerosis (GS) in allografts.

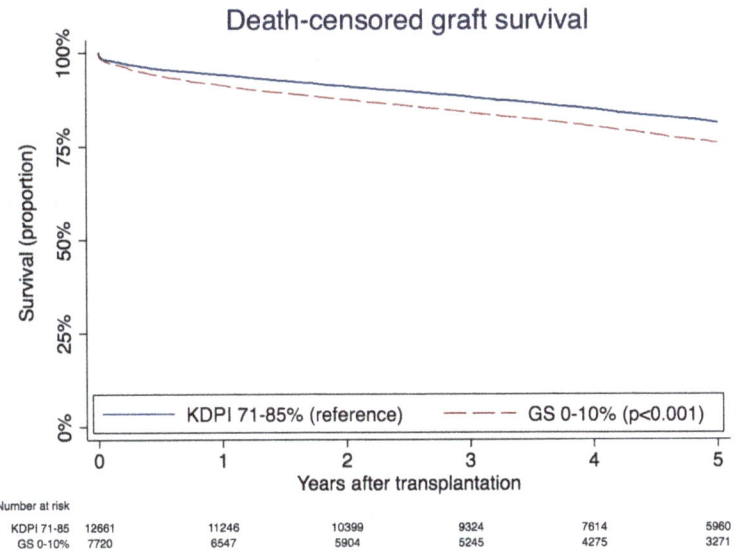

Figure 3. Kaplan–Meier death-censored graft survival curves between the kidney donor profile index (KDPI) 71–85% group and the KDPI >85% with 0–10% percent glomerulosclerosis (GS) group.

4. Discussion

Over 700,000 patients in the United States have ESKD, with the United States having the second-highest incidence rate of treated ESKD in the world [30]. Despite an improvement in dialysis care over the last 15 years, the overall survival on dialysis remains dismal with 22% at one year, 43% at three years and 58% at five years [31]. The risk of death is reduced by up to 66% with kidney transplantation [31]. A major limitation to increasing the number of kidney transplantations is the number of donors. It is thus of paramount importance to decrease the discard rates of high KDPI kidneys, which is estimated to be as high as 50% [8,32].

Our study showed that procurement biopsies are becoming increasingly common in marginal deceased donors in the United States. Ninety-one percent of KDPI >85% kidneys were biopsied on procurement during this study period compared to 85% between 2000 and 2003 in the United States [33]. The utility of procurement biopsies has been debated as they can delay decisions, require high resources, prolong duration of cold ischemia, and lead to unnecessary kidney discard [21,22]. Furthermore, the reliability of GS degree in predicting graft outcomes has been questioned [8,32]. While several studies have reported increased delayed graft function risk, leading to poor outcomes in kidneys with GS > 20% [19,25,28,34,35], and other studies have conversely reported similar prognoses in kidneys with GS > 20% compared to kidneys with lower GS [24,26,27,29]. Banff guidelines for procurement biopsies therefore discourage the use of rigidly defined histologic cutoffs for organ decision and allocation [19].

Using the UNOS database, we demonstrated that GS > 10% is an independent prognostic factor for graft failure in >85% KDPI kidneys, with an adjusted 1.28-fold increased risk of graft failure at 5 years when compared to kidneys with 0–10% GS. The findings of our study suggest that the use of GS percentage in procurement biopsy of >85% KDPI kidneys may improve risk stratification for recipient allograft survival. While GS > 10% was associated with a higher risk of graft failure in >85% KDPI kidneys, we did not find a difference in death-censored graft survival between allografts with 11–20% GS and >20% GS. This may suggest that >10% GS in procurement biopsies can potentially be utilized as a cutoff for risk prediction in clinical practice. Given that the presence of GS > 10% in >85% KDPI kidneys had no significant impact on delayed graft function rate, acute rejection, or patient survival, the underlying explanation for higher graft failure in GS > 10% kidneys is likely due to the progressive kidney aging process in a kidney with less residual function. As the phenotype of GS is associated with podocyte detachment and a reduced number of functioning and viable glomeruli, this leads to increasing ESKD prevalence [36,37]. It has been estimated that an allocation strategy based on pretransplant donor biopsy would increase the incidence of marginal KDPI (80% to 100%) renal transplants by over 20%, which would translate into an overall increase of 4% for the entire pool of donors [38]. Our study supports the clinical utility of the pretransplant biopsy.

This data should not discourage the use of >85% KDPI kidneys with >10% GS. There is an organ shortage with a growing number of individuals who develop ESKD every year [39] combined with a non-proportional limited supply of potential donors [32]. Overall, one-year post-transplant outcomes have improved since 2007, when the Centers for Medicare and Medicaid Services (CMS) solid organ transplant regulation was first implemented [40]. However, there is still a lack of long term graft and survival outcomes [41–44]. Although transplantation with KDPI > 85% kidneys might be associated with an increased delayed graft function rate and reduced graft survival [45], it is clearly evident based on the lower mortality rate that recipients benefit from transplantation of high-KDPI kidneys when compared with those who wait for low-KDPI kidneys [46,47]. Thus, instead of discarding >85% KDPI kidneys with >10% GS due to a higher risk of allograft loss, future studies are needed to identify techniques and strategies to improve the use and outcome of these "marginal" transplantable kidneys safely. Certain strategies are already being used, such as dual transplantation (both kidneys from one donor into the same recipient) [38,48–52] or creation of a protocol designed to timely identify and match suitable patient characteristics with these "marginal" kidneys (e.g., balancing the number of viable nephrons supplied within the graft versus the metabolic demand of the recipient [32]). For example, a >85% KDPI kidney with >10% GS recovered from a female donor with a low BMI may not be the best option for a male candidate with a BMI>35 kg/m^2 [53]; further studies are needed to identify other patient and donor characteristics that would yield optimal outcomes.

Although our study aimed to assess the impact of GS degree on >85% KDPI graft outcomes, the findings of our study cannot be generalized to lower KDPI kidneys. We did compare graft outcomes between KDPI >85% kidneys with 0–10% GS to the overall KDPI 71–85% kidneys. This demonstrated that graft outcomes of KDPI >85% kidneys with 0–10% GS were inferior to KDPI 71–85% kidneys, suggesting a stronger impact of KDPI-related factors on graft outcomes over the percentage of GS on procurement biopsies. As KDPI is comprised of several clinically important donor characteristics that impact outcomes [11], it is hypothesized that these characteristics would similarly have an impact on biopsy pathology that is not limited to GS. Thus, GS percentage should not be used in isolation from other biopsy findings for individualized organ acceptance decisions. In addition, the impact GS on graft outcomes of lower KDPI scores remains unclear, since many lower KDPI kidneys are not biopsied [17–19].

Although our study using the UNOS database is among the largest cohorts investigating procurement biopsies with KDPI > 85%, there are some major limitations. First, there is a lack of uniform criteria for procuring, processing and interpreting procurement graft biopsies [19,54]. Core needle biopsies (during reperfusion) are usually superior to wedge biopsies (during procurement), as wedge biopsies primarily obtain sub capsular tissue, which can overestimate the amount of GS [24,26,32]. Specimens are frozen sections as opposed to paraffin-embedded tissue obtained for regular kidney biopsies or biopsies at reperfusion [21,32]. Procurement biopsies are also often interpreted by on-call general pathologists rather than nephro-pathologists. Unfortunately, the numbers of glomeruli in samples or type of pathologist were not reported in the registry. Thus, more studies aimed at optimizing assessment of procurement biopsy samples to optimally allocate organs are needed. Second, data on other important biopsy parameters in the UNOS database, such as interstitial fibrosis, tubular atrophy, and arteriosclerosis, were limited. Only 30 patients in our cohort had available reports on the degree of interstitial fibrosis, tubular atrophy, or arteriosclerosis. Therefore, future studies evaluating the predictive role of a complete histological evaluation [55], including glomerular, tubular, interstitial, and vascular compartments of >85% KDPI kidneys, are required. Furthermore, GS percentage was reported in the database as 0–10%, 11–20%, and >20%. Thus, kidney transplant outcomes using a higher cut-off of GS percentage could not be evaluated and required future studies. Furthermore, given the differences between procurement biopsies and reperfusion biopsies [18], the findings of our study cannot be generalized to reperfusion biopsies for >85% KDPI kidneys. Finally, the registry may be subjected to selection bias. Kidneys from donors that did not undergo biopsy tended to have less unfavorable clinical characteristics, than those with biopsy as demonstrated in our study (kidney donors in the no biopsy group were younger and had a lower prevalence of diabetes and hypertension), and thus had comparable graft survival rate when compared to the 0–10% GS group, but superior to the >10% GS group. Kidneys with a higher degree of GS were likely to be more carefully selected for unreported factors, including other biopsy characteristics. Alternatively, the kidney discards in each GS percentage cohort may have been impacted by other non-reported factors that influenced study outcomes.

In conclusion, we demonstrated that procurement biopsies for >85% KDPI kidneys are very commonly obtained in the United States, at a rate of 91.2%. A higher percentage of GS in >85% KDPI kidney biopsies are associated with an increased discard rate. Among KDPI >85% kidneys, GS >10% is an independent risk factor for allograft failure. However, graft survival from 0–10% GS kidneys is still inferior to kidneys with KDPI 71–85%, suggesting a stronger impact of KDPI on graft outcomes. Instead of discarding kidneys, future studies are needed to identify strategies to optimally utilize these "marginal" kidneys safely.

Supplementary Materials: The following are available online at http://www.mdpi.com/2077-0383/9/5/1469/s1, Figure S1: Procurement cohort, Figure S2: Kidney transplant recipient cohort, Table S1: Univariable and multivariable cox regression analyses for post-transplant outcomes between Glomerulosclerosis >20% vs. 11–20%, Table S2: Univariable and multivariable cox regression analyses for post-transplant outcomes between Glomerulosclerosis >10% vs. 0–10%.

Author Contributions: Conceptualization, W.C., C.T., P.K.V., S.K., L.S.C., E.I., J.F. and N.L.; Data curation, W.C. and N.L.; Formal analysis, W.C., A.C. and N.L.; Investigation, W.C., C.T. and N.L.; Methodology, W.C., C.T. and N.L.; Project administration, T.B.; Resources, T.B. and N.L.; Software, N.L.; Supervision, C.T., F.L.K., M.A.M., T.B., S.A.S., S.K., L.S.C., E.I., J.F. and N.L.; Validation, W.C., C.T., A.C., P.H., F.L.K., M.A.M., S.A.S. and N.L.; Visualization, W.C. and C.T.; Writing—original draft, W.C.; Writing—review & editing, W.C., C.T., P.K.V., A.C., P.H., F.L.K., M.A.M., T.B., S.A.S., S.K., L.S.C., E.I., J.F. and N.L. W.C., C.T., P.K.V., A.C., P.H., F.L.K., M.A.M., T.B., S.A.S., S.K., L.S.C., E.I., J.F. and N.L. All authors have read and agreed to the published version of the manuscript.

Acknowledgments: None. All authors had access to the data and played essential roles in writing of the manuscript.

Conflicts of Interest: The authors declare no conflict of interest.

References

1. Hart, A.; Smith, J.M.; Skeans, M.A.; Gustafson, S.K.; Wilk, A.R.; Robinson, A.; Wainright, J.L.; Haynes, C.R.; Snyder, J.J.; Kasiske, B.L. OPTN/SRTR 2016 annual data report: Kidney. *Am. J. Transp.* **2018**, *18*, 18–113. [CrossRef] [PubMed]
2. Papadopoulos, E.B.; Ladanyi, M.; Emanuel, D.; Mackinnon, S.; Boulad, F.; Carabasi, M.H.; Castro-Malaspina, H.; Childs, B.H.; Gillio, A.P.; Small, T.N.; et al. Infusions of donor leukocytes to treat Epstein-Barr virus-associated lymphoproliferative disorders after allogeneic bone marrow transplantation. *N. Engl. J. Med.* **1994**, *330*, 1185–1191. [CrossRef]
3. Gupta, M.; Abt, P.L. Trends among kidney transplant candidates in the United States: Sifting through the tea leaves. *Am. J. Transp.* **2019**, *19*, 313–314. [CrossRef] [PubMed]
4. Cecka, J.M. Kidney transplantation in the United States. *Clin. Transp.* **2008**, 1–18.
5. Andre, M.; Huang, E.; Everly, M.; Bunnapradist, S. The UNOS renal transplant registry: Review of the last decade. *Clin Transp.* **2014**, 1–12.
6. Hart, A.; Smith, J.M.; Skeans, M.A.; Gustafson, S.K.; Stewart, D.E.; Cherikh, W.S.; Wainright, J.L.; Kucheryavaya, A.; Woodbury, M.; Snyder, J.J.; et al. OPTN/SRTR 2015 annual data report: Kidney. *Am. J. Transp.* **2017**, *17*, 21–116. [CrossRef]
7. United States Renal Data System. *2015 USRDS Annual Data Report: Epidemiology of Kidney Disease in the United States*; National Institutes of Health, National Institute of Diabetes and Digestive: Bethesda, MD, USA, 2015.
8. Mohan, S.; Chiles, M.C.; Patzer, R.E.; Pastan, S.O.; Husain, S.A.; Carpenter, D.J.; Dube, G.K.; Crew, R.J.; Ratner, L.E.; Cohen, D.J. Factors leading to the discard of deceased donor kidneys in the United States. *Kidney Int.* **2018**, *94*, 187–198. [CrossRef]
9. Lentine, K.L.; Naik, A.S.; Schnitzler, M.A.; Randall, H.; Wellen, J.R.; Kasiske, B.L.; Marklin, G.; Brockmeier, D.; Cooper, M.; Xiao, H.; et al. Variation in use of procurement biopsies and its implications for discard of deceased donor kidneys recovered for transplantation. *Am. J. Transp.* **2019**, *19*, 2241–2251. [CrossRef]
10. Metzger, R.A.; Delmonico, F.L.; Feng, S.; Port, F.K.; Wynn, J.J.; Merion, R.M. Expanded criteria donors for kidney transplantation. *Am. J. Transp.* **2003**, *4*, 114–125. [CrossRef]
11. Israni, A.K.; Salkowski, N.; Gustafson, S.; Snyder, J.J.; Friedewald, J.J.; Formica, R.N.; Wang, X.; Shteyn, E.; Cherikh, W.; Stewart, D.; et al. New national allocation policy for deceased donor kidneys in the United States and possible effect on patient outcomes. *J. Am. Soc. Nephrol.* **2014**, *25*, 1842–1848. [CrossRef]
12. Hart, A.; Smith, J.M.; Skeans, M.A.; Gustafson, S.K.; Wilk, A.R.; Castro, S.; Robinson, A.; Wainright, J.L.; Snyder, J.J.; Kasiske, B.L.; et al. OPTN/SRTR 2017 annual data report: Kidney. *Am. J. Transp.* **2019**, *19*, 19–123. [CrossRef] [PubMed]
13. Reese, P.P.; Harhay, M.N.; Abt, P.L.; Levine, M.H.; Halpern, S.D. New solutions to reduce discard of kidneys donated for transplantation. *J. Am. Soc. Nephrol.* **2016**, *27*, 973–980. [CrossRef] [PubMed]
14. Bae, S.; Massie, A.B.; Luo, X.; Anjum, S.; Desai, N.M.; Segev, D.L. Changes in discard rate after the introduction of the kidney donor profile index (KDPI). *Am. J. Transp.* **2016**, *16*, 2202–2207. [CrossRef] [PubMed]
15. Narvaez, J.R.F.; Nie, J.; Noyes, K.; Leeman, M.; Kayler, L.K. Hard-to-place kidney offers: Donor- and system-level predictors of discard. *Am. J. Transp.* **2018**, *18*, 2708–2718. [CrossRef]
16. Cohen, J.B.; Shults, J.; Goldberg, D.S.; Abt, P.L.; Sawinski, D.L.; Reese, P.P. Kidney allograft offers: Predictors of turndown and the impact of late organ acceptance on allograft survival. *Am. J. Transp.* **2018**, *18*, 391–401. [CrossRef] [PubMed]

17. Mohan, S.; Campenot, E.; Chiles, M.C.; Santoriello, D.; Bland, E.; Crew, R.J.; Rosenstiel, P.; Dube, G.; Batal, I.; Radhakrishnan, J.; et al. Association between reperfusion renal allograft biopsy findings and transplant outcomes. *J. Am. Soc. Nephrol.* **2017**, *28*, 3109–3117. [CrossRef]
18. Carpenter, D.; Husain, S.A.; Brennan, C.; Batal, I.; Hall, I.E.; Santoriello, D.; Rosen, R.; Crew, R.J.; Campenot, E.; Dube, G.K.; et al. Procurement biopsies in the evaluation of deceased donor kidneys. *Clin. J. Am. Soc. Nephrol.* **2018**, *13*, 1876–1885. [CrossRef]
19. Liapis, H.; Gaut, J.P.; Klein, C.; Bagnasco, S.; Kraus, E.; Farris, A.B., 3rd; Honsova, E.; Perkowska-Ptasinska, A.; David, D.; Goldberg, J.; et al. Banff histopathological consensus criteria for preimplantation kidney biopsies. *Am. J. Transp.* **2017**, *17*, 140–150. [CrossRef]
20. Hall, I.E.; Parikh, C.R.; Schroppel, B.; Weng, F.L.; Jia, Y.; Thiessen-Philbrook, H.; Reese, P.P.; Doshi, M.D. Procurement biopsy findings versus kidney donor risk index for predicting renal allograft survival. *Transp. Direct* **2018**, *4*, e373. [CrossRef]
21. Kasiske, B.L.; Stewart, D.E.; Bista, B.R.; Salkowski, N.; Snyder, J.J.; Israni, A.K.; Crary, G.S.; Rosendale, J.D.; Matas, A.J.; Delmonico, F.L. The role of procurement biopsies in acceptance decisions for kidneys retrieved for transplant. *Clin. J. Am. Soc. Nephrol.* **2014**, *9*, 562–571. [CrossRef]
22. Stewart, D.E.; Garcia, V.C.; Rosendale, J.D.; Klassen, D.K.; Carrico, B.J. Diagnosing the decades-long rise in the deceased donor kidney discard rate in the United States. *Transplantation* **2017**, *101*, 575–587. [CrossRef] [PubMed]
23. Wang, C.J.; Wetmore, J.B.; Crary, G.S.; Kasiske, B.L. The donor kidney biopsy and its implications in predicting graft outcomes: A systematic review. *Am. J. Transp.* **2015**, *15*, 1903–1914. [CrossRef]
24. Sung, R.S.; Christensen, L.L.; Leichtman, A.B.; Greenstein, S.M.; Distant, D.A.; Wynn, J.J.; Stegall, M.D.; Delmonico, F.L.; Port, F.K. Determinants of discard of expanded criteria donor kidneys: Impact of biopsy and machine perfusion. *Am. J. Transp.* **2008**, *8*, 783–792. [CrossRef] [PubMed]
25. Escofet, X.; Osman, H.; Griffiths, D.F.; Woydag, S.; Adam Jurewicz, W. The presence of glomerular sclerosis at time zero has a significant impact on function after cadaveric renal transplantation. *Transplantation* **2003**, *75*, 344–346. [CrossRef] [PubMed]
26. Malek, S.K. Procurement biopsies in kidneys retrieved for transplantation. *Clin. J. Am. Soc. Nephrol.* **2014**, *9*, 443–444. [CrossRef]
27. Bajwa, M.; Cho, Y.W.; Pham, P.T.; Shah, T.; Danovitch, G.; Wilkinson, A.; Bunnapradist, S. Donor biopsy and kidney transplant outcomes: An analysis using the organ procurement and transplantation network/united network for organ sharing (OPTN/UNOS) database. *Transplantation* **2007**, *84*, 1399–1405. [CrossRef]
28. Edwards, E.B.; Posner, M.P.; Maluf, D.G.; Kauffman, H.M. Reasons for non-use of recovered kidneys: The effect of donor glomerulosclerosis and creatinine clearance on graft survival. *Transplantation* **2004**, *77*, 1411–1415. [CrossRef]
29. Cicciarelli, J.; Cho, Y.; Mateo, R.; El-Shahawy, M.; Iwaki, Y.; Selby, R. Renal biopsy donor group: The influence of glomerulosclerosis on transplant outcomes. *Transplant. Proc.* **2005**, *37*, 712–713. [CrossRef]
30. Barlesi, F.; Vansteenkiste, J.; Spigel, D.; Ishii, H.; Garassino, M.; de Marinis, F.; Özgüroğlu, M.; Szczesna, A.; Polychronis, A.; Uslu, R.; et al. Avelumab versus docetaxel in patients with platinum-treated advanced non-small-cell lung cancer (JAVELIN Lung 200): An open-label, randomised, phase 3 study. *Lancet Oncol.* **2018**, *19*, 1468–1479. [CrossRef]
31. Hanna, R. Acute kidney injury after pembrolizumab-induced adrenalitis and adrenal insufficiency. *Case Rep. Nephrol. Dial.* **2018**, *8*, 238. [CrossRef]
32. Angeletti, A.; Cravedi, P. Making procurement biopsies important again for kidney transplant allocation. *Nephron* **2019**, *142*, 34–39. [CrossRef] [PubMed]
33. Cecka, J.M.; Cohen, B.; Rosendale, J.; Smith, M. Could more effective use of kidneys recovered from older deceased donors result in more kidney transplants for older patients? *Transplantation* **2006**, *81*, 966–970. [CrossRef] [PubMed]
34. Gaber, L.W.; Moore, L.W.; Alloway, R.R.; Amiri, M.H.; Vera, S.R.; Gaber, A.O. Glomerulosclerosis as a determinant of posttransplant function of older donor renal allografts. *Transplantation* **1995**, *60*, 334–339. [CrossRef] [PubMed]

35. Randhawa, P.S.; Minervini, M.I.; Lombardero, M.; Duquesnoy, R.; Fung, J.; Shapiro, R.; Jordan, M.; Vivas, C.; Scantlebury, V.; Demetris, A. Biopsy of marginal donor kidneys: Correlation of histologic findings with graft dysfunction. *Transplantation* **2000**, *69*, 1352–1357. [CrossRef]
36. Hodgin, J.B.; Bitzer, M.; Wickman, L.; Afshinnia, F.; Wang, S.Q.; O'Connor, C.; Yang, Y.; Meadowbrooke, C.; Chowdhury, M.; Kikuchi, M.; et al. Glomerular aging and focal global glomerulosclerosis: A podometric perspective. *J. Am. Soc. Nephrol.* **2015**, *26*, 3162–3178. [CrossRef]
37. Rowland, J.; Akbarov, A.; Maan, A.; Eales, J.; Dormer, J.; Tomaszewski, M. Tick-tock chimes the kidney clock—From biology of renal ageing to clinical applications. *Kidney Blood Press. Res.* **2018**, *43*, 55–67. [CrossRef]
38. Gandolfini, I.; Buzio, C.; Zanelli, P.; Palmisano, A.; Cremaschi, E.; Vaglio, A.; Piotti, G.; Melfa, L.; La Manna, G.; Feliciangeli, G.; et al. The Kidney Donor Profile Index (KDPI) of marginal donors allocated by standardized pretransplant donor biopsy assessment: Distribution and association with graft outcomes. *Am. J. Transp.* **2014**, *14*, 2515–2525. [CrossRef]
39. McCullough, K.P.; Morgenstern, H.; Saran, R.; Herman, W.H.; Robinson, B.M. Projecting ESRD incidence and prevalence in the United States through 2030. *J. Am. Soc. Nephrol.* **2019**, *30*, 127–135. [CrossRef]
40. Jay, C.; Schold, J.D. Measuring transplant center performance: The goals are not controversial but the methods and consequences can be. *Curr. Transp.* **2017**, *4*, 52–58. [CrossRef]
41. Thongprayoon, C.; Hansrivijit, P.; Leeaphorn, N.; Acharya, P.; Torres-Ortiz, A.; Kaewput, W.; Kovvuru, K.; Kanduri, S.R.; Bathini, T.; Cheungpasitporn, W. Recent advances and clinical outcomes of kidney transplantation. *J. Clin. Med.* **2020**, *9*, 1193. [CrossRef]
42. Thongprayoon, C.; Kaewput, W.; Kovvuru, K.; Hansrivijit, P.; Kanduri, S.R.; Bathini, T.; Chewcharat, A.; Leeaphorn, N.; Gonzalez-Suarez, M.L.; Cheungpasitporn, W. Promises of big data and artificial intelligence in nephrology and transplantation. *J. Clin. Med.* **2020**, *9*, 1107. [CrossRef] [PubMed]
43. Leeaphorn, N.; Thongprayoon, C.; Chon, W.J.; Cummings, L.S.; Mao, M.A.; Cheungpasitporn, W. Outcomes of kidney retransplantation after graft loss as a result of BK virus nephropathy in the era of newer immunosuppressant agents. *Am. J. Transp.* **2020**, *20*, 1334–1340. [CrossRef] [PubMed]
44. Cheungpasitporn, W.; Kremers, W.K.; Lorenz, E.; Amer, H.; Cosio, F.G.; Stegall, M.D.; Gandhi, M.J.; Schinstock, C.A. De novo donor-specific antibody following BK nephropathy: The incidence and association with antibody-mediated rejection. *Clin. Transp.* **2018**, *32*, e13194. [CrossRef] [PubMed]
45. Zens, T.J.; Danobeitia, J.S.; Leverson, G.; Chlebeck, P.J.; Zitur, L.J.; Redfield, R.R.; D'Alessandro, A.M.; Odorico, S.; Kaufman, D.B.; Fernandez, L.A. The impact of kidney donor profile index on delayed graft function and transplant outcomes: A single-center analysis. *Clin. Transp.* **2018**, *32*, e13190. [CrossRef] [PubMed]
46. Jay, C.L.; Washburn, K.; Dean, P.G.; Helmick, R.A.; Pugh, J.A.; Stegall, M.D. Survival benefit in older patients associated with earlier transplant with high KDPI kidneys. *Transplantation* **2017**, *101*, 867–872. [CrossRef]
47. Massie, A.B.; Luo, X.; Chow, E.K.; Alejo, J.L.; Desai, N.M.; Segev, D.L. Survival benefit of primary deceased donor transplantation with high-KDPI kidneys. *Am. J. Transp.* **2014**, *14*, 2310–2316. [CrossRef]
48. Ruggenenti, P.; Silvestre, C.; Boschiero, L.; Rota, G.; Furian, L.; Perna, A.; Rossini, G.; Remuzzi, G.; Rigotti, P. Long-term outcome of renal transplantation from octogenarian donors: A multicenter controlled study. *Am. J. Transp.* **2017**, *17*, 3159–3171. [CrossRef]
49. Moore, P.S.; Farney, A.C.; Sundberg, A.K.; Rohr, M.S.; Hartmann, E.L.; Iskandar, S.S.; Gautreaux, M.D.; Rogers, J.; Doares, W.; Anderson, T.K.; et al. Dual kidney transplantation: A case-control comparison with single kidney transplantation from standard and expanded criteria donors. *Transplantation* **2007**, *83*, 1551–1556. [CrossRef]
50. Gill, J.; Cho, Y.W.; Danovitch, G.M.; Wilkinson, A.; Lipshutz, G.; Pham, P.T.; Gill, J.S.; Shah, T.; Bunnapradist, S. Outcomes of dual adult kidney transplants in the United States: An analysis of the OPTN/UNOS database. *Transplantation* **2008**, *85*, 62–68. [CrossRef]
51. Remuzzi, G.; Cravedi, P.; Perna, A.; Dimitrov, B.D.; Turturro, M.; Locatelli, G.; Rigotti, P.; Baldan, N.; Beatini, M.; Valente, U.; et al. Long-term outcome of renal transplantation from older donors. *N. Engl. J. Med.* **2006**, *354*, 343–352. [CrossRef]
52. Lee, K.W.; Park, J.B.; Cha, S.R.; Lee, S.H.; Chung, Y.J.; Yoo, H.; Kim, K.; Kim, S.J. Dual kidney transplantation offers a safe and effective way to use kidneys from deceased donors older than 70 years. *BMC Nephrol.* **2020**, *21*, 3. [CrossRef] [PubMed]

53. Foley, D.P.; Sawinski, D. Personalizing donor kidney selection: Choosing the right donor for the right recipient. *Clin. J. Am. Soc. Nephrol.* **2019**, *15*, 418–420. [CrossRef] [PubMed]
54. Naesens, M. Zero-time renal transplant biopsies: A comprehensive review. *Transplantation* **2016**, *100*, 1425–1439. [CrossRef] [PubMed]
55. Karpinski, J.; Lajoie, G.; Cattran, D.; Fenton, S.; Zaltzman, J.; Cardella, C.; Cole, E. Outcome of kidney transplantation from high-risk donors is determined by both structure and function. *Transplantation* **1999**, *67*, 1162–1167. [CrossRef]

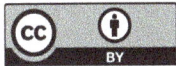

© 2020 by the authors. Licensee MDPI, Basel, Switzerland. This article is an open access article distributed under the terms and conditions of the Creative Commons Attribution (CC BY) license (http://creativecommons.org/licenses/by/4.0/).

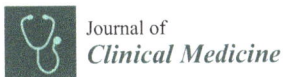

Article

Erythropoietin, Fibroblast Growth Factor 23, and Death After Kidney Transplantation

Michele F. Eisenga [1,*], Maarten A. De Jong [1], David E. Leaf [2], Ilja M. Nolte [3], Martin H. De Borst [1], Stephan J. L. Bakker [1] and Carlo A. J. M. Gaillard [1,4]

1. Division of Nephrology, Department of Internal Medicine, University of Groningen, University Medical Center Groningen, 9700 RB Groningen, The Netherlands; m.a.de.jong03@umcg.nl (M.A.D.J.); m.h.de.borst@umcg.nl (M.H.D.B.); s.j.l.bakker@umcg.nl (S.J.L.B.)
2. Division of Renal Medicine, Brigham and Women's Hospital, Harvard Medical School, Boston, MA 02215, USA; deleaf@bwh.harvard.edu
3. Department of Epidemiology, University of Groningen, University Medical Center Groningen, 9700 RB Groningen, The Netherlands; i.m.nolte@umcg.nl
4. Department of Internal Medicine and Dermatology, University of Utrecht, University Medical Center Utrecht, 3508 GA Utrecht, The Netherlands; C.A.J.M.Gaillard@umcutrecht.nl
* Correspondence: m.f.eisenga@umcg.nl; Tel.: +31-50-361-0165

Received: 30 April 2020; Accepted: 3 June 2020; Published: 4 June 2020

Abstract: Elevated levels of erythropoietin (EPO) are associated with an increased risk of death in renal transplant recipients (RTRs), but the underlying mechanisms remain unclear. Emerging data suggest that EPO stimulates production of the phosphaturic hormone fibroblast growth factor 23 (FGF23), another strong risk factor for death in RTRs. We hypothesized that the hitherto unexplained association between EPO levels and adverse outcomes may be attributable to increased levels of FGF23. We included 579 RTRs (age 51 ± 12 years, 55% males) from the TransplantLines Insulin Resistance and Inflammation Cohort study (NCT03272854). During a follow-up of 7.0 years, 121 RTRs died, of which 62 were due to cardiovascular cause. In multivariable Cox regression analysis, EPO was independently associated with all-cause (HR, 1.66; 95% CI 1.16–2.36; $P = 0.005$) and cardiovascular death (HR, 1.87; 95% CI 1.14–3.06; $P = 0.01$). However, the associations were abrogated following adjustment for FGF23 (HR, 1.28; 95% CI 0.87–1.88; $P = 0.20$, and HR, 1.45; 95% CI 0.84–2.48; $P = 0.18$, respectively). In subsequent mediation analysis, FGF23 mediated 72% and 50% of the association between EPO and all-cause and cardiovascular death, respectively. Our results underline the strong relationship between EPO and FGF23 physiology, and provide a potential mechanism underlying the relationship between increased EPO levels and adverse outcomes in RTRs.

Keywords: erythropoietin; fibroblast growth factor 23; death; kidney transplantation

---

1. Introduction

Renal transplant recipients (RTRs) have a high residual risk of all-cause and cardiovascular death, compared to the general population [1]. Previous studies demonstrated an independent association between higher circulating endogenous erythropoietin (EPO) levels and risk of all-cause and cardiovascular death among RTRs, similar to other patient populations such as chronic heart failure patients and the elderly [2–4]. In addition, administration of exogenous EPO may increase the risk of cardiovascular events in patients with chronic kidney disease (CKD) and end stage renal disease (ESRD) [5,6]. However, the underlying mechanisms responsible for the link between endogenous and exogenous EPO and adverse outcomes are unknown.

Studies from our group and others suggest that EPO is prominently involved in fibroblast growth factor-23 (FGF23) physiology [7–10]. FGF23 is an osteocyte-derived hormone that plays an essential role in regulating phosphate and vitamin D metabolism. In RTRs, increased FGF23 levels post-transplant are independently associated with an increased risk of graft failure and death [11,12]. Hypoxia, the main stimulus for EPO synthesis, stabilizes hypoxia-inducible factor (HIF)-1α, which is a heterodimeric transcription factor that regulates oxygen homeostasis [13,14]. Subsequently, stabilized HIF1-α upregulates FGF23 production while concomitantly increasing FGF23 cleavage into inactive fragments, resulting in elevated total FGF23 levels but normal levels of intact, bioactive FGF23 [15–18].

In the current study, we hypothesized that the previously established, but hitherto unexplained association between EPO levels and adverse outcomes may be attributable to increased levels of total FGF23. Therefore, we investigated the associations between EPO and total FGF23 levels and prospective outcomes in our RTRs cohort.

2. Methods

2.1. Patient Population

All RTRs (aged ≥ 18 years) who were at least 1-year post-transplantation were approached for participation in the current study during outpatient clinic visits between 2001 and 2003. All RTRs were transplanted in the University Medical Center Groningen (Groningen, the Netherlands). The study has been described in detail previously [19]. Among 847 RTRs approached for participation, 606 RTRs agreed to participate and were included. All patients provided written informed consent and the study protocol was approved by the local medical ethical committee (METc 2001/039). The study protocol adhered to principles of the Declaration of Helsinki and the Declaration of Istanbul. The co-primary endpoints of the study were all-cause and cardiovascular death. Cause of death was obtained by linking the number of the death certificate to the primary cause of death as coded by a physician from the Central Bureau of Statistics according to the International Classification of Diseases, 9th revision (ICD-9; https://icd.codes/icd9cm). CV death was defined as deaths in which the principal cause of death was cardiovascular in nature, using ICD-9 codes 410 to 447. Secondary endpoint constituted death-censored graft failure (DCGF). DCGF was defined as return to dialysis or re-transplantation. For the current analyses, we excluded RTRs who did not have plasma samples available for measuring EPO levels ($n = 14$) and RTRs who used exogenous EPO ($n = 13$) due to positive interference in EPO measurement, resulting in 579 RTRs eligible for analyses. Median follow-up time from inclusion to endpoint was 7.0 (interquartile range (IQR), 6.2 to 7.4) years. Data on the co-primary and secondary endpoints were available in all 579 participants. There was no loss-to-follow-up in the current study.

2.2. Data Collection

Relevant donor, recipient, and transplant characteristics at baseline were extracted from the Groningen Renal Transplant Database, as described in detail previously [19]. Information on medical history and medication use was obtained from patient records. Participants' height and weight were measured with participants wearing light indoor clothing without shoes. Blood pressure was measured according to a strict protocol as previously described [19]. Alcohol consumption and smoking behavior were recorded using a self-reported questionnaire. Smoking behavior was classified as never, former, or current smoker.

2.3. Laboratory Procedures

Blood samples were drawn during the next outpatient clinic visit after agreeing to participate. Blood was drawn in the morning after an 8–12 h overnight fast, and all measurements were performed in samples of the same timepoint. In plasma EDTA samples frozen at −80°C, we measured plasma EPO levels using an immunoassay based on chemiluminescence (Immulite, Los Angeles, CA) [20]. We measured plasma total FGF23 levels with a human FGF23 (C-terminal) enzyme-linked immunosorbent assay (ELISA; Quidel Corp., San Diego, CA, USA) with intra-assay and interassay coefficients (CVs) of variation of <5% and <16% in blinded replicated samples, respectively [21].

The total FGF23 immunometric assay uses two antibodies directed against different epitopes within the C-terminal part of FGF23, and as such the assay detects both the intact hormone as well as C-terminal cleavage products, and therefore measures total FGF23 levels. We measured plasma ferritin levels using an electrochemiluminescence immunoassay (Modular analytics E170, Roche diagnostics, Mannheim, Germany). Renal function was determined by estimating GFR by applying the Chronic Kidney Disease Epidemiology Collaboration equation [22]. Proteinuria was defined as urinary protein excretion ≥ 0.5 g/24 h in 24-h urine collection. Serum cholesterol was measured using standard laboratory procedures. Serum creatinine was assessed using a modified version of the Jaffé method (MEGA AU 510; Merck Diagnostica, Darmstadt, Germany). Erythrocytosis was defined as hemoglobin level higher than 16.0 g/dL for women, and higher than 16.5 g/dL for men [23].

2.4. Statistical Analyses

Data were analyzed using IBM SPSS software, version 23.0 (SPSS Inc., Chicago, IL), R version 3.2.3 (Vienna, Austria) and STATA 14.1 (STATA Corp., College Station, TX). Data are expressed as mean ± standard deviation [SD] for normally distributed variables and as median (25th–75th interquartile range (IQR)) for variables with a skewed distribution. Categorical data are expressed as numbers (percentages). Co-linearity was tested by means of variance inflation factor (VIF) calculation, with a VIF score of lower than 5 indicating no evidence for co-linearity. We used Cox proportional hazards regression analysis to investigate the association between EPO levels and prospective outcomes. Assumptions of proportionality in Cox regression analyses were checked using Schoenfeld residuals plots and checking nonsignificance of covariates and with the global test (Model 1; EPO with death and CV death; $P > 0.30$ for global test). In these Cox regression analyses, we adjusted for potential confounders based on univariable associations or for factors of known biologic importance. We adjusted for age, sex, body surface area (BSA), eGFR, proteinuria, time since transplantation, presence of diabetes, systolic blood pressure (SBP), total cholesterol, and use of calcineurin inhibitors, proliferation inhibitors, and angiotensin-converting enzyme (ACE)-inhibitors and angiotensin II-receptor blockers (ARBs) (Model 1). We subsequently adjusted for potential mediators in the pathway between EPO and death, i.e., hemoglobin levels (Model 2); for ferritin (Model 3), high-sensitive C-reactive protein (hs-CRP) (Model 4), and finally for total FGF23 (Model 5). Due to skewed distribution, EPO, ferritin, hs-CRP, and total FGF23 were natural log-transformed. We repeated the Cox regression analyses between EPO and outcomes with EPO levels being divided in quartiles. Furthermore, we generated Kaplan–Meier curves to visually show the effect of increased risk of death and cardiovascular death while being in the highest EPO quartile. A log-rank test for trend was used to compare rates of death across quartiles. We also assessed the association between FGF23 levels and prospective outcomes adjusting for all potential confounders according to Model 1 and including EPO. To reflect the contribution of covariates in the different Cox regression models, we generated Supplementary Tables S1–S4 showing the strength of covariates in univariable and multivariable models. To allow comparability between the hazard ratios (HR) of covariates, HR of continuous variables in Supplementary Tables S1–S4 are shown as expressed per SD. As sensitivity analysis, we assessed the prevalence of different etiologies of CKD in total cohort and across EPO quartiles, and we adjusted the association between EPO and all-cause and cardiovascular death for etiology of CKD. Subsequently, we calculated the percentage of change in HR before and after adjustment for FGF23. Percentage change in HR was calculated as—(HR without adjustment − HR with adjustment)/(HR without adjustment − 1) × 100% [24]. Hereafter, we performed mediation analyses with the methods as previously described by Preacher and Hayes, which are based on logistic regression [25,26]. These analyses allow for testing significance and magnitude of mediation on the association between EPO and outcomes [25,26]. Overall, 0.4% of demographic data were missing and these data were imputed using regressive switching [27]. Five datasets were multiply-imputed, and results were pooled and analyzed according to Rubin's rules [28]. In all analyses, a two-sided p-value < 0.05 was considered significant.

3. Results

3.1. Baseline Characteristics

We included 579 RTRs (mean age of 51 ± 12 years; 55% male) at a median of 6.0 (2.6–11.6) years after transplantation. Erythrocytosis was present in 27 (5%) of the included RTRs. Further demographics and clinical baseline characteristics across quartiles of EPO are shown in Table 1.

Table 1. Baseline characteristics of the included 579 renal transplant recipients (RTRs) across erythropoietin (EPO) quartiles.

		Quartiles of EPO (IU/L)				
	All Patients (n = 579)	Q1 (n = 146) [4.0–11.9]	Q2 (n = 143) [12.0–17.2]	Q33 (n = 145) [17.3–23.9]	Q4 (n = 145) [24.2–182.0]	P-value
Age (years)	51 ± 12	47 ± 13	50 ± 12	53 ± 11	54 ± 11	<0.001
Male sex (n, %)	317 (55)	92 (63)	78 (55)	73 (50)	74 (51)	0.11
Body surface area, m^2	1.87 ± 0.19	1.86 ± 0.19	1.86 ± 0.20	1.87 ± 0.18	1.88 ± 0.20	0.81
Alcohol use (n, %)	290 (50)	77 (52)	73 (51)	64 (44)	76 (52)	0.35
Smoking status						0.29
Never smoker (n, %)	205 (35)	47 (32)	49 (34)	59 (41)	50 (35)	
Former smoker (n, %)	246 (43)	64 (44)	68 (48)	59 (41)	55 (38)	
Current smoker (n, %)	126 (22)	35 (24)	25 (18)	27 (19)	39 (27)	
Time since Tx (yrs)	6.0 (2.6–11.6)	4.6 (2.1–9.2)	5.7 (3.1–11.2)	6.5 (3.3–12.4)	7.0 (2.8–13.7)	0.007
Diabetes mellitus (n, %)	102 (18)	25 (17)	21 (15)	27 (19)	29 (20)	0.67
SBP (mmHg)	153 ± 23	150 ± 20	151 ± 21	153 ± 22	157 ± 26	0.05
DBP (mmHg)	90 ± 10	90 ± 9	90 ± 9	90 ± 10	90 ± 11	0.91
Laboratory measurements						
FGF23 (RU/mL)	137 (94–212)	115 (81–168)	125 (88–184)	138 (95–212)	195 (115–363)	<0.001
Hemoglobin (g/dL)	13.9 ± 1.5	14.2 ± 1.5	14.0 ± 1.5	13.8 ± 1.5	13.5 ± 1.5	0.001
Erythrocytosis (n, %)‡	27 (5)	11 (8)	8 (6)	5 (3)	3 (2)	0.13
MCV (fL)	91 ± 6	89 ± 4	91 ± 6	92 ± 6	92 ± 8	<0.001
Ferritin (µg/L)	154 (76–282)	154 (76–320)	164 (100–305)	159 (89–283)	118 (61–240)	0.02
Total cholesterol (mmol/L)	5.6 ± 1.1	5.7 ± 0.9	5.7 ± 1.3	5.6 ± 1.0	5.6 ± 1.1	0.78
Phosphate (mmol/L)	1.1 ± 0.2	1.05 ± 0.21	1.07 ± 0.21	1.05 ± 0.19	1.07 ± 0.22	0.85
Calcium (mmol/L)	2.39 ± 0.16	2.39 ± 0.16	2.38 ± 0.16	2.39 ± 0.18	2.41 ± 0.15	0.51
Vit. 25(OH) D, nmol/l *	53 ± 23	52 ± 24	51 ± 21	57 ± 21	53 ± 25	0.33
Vit. 1,25(OH)$_2$ D, pmol/L*	109 ± 46	106 ± 50	112 ± 46	107 ± 40	110 ± 47	0.80
PTH (pmol/L)	9.1 (6.0–13.4)	8.8 (6.2–13.2)	9.6 (5.8–13.9)	9.2 (6.0–13.7)	8.9 (6.0–14.0)	0.93
eGFR (ml/min/1.73m^2)	48 ± 15	50 ± 16	48 ± 14	47 ± 15	46 ± 16	0.16
Creatinine (µmol/L)	144 ± 52	145 ± 51	139 ± 40	142 ± 51	148 ± 62	0.50
Proteinuria (>0.5g) (n, %)	155 (27)	34 (23)	32 (22)	39 (27)	50 (35)	0.07
hs-CRP (mg/L)	2.0 (0.8–4.8)	1.4 (0.6–3.8)	2.0 (0.7–4.1)	2.1 (1.0–4.2)	3.2 (1.2–7.2)	<0.001
Treatment						
ACE-i/AII-antagonists (n, %)	190 (33)	65 (45)	50 (35)	37 (26)	38 (26)	0.001
ACE-I (n, %)	154 (27)	53 (36)	37 (26)	31 (24)	33 (23)	
AII-antagonists (n,%)	36 (6)	12 (8)	13 (9)	6 (4)	5 (3)	
Bèta-blocker (n, %)	356 (62)	88 (63)	96 (67)	81 (56)	91 (63)	0.26
Ca^{2+} channel blockers (n, %)	220 (39)	56 (38)	52 (36)	51 (35)	61 (42)	0.45
Diuretic use (n, %)	250 (43)	52 (36)	62 (43)	60 (41)	76 (52)	0.04
Proliferation inhibitor (n, %)	428 (74)	95 (65)	99 (69)	115 (79)	119 (82)	0.002
Azathioprine (n, %)	187 (32)	18 (12)	42 (29)	55 (38)	72 (50)	
Mycophenolic acid (n, %)	241 (42)	77 (53)	57 (40)	60 (41)	47 (32)	
Calcineurin inhibitor (n, %)	457 (79)	131 (90)	120 (84)	103 (71)	103 (71)	<0.001
Ciclosporin (n,%)	376 (65)	108 (78)	101 (71)	81 (56)	86 (59)	
Tacrolimus (n, %)	81 (14)	23 (16)	19 (13)	22 (15)	17 (12)	

‡ Erythrocytosis defined as hemoglobin level >16 g/dL (F) and >16.5 g/dL (M) * Only available in a subset cohort of 415 RTRs. Values are means ± standard deviation, medians (interquartile range) or proportions (%). Diabetes mellitus was defined as serum glucose > 7 mmol/L or the use of antidiabetic drugs. Abbreviations—ACE-i, angiotensin converting enzyme inhibitors; DBP, diastolic blood pressure; eGFR, estimated glomerular filtration rate; FGF23, fibroblast growth factor 23; hs-CRP, high-sensitivity C-reactive protein; MCV, mean corpuscular volume; SBP, systolic blood pressure; Tx, transplantation.

Median plasma EPO levels were 17.4 (11.9–24.2) IU/L and median FGF23 levels were 137 (94–212) RU/mL. Increased FGF23 levels were noted across EPO quartiles (115 (81–168) RU/mL; 125 (88–184) RU/mL; 138 (95–212) RU/mL; and 195 (115–363) RU/mL respectively, $P < 0.001$). FGF23 levels were positively correlated with EPO levels ($r = 0.28$, $P < 0.001$), with a VIF of 1.15, indicating very minimal co-linearity.

3.2. EPO, FGF23, and Death

During a median follow-up of 7.0 (6.2–7.4) years, 121 RTRs died. Of the 121 deceased RTRs, 62 RTRs (51%) died from cardiovascular causes. Other causes of death were infection (18%), malignancy (24%), and miscellaneous causes (8%).

In univariable Cox regression analyses, higher EPO levels were associated with an increased risk of all-cause death (HR per 1 ln IU/L increase, 1.74; 95% confidence interval (CI), 1.29–2.34; $P < 0.001$). A full list of HRs for covariates univariably with death are described in Supplementary Table S1.

In multivariable Cox regression analyses, the association between EPO and all-cause death remained significant (HR, 1.66; 95% CI, 1.16-2.36; P=0.005) independent of adjustment for age, sex, BSA, eGFR, proteinuria, time since transplantation, presence of diabetes, SBP, total cholesterol, use of calcineurin inhibitors, proliferation inhibitors, ACE-inhibitors or ARB (Model 1). Further adjustment for hemoglobin, ferritin, or hs-CRP levels did not materially alter the results. However, further adjustment for FGF23 levels attenuated the association between EPO and all-cause death such that the association no longer remained significant (HR, 1.28; 95% CI, 0.87–1.88; $P = 0.20$) (Table 2). A full list of HRs for covariates in the multivariable model can be found in Supplementary Table S2.

Table 2. Association between erythropoietin levels and risk of all-cause and cardiovascular death.

	EPO (IU/L)	
All–cause death	HR (95% CI) *	P-value
Univariable	1.74 (1.29–2.34)	<0.001
Model 1	1.66 (1.16–2.36)	0.005
Model 2	1.72 (1.21–2.46)	0.003
Model 3	1.80 (1.25–2.60)	0.002
Model 4	1.60 (1.12–2.29)	0.01
Model 5	1.28 (0.87–1.88)	0.20
Cardiovascular death	**HR (95% CI) ***	**P-value**
Univariable	1.70 (1.12–2.58)	0.01
Model 1	1.87 (1.14–3.06)	0.01
Model 2	1.90 (1.16–3.12)	0.01
Model 3	2.05 (1.22–3.44)	0.006
Model 4	1.87 (1.14–3.06)	0.01
Model 5	1.45 (0.84–2.48)	0.18

* Hazard ratios are shown per 1 ln IU/L increase in EPO levels; Model 1: Adjusted for age, sex, body surface area, eGFR, proteinuria, time since transplantation, presence of diabetes, systolic blood pressure, total cholesterol, use of calcineurin inhibitors, proliferation inhibitors, and ACE-inhibitors or ARB; Model 2: Model 1 + adjustment for hemoglobin; Model 3: Model 1 + adjustment for ferritin; Model 4: Model 1 + adjustment for hs-CRP; Model 5: Model 1 + adjustment for FGF23. Ferritin, hs-CRP, and FGF23 were naturally log transformed before adding to the Cox regression analysis due to skewed distribution. Abbreviations—ACE, angiotensin-converting enzyme; ARB, angiotensin-receptor blockers; FGF23, fibroblast growth factor 23; CI, confidence interval; eGFR, estimated glomerular filtration rate; HR, hazard ratio; hs-CRP, high-sensitive C-reactive protein.

We identified similar results when subdividing EPO levels into quartiles (Table 3; Figure 1 with Kaplan–Meier curves showing the univariably increased risk of death across EPO quartiles).

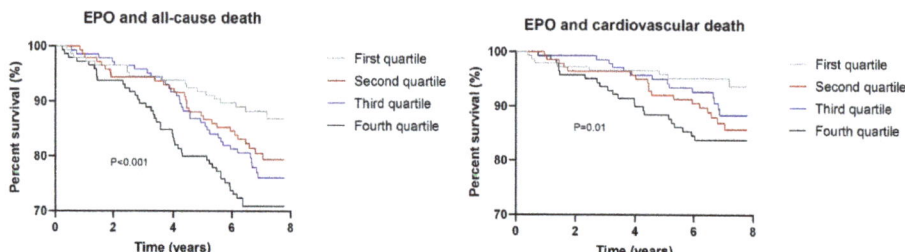

Figure 1. Kaplan–Meier Curves depicting the association between EPO quartiles and risk of all-cause (left panel) and cardiovascular death (right panel). Reported p-values have been calculated with the log-rank test for trend.

Table 3. Association between erythropoietin quartiles and risk of all-cause and cardiovascular death.

	Quartiles of EPO (IU/L)			
	Q1	Q2	Q3	Q4
All–cause death	Ref	HR (95% CI)	HR (95% CI)	HR (95% CI)
Univariable	1.00	1.64 (0.91–2.97)	1.93 (1.08–3.42)	2.62 (1.51–4.55)
Model 1	1.00	1.57 (0.85–2.89)	1.47 (0.81–2.69)	2.11 (1.15–3.86)
Model 2	1.00	1.54 (0.83–2.84)	1.51 (0.83–2.75)	2.19 (1.19–4.05)
Model 3	1.00	1.65 (0.88–3.11)	1.57 (0.84–2.93)	2.29 (1.21–4.31)
Model 4	1.00	1.55 (0.85–2.85)	1.42 (0.78–2.58)	1.99 (1.09–3.65)
Model 5	1.00	1.63 (0.89–3.01)	1.41 (0.77–2.57)	1.55 (0.82–2.91)
Cardiovascular Death	Ref	HR (95% CI)	HR (95% CI)	HR (95% CI)
Univariable	1.00	2.38 (1.04–5.48)	1.85 (0.78–4.40)	3.08 (1.37–6.92)
Model 1	1.00	2.73 (1.15–6.45)	1.69 (0.68–4.18)	3.34 (1.36–8.20)
Model 2	1.00	2.58 (1.08–6.16)	1.71 (0.69–4.25)	3.41 (1.31–8.47)
Model 3	1.00	2.91 (1.17–7.23)	1.77 (0.68–4.59)	3.57 (1.39–9.20)
Model 4	1.00	2.65 (1.12–6.25)	1.60 (0.65–3.95)	3.10 (1.27–7.60)
Model 5	1.00	2.90 (1.22–6.91)	1.65 (0.66–4.08)	2.47 (0.97–6.31)

Model 1: Adjusted for age, sex, body surface area, eGFR, proteinuria, time since transplantation, presence of diabetes, systolic blood pressure, total cholesterol, use of calcineurin inhibitors, proliferation inhibitors, and ACE-inhibitors or ARB. Model 2: Model 1 + adjustment for hemoglobin; Model 3: Model 1 + adjustment for ferritin; Model 4: Model 1 + adjustment for hs-CRP; Model 5: Model 1 + adjustment for FGF23. Ferritin, hs-CRP, and FGF23 were naturally log transformed before adding to the Cox regression analysis due to skewed distribution. Abbreviations—ACE, angiotensin-converting enzyme; ARB, angiotensin-receptor blockers; FGF23, fibroblast growth factor 23; CI, confidence interval; eGFR, estimated glomerular filtration rate; HR, hazard ratio; hs-CRP, high-sensitive C-reactive protein.

In multivariable Cox regression analysis, RTRs in the upper quartile of EPO had a more than two times higher risk of death (HR, 2.11; 95% CI, 1.15–3.86), when compared to RTRs in the lowest quartile, independent of potential confounders. In line with the association between EPO as continuous variable and death, further adjustment for FGF23 levels attenuated the association between the upper EPO quartile and risk of death (HR, 1.55; 95% CI, 0.82–2.91; Table 3; Figure 2A). A full list of HRs for covariates in the multivariable model for EPO divided in quartiles can be found in Supplementary Table S3.

When we assessed the associations between EPO and cardiovascular death, we found similar findings. Higher EPO levels were associated with an increased risk of cardiovascular death in univariable analyses (Figure 1) and in all subsequent models (Table 2). However, the association no longer remained significant, both as a continuous variable and as divided in quartiles, after further adjustment for FGF23 (Tables 2 and 3; Figure 2B).

In contrast, FGF23 levels per se were strongly associated with all-cause death independent of adjustment for potential confounders including EPO (HR per RU/mL, 1.76; 95% CI, 1.33–2.34; $P < 0.001$). Likewise, FGF23 levels per se were also strongly associated with cardiovascular death independent of adjustment for potential confounders including EPO (HR, 1.84; 95% CI, 1.23–2.76; P = 0.003). A full list of HRs for covariates can be found in Supplementary Table S4.

As sensitivity analysis, we assessed the prevalence of different etiologies of CKD in the total cohort and across quartiles of EPO (Supplementary Table S5). The most prevalent etiologies of CKD were primary glomerular disease (28%), polycystic disease (18%), and tubulo-interstitial disease (16%). Following adjustment for etiology of CKD additive to model 1, the association between EPO and all-cause death (HR, 1.57; 95% CI, 1.09–2.26; P = 0.02) and between EPO and cardiovascular death (HR, 1.75; 95% CI, 1.05–2.90; P = 0.03) remained materially unchanged.

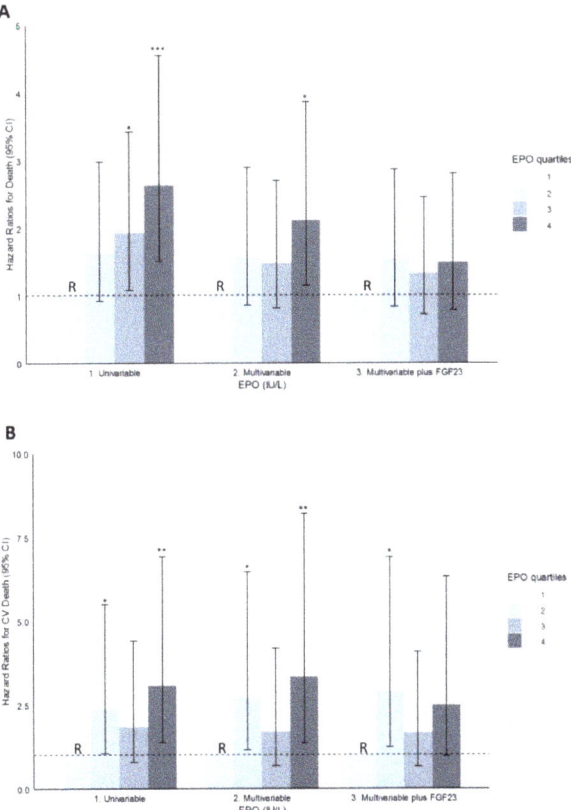

Figure 2. Hazard ratios and corresponding 95% confidence intervals are depicted for risk of death, both all-cause (**A**) and cardiovascular death (**B**), according to quartiles of erythropoietin levels. First, the univariate association is shown. Second, the multivariable adjustment is performed with adjustment for age, sex, body surface area (BSA), eGFR, proteinuria, time since transplantation, presence of diabetes, systolic blood pressure (SBP), total cholesterol, and use of calcineurin inhibitors, proliferation inhibitors, and angiotensin-converting enzyme (ACE)-inhibitors and angiotensin II-receptor blockers (ARBs). Third, adjustment for FGF23 is performed following the multivariable adjustment. The first quartile was chosen as a reference group in all analyses. Significance levels are indicated by numbers of asterisks, i.e., *** <0.001, ** <0.01, * <0.05; Abbreviations—BSA, body surface area; CI, confidence interval; eGFR, estimated glomerular filtration rate.

3.3. EPO, FGF23, and Graft Failure

During a median follow-up of 6.9 (6.1–7.4) years, 46 RTRs developed DCGF. When we assessed the associations between EPO and DCGF, we did not find an association (HR, 0.82; 95% CI, 0.48–1.41; $P = 0.48$). Further adjustment for potential confounders did not ameliorate the association between EPO and DCGF. In contrast, FGF23 levels were univariately associated with DCGF (HR, 3.07; 95% CI, 2.22–4.24; $P < 0.001$). However, after adjustment for potential confounders including EPO, FGF23 was no longer associated with DCGF (HR, 1.57; 95% CI, 0.94–2.64; $P = 0.09$).

3.4. Percentage Change HR and Mediation Analyses

Adjustment for FGF23 caused a large reduction in HR in the Cox Regression analysis in the association between EPO and all-cause and cardiovascular death (58% reduction in HR between EPO and all-cause death; and 48% reduction in HR between EPO and cardiovascular death). In subsequent mediation analyses, we identified that FGF23 was a significant mediator of the association between EPO and all-cause death (P value for indirect effect <0.05; 72% of the association was explained by FGF23; Table 4). Similarly, FGF23 explained 50% of the association between EPO and cardiovascular death (P value for indirect effect <0.05; Table 4).

Table 4. Mediation analysis of FGF23 on the association between EPO and all-cause and cardiovascular death in renal transplant recipients.

Potential Mediator	Outcome	Effect (path) *	Multivariable Model **	
			Coefficient (95% CI, bc) †	Proportion Mediated ***
FGF23	All-cause death	Indirect effect (ab path)	0.090 (0.044; 0.139)	72%
		Total effect (ab + c′ path)	0.124 (−0.011; 0.255)	
		Unstandardized total effect ‡	0.120 (−0.385; 0.624)	
FGF23	Cardiovascular death	Indirect effect (ab path)	0.065 (0.015; 0.122)	50%
		Total effect (ab + c′ path)	0.129 (−0.040; 0.290)	
		Unstandardized total effect ‡	0.218 (−0.405; 0.840)	

* The coefficients of the indirect ab path and the total $ab + c'$ path are standardized for the standard deviations of EPO, FGF23, all-cause and cardiovascular death. **All coefficients are adjusted for age, sex, body surface area, eGFR, proteinuria, time since transplantation, presence of diabetes, systolic blood pressure, total cholesterol, use of calcineurin inhibitors, proliferation inhibitors, ACE-inhibitors or ARB. *** The size of the significant mediated effect is calculated as the standardized indirect effect divided by the standardized total effect multiplied by 100, e.g., 0.090 divided by 0.124 multiplied by 100 constitutes 72% as percentage of mediation ‡ Odds ratios for risk of outcomes can be calculated by taking the exponent of the unstandardized total effect. For example, the unstandardized coefficient of the direct effect of EPO on all-cause death while adjusting for FGF23 is 0.120, which can be calculated to an OR by taking the exponent of this regression coefficient, i.e., $e^{0.120} = 1.12$, which corresponds to the HR of 1.28 (see Table 2). The discrepancy between the ratios is due to taking into account time-to-event with HR in contrast to OR. †95% CIs for the indirect and total effects were bias-corrected confidence intervals after running 2000 bootstrap samples. Abbreviations—ACE, angiotensin converting enzyme; ARB, angiotensin receptor blockers; Bc, bias corrected; CI, confidence interval; eGFR, estimated glomerular filtration rate; FGF23, fibroblast growth factor 23.

4. Discussion

In this study, we show that higher endogenous EPO levels are associated with an increased risk of all-cause and cardiovascular death in RTRs, and that these associations are largely explained by variation in FGF23 levels. This study confirms recent studies about the essential role of EPO in FGF23 physiology in experimental and human models [7–10], extends these findings to RTRs, and support the notion that FGF23 is an important mediator in the association between EPO and risk of death.

EPO, a hormone mainly produced in the kidney in response to hypoxia, is essential for erythropoiesis [29]. EPO controls proliferation, maturation, and also survival of erythroid progenitor cells [30]. Previously, it has been shown that high endogenous EPO levels were associated with an increased risk of all-cause and cardiovascular death in RTRs [2,3]. Similarly, in the setting of CKD and ESRD, correction of anemia with recombinant EPO led an increased risk of cardiovascular morbidity and death [5,6]. The mechanisms responsible for these adverse effects of both endogenous as exogenous EPO are unknown. In the Correction of Hemoglobin and Outcomes in Renal Insufficiency (CHOIR) trial, the highest risk of cardiovascular death was seen in patients with the highest EPO dose, suggesting that EPO resistance through inflammation and/or functional iron deficiency might be a possible link [6]. However, in the current study, the association between endogenous EPO levels and death was independent of adjustment for inflammation as well as independent of iron parameters, renal function, and standard classical cardiovascular risk factors including systolic blood pressure and cholesterol levels. Although there was a difference in prevalence of use of calcineurin and proliferation inhibitors across EPO quartiles, the association between EPO and death remained independent of adjustment for calcineurin and proliferation inhibitors. In contrast, adjustment for FGF23 markedly attenuated the association between EPO and death.

Elevated total FGF23 levels have previously been shown to be associated with increased risk of death in RTRs, as well as in various other patient groups including postoperative acute kidney injury, nondialysis CKD, and ESRD [31–35]. FGF23 regulation is determined by a complex interplay between parathyroid hormone, 1,25-dihydroxyvitamin D, klotho, glucocorticoids, calcium, and phosphate [36,37]. In recent years, iron deficiency has been identified as an important regulator of FGF23 [38–40]. In addition, recent studies demonstrated that EPO stimulates murine and human FGF23 [7,8]. Clinkenbeard and colleagues reported increased FGF23 mRNA expression in vitro, ex vivo, and in vivo due to EPO treatment in UMR-106 cells, in isolated bone marrow cells, and in marrow from mice, respectively [7]. In addition, Rabadi et al. showed in experimental animal models that an acute loss of 10% blood volume led to an increase in total FGF23 and EPO levels within six hours. Furthermore, exogenous administration of EPO resulted in an acute increase in plasma total FGF23 levels similar to those seen in acute blood loss [8]. Similarly, Flamme et al. described in animal models an increase in plasma total FGF23 both after injection of recombinant human EPO and after HIF-proline hydroxylase inhibitor [41]. The present findings in our study underscore these observations and emphasize the important role of EPO in FGF23 physiology. Importantly, the current study is the first to show that prospective associations between EPO and adverse outcomes in RTRs seem to be, at least to large extent, related to increased levels of total FGF23.

The mechanisms through which EPO, as reflection of tissue hypoxia, lead to increased bone marrow FGF23 transcription are currently unknown and require additional investigation. The previously performed studies showed that EPO acutely increases total FGF23 levels out of proportion to intact FGF23 (iFGF23), suggesting an upregulated FGF23 production with concomitantly increased cleavage, with as a result an increase in C-terminal FGF23 fragments. To date, it remains incompletely understood how EPO increases post-translational cleavage. Results from our group and collaborators found previously in EPO-overexpressing mice a decreased GalNT3 bone marrow mRNA expression, without differences in Fam20C or furin expression, implying that a decreased GalNT3 might play a possible role [9]. However, more investigation is imperative to unravel this mechanistic link.

The downstream consequences of elevated levels of FGF23 and the subsequent excess risk of death have not been fully elucidated yet. Several previous reports have shown that iFGF23 has biologic activity through binding to several FGF23 receptors. Besides the well-known functions of iFGF23 in the regulation of renal phosphate handling and vitamin D metabolism, recent studies have shown a myriad "off-target" effects of iFGF23 on the heart and other organs. Preclinical studies demonstrated that FGF23 can lead to left ventricular hypertrophy in cardiac myocytes, and promote endothelial dysfunction [42,43]. In addition, FGF23 stimulates renal fibrosis [44], exerts pro-inflammatory effects [45], and disrupts normal immune function [46]. Most likely, the increased death risk due to elevated levels of FGF23 is attributable to a combination of these effects. Although the biologic activity of iFGF23 has unequivocally been demonstrated, the biologic activity of C-terminal FGF23 fragments remains uncertain. Previously, it has been shown that C-terminal FGF23 may function as an iFGF23 antagonist, by competing with iFGF23 for binding to its receptor, which may reduce phosphaturia and aggravate soft tissue calcification [47]. In addition, Courbabaisse et al. has shown, at least in vitro, that C-terminal FGF23 increases adult rat ventricular cardiomyocyte size by stimulation of FGF receptor

4 in the absence of co-stimulatory factor alpha-klotho, and in sickle cell disease patients that elevated cleaved FGF23 levels were associated with heart hypertrophy [48].

Our study has multiple strengths as well as limitations. The major strength of the current study is the large prospective cohort of stable RTRs with detailed clinical and laboratory data available, including EPO, FGF23, hs-CRP, and ferritin levels. Additionally, no participants were lost to follow-up with respect to the endpoints, despite a considerable follow-up period. Limitations of the current study include that, due to the observational status of our single center study, we cannot exclude the possibility of residual confounding, and conclusions about causality cannot be drawn. Furthermore, we were unable to measure iFGF23 levels, since samples were not stored with protease inhibitors, and iFGF23 has been shown to be susceptible to degradation with long-term storage [49]. This precludes us to discern whether the elevated total FGF23 levels are the result of increased iFGF23 levels or due to an increase in allegedly assumed inactive C-terminal fragments. Another limitation of the study is that we only used CRP levels as inflammatory parameter, other markers of inflammation (e.g., cytokines, cell subtypes) were not available, but could possibly have contributed to the results. In addition, another limitation of current study is the use of single-time measurements hampering the possibility to track the levels of EPO and FGF23 over time with respect to each other and with respect to risk of death. However, it should be realized that most epidemiological studies use a single baseline measurement to investigate associations of variables with outcomes, which adversely affects the strength and significance of the association of these variables with outcomes. If intraindividual variability of variables is taken into account, this results in strengthening of associations that also existed for single measurements of these variables [50,51]. Finally, we want to emphasize that the mediation analyses that we performed are plain straightforward mediation analyses. Although based on literature, we have strong evidence that FGF23 is a mediator in the association of EPO with risk of death, we cannot exclude that an unmeasured cause of mortality or alternative potential mediators has influenced the currently identified results.

In conclusion, we identified that elevated levels of EPO were independently associated with an increased risk of death in RTRs, and that this association was to a large extent explained by variation in FGF23 levels. Further research is needed to fully elucidate the mechanism through which this ensues and to unravel whether the currently identified results can be extrapolated to exogenous EPO in RTRs.

Supplementary Materials: The following are available online at http://www.mdpi.com/2077-0383/9/6/1737/s1, Supplementary Table S1: Univariable associations of variables with prospective outcomes (i.e., all-cause death and cardiovascular death), Supplementary Table S2: Reporting of all hazard ratios of all covariates included in the Cox Regression Analyses for the association between erythropoietin as continuous variable and risk of all-cause and cardiovascular death (according to model 5 [including FGF23]), Supplementary Table S3: Reporting of all hazard ratios of all covariates included in the Cox Regression Analyses for the association between quartiles of erythropoietin and risk of all-cause and cardiovascular death (according to model 5 [including FGF23]), Supplementary Table S4: Reporting of all hazard ratios of all covariates included in the Cox Regression Analyses for the association between FGF23 as continuous variable and risk of all-cause and cardiovascular death (multivariable excluding erythropoietin [Supplementary Table S2 includes erythropoietin]), Supplementary Table S5: Prevalence of the different etiologies of CKD described in the total cohort of 579 RTRs and across the quartiles of erythropoietin levels.

Author Contributions: Conceptualization, M.F.E.; Data curation, M.H.D.B. and S.J.L.B.; Formal analysis, M.F.E., M.A.D.J., D.E.L. and I.M.N.; Investigation, S.J.L.B.; Methodology, M.F.E., M.H.D.B., S.J.L.B. and C.A.J.M.G.; Supervision, S.J.L.B. and C.A.J.M.G.; Visualization, M.F.E.; Writing—original draft, M.F.E.; Writing—review and editing, M.A.D.J., D.E.L., I.M.N., M.H.D.B., S.J.L.B. and C.A.J.M.G. All authors have read and agreed to the published version of the manuscript.

Funding: This research received no external funding

Acknowledgments: The current study was based on TransplantLines Insulin Resistance and Inflammation (TxL-IRI) Cohort Study (NCT03272854).

Conflicts of Interest: The authors declare no conflict of interest.

References

1. Jardine, A.; Gaston, R.S.; Fellström, B.C.; Holdaas, H. Prevention of cardiovascular disease in adult recipients of kidney transplants. *Lancet* **2011**, *378*, 1419–1427. [CrossRef]
2. Sinkeler, S.J.; Zelle, D.M.; van der Heide, J.J.H.; Gans, R.; Navis, G.; Bakker, S.J.L. Endogenous plasma erythropoietin, cardiovascular mortality and all-cause mortality in renal transplant recipients. *Arab. Archaeol. Epigr.* **2011**, *12*, 485–491. [CrossRef] [PubMed]
3. Molnar, M.Z.; Tabak, A.G.; Alam, A.; Czira, M.E.; Rudas, A.; Ujszaszi, A.; Beko, G.; Novak, M.; Kalantar-Zadeh, K.; Kovesdy, C.P.; et al. Serum erythropoietin level and mortality in kidney transplant recipients. *Clin. J. Am. Soc. Nephrol.* **2011**, *6*, 2879–2886. [CrossRef] [PubMed]
4. Den Elzen, W.P.; Willems, J.M.; Westendorp, R.G.; de Craen, A.J.; Blauw, G.J.; Ferrucci, L.; Assendelft, W.J.; Gussekloo, J. Effect of erythropoietin levels on mortality in old age: The leiden 85-plus study. *Can. Med. Assoc. J.* **2010**, *182*, 1953–1958. [CrossRef]
5. Pfeffer, M.A.; Burdmann, E.; Chen, C.-Y.; E Cooper, M.; de Zeeuw, D.; Eckardt, K.-U.; Ivanovich, P.; KewalRamani, R.; Levey, A.S.; Lewis, E.F.; et al. Baseline characteristics in the trial to reduce cardiovascular events with aranesp therapy (TREAT). *Am. J. Kidney Dis.* **2009**, *54*, 59–69. [CrossRef] [PubMed]
6. Singh, A.K.; Szczech, L.; Tang, K.L.; Barnhart, H.; Sapp, S.; Wolfson, M.; Reddan, D.; CHOIR Investigators. Correction of anemia with epoetin alfa in chronic kidney disease. *New Engl. J. Med.* **2006**, *355*, 2085–2098. [CrossRef]
7. Clinkenbeard, E.L.; Hanudel, M.R.; Stayrook, K.R.; Appaiah, H.N.; Farrow, E.G.; Cass, T.A.; Summers, L.J.; Ip, C.S.; Hum, J.M.; Thomas, J.C.; et al. Erythropoietin stimulates murine and human fibroblast growth factor-23, revealing novel roles for bone and bone marrow. *Haematologica* **2017**, *102*, e427–e430. [CrossRef]
8. Rabadi, S.; Udo, I.; Leaf, D.E.; Waikar, S.S.; Christov, M. Acute blood loss stimulates fibroblast growth factor 23 production. *Am. J. Physiol. Ren. Physiol.* **2017**, *314*, F132–F139. [CrossRef]
9. Hanudel, M.R.; Eisenga, M.; Rappaport, M.; Chua, K.; Qiao, B.; Jung, G.; Gabayan, V.; Gales, B.; Ramos, G.; A De Jong, M.; et al. Effects of erythropoietin on fibroblast growth factor 23 in mice and humans. *Nephrol. Dial. Transpl.* **2018**, *34*, 2057–2065. [CrossRef]
10. Toro, L.; Barrientos, V.; León, P.; Rojas, M.; González, M.; González-Ibáñez, A.; Illanes, S.; Sugikawa, K.; Abarzúa, N.; Bascuñán, C.; et al. Erythropoietin induces bone marrow and plasma fibroblast growth factor 23 during acute kidney injury. *Kidney Int.* **2018**, *93*, 1131–1141. [CrossRef]
11. Baia, L.C.; Humalda, J.K.; Vervloet, M.G.; Navis, G.; Bakker, S.J.; De Borst, M.H. Fibroblast growth factor 23 and cardiovascular mortality after kidney transplantation. *Clin. J. Am. Soc. Nephrol.* **2013**, *8*, 1968–1978. [CrossRef] [PubMed]
12. Wolf, M.; Molnar, M.Z.; Amaral, A.P.; Czira, M.E.; Rudas, A.; Ujszaszi, A.; Kiss, I.; Rosivall, L.; Kosa, J.; Lakatos, P.; et al. Elevated fibroblast growth factor 23 is a risk factor for kidney transplant loss and mortality. *J. Am. Soc. Nephrol.* **2011**, *22*, 956–966. [CrossRef]
13. Stockmann, C.; Fandrey, J. Hypoxia-Induced erythropoietin production: A paradigm for oxygen-regulated gene expression. *Clin. Exp. Pharmacol. Physiol.* **2006**, *33*, 968–979. [CrossRef] [PubMed]
14. Ziello, J.E.; Jovin, I.S.; Huang, Y. Hypoxia-Inducible factor (HIF)-1 regulatory pathway and its potential for therapeutic intervention in malignancy and ischemia. *Yale J. Boil. Med.* **2007**, *80*, 51–60.
15. Hamrick, S.E.G.; McQuillen, P.S.; Jiang, X.; Mu, D.; Madan, A.; Ferriero, D.M. A role for hypoxia-inducible factor-1α in desferoxamine neuroprotection. *Neurosci. Lett.* **2005**, *379*, 96–100. [CrossRef] [PubMed]
16. McMahon, S.; Grondin, F.; McDonald, P.P.; Richard, D.E.; Dubois, C.M. Hypoxia-enhanced expression of the proprotein convertase furin is mediated by hypoxia-inducible factor-1: Impact on the bioactivation of proproteins. *J. Biol. Chem.* **2005**, *280*, 6561–6569. [CrossRef] [PubMed]
17. Wolf, M.; White, K.E. Coupling fibroblast growth factor 23 production and cleavage. *Curr. Opin. Nephrol. Hypertens.* **2014**, *23*, 411–419. [CrossRef]
18. Hanudel, M.R.; Wesseling-Perry, K.; Gales, B.; Ramos, G.; Campbell, V.; Ethridge, K.; Scotti, M.; Elashoff, D.A.; Alejos, J.; Reemtsen, B.; et al. Effects of acute kidney injury and chronic hypoxemia on fibroblast growth factor 23 levels in pediatric cardiac surgery patients. *Pediatr. Nephrol.* **2015**, *31*, 661–669. [CrossRef]
19. De Vries, A.; Bakker, S.J.L.; van Son, W.J.; van der Heide, J.J.H.; Ploeg, R.J.; The, H.T.; de Jong, P.E.; Gans, R.O.B. Metabolic syndrome is associated with impaired long-term renal allograft function; Not all component criteria contribute equally. *Arab. Archaeol. Epigr.* **2004**, *4*, 1675–1683. [CrossRef]

20. Benson, E.W.; Hardy, R.; Chaffin, C.; Robinson, C.A.; Konrad, R.J. New automated chemiluminescent assay for erythropoietin. *J. Clin. Lab. Anal.* **2000**, *14*, 271–273. [CrossRef]
21. Heijboer, A.C.; Levitus, M.; Vervloet, M.; Lips, P.; Wee, P.M.T.; Dijstelbloem, H.M.; Blankenstein, M. Determination of fibroblast growth factor 23. *Ann. Clin. Biochem. Int. J. Lab. Med.* **2009**, *46*, 338–340. [CrossRef] [PubMed]
22. Levey, A.S.; Stevens, L.A.; Schmid, C.H.; Zhang, Y.L.; Castro, A.F., 3rd; Feldman, H.I.; Kusek, J.W.; Eggers, P.; Van Lente, F.; Greene, T.; et al. A new equation to estimate glomerular filtration rate. *Ann. Intern. Med.* **2009**, *150*, 604–612. [CrossRef] [PubMed]
23. Arber, D.A.; Orazi, A.; Hasserjian, R.; Thiele, J.; Borowitz, M.J.; Beau, M.M.L.; Bloomfield, C.D.; Cazzola, M.; Vardiman, J.W. The 2016 revision to the World Health Organization classification of myeloid neoplasms and acute leukemia. *Blood* **2016**, *127*, 2391–2405. [CrossRef] [PubMed]
24. Oterdoom, L.H.; de Vries, A.; van Ree, R.M.; Gansevoort, R.T.; van Son, W.J.; van der Heide, J.J.H.; Navis, G.; de Jong, P.E.; Gans, R.O.; Bakker, S.J. N-Terminal Pro-B-Type natriuretic peptide and mortality in renal transplant recipients versus the general population. *Transplantation* **2009**, *87*, 1562–1570. [CrossRef]
25. Preacher, K.J.; Hayes, A.F. SPSS and SAS procedures for estimating indirect effects in simple mediation models. *Behav. Res. Methods Instrum. Comput.* **2004**, *36*, 717–731. [CrossRef]
26. Hayes, A.F. Beyond baron and kenny: Statistical mediation analysis in the new millennium. *Commun. Monogr.* **2009**, *76*, 408–420. [CrossRef]
27. White, I.R.; Wood, A.M.; Royston, P. Multiple imputation using chained equations: Issues and guidance for practice. *Stat. Med.* **2010**, *30*, 377–399. [CrossRef]
28. Rubin, D.B. *Multiple Imputation for Nonresponse in Surveys*; Wiley: New York, NY, USA, 1987.
29. Jelkmann, W. Regulation of erythropoietin production. *J. Physiol.* **2010**, *589*, 1251–1258. [CrossRef]
30. Rossert, J.; Eckardt, K.-U. Erythropoietin receptors: Their role beyond erythropoiesis. *Nephrol. Dial. Transpl.* **2005**, *20*, 1025–1028. [CrossRef]
31. Gutierrez, O.M.; Mannstadt, M.; Isakova, T.; Rauh-Hain, J.A.; Tamez, H.; Shah, A.; Smith, K.; Lee, H.; Thadhani, R.; Jüppner, H.; et al. Fibroblast growth factor 23 and mortality among patients undergoing hemodialysis. *New Engl. J. Med.* **2008**, *359*, 584–592. [CrossRef]
32. Isakova, T.; Xie, H.; Yang, W.; Xie, D.; Anderson, A.H.; Sciallia, J.; Wahl, P.; Gutierrez, O.M.; Steigerwalt, S.; He, J.; et al. Chronic renal insufficiency cohort (CRIC) study group fibroblast growth factor 23 and risks of mortality and end-stage renal disease in patients with chronic kidney disease. *J. Am. Med. Assoc.* **2011**, *305*, 2432–2439. [CrossRef] [PubMed]
33. Leaf, D.E.; Christov, M.; Jüppner, H.; Siew, E.; Ikizler, T.A.; Bian, A.; Chen, G.; Sabbisetti, V.S.; Bonventre, J.V.; Cai, X.; et al. Fibroblast growth factor 23 levels are elevated and associated with severe acute kidney injury and death following cardiac surgery. *Kidney Int.* **2016**, *89*, 939–948. [CrossRef] [PubMed]
34. Kendrick, J.; Cheung, A.K.; Kaufman, J.S.; Greene, T.; Roberts, W.L.; Smits, G.; Chonchol, M.; HOST Investigators. FGF-23 associates with death, cardiovascular events, and initiation of chronic dialysis. *J. Am. Soc. Nephrol.* **2011**, *22*, 1913–1922. [CrossRef] [PubMed]
35. Mendoza, J.M.; Isakova, T.; Cai, X.; Bayes, L.Y.; Faul, C.; Sciallia, J.J.; Lash, J.P.; Chen, J.; He, J.; Navaneethan, S.; et al. CRIC study investigators inflammation and elevated levels of fibroblast growth factor 23 are independent risk factors for death in chronic kidney disease. *Kidney Int.* **2017**, *91*, 711–719. [CrossRef]
36. Nguyen-Yamamoto, L.; Karaplis, A.C.; St-Arnaud, R.; Goltzman, D. Fibroblast growth factor 23 regulation by systemic and local osteoblast-synthesized 1,25-Dihydroxyvitamin D. *J. Am. Soc. Nephrol.* **2016**, *28*, 586–597. [CrossRef]
37. Kovesdy, C.P.; Quarles, L.D. Fibroblast growth factor-23: What we know, what we don't know, and what we need to know. *Nephrol. Dial. Transpl.* **2013**, *28*, 2228–2236. [CrossRef]
38. Eisenga, M.; van Londen, M.; Leaf, D.E.; Nolte, I.M.; Navis, G.; Bakker, S.J.; De Borst, M.H.; Gaillard, C.A. C-Terminal fibroblast growth factor 23, iron deficiency, and mortality in renal transplant recipients. *J. Am. Soc. Nephrol.* **2017**, *28*, 3639–3646. [CrossRef]
39. Wolf, M.; Koch, T.A.; Bregman, D.B. Effects of iron deficiency anemia and its treatment on fibroblast growth factor 23 and phosphate homeostasis in women. *J. Bone Miner. Res.* **2013**, *28*, 1793–1803. [CrossRef]
40. David, V.; Martin, A.; Isakova, T.; Spaulding, C.; Qi, L.; Ramirez, V.; Zumbrennen-Bullough, K.B.; Sun, C.C.; Lin, H.Y.; Babitt, J.L.; et al. Inflammation and functional iron deficiency regulate fibroblast growth factor 23 production. *Kidney Int.* **2016**, *89*, 135–146. [CrossRef]

41. Flamme, I.; Ellinghaus, P.; Urrego, D.; Krüger, T. FGF23 expression in rodents is directly induced via erythropoietin after inhibition of hypoxia inducible factor proline hydroxylase. *PLoS ONE* **2017**, *12*, e0186979. [CrossRef]
42. Silswal, N.; Touchberry, C.; Daniel, D.R.; McCarthy, D.L.; Zhang, S.; Andresen, J.; Stubbs, J.R.; Wacker, M.J. FGF23 directly impairs endothelium-dependent vasorelaxation by increasing superoxide levels and reducing nitric oxide bioavailability. *Am. J. Physiol. Metab.* **2014**, *307*, E426–E436. [CrossRef]
43. Faul, C.; Amaral, A.P.; Oskouei, B.; Hu, M.-C.; Sloan, A.; Isakova, T.; Gutierrez, O.M.; Aguillon-Prada, R.; Lincoln, J.; Hare, J.M.; et al. FGF23 induces left ventricular hypertrophy. *J. Clin. Investig.* **2011**, *121*, 4393–4408. [CrossRef]
44. Smith, E.R.; Tan, S.-J.; Holt, S.G.; Hewitson, T. FGF23 is synthesised locally by renal tubules and activates injury-primed fibroblasts. *Sci. Rep.* **2017**, *7*, 3345. [CrossRef] [PubMed]
45. Singh, S.; Grabner, A.; Yanucil, C.; Schramm, K.; Czaya, B.; Krick, S.; Czaja, M.J.; Bartz, R.; Abraham, R.; Marco, G.S.D.; et al. Fibroblast growth factor 23 directly targets hepatocytes to promote inflammation in chronic kidney disease. *Kidney Int.* **2016**, *90*, 985–996. [CrossRef] [PubMed]
46. Rossaint, J.; Oehmichen, J.; van Aken, H.; Reuter, S.; Pavenstädt, H.J.; Meersch, M.; Unruh, M.L.; Zarbock, A. FGF23 signaling impairs neutrophil recruitment and host defense during CKD. *J. Clin. Investig.* **2016**, *126*, 962–974. [CrossRef] [PubMed]
47. Goetz, R.; Nakada, Y.; Hu, M.C.; Kurosu, H.; Wang, L.; Nakatani, T.; Shi, M.; Eliseenkova, A.V.; Razzaque, M.S.; Moe, O.W.; et al. Isolated C-terminal tail of FGF23 alleviates hypophosphatemia by inhibiting FGF23-FGFR-Klotho complex formation. *Proc. Natl. Acad. Sci. USA* **2009**, *107*, 407–412. [CrossRef]
48. Courbebaisse, M.; Mehel, H.; Petit-Hoang, C.; Ribeil, J.-A.; Sabbah, L.; Tuloup-Minguez, V.; Bergerat, D.; Arlet, J.-B.; Stanislas, A.; Souberbielle, J.-C.; et al. Carboxy-terminal fragment of fibroblast growth factor 23 induces heart hypertrophy in sickle cell disease. *Haematologica* **2016**, *102*, e33–e35. [CrossRef]
49. El-Maouche, D.; Dumitrescu, C.E.; Andreopoulou, P.; Gafni, R.I.; Brillante, B.A.; Bhattacharyya, N.; Fedarko, N.S.; Collins, M.T. Stability and degradation of fibroblast growth factor 23 (FGF23): The effect of time and temperature and assay type. *Osteoporos. Int.* **2016**, *27*, 2345–2353. [CrossRef]
50. Koenig, W.; Sund, M.; Fröhlich, M.; Löwel, H.; Hutchinson, W.L.; Pepys, M.B. Refinement of the association of serum C-reactive protein concentration and coronary heart disease risk by correction for within-subject variation over time: The MONICA Augsburg studies, 1984 and 1987. *Am. J. Epidemiol.* **2003**, *158*, 357–364. [CrossRef]
51. Danesh, J.; Wheeler, J.G.; Hirschfield, G.; Eda, S.; Eiriksdottir, G.; Rumley, A.; Lowe, G.; Pepys, M.B.; Gudnason, V. C-Reactive protein and other circulating markers of inflammation in the prediction of coronary heart disease. *New Engl. J. Med.* **2004**, *350*, 1387–1397. [CrossRef] [PubMed]

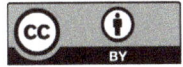

© 2020 by the authors. Licensee MDPI, Basel, Switzerland. This article is an open access article distributed under the terms and conditions of the Creative Commons Attribution (CC BY) license (http://creativecommons.org/licenses/by/4.0/).

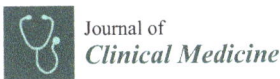

Article

Weekend Effect and in-Hospital Mortality in Elderly Patients with Acute Kidney Injury: A Retrospective Analysis of a National Hospital Database in Italy

Fabio Fabbian [1,2,*], Alfredo De Giorgi [1], Emanuele Di Simone [1], Rosaria Cappadona [2], Nicola Lamberti [3], Fabio Manfredini [3,4], Benedetta Boari [1], Alda Storari [5] and Roberto Manfredini [1,2]

1. Clinica Medica Unit, Azienda Ospedaliero-Universitaria, I-44121 Ferrara, Italy; degiorgialfredo@libero.it (A.D.G.); emanuele.disimone@uniroma1.it (E.D.S.); benedetta.boari@unife.it (B.B.); roberto.manfredini@unife.it (R.M.)
2. Department of Medical Sciences, University of Ferrara, I-44121 Ferrara, Italy; rosaria.cappadona@unife.it
3. Department of Biomedical and Specialty Surgical Sciences, University of Ferrara, I-44121 Ferrara, Italy; nicola.lamberti@unife.it (N.L.); fabio.manfredini@unife.it (F.M.)
4. Neuroscience and Rehabilitation Department, Azienda Ospedaliero-Universitaria, I-44121 Ferrara, Italy
5. Nephrology and Dialysis Unit, Azienda Ospedaliero-Universitaria, I-44121 Ferrara, Italy; a.storari@ospfe.it
* Correspondence: f.fabbian@ospfe.it; Tel.: +39-053-223-7071

Received: 7 May 2020; Accepted: 9 June 2020; Published: 11 June 2020

Abstract: Background: The aim of this study was to relate the weekend (WE) effect and acute kidney injury (AKI) in elderly patients by using the Italian National Hospital Database (NHD). Methods: Hospitalizations with AKI of subjects aged ≥ 65 years from 2000–2015 who were identified by the ICD-9-CM were included. Admissions from Friday to Sunday were considered as WE, while all the other days were weekdays (WD). In-hospital mortality (IHM) was our outcome, and the comorbidity burden was calculated by the modified Elixhauser Index (mEI), based on ICD-9-CM codes. Results: 760,664 hospitalizations were analyzed. Mean age was 80.5 ± 7.8 years and 52.2% were males. Of the studied patients, 9% underwent dialysis treatment, 24.3% were admitted during WE, and IHM was 27.7%. Deceased patients were more frequently comorbid males, with higher age, treated with dialysis more frequently, and had higher admission during WE. WE hospitalizations were more frequent in males, and in older patients with higher mEI. IHM was independently associated with dialysis-dependent AKI (OR 2.711; 95%CI 2.667–2.755, $p < 0.001$), WE admission (OR 1.113; 95%CI 1.100–1.126, $p < 0.001$), and mEI (OR 1.056; 95% CI 1.055–1.057, $p < 0.001$). Discussion: Italian elderly patients admitted during WE with AKI are exposed to a higher risk of IHM, especially if they need dialysis treatment and have high comorbidity burden.

Keywords: acute kidney injury; weekend effect; in-hospital mortality; comorbidity; dialysis; elderly

1. Introduction

The negative clinical impact of the so-called weekend (WE) effect has been a matter of debate since the past two decades. Different research groups have reported poorer outcomes for patients admitted on WE compared to weekdays (WD). A milestone study published in 2001, conducted on almost 4 million acute care admissions from emergency departments in Ontario, Canada, found that patients with some serious medical conditions had higher in-hospital mortality (IHM) if they were admitted on a WE than on a WD [1]. A few years later, Cram et al. confirmed a modest increase in mortality after WE admission for all admissions, either unscheduled or emergency department admissions [2]. Our group also documented a higher IHM for some cardiovascular events, such as acute heart failure (OR 1.33) [3], and acute pulmonary embolism (OR 1.18) [4]. A systematic review evaluated 97 studies enrolling more than 51 million subjects, and patients admitted on WE had a significantly higher overall mortality, independent of factors including the levels of staffing, procedure rates and delays, and illness severity [5]. Another systematic review and meta-analysis focused on United Kingdom (UK) hospitals confirmed that WE admissions had higher odds of mortality than those admitted during WD, as well as when measures of case mix severity were included in the models. On the other hand, the WE effect was not significant when clinical registry data was used [6]. Finally, Chen et al. performed a large meta-analysis (68 studies, 640 million admissions), and found that risk of mortality during all WE admissions was 1.16, although it was greater for elective admissions than emergency ones [7]. A first consideration is that differences in hospital care associated with the day of the week (measured by indicators including short term mortality) can vary depending on the place, time, and reason for hospital admission [8]. On one hand, medical and nursing understaffing, shortage of diagnostic or procedural services, and the presence of inexperienced residents have been suggested as possible causes [9]. On the other, temporal aspects of onset of acute vascular diseases may also play a role, and it is possible that these diseases do not present with equal severity relative to time, that is, day of the week or hour of the day [10,11]. A single-center study on acute coronary syndromes (ACSs) showed that although there were fewer ACS admissions than expected on nights and WE, the proportion of patients with ACS presenting with ST-elevation myocardial infarctions was 64% higher on WE [12]. Again, in their large study on pulmonary embolism admissions, Nanchal et al. reported a 19% increase in patients admitted on WE [13], but WE admissions showed significantly worse parameters of severity, such as the need for mechanical ventilation, thrombolytic therapy use, and the use of vasopressors. A further confirmation to this hypothesis comes from the results of a study conducted on more than 500,000 unselected emergency admissions in the UK, evaluating and adjusting for multiple confounders including demographics, comorbidities, and admission characteristics, and common hematology and biochemistry test results. Hospital workload was not associated with mortality, suggesting that the WE effect could be associated with patient-level differences at admission rather than reduced hospital staffing or services [14]. Therefore, the debate about clinical impact of the WE effect is still open. Acute kidney injury (AKI) is a frequent finding in hospitalized subjects, especially in people who are 65 years old or older [15–17]. However, available data about admissions due to renal diseases are scarce; therefore, we wanted to explore the possible relationship between the WE effect and AK by using the National Hospital Database (NHD).

2. Experimental Section

2.1. Patient Selection and Eligibility

This retrospective study was conducted in agreement with the Declaration of Helsinki of 1975, revised in 2013. Subject identifiers were deleted before data analysis with the aim of maintaining data anonymity and confidentiality; therefore, none of the patients could be identified, either in this paper or in the database. The study was conducted in agreement with the existent Italian disposition-by-law (G.U. n.76, 31 March 2008), and due to the study design, ethics committee approval was not necessary.

We accessed the National Hospital Database (NHD), provided by the Italian Ministry of Health (SDO Database, Ministry of Health, General Directorate for Health Planning), selecting all hospitalizations complicated by AKI between 1 January 2000, and 31 December 2015. This database stores data of all hospitalizations both in public and private Italian hospitals. Based on the International Classification of Diseases, 9th Revision, Clinical Modification (ICD-9-CM), the hospital discharge record files contain information such as gender, age, date and department of admission and discharge, vital status at discharge (in-hospital death vs. discharged alive), main diagnosis, up to five co-morbidities, and up to six procedures/interventions. For this analysis, patients' names and all other potential identifiers were removed by the Ministry of Health from the database, following the national disposition-by-law in terms of privacy. A consecutive number for each patient was the only identifier. Although in clinical settings the term AKI has replaced the term acute renal failure, in administrative database codes the latter term is usually the reference term. We selected patients aged ≥65 years in whom the ICD-9-CM code 584.xx identified AKI when used as a first or second discharge diagnosis. As for a temporal definition, midnight Friday to midnight Sunday was considered as WE, while all the other days were assumed as WD. The nine main national festive days in Italy (1 January, 25 April, 1 May, 2 June, 15 August, 2 November, 8 December, 25 December, and 26 December), when occurring on WD, were considered as WE.

2.2. Data Analysis

In-hospital mortality (IHM) was the hard clinical outcome indicator. In order to evaluate the comorbidity burden, a novel score from our group, a modified Elixhauser Index (mEI) [18], was calculated based on the guidelines set by Quan et al [19]. To calculate the score, the following conditions were considered: age, gender, presence of chronic kidney disease (CKD), neurological disorders, lymphoma, solid tumor with metastasis, ischemic heart disease, congestive heart disease, coagulopathy, fluid and electrolyte disorders, liver disease, weight loss, and metastatic cancer. The original score was corrected, removing the diagnosis of previous AKI; therefore, the points assigned to renal diseases were considered only if CKD was recorded. The points for each condition ranged from 0 to 16, and the total score calculated could vary between 0 and 89. When the score was >40, the risk of IHM was >60%. The score, based on administrative data, was calculated automatically. Table 1 reports single items and relative score. Finally, dialysis treatment was also taken into consideration (code ICD-9-CM 39.95).

Table 1. Items and relative assigned score to calculate in-hospital mortality (IHM).

Items	Score
Age 0–60 (years)	0
Age 61–70 (years)	3
Age 71–80 (years)	7
Age 81–90 (years)	11
Age 91+ (years)	16
Chronic kidney disease	1
Male gender	2
Neurological disorders	3
Lymphoma	4
Solid tumor without metastasis	4
Ischemic heart disease	5
Congestive heart failure	5
Coagulopathy	8
Fluid and electrolyte disorders	8
Liver disease	10
Cachexia	11
Metastatic cancer	12

2.3. Statistical Analysis

A descriptive analysis of the whole population, i.e., absolute numbers, percentages, and means ± SD, was performed. Univariate analysis was carried out by using the Chi-Squared test, Student t-tests, Mann–Whitney U-test, and ANOVA as appropriate, comparing survivors and deceased subjects, and AKI patients admitted during the WE or WD. Moreover, in order to evaluate the relationship between the WE effect and IHM, the latter was considered as the dependent variable in a logistic regression analysis, while demography, comorbidity score, and dialysis-dependent AKI were considered as independent variables. Odds ratios (ORs) with their 95% confidence intervals (95% CI) were reported. All p-values were 2-tailed, and p-value <0.5 was considered significant. SPSS 13.0 for Windows (SPSS IN., Chicago, IL, USA, 2004) was used for statistical analysis.

3. Results

The total sample consisted of 760,664 hospitalizations due to AKI, 52.2% were men, with a mean age of 80.5 ± 7.8 years, and 9% underwent dialysis treatment. Of these patients, 24.3% were admitted during WE and 27.7% died during hospitalization (Table 2).

Table 2. Demographic features of the considered sample (AKI: acute kidney injury, WE: weekend effect).

Total Number of Records	760,664
Men (n (%))	397,174 (52.2)
Women (n (%))	361,490 (47.8)
Age (years)	80.5 ± 7.8
Comorbidity score	14.57 ± 6.21
Dialysis dependent AKI (n (%))	68,563 (9)
Patients admitted during WE (n (%))	184,727 (24.3)
Deceased subjects (n (%))	210,661 (27.7)

IHM was significantly higher in men (51.8% vs. 48.2%, $p < 0.001$). Deceased subjects were more likely to be older (81.9 ± 7.9 vs. 80 ± 7.7 years, $p < 0.001$), to have higher comorbidity score (15.96 ± 6.48 vs. 14.04 ± 6.02, $p < 0.001$), to be treated with dialysis (17.7% vs. 6.8%, $p < 0.001$), and to show higher admission during WE (25.8% vs. 23.7%, $p < 0.001$), compared to survivors (Table 3).

Table 3. Comparison between survivors and deceased subjects.

	Survivors n = 550,003	Deceased n = 210,661	p
Men (n (%))	288,120 (52.4)	109,054 (51.8)	<0.001
Women (n (%))	261,883 (47.6)	101,607 (48.2)	
Age (years)	80 ± 7.7	81.9 ± 7.9	<0.001
Comorbidity score	14.04 ± 6.02	15.96 ± 6.48	<0.001
Dialysis dependent AKI (n (%))	37,598 (6.8)	31,055 (17.7)	<0.001
Patients admitted during WE (n (%))	130,318 (23.7)	54,409 (25.8)	<0.001

Patients admitted during WE were more likely to be male (51.5% vs. 48.5%, $p < 0.001$), older (mean age 81 ± 7.8 vs. 80.4 ± 7.8 years, $p < 0.001$), and had a higher comorbidity score (14.75 ± 6.2 vs. 14.52 ± 6.22, $p < 0.001$). No difference was found for prevalence of dialysis dependent AKI (Table 4).

Table 4. Comparison between subjects admitted during weekdays (WD) or weekends (WE).

	WD Admissions n = 575,937	WE Admissions n = 184,727	p
Men (n (%))	302,010 (52.4)	95,164 (51.5)	<0.001
Women (n (%))	273,927 (47.6)	89,563 (48.5)	
Age (years)	80.4 ± 7.8	81 ± 7.8	<0.001
Dialysis dependent AKI (n (%))	52,075 (9)	16,578 (9)	NS
Comorbidity score	14.52 ± 6.22	14.75 ± 6.2	<0.001

NS: non-significant.

At the logistic regression analysis, IHM was independently associated, in decreasing order, with dialysis-dependent AKI, WE admission, and comorbidity score (Table 5). As for the comorbidity score, the risk of death raised of 5.6% for every 1-point increase.

Table 5. Logistic regression analysis showing factors independently associated with in-hospital mortality. OR: Odds Ratio; 95%CI: 95% confidence intervals; WE: weekend.

	OR	95% Confidence Intervals	p
Dialysis dependent AKI	2.711	2.667–2.755	<0.001
WE admission	1.113	1.100–1.126	<0.001
Comorbidity score	1.056	1.055–1.057	<0.001

4. Discussion

In this study, based on a large national database of hospitalizations, the day of admission had a significant clinical impact on elderly subjects with AKI. The WE effect was independently associated with IHM, along with dialysis treatment and comorbidity burden. The OR for IHM was 1.113, and this finding confirmed previous results from our group, also drawn by analysis of the NHD records, regarding pulmonary embolism (OR 1.15) [20], and acute aortic dissection or rupture (OR 1.34) [21]. The importance of a diverse level of emergency has been underlined by previous studies. Concha et al. studied the 7-day post-admission time patterns of excess mortality following WE admission to investigate whether the phenomenon could be due to poorer quality of care or a case selection. After evaluation of mortality risk for WE and WD, adjusting for age, sex, Charlson Comorbidity Index (CCI), and diagnostic group, they found that WE mortality was diverse for different diagnostic groups, and concluded that the WE effect is probably not a uniform phenomenon, but rather a complex cluster of different causal pathways, even associated with quite different risk profiles [22]. Similar results were reported by Roberts et al., who evaluated 30-day mortality for WE admissions in England and Wales. The WE effect was more evident for disorders with high mortality during the acute phase, and negligible for less acute ones [23].

Moreover, the presence of comorbidities plays a primary role in determining IHM. In the present study, in fact, the OR of comorbidity score is lower than that of presence of dialysis and age, but the risk of death raised of 4.2% for every 1-point increase. In a previous study conducted by our group, we showed that CCI was significantly higher in subjects admitted during WE, and significantly contributed to clinical outcome, along with gender and age. In logistic regression analysis, in fact, admission on WE, CCI, male sex, and age were significantly associated with IHM [24].

To the best of our knowledge, this is the first study considering the relationship between the WE effect and IHM in elderly patients hospitalized because of AKI. The question of whether the WE effect also exists in renal diseases is still matter of debate, because the number of available studies is limited, and results are not univocal. We are aware of only three studies considered the relationship between WE admission and AKI, conducted in the United States (USA), United Kingdom (UK), and Wales, respectively. James et al. analyzed data from the U.S. Nationwide Inpatient Sample and selected more than 200,000 admissions reporting AKI as the primary diagnosis. The prevalence of WE admission was 21% and WE hospitalizations were independently associated with IHM [25]. Kolhe et al. conducted a study on more than 53,000 dialysis-dependent AKI patients. The prevalence of WE admission was 23%, and WE admissions were significantly associated with higher mortality in the unadjusted model, but not in the multivariable analysis [26]. Finally, Holmes et al. did not find any WE effect for mortality associated with hospital-acquired AKI [27]. None of these studies, however, included comorbidity analysis.

A higher interest in the WE effect has been shown to investigate possible negative outcomes in renal transplantation, but results have not demonstrated any negative outcome thus far. In the U.S., Baid-Agrawal et al. did not confirm the hypothesis that kidney transplants performed during WE could have worse outcomes than those performed during WD. In fact, the day of surgery did not affect death, length of hospitalization after transplantation, delayed allograft function, acute rejection within the first year of transplant, and patient and allograft survival at 1 month and at 1 year after transplantation [28]. In Germany, Schütte-Nütgen et al. found no differences between subjects transplanted on WD or WE in terms of 3-year patient and graft survival, frequencies of delayed graft function, acute rejections, 1-year estimated glomerular filtration rate, and length of hospital stay [29]. Again, in England, Anderson et al. did not confirm the relationship between WE and mortality, rehospitalization, and kidney allograft failure/rejection [30]. Moreover, a study of the Australia and New Zealand Dialysis and Transplant registry concluded that timing of transplantation did not impact on allograft outcome [31]. Also, our group tested this hypothesis on all cases of the Emilia-Romagna region, but did not find any risk of adverse outcome related to the WE effect, observing only that WE admissions were characterized by longer duration of hospitalization [32].

On the other hand, WE admission seems to negatively influence outcomes in dialysis patients, although the available evidence is strictly limited to a couple of studies. In the U.S., Sakhuja et al. reported that WE admissions were more likely to have higher IHM, higher mortality during the first 3 days of admission, longer hospital stays, and less likely to be discharged to home. Moreover, time to death was shorter compared with WD admissions [33]. Finally, data from the Australia and New Zealand Dialysis and Transplant Registry reported higher rates of hospitalization secondary to peritonitis on WE compared to WD [34].

In our present study, dialysis-dependent AKI and the WE effect were independently associated with IHM; it could be that the two factors negatively impact patients' survival and complications.

Limitations

We are aware that a major limitation is introduced by the study design: retrospective, based on administrative data, and with no possibility to assess whether AKI was cause or complication of hospitalization. We observed that day-of-week of hospital admission has a significant impact on outcome, but we cannot extrapolate from the administrative database some important items, such as cause of admission and death, intensive care level or hospitals' facilities, device use, type of treatment, and impact of clinical or biochemical parameters. It is known that administrative databases, born to be used for other reasons (i.e., reimbursement), lack specific clinical information and may cause possible misclassification of outcomes, thereby generating confounding factors [35]. Moreover, we did not identify AKI on the basis of international Kidney Disease Improving Global Outcomes (KDIGO) guidelines [36], nor differentiate patients on the basis of the cause of AKI and the treatment setting, with the exception of dialysis treatment.

We previously stated that medical and nursing understaffing, shortage of diagnostic or procedural services, and the presence of inexperienced residents could be related to WE effect [9]. Unfortunately, administrative databases do not allow us investigate these aspects, being conceived for financial reasons.

Some years ago, concerns about WE effect were raised due to three main potential limitations of administrative databases: (1) coding mistakes, (2) insufficient consideration of comorbidity, and (3) failure to consider the severity or acuity of patients [37]. According to several authors, the performance of ICD-9-CM for diagnosis of acute renal failure showed poor sensitivity, and high specificity, while positive and negative predictive value could differ [38–41]. However, Grams et al. underlined that sensitivity was significantly higher when the selected individuals were aged ≥ 65 years; moreover, AKI diagnosed by administrative data detected more severe disease and higher IHM mortality [41]. Due to this reason, we decided to focus on patients aged > 65 years. Finally, we also have to underline some strengths of our study: (1) a high number of records derived from a national database, (2) the long period of time analyzed, and (3) the utilization of a hard outcome indicator, such as IHM.

5. Conclusions

The global population is ageing, and the prevalence of elderly subjects is increasing. Older adults are projected to increase enormously by 2050, rising to more than 400 million [42]. Chronic illnesses and disability causing hospitalization are frequent in the last decades of life and AKI is a frequent cause of morbidity and mortality as shown by the U.S. Renal Data Services (USRDS) 2018 [43]. The latter data demonstrated an increasing incidence rate of AKI over the past several years, in the elderly population.

Patients over the age of 65 who required dialysis continued to have substantially higher mortality compared to general population [43]. Last year, our group demonstrated that in-hospital mortality was a frequent complication in elderly subjects with AKI discharge codes, involving more than a quarter of admissions. The increasing burden of comorbidity, dialysis-dependent AKI, and sepsis were the major risk factors for mortality [16]. Comorbidity is a well-known risk factor affecting survival in dialysis patients [44]; however, predictors of short-term survival in renal patients are still a matter of debate.

Multi-morbidity is crucial for defining the prognosis of the aged population [45], and our findings suggest that pre-existing diseases diagnosed prior to admission may be associated with the outcome of an acute condition such as AKI (especially if AKI needs dialysis treatment). In elderly hospitalized subjects with AKI, WE effect seems to be a risk factor for IHM, even adjusting for comorbidity and advanced AKI stage. Thus, elderly patients admitted on Saturday or Sunday should deserve careful attention and evaluation, and consideration should be taken of their higher risk of IHM.

Author Contributions: Conceptualization, A.D.G., F.F., and R.M..; methodology, F.F, A.D.G., E.D.S., N.L. and F.M.; software, A.D.G., and E.D.S.; validation, E.D.S., N.L., F.M, and A.S.; formal analysis, F.F., A.D.G., N.L., and F.M.; investigation, E.D.S., B.B.; and A.S.; resources, R.C., A.S., and R.M.; data curation, A.D.G., E.D.S., R.C., N.L., and F.M.; writing—original draft preparation, F.F., and B.B.; writing—review and editing, F.F., and R.M.; visualization, A.D.G., R.C., and B.B.; supervision, F.F., B.B., A.S., and R.M.; project administration, R.C., B.B., and R.M; funding acquisition, F.F., and R.M. All authors have read and agreed to the published version of the manuscript.

Funding: This work has been supported, in part, by a research grant from the University of Ferrara (Fondo Ateneo Ricerca—FAR 2019, Fabio Fabbian).

Acknowledgments: We thank Massimo Gallerani, head of Medical Department, Azienda Ospedaliero-Universitaria "S.Anna", Ferrara, Italy, for precious help in obtaining data from the Italian Ministry of Health.

Conflicts of Interest: The authors declare no conflict of interest. The funders had no role in the design of the study; in the collection, analyses, or interpretation of data; in the writing of the manuscript, or in the decision to publish the results.

References

1. Bell, C.M.; Redelmeier, D.A. Mortality among Patients Admitted to Hospitals on Weekends as Compared with Weekdays. *N. Engl. J. Med.* **2001**, *345*, 663–668. [CrossRef] [PubMed]
2. Cram, P.; Hillis, S.L.; Barnett, M.; E Rosenthal, G. Effects of weekend admission and hospital teaching status on in-hospital mortality. *Am. J. Med.* **2004**, *117*, 151–157. [CrossRef] [PubMed]
3. Gallerani, M.; Boari, B.; Manfredini, F.; Mari, E.; Maraldi, C.; Manfredini, R. Weekend versus weekday hospital admissions for acute heart failure. *Int. J. Cardiol.* **2011**, *146*, 444–447. [CrossRef] [PubMed]
4. Imberti, D.; Ageno, W.; Dentali, F.; Manfredini, R.; Gallerani, M. Higher mortality rate in patients hospitalised for acute pulmonary embolism during weekends. *Thromb. Haemost.* **2011**, *106*, 83–89. [CrossRef] [PubMed]
5. Pauls, L.; Johnson-Paben, R.; Mcgready, J.; Murphy, J.; Pronovost, P.J.; Wu, C. The Weekend Effect in Hospitalized Patients: A Meta-Analysis. *J. Hosp. Med.* **2017**, *12*, 760–766. [CrossRef] [PubMed]
6. Honeyford, K.; Cecil, E.; Lo, M.; Bottle, A.; Aylin, P. The weekend effect: Does hospital mortality differ by day of the week? A systematic review and meta-analysis. *BMC Heal. Serv. Res.* **2018**, *18*, 870. [CrossRef]
7. Chen, Y.-F.; Armoiry, X.; Higenbottam, C.; Cowley, N.; Basra, R.; Watson, S.I.; Tarrant, C.; Boyal, A.; Sutton, E.; Wu, C.-W.; et al. Magnitude and modifiers of the weekend effect in hospital admissions: A systematic review and meta-analysis. *BMJ Open* **2019**, *9*, e025764. [CrossRef] [PubMed]
8. Fedeli, U.; Gallerani, M.; Manfredini, R. Factors Contributing to the Weekend Effect. *JAMA* **2017**, *317*, 1582. [CrossRef] [PubMed]
9. Kostis, W.J.; Demissie, K.; Marcella, S.W.; Shao, Y.-H.; Wilson, A.C.; E Moreyra, A. Weekend versus Weekday Admission and Mortality from Myocardial Infarction. *N. Engl. J. Med.* **2007**, *356*, 1099–1109. [CrossRef] [PubMed]
10. Manfredini, R.; Salmi, R.; Gallerani, M. Weekend effect for pulmonary embolism and other acute cardiovascular diseases. *Chest* **2013**, *143*, 275–276. [CrossRef]
11. Manfredini, R.; Manfredini, F.; Salmi, R.; Gallerani, M. Weekend admissions and increased risk for mortality: Less urgent treatments only? *JAMA Neurol.* **2013**, *70*, 131–132. [CrossRef] [PubMed]

12. LaBounty, T.; Eagle, K.A.; Manfredini, R.; Fang, J.; Tsai, T.; Smith, D.; Rubenfire, M. The impact of time and day on the presentation of acute coronary syndromes. *Clin. Cardiol.* **2006**, *29*, 542–546. [CrossRef] [PubMed]
13. Nanchal, R.; Kumar, G.; Taneja, A.; Patel, J.; Deshmukh, A.; Tarima, S.; Jacobs, E.R.; Whittle, J. From the Milwaukee Initiative in Critical Care Outcomes Research (MICCOR) Group of Investigators Pulmonary embolism: The weekend effect. *Chest* **2012**, *142*, 690–696. [CrossRef] [PubMed]
14. Walker, A.S.; Mason, A.M.; Quan, T.P.; Fawcett, N.J.; Watkinson, P.; Llewelyn, M.J.; Stoesser, N.; Finney, J.; Davies, J.; Wyllie, D.H.; et al. Mortality risks associated with emergency admissions during weekends and public holidays: An analysis of electronic health records. *Lancet* **2017**, *390*, 62–72. [CrossRef]
15. Gameiro, J.; Fonseca, J.A.; Jorge, S.; Lopes, J.A. Acute Kidney Injury Definition and Diagnosis: A Narrative Review. *J. Clin. Med.* **2018**, *7*, 307. [CrossRef]
16. Fabbian, F.; Savriè, C.; De Giorgi, A.; Cappadona, R.; Simone, D.; Boari, B.; Storari, A.; Gallerani, M.; Manfredini, R.; De Giorgi, A.; et al. Acute Kidney Injury and In-Hospital Mortality: A Retrospective Analysis of a Nationwide Administrative Database of Elderly Subjects in Italy. *J. Clin. Med.* **2019**, *8*, 1371. [CrossRef]
17. Thongprayoon, C.; Hansrivijit, P.; Kovvuru, K.; Kanduri, S.R.; Torres-Ortiz, A.; Acharya, P.; Gonzalez-Suarez, M.L.; Kaewput, W.; Bathini, T.; Cheungpasitporn, W. Diagnostics, Risk Factors, Treatment and Outcomes of Acute Kidney Injury in a New Paradigm. *J. Clin. Med.* **2020**, *9*, 1104. [CrossRef]
18. Fabbian, F.; De Giorgi, A.; Maietti, E.; Gallerani, M.; Pala, M.; Cappadona, R.; Manfredini, R.; Fedeli, U. A modified Elixhauser score for predicting in-hospital mortality in internal medicine admissions. *Eur. J. Intern. Med.* **2017**, *40*, 37–42. [CrossRef]
19. Quan, H.; Sundararajan, V.; Halfon, P.; Fong, A.; Burnand, B.; Luthi, J.-C.; Saunders, L.D.; Beck, C.A.; Feasby, T.E.; Ghali, W.A. Coding Algorithms for Defining Comorbidities in ICD-9-CM and ICD-10 Administrative Data. *Med Care* **2005**, *43*, 1130–1139. [CrossRef]
20. Gallerani, M.; Fedeli, U.; Pala, M.; De Giorgi, A.; Fabbian, F.; Manfredini, R. Weekend Versus Weekday Admission and In-Hospital Mortality for Pulmonary Embolism: A 14-Year Retrospective Study on the National Hospital Database of Italy. *Angiology* **2017**, *69*, 236–241. [CrossRef]
21. Gallerani, M.; Volpato, S.; Boari, B.; Pala, M.; De Giorgi, A.; Fabbian, F.; Gasbarro, V.; Bossone, E.; Eagle, K.; Carle, F.; et al. Outcomes of weekend versus weekday admission for acute aortic dissection or rupture: A retrospective study on the Italian National Hospital Database. *Int. J. Cardiol.* **2013**, *168*, 3117–3119. [CrossRef] [PubMed]
22. Concha, O.P.; Gallego, B.; Hillman, K.; Delaney, G.P.; Coiera, E. Do variations in hospital mortality patterns after weekend admission reflect reduced quality of care or different patient cohorts? A population-based study. *BMJ Qual. Saf.* **2013**, *23*, 215–222. [CrossRef] [PubMed]
23. Roberts, E.S.; Thorne, K.; Akbari, A.; Samuel, D.G.; Williams, J.G. Weekend emergency admissions and mortality in England and Wales. *Lancet* **2015**, *385*, 1829. [CrossRef]
24. De Giorgi, A.; Fabbian, F.; Tiseo, R.; Misurati, E.; Boari, B.; Zucchi, B.; Signani, F.; Salmi, R.; Gallerani, M.; Manfredini, R. Weekend hospitalization and inhospital mortality: A gender effect? *Am. J. Emerg. Med.* **2015**, *33*, 1701–1703. [CrossRef] [PubMed]
25. James, M.T.; Wald, R.; Bell, C.M.; Tonelli, M.; Hemmelgarn, B.R.; Waikar, S.S.; Chertow, G.M. Weekend hospital admission, acute kidney injury, and mortality. *J. Am. Soc. Nephrol.* **2010**, *21*, 845–851. [CrossRef]
26. Kolhe, N.V.; Fluck, R.J.; Taal, M.W. Effect of weekend admission on mortality associated with severe acute kidney injury in England: A propensity score matched, population-based study. *PLoS ONE* **2017**, *12*, e0186048. [CrossRef]
27. Holmes, J.; Rainer, T.; Geen, J.; Williams, J.D.; Phillips, A.O. Welsh AKI Steering Group Adding a new dimension to the weekend effect: An analysis of a national data set of electronic AKI alerts. *Qjm Int. J. Med.* **2018**, *111*, 249–255. [CrossRef]
28. Baid-Agrawal, S.; Martus, P.; Feldman, H.; Kramer, H. Weekend versus weekday transplant surgery and outcomes after kidney transplantation in the USA: A retrospective national database analysis. *BMJ Open* **2016**, *6*, e010482. [CrossRef]
29. Schütte-Nütgen, K.; Thölking, G.; Dahmen, M.; Becker, F.; Kebschull, L.; Schmidt, R.; Pavenstädt, H.; Suwelack, B.; Reuteret, S. Is there a "weekend effect" in kidney transplantation? *PLoS ONE* **2017**, *12*, e0190227. [CrossRef]
30. Anderson, B.M.; Mytton, J.L.; Evison, F.; Ferro, C.J.; Sharif, A. Outcomes After Weekend Admission for Deceased Donor Kidney Transplantation. *Transplantation* **2017**, *101*, 2244–2252. [CrossRef]

31. Lim, W.H.; Coates, P.T.; Russ, G.R.; Russell, C.; He, B.; Jaques, B.; Pleass, H.; Chapman, J.R.; Wong, G. Weekend effect on early allograft outcome after kidney transplantation- a multi-centre cohort study. *Transpl. Int.* **2018**, *32*, 387–398. [CrossRef] [PubMed]
32. Manfredini, R.; Gallerani, M.; De Giorgi, A.; Boari, B.; Lamberti, N.; Manfredini, F.; Storari, A.; La Manna, G.; Fabbian, F. Lack of a "Weekend Effect" for Renal Transplant Recipients: The Hospital Database of the Emilia-Romagna Region of Italy. *Angiology* **2017**, *68*, 366–373. [CrossRef] [PubMed]
33. Sakhuja, A.; Schold, J.D.; Kumar, G.; Dall, A.; Sood, P.; Navaneethan, S.D. Outcomes of Patients Receiving Maintenance Dialysis Admitted Over Weekends. *Am. J. Kidney Dis.* **2013**, *62*, 763–770. [CrossRef] [PubMed]
34. Johnson, D.W.; Clayton, P.; Cho, Y.; Badve, S.V.; Hawley, C.; McDonald, S.; Boudville, N.; Wiggins, K.J.; Bannister, K.; Brown, F. Weekend Compared with Weekday Presentations of Peritoneal Dialysis–Associated Peritonitis. *Perit. Dial. Int.* **2012**, *32*, 516–524. [CrossRef] [PubMed]
35. Mazzali, C.; Duca, P. Use of administrative data in health care research. *Intern. Emerg. Med.* **2015**, *10*, 517–524. [CrossRef] [PubMed]
36. Clinical Practice Guideline for Acute Kidney Injury. Available online: https://kdigo.org/wp-content/uploads/2016/10/KDIGO-2012-AKI-Guideline-English.pdf (accessed on 8 June 2020).
37. Black, N. Higher Mortality in Weekend Admissions to the Hospital. *JAMA* **2016**, *316*, 2593–2594. [CrossRef]
38. Waikar, S.S.; Wald, R.; Chertow, G.M.; Curhan, G.C.; Winkelmayer, W.C.; Liangos, O.; Sosa, M.A.; Jaber, B.L. Validity of International Classification of Diseases, Ninth Revision, Clinical Modification Codes for Acute Renal Failure. *J. Am. Soc. Nephrol.* **2006**, *17*, 1688–1694. [CrossRef]
39. Vlasschaert, M.E.; Bejaimal, S.A.; Hackam, D.G.; Quinn, R.; Cuerden, M.S.; Oliver, M.J.; Iansavichus, A.; Sultan, N.; Mills, A.; Garg, A.X. Validity of Administrative Database Coding for Kidney Disease: A Systematic Review. *Am. J. Kidney Dis.* **2011**, *57*, 29–43. [CrossRef]
40. Tomlinson, L.A.; Riding, A.M.; Payne, R.A.; Abel, G.A.; Tomson, C.R.; Wilkinson, I.B.; Roland, M.O.; Chaudhry, A.N. The accuracy of diagnostic coding for acute kidney injury in England—A single centre study. *BMC Nephrol.* **2013**, *14*, 58. [CrossRef]
41. Grams, M.E.; Waikar, S.S.; MacMahon, B.; Whelton, S.; Ballew, S.; Coresh, J. Performance and Limitations of Administrative Data in the Identification of AKI. *Clin. J. Am. Soc. Nephrol.* **2014**, *9*, 682–689. [CrossRef]
42. Available online: www.who.int/ageing/population/global_health.pdf (accessed on 8 June 2020).
43. Saran, R.; Robinson, B.; Abbott, K.C.; Bragg-Gresham, J.; Chen, X.; Gipson, D.; Gu, H.; Hirth, R.A.; Hutton, D.; Jin, Y.; et al. US Renal Data System 2019 Annual Data Report: Epidemiology of Kidney Disease in the United States. *Am. J. Kidney Dis.* **2019**, *75*, A6–A7. [CrossRef] [PubMed]
44. Floege, J.; Gillespie, I.; Kronenberg, F.; Anker, S.D.; Gioni, I.; Richards, S.; Pisoni, R.L.; Robinson, B.M.; Marcelli, D.; Froissart, M.; et al. Development and validation of a predictive mortality risk score from a European hemodialysis cohort. *Kidney Int.* **2015**, *87*, 996–1008. [CrossRef] [PubMed]
45. Barnett, K.; Mercer, S.; Norbury, M.; Watt, G.; Wyke, S.; Guthrie, B. Epidemiology of multimorbidity and implications for health care, research, and medical education: A cross-sectional study. *Lancet* **2012**, *380*, 37–43. [CrossRef]

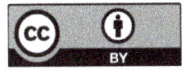

© 2020 by the authors. Licensee MDPI, Basel, Switzerland. This article is an open access article distributed under the terms and conditions of the Creative Commons Attribution (CC BY) license (http://creativecommons.org/licenses/by/4.0/).

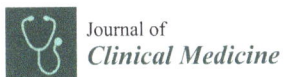

Review

Artificial Intelligence in Acute Kidney Injury Risk Prediction

Joana Gameiro [1,*], Tiago Branco [2] and José António Lopes [1]

[1] Division of Nephrology and Renal Transplantation, Department of Medicine, Centro Hospitalar Lisboa Norte, EPE, Av. Prof. Egas Moniz, 1649-035 Lisboa, Portugal; jalopes93@hotmail.com
[2] Department of Medicine, Centro Hospitalar Lisboa Norte, EPE, Av. Prof. Egas Moniz, 1649-035 Lisboa, Portugal; tiagobranco.md@gmail.com
* Correspondence: joana.estrelagameiro@gmail.com

Received: 27 January 2020; Accepted: 28 February 2020; Published: 3 March 2020

Abstract: Acute kidney injury (AKI) is a frequent complication in hospitalized patients, which is associated with worse short and long-term outcomes. It is crucial to develop methods to identify patients at risk for AKI and to diagnose subclinical AKI in order to improve patient outcomes. The advances in clinical informatics and the increasing availability of electronic medical records have allowed for the development of artificial intelligence predictive models of risk estimation in AKI. In this review, we discussed the progress of AKI risk prediction from risk scores to electronic alerts to machine learning methods.

Keywords: acute kidney injury; risk prediction; artificial intelligence

1. Introduction

Acute kidney injury (AKI) is a complex syndrome caused by multiple etiologies and characterized by a sudden decrease in kidney function, defined by an increase in serum creatinine or a decrease in urine output [1,2]. AKI is a frequent complication in hospitalized patients, which is associated with worse short- and long-term outcomes, namely, increased length of hospital stay, increased health care costs, increased risk of in-hospital and long-term mortality, long-term progression to chronic kidney disease, and long-term risk of cardiovascular events [3–7].

The incidence of AKI has increased in the past decades due to the population aging and rising incidence of comorbidities, such as chronic kidney disease, diabetes, and hypertension [2,8–10]. Furthermore, the development of a standardized definition for AKI and the acknowledgment of the impact of AKI on patient outcomes are also responsible for the increased recognition of this syndrome [2]. Despite the decrease in mortality rates associated with AKI, these remain significant, ranging from 15% among hospitalized patients to more than 50% in critically ill patients [11–13].

Considering the impact of AKI on short and long-term outcomes, it is of high importance to develop methods to identify patients at risk for AKI and to diagnose subclinical AKI in order to improve patient outcomes [4]. The advances in clinical informatics and the increasing availability of electronic medical records (EMR) have allowed for the development of predictive models of risk estimation in AKI [14].

In this review, we discussed the progress of AKI risk prediction from risk scores to electronic alerts to machine learning (ML) methods.

2. AKI Definition and Biomarkers

The Kidney Disease Improving Global Outcomes workgroup defines AKI as an increase in serum creatinine (SCr) of at least 0.3 mg/dL within 48 h, or an increase in SCr to more than 1.5 times of baseline level, which is known or presumed to have occurred within the prior 7 days, or a urine output (UO) decrease to less than 0.5 mL/kg/h for 6 h [15].

Despite the importance of the development and use of this standardized classification in the epidemiology of AKI, SCr and UO are insensitive and unspecific markers of AKI, which do not account for the duration or cause of AKI [16]. Values of SCr are influenced by age, gender, muscle mass, fluid balance, and medications, which limit its secretion, and values of UO are influenced by patient volemic status and diuretic use. Baseline SCr is frequently unknown, and UO assessment is complex without a urinary catheter.

Novel biomarkers have been investigated in multiple settings to increase diagnostic accuracy, which so far include cystatin C (Cys-C), neutrophil gelatinase-associated lipocalin (NGAL), N-acetyl-glucosaminidase (NAG), kidney injury molecule 1 (KIM-1), interleukin-6 (IL-6), interleukin-8 (IL-8), interleukin 18 (IL-18), liver-type fatty acid-binding protein (L-FABP), calprotectin, urine angiotensinogen (AGT), urine microRNAs, insulin-like growth factor-binding protein 7 (IGFBP7), and tissue inhibitor of metalloproteinases-2 (TIMP-2) [17–27].

Important weaknesses have limited the generalization of the use of these biomarkers in clinical practice [19]. These have not consistently distinguished pre-renal from renal AKI; several patient characteristics and comorbidities can produce range variations that limit their validity; cost-effectiveness is limited due to the increased costs associated with these biomarkers and need for multiple assessments, and evidence of outcome improvement is still lacking [28,29]. Given the complexity of AKI, perhaps the use of a panel of several biomarkers covering different stages of the syndrome could provide a better understanding of its pathophysiology and identify future treatment targets [29,30].

3. AKI Risk Factors

Several investigators have focused on determining significant risk factors for AKI [31–33]. Both patient susceptibilities and exposures are important risk factors for AKI. Patient age is an important non-modifiable risk factor [34–36]. The loss of renal reserve and physiologic decline of glomerular filtration rate (GFR) may place older patients at risk for AKI [37,38].

Chronic kidney disease (CKD) is another major risk factor for AKI [38] The loss of autoregulation, abnormal vasodilation, susceptibility to antihypertensive agents and nephrotoxins, and the side effects of medication contribute to the development of AKI in CKD patients [38].

Patient comorbidities, such as diabetes mellitus, hypertension, cardiovascular disease, chronic liver disease, and chronic obstructive pulmonary disease, have also been identified as important AKI predictors [15,31–33,36,39,40]. It is also important to note that HIV infection is a risk factor, predisposing patients to AKI, given the increasing incidence of HIV-infected patients in the past decades. Furthermore, AKI remains an important predictor of mortality in these patients despite the decrease in the incidence of AKI with the widespread use of antiretroviral therapy [41,42].

Exposure to sepsis, surgery, nephrotoxins, and shock are specific modifiable factors, which contribute to AKI [8,15]. Large cohort studies focusing on critically ill patients report that the two most important causes of AKI are sepsis and surgery [9,10,43–45].

More recent research has reported that hyperuricemia, hypoalbuminemia, obesity, anemia, and hyperglycemia may be new predictors of AKI [36].

Uric acid can contribute to AKI in several settings due to intratubular crystal precipitation, but also by inducing renal vasoconstriction and impairing autoregulation, and due to proinflammatory and antiangiogenic effects [46–49].

Hypoalbuminemia has been used as a nonspecific marker of patient nutrition, inflammation, hepatic function, and catabolic state and has been reported as an independent predictor of AKI in multiple settings [50–54].

The increasing incidence of obesity has raised the interest to study its association with AKI. Although the exact mechanisms are still uncertain, there is substantial evidence that obesity is an independent predictor of AKI in multiple medical and surgical settings [55–58].

Anemia has been associated with increased AKI risk, mainly in the surgical setting [59,60]. Furthermore, transfusions of red blood cells are also associated with increased risk of AKI [61,62]. The mechanisms are likely multifactorial, including reduced renal oxygen delivery, worsening oxidative stress, systemic inflammation, and impaired hemostasis [36,59,63]. Stored red blood cells have an impaired ability to carry oxygen and proinflammatory effects, associated with the direct toxic effect of by-products of red blood cell storage, contributing to organ failure in critically ill patients [59,64].

Hyperglycemia is another novel risk factor, which has been associated with increased AKI development [65–70]. However, the target level of glucose to decrease AKI risk has not been determined. The exact mechanism is still uncertain, but hyperglycemia might contribute to AKI through stimulation of oxidative stress, vasoconstriction and reduced renal oxygen delivery, and volume depletion due to osmotic diuresis [68,70].

4. AKI Risk Scores

A precise risk prediction score should be able to identify at-risk patients and guide clinicians on performing further diagnostic tests and prompting preventive and/or treatment measures. A risk score is produced by the combination of independent predictors of AKI and assigning relative impact, ideally with external validation analysis [14].

Risk prediction scores for AKI have been reported in several clinical settings, mostly in critical care, surgery, and contrast-induced nephropathy [71–77]. Still, most AKI cases are reported in general hospital wards, and risk scores in this setting are scarce [78–81].

Most models include age, gender, baseline kidney function, comorbidities, such as chronic kidney disease, diabetes, liver failure, and heart failure, medication history, namely, diuretics, angiotensin-converting-enzyme inhibitors and angiotensin-receptor blockers, and intra-procedure data to predict the risk of AKI [76,82]. An ideal risk prediction score for AKI should include a combination of demographic, clinical, and biological factors, along with biomarkers [76,77].

Malhotra et al. developed an easily calculated risk prediction score for AKI in critical care patients [77]. This risk score combines chronic kidney disease, chronic liver disease, congestive heart failure, hypertension, atherosclerotic coronary vascular disease, acidemia, nephrotoxin exposure, sepsis, mechanical ventilation, and anemia and has demonstrated good calibration in the test and external validation cohorts [77].

Flechet et al. developed four prediction scores, which can be used successively, based on the clinical information available [83]. The variables included in the baseline risk score are age, baseline SCr, surgical or medical category, diabetes, and planned admission. For the admission risk score, it includes blood glucose, suspected sepsis, hemodynamic support, and previous risk score variables. On day 1, the risk score includes SCr, Acute Physiology And Chronic Health Evaluation (APACHE) II score, maximum lactate, bilirubin, hours of ICU stay, and previous risk score variables. The risk score to be used after the first day includes the previous risk score variables and the total amount of urine, urine slope, mean arterial pressure, and hemodynamic support. One of the main strong points of this study is the availability of the online calculator of this risk score, which enhances its use in clinical practice and promotes further validation [83].

The most widely validated risk prediction score for AKI in cardiac surgery was developed by Thakar et al. and comprises 13 pre-operative variables, namely, gender, heart failure, left ventricular ejection fraction, preoperative use of intra-aortic balloon pump, chronic obstructive pulmonary disease, diabetes, previous cardiac surgery, emergency setting, type of surgery, and pre-operative SCr [84].

The clinical application of these risk prediction scores has been limited by the lack of external validation of several studies, the use of heterogeneous definitions of AKI, the difficulty in assessing baseline renal function, and importantly the lack of impact analysis studies and lack of evidence of clinical use [14,76].

5. Automated Electronic Alerts

The use of automated electronic alerts (E-alerts) has received considerable consideration in the past years [85]. E-alerts consist of algorithms configured from patients' EMRs and clinical information to notify early or imminent AKI, prompting an earlier clinical evaluation and prompt prevention and treatment strategies [86,87].

Theoretically, this would prompt early treatment and improve patient outcomes. Nevertheless, a recent systematic review of randomized AKI E-alert trials pooled data from six studies and 10,165 patients and found that these did not reduce mortality (OR 1.05; 95% CI, 0.84–1.31), need for renal replacement therapy (OR 1.20; 95% CI, 0.91–1.57), or change patient care practices (OR 2.18; 95% CI, 0.46–10.31) [88]. In these studies, E-alerts were issued within one hour, following the detection of changes in SCr; however, there was significant variability in study design, alert format, and targeted providers [88].

Beyond the limitations of SCr as a marker of AKI, other important challenges of the use of E-alerts are the distinction of community and hospital-acquired AKI cases, the presence of multiple alerts per patient, the assessment of significance of small SCr changes in patients with CKD, and the limitations on cases without baseline renal function [14].

A care bundle is a group of evidence-based and easily applicable interventions that have a better outcome when performed together than if performed individually [14]. There is no current specific treatment for AKI, and the most recent guidelines suggest supportive management, including treatment of sepsis, shock, and hypovolemia, avoidance of nephrotoxins, appropriate investigations, and referral to specialists when indicated [15].

Kolhe et al. demonstrated that implementing a care bundle with E-alerts improved outcomes in patients with AKI in two cohort studies. The care bundle consists of standardized investigations and interventions, namely, Assessment of history and examination, Urinalysis, establishing a clinical Diagnosis of AKI, plan Investigations, and Treatment and Seeking advice from a nephrologist (AUDITS) [89,90].

These findings were also reported in a study by Chandrasekar et al., in which an E-alert was combined with a care bundle consisting of treatment of Acute complications, Blood pressure control, Catheterization, review Drug prescription, Investigate the cause, and Treat the underlying cause (ABCD-IT) [91]. The authors reported a decrease in mortality and length of stay [91].

A recent study by Hodgson et al. evaluated the impact of combining care bundles to a risk prediction score and to E-alerts. This study demonstrated a decrease in hospital-acquired AKI and a decrease in AKI-associated mortality [92].

Therefore, it may not be enough to merely alert for the presence of AKI but important to initiate appropriate care to lead to improved outcomes [14].

We believe that it is essential to incorporate these scientific advances in daily clinical practice in the near future.

6. The Era of Artificial Intelligence

The past decade has seen significant development of electronic technology in medicine, namely, in EMR, data registries and management, and analytic methodologies [93].

Indeed, a new era of AKI prediction and detection has started with the increasing use of risk prediction scores and E-alerts [93]. More recently, artificial intelligence (AI), namely, ML techniques, has been reported to identify AKI predictors [94].

AI is a branch of engineering, generally defined as the ability of a machine to reason, communicate, and function with the minimal human intervention [95]. In the medical field, AI can be applied as two branches: physical or virtual [95]. The physical branch includes medical devices and sophisticated robots, which contribute to the delivery of care [95]. The virtual branch refers to ML, which includes the algorithms and statistical models that learn from data from which they are able to recognize and deduce patterns [95].

There are numerous types of ML algorithms, which have the ability to find patterns, to classify and predict algorithms based on previous examples, and to create a strategy for prediction by sequences of rewards and punishments [94–98]. The dynamic ability of these algorithms is key to identify and integrate variables from numerous electronic data [94]. Thus, ML techniques can be used alone or combined to analyze datasets and determine AKI predictors. The description of each available ML algorithm is out of the scope of this review.

Currently, logistic regression is the most frequently used statistical algorithm of multivariate analysis to determine risk predictors in the short-term [99]. In complex settings in which clinical features and outcomes have a non-linear relationship and for big data analysis, many investigators support the use of more advanced ML algorithms in detriment of logistic regression to develop predictive models [100].

Considering that AKI can be determined from the calculation of SCr levels and the increasing integration of the available EMRs, ML algorithms are promising in the development of AKI risk prediction models.

The development of risk prediction models has flourished in recent years. However, inefficient statistical methods, the use of small samples, missing data, and lack of validation are common faults, which limit the use of these models [99]. The development of risk prediction models should include internal validation within the original study sample to quantify the predictive ability of the model and should preferably also include external validation to evaluate the predictive ability of the model in other participant data [99]. To improve the quality of reporting of published prediction model studies, the Transparent Reporting of a multivariable prediction model for Individual Prognosis or Diagnosis (TRIPOD) Statement produced a checklist of items to include in studies developing or validating a multivariable prediction model [99].

Furthermore, it is important to consider the specificity and sensitivity of these models, which will have a clinical impact [101]. High specificity values lead to fewer false-positive results, and high sensitivity values lead to fewer false negatives [101]. This has an important impact on prognostic modeling and decision-making, namely, high specificity would trigger less often to prompt interventions with higher risk, and high sensitivity would trigger more often to prompt interventions with lower risk [101].

The first study to compare logistic regression models and ML algorithms was a retrospective study by Kate et al., who analyzed EMRs of 25,521 hospital stays of elderly patients and aimed to predict within the first 24 h of admission whether a patient would develop AKI during hospitalization. This study demonstrated only modest performance in all ML models (support vector machines, decision trees, and naïve Bayes), with an area under the receiver operating characteristic curve (AUROC) ranging from 0.621–0.664, and better performance of logistic regression with an AUROC of 0.743 [102].

A research group led by Bihorac performed a retrospective study of 50,318 adult surgical patients and compared four predictive ML modeling approaches for two major postoperative complications, using data from EMRs [103]. This study demonstrated that the choice of predictive modeling approach affected the risk prediction performance for postoperative AKI and sepsis; specifically, generalized additive models showed the best performance with an AUROC of 0.858 [103].

Davis et al. also compared several ML models (random forest, neural network, and naïve Bayes) and logistic regression methods to predict AKI in a retrospective study of 2003 patients [104]. Both methods had a good performance in detecting AKI, but importantly, over-time logistic regression methods required more updates than random forest or neural network methods to compensate overprediction [104].

Cheng et al. developed ML-based AKI prediction models using EMRs from 48,955 hospital admissions and concluded that the best model for predicting AKI within 24 h had an AUROC of 0.76 achieved by a random forest algorithm [105]. Indeed, this ML algorithm could predict AKI 2-days with AUC of 0.73 and 3-days prior with AUC of 0.700 [105].

Ibrahim et al. developed a clinical and proteomics AKI risk predictor with an ML approach (least absolute shrinkage and selection operator (LASSO) with logistic regression) in a prospective study of 889 patients undergoing coronary angiography [106]. The risk predictor included a history of diabetes, blood urea nitrogen/creatinine ratio, c-reactive protein, osteopontin, CD5 antigen-like, and Factor VII and had an AUROC of 0.790 for predicting procedural AKI [106].

Koola et al. analyzed a retrospective cohort of 504 cirrhotic patients and compared the ability of ML methods (logistic regression, naïve Bayes, support vector machines, random forest, and gradient boosting) to predict hepatorenal syndrome (HRS) [107]. This study demonstrated the ability to create a high-performance risk prediction algorithm to detect cases of HRS, with AUROC ranging between 0.730–0.930 [107].

Another mortality prediction model was constructed using the random forest algorithm in 19,044 AKI patients by Lin and colleagues [100]. Urine output, systolic blood pressure, age, serum bicarbonate, and heart rate were the most significant variables, predicting AKI-associated mortality [100]. This model had a great performance with an AUROC of 0.866 and could prove useful in avoiding delays of AKI treatment in high-mortality risk patients [100].

Koyner et al. developed a gradient boosting model, which could predict AKI in the emergency department, wards, and ICU [108]. Their model included data from 121,158 admissions, such as patient demographics, vital signs, laboratories, clinical interventions, and diagnostics, and demonstrated increasing accuracy across AKI severity, providing AUROC greater than 0.900 for renal replacement therapy requirement within 72 h [108].

Huang et al. performed a retrospective study of 947,091 patients submitted to percutaneous coronary intervention and compared logistic regression and gradient descent boosting to detect if ML algorithms could enhance AKI prediction [109]. Their algorithm had a good performance in detecting AKI with an AUROC 0.728 [109]. The risk prediction model included 12 variables, namely, age, heart failure, cardiogenic shock within 24 h, cardiac arrest within 24 h, diabetes, coronary artery disease, baseline renal function, admission source, body mass index, emergency status, and left ventricular ejection fraction [109].

In another retrospective study of 2,076,694 patients submitted to percutaneous coronary intervention, Huang et al. applied an ML method to predict AKI risk according to contrast volume [110]. The generalized additive model produced an AUROC of 0.777 (95% CI, 0.775–0.779) for predicting the risk of a creatinine level increase of at least 0.3 mg/dL [110]. The model was developed from a random 50% of the cohort, and performance was evaluated in the remaining 50% of the cohort. The association of contrast volume with AKI risk was nonlinear, and this model proved useful to quantify individual risk and adjust contrast volume to decrease AKI risk [110].

Tomasev et al. developed a recurrent neural network model, which predicted 55.8% of all inpatient episodes of AKI and 90.2% of all dialysis, requiring AKI up to 48 h in advance in 703,782 adult patients from inpatient and outpatient sites [111]. This ML model had a great performance with an AUROC of 0.921, and, at each time point, this model outputted the risk of AKI occurrence within the next 48 h, thus allowing for the prompt implementation of preventive and treatment strategies [111].

MySurgeryRisk is an ML algorithm recently developed and internally validated from a retrospective single-center cohort of 2911 adults who underwent surgery [112]. This random forest model combined preoperative and intraoperative variables and had an AUROC of 0.860 to predict the risk of developing postoperative AKI [112].

Flechet et al. conducted a prospective observational study of 252 critically ill patients and compared the AKI predictions by physicians and a random forest method, *AKIpredictor* [113]. There was no statistically significant difference in discrimination between physicians and *AKIpredictor*; however, physicians overestimated the risk, and *AKIpredictor* allowed for the selection of high-risk patients or reducing false positives, and *AKIpredictor* provided its prediction earlier than physicians [113].

Parreco et al. developed and compared different ML models (gradient boosted trees, logistic regression, and deep learning) to predict AKI from the laboratory values, vital signs, and slopes in

151,098 ICU admissions [114]. Gradient boosted trees method was the most accurate model with an AUROC of 0.834, for which the most important variable was the slope of the minimum creatinine [114].

Xu et al. investigated ML models (logistic regression, random forest. and gradient boosting decision tree) for predicting the mortality risk of 58,976 AKI patients admitted to an ICU, stratified according to AKI severity stages [115]. Gradient boosting decision tree presented a better performance than other models for mortality prediction [115].

Tran et al. developed an ML method (k-nearest neighbor) to predict AKI in 50 burn patients, which included measurements of neutrophil gelatinase-associated lipocalin (NGAL), UO, SCr, and N-terminal B-type natriuretic peptide (NT-proBNP) measured within the first 24 h of admission. This method performed greatly with an AUROC of 0.920 and achieved a 90%–100% accuracy for identifying AKI, with a mean time-to-AKI recognition within 18 h [116].

In 6682 critical care patients, Zhang et al. identified predictors of volume responsive AKI, such as age, urinary creatinine concentration, maximum blood urea nitrogen concentration, and albumin using ML methods [117]. Their model (gradient boosting) had an AUROC of 0.860 and could prove useful to stratify patients with oliguria responsive to fluids and prompt immediate therapeutic measures [117].

Zimmerman et al. conducted a retrospective cohort of 23,950 adult critical care patients and developed a predictive model by logistic regression for early prediction of AKI in the first 72 h. following ICU admission with an AUROC of 0.783 [118]. Their model included first-day measurements of physiologic variables but not medications and procedures, in order to detect which deterioration of patients' physiologic baselines are predictive of AKI [118]. This was cross-validated with ML algorithms, demonstrating an accurate and early prediction of AKI with their risk prediction score [118].

Rashidi and colleagues developed, internally validated, and compared ML models for early recognition of AKI in 50 burn and 51 trauma patients, including NGAL, NT-proBNP, SCr, and UO into the predictive model [119]. Their models were able to accurately predict AKI 62 h in advance [119].

Overall, ML algorithms have performed impressively, and sensitivity is favored over specificity in order to early detect as many cases of AKI, allowing for a higher number of false positives. The ML algorithms have also performed better than the currently used logistic regression in the majority of studies. These studies are summarized in Table 1.

Table 1. Machine learning studies on acute kidney injury (AKI) prediction.

Study	Design	Setting	N	AKI Definition	Timing of AKI	ML Algorithm	Predictive Ability	Sensitivity; Specificity; Confidence Interval	External Validation
Kate et al. (2016)	retrospective	medical and surgical	25,521	AKIN	during hospitalization	naïve Bayes; support vector machine; decision trees; logistic regression	AUROC 0.654 AUROC 0.621 AUROC 0.639 AUROC 0.660	75%; 61%; -	no
Thottakkara et al. (2016)	retrospective	surgical	50,318	KDIGO	post surgery	naïve Bayes; generalized additive model; logistic regression; support vector machine	AUROC 0.819 AUROC 0.858 AUROC 0.853 AUROC 0.857	77%; -; -	no
Davis et al. (2017)	retrospective	medical and surgical	2003	KDIGO	during hospitalization	random forest; neural network; naïve Bayes; logistic regression	AUROC 0.730 AUROC 0.720 AUROC 0.690 AUROC 0.780	-; -; 95% CI	no
Cheng et al. (2018)	retrospective	medical and surgical	60,534	KDIGO, AKIN, RIFLE	during hospitalization	random forest; AdaBoostM1; logistic regression	AUROC 0.765 AUROC 0.751 AUROC 0.763	69%; 71%; -	no
Ibrahim et al. (2018)	prospective	contrast	889	KDIGO	pre and post intervention	logistic regression	AUROC 0.790	77%; 75%; -	no

Table 1. Cont.

Study	Design	Setting	N	AKI Definition	Timing of AKI	ML Algorithm	Predictive Ability	Sensitivity; Specificity; Confidence Interval	External Validation
Koola et al. (2018)	retrospective	medical and surgical	504	KDIGO	during hospitalization	logistic regression; naïve Bayes; support vector machines; random forest; gradient boosting	AUROC 0.930 AUROC 0.730 AUROC 0.900 AUROC 0.910 AUROC 0.880	87%; 76%; -	no
Lin et al. (2018)	retrospective	ICU	19,044	KDIGO	during hospitalization	support vector machine	AUROC 0.860	-	no
Koyner et al. (2018)	retrospective	medical and surgical	121,158	KDIGO	24 h post admission	gradient boosting	AUROC 0.900	95% CI	no
Huang et al. (2018)	retrospective	PCI	947,091	AKIN	during hospitalization	gradient boost; logistic regression	AUROC 0.728 AUROC 0.717	-; -; 95% CI	no
Huang et al. (2019)	retrospective	PCI	2,076,694	AKIN	pre and post intervention	generalized additive model	AUROC 0.777	-; -; 95% CI	no
Tomašev et al. (2019)	retrospective	medical and surgical	703,782	KDIGO	during hospitalization	recurrent neural network	AUROC 0.921	95%; 70.3%; -	no
Adhikari et al. (2019)	retrospective	surgical	2901	KDIGO	post surgery	random forest	AUROC 0.860	68%; -; -	no
Flechet et al. (2019)	prospective	ICU	252	KDIGO	during hospitalization	random forest	AUROC 0.780	-; -; 95% CI	no

Table 1. Cont.

Study	Design	Setting	N	AKI Definition	Timing of AKI	ML Algorithm	Predictive Ability	Sensitivity; Specificity; Confidence Interval	External Validation
Parreco et al. (2019)	retrospective	medical and surgical	151,098	KDIGO	during hospitalization	gradient boosting; logistic regression; deep learning	AUROC 0.834 AUROC 0.827 AUROC 0.817	-; -; 95% CI	no
Xu et al. (2019)	retrospective	medical and surgical	58,976	KDIGO	during hospitalization	gradient boosting	AUROC 0.749	-	no
Tran et al. (2019)	prospective	burn	50	KDIGO	during hospitalization	k-nearest neighbor	AUROC 0.920	90%; -; -	no
Zhang et al. (2019)	retrospective	ICU	6682	KDIGO	24 h post admission	gradient boosting	AUROC 0.860	-; -; 95% CI	no
Zimmerman et al. (2019)	retrospective	ICU	46,000	KDIGO	72 h post admission	logistic regression; random forest; neural network	AUROC 0.783 AUROC 0.779 AUROC 0.796	68%; 34%; -	no
Rashidi et al. (2020)	retrospective and prospective	burn and trauma	50/51	KDIGO vs New Biomarkers	1st week post ICU admission	recurrent neural network	AUROC 0.920	-; -; 92% CI	no

AKI-acute kidney injury, AKIN-acute kidney injury network, AUROC-area under the receiver operating characteristic curve, ICU-intensive care unit, KDIGO-kidney disease improving global outcomes, ML-machine learning, PCI-percutaneous coronary intervention, RIFLE-risk, injury, failure, loss of kidney function, end-stage kidney disease.

These studies have demonstrated the efficacy of ML algorithms to detect clinical and laboratory characteristics associated with AKI risk and detection in big data studies. The future widespread use of ML algorithms could improve risk stratification of patients, early detection of AKI, and provide decision aid on treatment, ultimately improving patient care and increasing time and cost-efficiency. Furthermore, these algorithms could predict further adverse events and long-term prognosis, therefore, providing useful information to establish an individualized follow-up plan.

Despite the promising results, important limitations have to be considered [82]. Firstly, most ML approaches have performed positively in retrospective cohorts, and prospective implementation of these methods is still challenging [95,101]. None of these studies have external validation, and the variability in the availability of EMRs across centers limits the widespread use of these models [95,101]. The development of these risk prediction models requires a substantial amount of data from EMRs and computer-assisted risk prediction [82]. Furthermore, to guarantee detailed information on comorbidities, physiological and laboratory parameters and medication, and electronic connections between community and hospital data are necessary [82]. Logistic regression models are more familiar to clinicians than ML models, limiting data interpretation [103]. It is also important to note that neural networks are developed and tested in the same dataset, which limits generalizability [95,101]. Additionally, from a legal and ethical perspective, the inability to clarify what contributes to decision-making in neural networks is an important restriction in these models, which is conflicting to general data protection requirements [95,101].

7. Conclusions

AKI has a significant negative impact on short and long-term outcomes; thus, it is crucial to develop methods to identify patients at risk for AKI and to diagnose subclinical AKI. The increasing amount of evidence is encouraging the real-time implementation of these ML risk models as this does not require additional AKI biomarker testing. Combining these risk prediction models with early care bundles in the future is likely to improve patient outcomes.

Author Contributions: The authors participated as follows: J.G. drafted the article, T.B. participated in the acquisition of data, J.A.L. revised the article and approved the final version to be submitted for publication. All authors have read and agreed to the published version of the manuscript.

Funding: There was no funding for this study.

Conflicts of Interest: There is no conflict of interest. The results presented in this paper have not been published previously in whole or part.

References

1. Kellum, J.A.; Prowle, J.R. Paradigms of acute kidney injury in the intensive care setting. *Nat. Rev. Nephrol.* **2018**, *14*, 217–230. [CrossRef] [PubMed]
2. Hoste, E.A.J.; Schurgers, M. Epidemiology of acute kidney injury: How big is the problem? *Crit. Care Med.* **2008**, *36* (Suppl. S36), S146–S151. [CrossRef] [PubMed]
3. Coca, S.G.; Yusuf, B.; Shlipak, M.G.; Garg, A.X.; Parikh, C.R. Long-term Risk of Mortality and Other Adverse Outcomes After Acute Kidney Injury: A Systematic Review and Meta-analysis. *Am. J. Kidney Dis.* **2009**, *53*, 961–973. [CrossRef] [PubMed]
4. Chertow, G.M.; Burdick, E.; Honour, M.; Bonventre, J.V.; Bates, D.W. Acute Kidney Injury, Mortality, Length of Stay, and Costs in Hospitalized Patients. *J. Am. Soc. Nephrol.* **2005**, *16*, 3365–3370. [CrossRef] [PubMed]
5. Chawla, L.S.; Bellomo, R.; Bihorac, A.; Goldstein, S.L.; Siew, E.D.; Bagshaw, S.M.; Bittleman, D.; Cruz, D.; Endre, Z.; Fitzgerald, R.L.; et al. Acute kidney disease and renal recovery: Consensus report of the Acute Disease Quality Initiative (ADQI) 16 Workgroup. *Nat. Rev. Nephrol.* **2017**, *13*, 241–257. [CrossRef] [PubMed]
6. Wald, R. Chronic Dialysis and Death Among Survivors of Acute Kidney Injury Requiring Dialysis. *JAMA* **2009**, *302*, 1179. [CrossRef] [PubMed]

7. De Corte, W.; Dhondt, A.; Vanholder, R.; De Waele, J.; Decruyenaere, J.; Sergoyne, V.; Vanhalst, J.; Claus, S.; Hoste, E.A. Long-term outcome in ICU patients with acute kidney injury treated with renal replacement therapy: A prospective cohort study. *Crit. Care* **2016**, *20*, 256. [CrossRef]
8. Susantitaphong, P.; Cruz, D.N.; Cerda, J.; Abulfaraj, M.; Alqahtani, F.; Koulouridis, I.; Jaber, B.L. Acute Kidney Injury Advisory Group of the American Society of Nephrology. World Incidence of AKI: A Meta-Analysis. *Clin. J. Am. Soc. Nephrol.* **2013**, *8*, 1482–1493. [CrossRef]
9. Uchino, S. Acute Renal Failure in Critically Ill PatientsA Multinational, Multicenter Study. *JAMA* **2005**, *294*, 813. [CrossRef]
10. Hoste, E.A.J.; Bagshaw, S.M.; Bellomo, R.; Cely, C.M.; Colman, R.; Cruz, D.N.; Edipidis, K.; Forni, L.G.; Gomersall, C.D.; Govil, D.; et al. Epidemiology of acute kidney injury in critically ill patients: The multinational AKI-EPI study. *Intensive Care Med.* **2015**, *41*, 1411–1423. [CrossRef]
11. Ympa, Y.P.; Sakr, Y.; Reinhart, K.; Vincent, J.-L. Has mortality from acute renal failure decreased? A systematic review of the literature. *Am. J. Med.* **2005**, *118*, 827–832. [CrossRef] [PubMed]
12. Waikar, S.S.; Curhan, G.C.; Wald, R.; McCarthy, E.P.; Chertow, G.M. Declining Mortality in Patients with Acute Renal Failure, 1988 to 2002. *J. Am. Soc. Nephrol.* **2006**, *17*, 1143–1150. [CrossRef] [PubMed]
13. Wald, R.; McArthur, E.; Adhikari, N.K.J.; Bagshaw, S.M.; Burns, K.E.; Garg, A.X.; Harel, Z.; Kitchlu, A.; Mazer, C.D.; Nash, D.M.; et al. Changing Incidence and Outcomes Following Dialysis-Requiring Acute Kidney Injury Among Critically Ill Adults: A Population-Based Cohort Study. *Am. J. Kidney Dis.* **2015**, *65*, 870–877. [CrossRef]
14. Hodgson, L.E.; Selby, N.; Huang, T.-M.; Forni, L.G. The Role of Risk Prediction Models in Prevention and Management of AKI. *Semin. Nephrol.* **2019**, *39*, 421–430. [CrossRef] [PubMed]
15. Khwaja, A. KDIGO Clinical Practice Guidelines for Acute Kidney Injury. *Nephron* **2012**, *120*, c179–c184. [CrossRef] [PubMed]
16. Thomas, M.E.; Blaine, C.; Dawnay, A.; Devonald, M.A.; Ftouh, S.; Laing, C.; Latchem, S.; Lewington, A.; Milford, D.V.; Ostermann, M. The definition of acute kidney injury and its use in practice. *Kidney Int.* **2015**, *87*, 62–73. [CrossRef] [PubMed]
17. Schinstock, C.A.; Semret, M.H.; Wagner, S.J.; Borland, T.M.; Bryant, S.C.; Kashani, K.B.; Larson, T.S.; Lieske, J.C. Urinalysis is more specific and urinary neutrophil gelatinase-associated lipocalin is more sensitive for early detection of acute kidney injury. *Nephrol. Dial. Transplant.* **2012**, *28*, 1175–1185. [CrossRef]
18. Han, W.K.; Bailly, V.; Abichandani, R.; Thadhani, R.; Bonventre, J.V. Kidney Injury Molecule-1 (KIM-1): A novel biomarker for human renal proximal tubule injury. *Kidney Int.* **2002**, *62*, 237–244. [CrossRef]
19. Ostermann, M.; Philips, B.J.; Forni, L.G. Clinical review: Biomarkers of acute kidney injury: Where are we now? *Crit. Care* **2012**, *16*, 233. [CrossRef]
20. Parikh, C.R.; Mishra, J.; Thiessen-Philbrook, H.; Dursun, B.; Ma, Q.; Kelly, C.; Dent, C.; Devarajan, P.; Edelstein, C.L. Urinary IL-18 is an early predictive biomarker of acute kidney injury after cardiac surgery. *Kidney Int.* **2006**, *70*, 199–203. [CrossRef]
21. Di Somma, S.; Magrini, L.; De Berardinis, B.; Marino, R.; Ferri, E.; Moscatelli, P.; Ballarino, P.; Carpinteri, G.; Noto, P.; Gliozzo, B.; et al. Additive value of blood neutrophil gelatinase-associated lipocalin to clinical judgement in acute kidney injury diagnosis and mortality prediction in patients hospitalized from the emergency department. *Crit. Care* **2013**, *17*, R29. [CrossRef] [PubMed]
22. Bennett, M.; Dent, C.L.; Ma, Q.; Dastrala, S.; Grenier, F.; Workman, R.; Syed, H.; Ali, S.; Barasch, J.; Devarajan, P. Urine NGAL Predicts Severity of Acute Kidney Injury After Cardiac Surgery: A Prospective Study. *Clin. J. Am. Soc. Nephrol.* **2008**, *3*, 665–673. [CrossRef] [PubMed]
23. Hall, I.E.; Yarlagadda, S.G.; Coca, S.G.; Wang, Z.; Doshi, M.; Devarajan, P.; Han, W.K.; Marcus, R.J.; Parikh, C.R. IL-18 and Urinary NGAL Predict Dialysis and Graft Recovery after Kidney Transplantation. *J. Am. Soc. Nephrol.* **2009**, *21*, 189–197. [CrossRef] [PubMed]
24. Jia, H.-M.; Huang, L.-F.; Zheng, Y.; Li, W.-X. Diagnostic value of urinary tissue inhibitor of metalloproteinase-2 and insulin-like growth factor binding protein 7 for acute kidney injury: A meta-analysis. *Crit. Care* **2017**, *21*. [CrossRef]
25. Bargnoux, A.-S.; Piéroni, L.; Cristol, J.-P. Analytical study of a new turbidimetric assay for urinary neutrophil gelatinase-associated lipocalin (NGAL) determination. *Clin. Chem. Lab. Med.* **2013**, *51*. [CrossRef]

26. Westhoff, J.H.; Tönshoff, B.; Waldherr, S.; Pöschl, J.; Teufel, U.; Westhoff, T.H.; Fichtner, A. Urinary Tissue Inhibitor of Metalloproteinase-2 (TIMP-2) • Insulin-Like Growth Factor-Binding Protein 7 (IGFBP7) Predicts Adverse Outcome in Pediatric Acute Kidney Injury. *PLoS ONE* **2015**, *10*, e0143628. [CrossRef]
27. Lima, C.; Macedo, E. Urinary Biochemistry in the Diagnosis of Acute Kidney Injury. *Dis. Markers* **2018**, *2018*, 1–7. [CrossRef]
28. Vanmassenhove, J.; Vanholder, R.; Nagler, E.; Van Biesen, W. Urinary and serum biomarkers for the diagnosis of acute kidney injury: An in-depth review of the literature. *Nephrol. Dial. Transplant.* **2012**, *28*, 254–273. [CrossRef]
29. Marx, D.; Metzger, J.; Pejchinovski, M.; Gil, R.B.; Frantzi, M.; Latosinska, A.; Belczacka, I.; Heinzmann, S.S.; Husi, H.; Zoidakis, J.; et al. Proteomics and Metabolomics for AKI Diagnosis. *Semin. Nephrol.* **2018**, *38*, 63–87. [CrossRef]
30. Kashani, K.; Cheungpasitporn, W.; Ronco, C. Biomarkers of acute kidney injury: The pathway from discovery to clinical adoption. *Clin. Chem. Lab. Med.* **2017**, *55*, 1074–1089. [CrossRef]
31. Cruz, D.N.; Ronco, C. Acute kidney injury in the intensive care unit: Current trends in incidence and outcome. *Crit. Care* **2007**, *11*, 149. [CrossRef] [PubMed]
32. Ali, T.; Khan, I.; Simpson, W.; Prescott, G.; Townend, J.; Smith, W.; Macleod, A. Incidence and Outcomes in Acute Kidney Injury: A Comprehensive Population-Based Study. *J. Am. Soc. Nephrol.* **2007**, *18*, 1292–1298. [CrossRef] [PubMed]
33. Lameire, N.H.; Bagga, A.; Cruz, D.; De Maeseneer, J.; Endre, Z.; Kellum, J.A.; Liu, K.D.; Mehta, R.L.; Pannu, N.; Van Biesen, W.; et al. Acute kidney injury: An increasing global concern. *Lancet* **2013**, *382*, 170–179. [CrossRef]
34. Grams, M.E.; Sang, Y.; Ballew, S.H.; Gansevoort, R.T.; Kimm, H.; Kovesdy, C.P.; Naimark, D.; Oien, C.; Smith, D.H.; Coresh, J.; et al. A Meta-analysis of the Association of Estimated GFR, Albuminuria, Age, Race, and Sex With Acute Kidney Injury. *Am. J. Kidney Dis.* **2015**, *66*, 591–601. [CrossRef] [PubMed]
35. De Zan, F.; Amigoni, A.; Pozzato, R.; Pettenazzo, A.; Murer, L.; Vidal, E. Acute Kidney Injury in Critically Ill Children: A Retrospective Analysis of Risk Factors. *Blood Purif.* **2019**, 1–7. [CrossRef] [PubMed]
36. Nie, S.; Tang, L.; Zhang, W.; Feng, Z.; Chen, X. Are There Modifiable Risk Factors to Improve AKI? *Biomed. Res. Int.* **2017**, *2017*, 1–9. [CrossRef]
37. Anderson, S.; Eldadah, B.; Halter, J.B.; Hazzard, W.R.; Himmelfarb, J.; Horne, F.M.; Kimmel, P.L.; Molitoris, B.A.; Murthy, M.; O'Hare, A.M.; et al. Acute Kidney Injury in Older Adults. *J. Am. Soc. Nephrol.* **2011**, *22*, 28–38. [CrossRef]
38. Chawla, L.S.; Eggers, P.W.; Star, R.A.; Kimmel, P.L. Acute Kidney Injury and Chronic Kidney Disease as Interconnected Syndromes. *N. Engl. J. Med.* **2014**, *371*, 58–66. [CrossRef]
39. Nie, S.; Feng, Z.; Xia, L.; Bai, J.; Xiao, F.; Liu, J.; Tang, L.; Chen, X. Risk factors of prognosis after acute kidney injury in hospitalized patients. *Front. Med.* **2017**, *11*, 393–402. [CrossRef]
40. Kane-Gill, S.L.; Sileanu, F.E.; Murugan, R.; Trietley, G.S.; Handler, S.M.; Kellum, J.A. Risk Factors for Acute Kidney Injury in Older Adults With Critical Illness: A Retrospective Cohort Study. *Am. J. Kidney Dis.* **2015**, *65*, 860–869. [CrossRef] [PubMed]
41. Gameiro, J.; Agapito Fonseca, J.; Jorge, S.; Lopes, J.A. Acute kidney injury in HIV-infected patients: A critical review. *HIV Med.* **2019**, *20*. [CrossRef] [PubMed]
42. Wyatt, C.M.; Arons, R.R.; Klotman, P.E.; Klotman, M.E. Acute renal failure in hospitalized patients with HIV: Risk factors and impact on in-hospital mortality. *AIDS* **2006**, *20*, 561–565. [CrossRef] [PubMed]
43. Singbartl, K.; Kellum, J.A. AKI in the ICU: Definition, epidemiology, risk stratification, and outcomes. *Kidney Int.* **2012**, *81*, 819–825. [CrossRef] [PubMed]
44. Lameire, N.; Van Biesen, W.; Vanholder, R. The changing epidemiology of acute renal failure. *Nat. Clin. Pract. Nephrol.* **2006**, *2*, 364–377. [CrossRef]
45. Liaño, F.; Junco, E.; Pascual, J.; Madero, R.; Verde, E. The spectrum of acute renal failure in the intensive care unit compared with that seen in other settings. The Madrid Acute Renal Failure Study Group. *Kidney Int. Suppl.* **1998**, *66*, S16–S24. [PubMed]
46. Ejaz, A.A.; Beaver, T.M.; Shimada, M.; Sood, P.; Lingegowda, V.; Schold, J.D.; Kim, T.; Johnson, R.J. Uric Acid: A Novel Risk Factor for Acute Kidney Injury in High-Risk Cardiac Surgery Patients? *Am. J. Nephrol.* **2009**, *30*, 425–429. [CrossRef] [PubMed]

47. Ejaz, A.A.; Kambhampati, G.; Ejaz, N.I.; Dass, B.; Lapsia, V.; Arif, A.A.; Asmar, A.; Shimada, M.; Alsabbagh, M.M.; Aiyer, R.; et al. Post-operative serum uric acid and acute kidney injury. *J. Nephrol.* **2012**, *25*, 497–505. [CrossRef]
48. Lapsia, V.; Johnson, R.J.; Dass, B.; Shimada, M.; Kambhampati, G.; Ejaz, N.I.; Arif, A.A.; Ejaz, A.A. Elevated Uric Acid Increases the Risk for Acute Kidney Injury. *Am. J. Med.* **2012**, *125*, 302.e9–302.e17. [CrossRef]
49. Guo, W.; Liu, Y.; Chen, J.-Y.; Chen, S.Q.; Li, H.L.; Duan, C.Y.; Liu, Y.H.; Tan, N. Hyperuricemia Is an Independent Predictor of Contrast-Induced Acute Kidney Injury and Mortality in Patients Undergoing Percutaneous Coronary Intervention. *Angiology* **2015**, *66*, 721–726. [CrossRef]
50. Kim, C.S.; Oak, C.Y.; Kim, H.Y.; Kang, Y.U.; Choi, J.S.; Bae, E.H.; Ma, S.K.; Kweon, S.S.; Kim, S.W. Incidence, Predictive Factors, and Clinical Outcomes of Acute Kidney Injury after Gastric Surgery for Gastric Cancer. *PLoS ONE* **2013**, *8*, e82289. [CrossRef]
51. Lee, E.-H.; Baek, S.-H.; Chin, J.-H.; Choi, D.K.; Son, H.J.; Kim, W.J.; Hahm, K.D.; Sim, J.Y.; Choi, I.C. Preoperative hypoalbuminemia is a major risk factor for acute kidney injury following off-pump coronary artery bypass surgery. *Intensive Care Med.* **2012**, *38*, 1478–1486. [CrossRef] [PubMed]
52. Wiedermann, C.J.; Wiedermann, W.; Joannidis, M. Hypoalbuminemia and acute kidney injury: A meta-analysis of observational clinical studies. *Intensive Care Med.* **2010**, *36*, 1657–1665. [CrossRef] [PubMed]
53. Delaney, A.P.; Dan, A.; McCaffrey, J.; Finfer, S. The role of albumin as a resuscitation fluid for patients with sepsis: A systematic review and meta-analysis. *Crit. Care Med.* **2011**, *39*, 386–391. [CrossRef] [PubMed]
54. Li, N.; Qiao, H.; Guo, J.-F.; Yang, H.Y.; Li, X.Y.; Li, S.L.; Wang, D.X.; Yang, L. Preoperative hypoalbuminemia was associated with acute kidney injury in high-risk patients following non-cardiac surgery: A retrospective cohort study. *BMC Anesthesiol.* **2019**, *19*, 171. [CrossRef] [PubMed]
55. Glance, L.G.; Wissler, R.; Mukamel, D.B.; Li, Y.; Diachun, C.A.; Salloum, R.; Fleming, F.J.; Dick, A.W. Perioperative Outcomes among Patients with the Modified Metabolic Syndrome Who Are Undergoing Noncardiac Surgery. *Anesthesiology* **2010**, *113*, 859–872. [CrossRef] [PubMed]
56. Kelz, R.R.; Reinke, C.E.; Zubizarreta, J.R.; Wang, M.; Saynisch, P.; Even-Shoshan, O.; Reese, P.P.; Fleisher, L.A.; Silber, J.H. Acute Kidney Injury, Renal Function, and the Elderly Obese Surgical Patient. *Ann. Surg.* **2013**, *258*, 359–363. [CrossRef]
57. Danziger, J.; Chen, K.P.; Lee, J.; Feng, M.; Mark, R.G.; Celi, L.A.; Mukamal, K.J. Obesity, Acute Kidney Injury, and Mortality in Critical Illness. *Crit. Care Med.* **2016**, *44*, 328–334. [CrossRef]
58. Billings, F.T.; Pretorius, M.; Schildcrout, J.S.; Mercaldo, N.D.; Byrne, J.G.; Ikizler, T.A.; Brown, N.J. Obesity and Oxidative Stress Predict AKI after Cardiac Surgery. *J. Am. Soc. Nephrol.* **2012**, *23*, 1221–1228. [CrossRef]
59. Karkouti, K.; Grocott, H.P.; Hall, R.; Jessen, M.E.; Kruger, C.; Lerner, A.B.; MacAdams, C.; Mazer, C.D.; de Medicis, É.; Myles, P.; et al. Interrelationship of preoperative anemia, intraoperative anemia, and red blood cell transfusion as potentially modifiable risk factors for acute kidney injury in cardiac surgery: A historical multicentre cohort study. *Can. J. Anesth. Can. d'anesthésie* **2014**, *62*, 377–384. [CrossRef]
60. Karkouti, K.; Wijeysundera, D.N.; Yau, T.M.; Callum, J.L.; Cheng, D.C.; Crowther, M.; Dupuis, J.Y.; Fremes, S.E.; Kent, B.; Laflamme, C.; et al. Acute Kidney Injury After Cardiac Surgery. *Circulation* **2009**, *119*, 495–502. [CrossRef]
61. Haase, M.; Bellomo, R.; Story, D.; Letis, A.; Klemz, K.; Matalanis, G.; Seevanayagam, S.; Dragun, D.; Seeliger, E.; Mertens, P.R.; et al. Effect of mean arterial pressure, haemoglobin and blood transfusion during cardiopulmonary bypass on post-operative acute kidney injury. *Nephrol. Dial. Transplant.* **2012**, *27*, 153–160. [CrossRef] [PubMed]
62. Lelubre, C.; Vincent, J.-L. Red blood cell transfusion in the critically ill patient. *Ann. Intensive Care* **2011**, *1*, 43. [CrossRef] [PubMed]
63. Koch, C.G.; Li, L.; Sessler, D.I.; Figueroa, P.; Hoeltge, G.A.; Mihaljevic, T.; Blackstone, E.H. Duration of Red-Cell Storage and Complications after Cardiac Surgery. *N. Engl. J. Med.* **2008**, *358*, 1229–1239. [CrossRef] [PubMed]
64. Tinmouth, A.; Fergusson, D.; Yee, I.C.; Hébert, P.C. Clinical consequences of red cell storage in the critically ill. *Transfusion* **2006**, *46*, 2014–2027. [CrossRef]
65. Moriyama, N.; Ishihara, M.; Noguchi, T.; Nakanishi, M.; Arakawa, T.; Asaumi, Y.; Kumasaka, L.; Kanaya, T.; Miyagi, T.; Nagai, T.; et al. Admission Hyperglycemia Is an Independent Predictor of Acute Kidney Injury in Patients With Acute Myocardial Infarction. *Circ. J.* **2014**, *78*, 1475–1480. [CrossRef]

66. Palomba, H.; de Castro, I.; Neto, A.L.C.; Lage, S.; Yu, L. Acute kidney injury prediction following elective cardiac surgery: AKICS Score. *Kidney Int.* **2007**, *72*, 624–631. [CrossRef]
67. Stolker, J.M.; McCullough, P.A.; Rao, S.; Inzucchi, S.E.; Spertus, J.A.; Maddox, T.M.; Masoudi, F.A.; Xiao, L.; Kosiborod, M. Pre-Procedural Glucose Levels and the Risk for Contrast-Induced Acute Kidney Injury in Patients Undergoing Coronary Angiography. *J. Am. Coll. Cardiol.* **2010**, *55*, 1433–1440. [CrossRef]
68. Giannini, F.; Latib, A.; Jabbour, R.J.; Ruparelia, N.; Aurelio, A.; Ancona, M.B.; Figini, F.; Mangieri, A.; Regazzoli, D.; Tanaka, A.; et al. Impact of post-procedural hyperglycemia on acute kidney injury after transcatheter aortic valve implantation. *Int. J. Cardiol.* **2016**, *221*, 892–897. [CrossRef]
69. Yoo, S.; Lee, H.-J.; Lee, H.; Ryu, H.-G. Association Between Perioperative Hyperglycemia or Glucose Variability and Postoperative Acute Kidney Injury After Liver Transplantation. *Anesth. Analg.* **2017**, *124*, 35–41. [CrossRef]
70. Shacham, Y.; Gal-Oz, A.; Leshem-Rubinow, E.; Arbel, Y.; Keren, G.; Roth, A.; Steinvil, A. Admission Glucose Levels and the Risk of Acute Kidney Injury in Nondiabetic ST Segment Elevation Myocardial Infarction Patients Undergoing Primary Percutaneous Coronary Intervention. *Cardiorenal Med.* **2015**, *5*, 191–198. [CrossRef]
71. Hoste, E.A.J.; Kellum, J.A.; Selby, N.M.; Arbel, Y.; Keren, G.; Roth, A.; Steinvil, A. Global epidemiology and outcomes of acute kidney injury. *Nat. Rev. Nephrol.* **2018**, *14*, 607–625. [CrossRef] [PubMed]
72. Kheterpal, S.; Tremper, K.K.; Englesbe, M.J.; O'Reilly, M.; Shanks, A.M.; Fetterman, D.M.; Rosenberg, A.L.; Swartz, R.D. Predictors of Postoperative Acute Renal Failure after Noncardiac Surgery in Patients with Previously Normal Renal Function. *Anesthesiology* **2007**, *107*, 892–902. [CrossRef] [PubMed]
73. Park, S.; Cho, H.; Park, S.; Lee, S.; Kim, K.; Yoon, H.J.; Park, J.; Choi, Y.; Lee, S.; Kim, J.H.; et al. Simple Postoperative AKI Risk (SPARK) Classification before Noncardiac Surgery: A Prediction Index Development Study with External Validation. *J. Am. Soc. Nephrol.* **2019**, *30*, 170–181. [CrossRef] [PubMed]
74. Silver, S.A.; Shah, P.M.; Chertow, G.M.; Harel, S.; Wald, R.; Harel, Z. Risk prediction models for contrast induced nephropathy: Systematic review. *BMJ* **2015**, h4395. [CrossRef]
75. Wilson, T.; Quan, S.; Cheema, K.; Zarnke, K.; Quinn, R.; de Koning, L.; Dixon, E.; Pannu, N.; James, M.T. Risk prediction models for acute kidney injury following major noncardiac surgery: Systematic review. *Nephrol. Dial. Transplant.* **2015**, gfv415. [CrossRef]
76. Hodgson, L.E.; Sarnowski, A.; Roderick, P.J.; Dimitrov, B.D.; Venn, R.M.; Forni, L.G. Systematic review of prognostic prediction models for acute kidney injury (AKI) in general hospital populations. *BMJ Open* **2017**, *7*, e016591. [CrossRef]
77. Malhotra, R.; Kashani, K.B.; Macedo, E.; Kim, J.; Bouchard, J.; Wynn, S.; Li, G.; Ohno-Machado, L.; Mehta, R. A risk prediction score for acute kidney injury in the intensive care unit. *Nephrol. Dial. Transplant.* **2017**, *32*, 814–822. [CrossRef]
78. Koyner, J.L.; Adhikari, R.; Edelson, D.P.; Churpek, M.M. Development of a Multicenter Ward–Based AKI Prediction Model. *Clin. J. Am. Soc. Nephrol.* **2016**, *11*, 1935–1943. [CrossRef]
79. Bedford, M.; Stevens, P.; Coulton, S.; Billings, J.; Farr, M.; Wheeler, T.; Kalli, M.; Mottishaw, T.; Farmer, C. Development of risk models for the prediction of new or worsening acute kidney injury on or during hospital admission: A cohort and nested study. *Health Serv. Deliv. Res.* **2016**, *4*, 1–160. [CrossRef]
80. Forni, L.G.; Dawes, T.; Sinclair, H.; Cheek, E.; Bewick, V.; Dennis, M.; Venn, R. Identifying the Patient at Risk of Acute Kidney Injury: A Predictive Scoring System for the Development of Acute Kidney Injury in Acute Medical Patients. *Nephron Clin. Pract.* **2013**, *123*, 143–150. [CrossRef]
81. Breidthardt, T.; Socrates, T.; Noveanu, M.; Klima, T.; Heinisch, C.; Reichlin, T.; Potocki, M.; Nowak, A.; Tschung, C.; Arenja, N.; et al. Effect and Clinical Prediction of Worsening Renal Function in Acute Decompensated Heart Failure. *Am. J. Cardiol.* **2011**, *107*, 730–735. [CrossRef] [PubMed]
82. Park, S.; Lee, H. Acute kidney injury prediction models. *Curr. Opin. Nephrol. Hypertens.* **2019**, *28*, 552–559. [CrossRef]
83. Flechet, M.; Güiza, F.; Schetz, M.; Wouters, P.; Vanhorebeek, I.; Derese, I.; Gunst, J.; Spriet, I.; Casaer, M.; Van den Berghe, G.; et al. AKIpredictor, an online prognostic calculator for acute kidney injury in adult critically ill patients: Development, validation and comparison to serum neutrophil gelatinase-associated lipocalin. *Intensive Care Med.* **2017**, *43*, 764–773. [CrossRef] [PubMed]
84. Thakar, C.V.; Arrigain, S.; Worley, S.; Yared, J.-P.; Paganini, E.P. A Clinical Score to Predict Acute Renal Failure after Cardiac Surgery. *J. Am. Soc. Nephrol.* **2005**, *16*, 162–168. [CrossRef] [PubMed]

85. Cheungpasitporn, W.; Kashani, K. Electronic Data Systems and Acute Kidney Injury. *Contrib. Nephrol.* **2016**, *187*, 73–83. [CrossRef] [PubMed]
86. James, M.T.; Hobson, C.E.; Darmon, M.; Mohan, S.; Hudson, D.; Goldstein, S.L.; Ronco, C.; Kellum, J.A.; Bagshaw, S.M. Acute Dialysis Quality Initiative (ADQI) Consensus Group. Applications for Detection of Acute Kidney Injury Using Electronic Medical Records and Clinical Information Systems: Workgroup Statements from the 15th ADQI Consensus Conference. *Can. J. Kidney Health Dis.* **2016**, *3*, 100. [CrossRef] [PubMed]
87. Selby, N.M.; Crowley, L.; Fluck, R.J.; McIntyre, C.W.; Monaghan, J.; Lawson, N.; Kolhe, N.V. Use of Electronic Results Reporting to Diagnose and Monitor AKI in Hospitalized Patients. *Clin. J. Am. Soc. Nephrol.* **2012**, *7*, 533–540. [CrossRef]
88. Lachance, P.; Villeneuve, P.-M.; Rewa, O.G.; Wilson, F.P.; Selby, N.M.; Featherstone, R.M.; Bagshaw, S.M. Association between e-alert implementation for detection of acute kidney injury and outcomes: A systematic review. *Nephrol. Dial. Transplant.* **2017**, gfw424. [CrossRef]
89. Kolhe, N.V.; Reilly, T.; Leung, J.; Fluck, R.J.; Swinscoe, K.E.; Selby, N.M.; Taal, M.W. A simple care bundle for use in acute kidney injury: A propensity score-matched cohort study. *Nephrol. Dial. Transplant.* **2016**, *31*, 1846–1854. [CrossRef]
90. Kolhe, N.V.; Staples, D.; Reilly, T.; Merrison, D.; Mcintyre, C.W.; Fluck, R.J.; Selby, N.M.; Taal, M.W. Impact of Compliance with a Care Bundle on Acute Kidney Injury Outcomes: A Prospective Observational Study. *PLoS ONE* **2015**, *10*, e0132279. [CrossRef]
91. Chandrasekar, T.; Sharma, A.; Tennent, L.; Wong, C.; Chamberlain, P.; Abraham, K.A. A whole system approach to improving mortality associated with acute kidney injury. *QJM Int. J. Med.* **2017**, *110*, 657–666. [CrossRef] [PubMed]
92. Hodgson, L.E.; Roderick, P.J.; Venn, R.M.; Yao, G.L.; Dimitrov, B.D.; Forni, L.G. The ICE-AKI study: Impact analysis of a Clinical prediction rule and Electronic AKI alert in general medical patients. *PLoS ONE* **2018**, *13*, e0200584. [CrossRef] [PubMed]
93. Sutherland, S.M.; Chawla, L.S.; Kane-Gill, S.L.; Hsu, R.K.; Kramer, A.A.; Goldstein, S.L.; Kellum, J.A.; Ronco, C.; Bagshaw, S.M. 15 ADQI Consensus Group. Utilizing Electronic Health Records to Predict Acute Kidney Injury Risk and Outcomes: Workgroup Statements from the 15 th ADQI Consensus Conference. *Can. J. Kidney Health Dis.* **2016**, *3*, 99. [CrossRef] [PubMed]
94. Sutherland, S.M.; Goldstein, S.L.; Bagshaw, S.M. Acute Kidney Injury and Big Data. *Contrib. Nephrol.* **2018**, *193*, 55–67. [CrossRef]
95. Hamet, P.; Tremblay, J. Artificial intelligence in medicine. *Metabolism* **2017**, *69*, S36–S40. [CrossRef] [PubMed]
96. Lee, J.-G.; Jun, S.; Cho, Y.-W.; Lee, H.; Kim, G.B.; Seo, J.B.; Kim, N. Deep Learning in Medical Imaging: General Overview. *Korean J. Radiol.* **2017**, *18*, 570. [CrossRef]
97. Kulikowski, C.A. Beginnings of Artificial Intelligence in Medicine (AIM): Computational Artifice Assisting Scientific Inquiry and Clinical Art—With Reflections on Present AIM Challenges. *Yearb. Med. Inform.* **2019**, *28*, 249–256. [CrossRef]
98. LeCun, Y.; Bengio, Y.; Hinton, G. Deep learning. *Nature* **2015**, *521*, 436–444. [CrossRef]
99. Collins, G.S.; Reitsma, J.B.; Altman, D.G.; Moons, K.G.M. Transparent Reporting of a multivariable prediction model for Individual Prognosis Or Diagnosis (TRIPOD): The TRIPOD Statement. *Ann. Intern. Med.* **2015**, *162*, 55. [CrossRef]
100. Lin, K.; Hu, Y.; Kong, G. Predicting in-hospital mortality of patients with acute kidney injury in the ICU using random forest model. *Int. J. Med. Inform.* **2019**, *125*, 55–61. [CrossRef]
101. Wilson, F.P. Machine Learning to Predict Acute Kidney Injury. *Am. J. Kidney Dis.* **2019**. [CrossRef]
102. Kate, R.J.; Perez, R.M.; Mazumdar, D.; Pasupathy, K.S.; Nilakantan, V. Prediction and detection models for acute kidney injury in hospitalized older adults. *BMC Med. Inform. Decis. Mak.* **2016**, *16*, 39. [CrossRef] [PubMed]
103. Thottakkara, P.; Ozrazgat-Baslanti, T.; Hupf, B.B.; Rashidi, P.; Pardalos, P.; Momcilovic, P.; Bihorac, A. Application of Machine Learning Techniques to High-Dimensional Clinical Data to Forecast Postoperative Complications. *PLoS ONE* **2016**, *11*, e0155705. [CrossRef] [PubMed]
104. Davis, S.E.; Lasko, T.A.; Chen, G.; Siew, E.D.; Matheny, M.E. Calibration drift in regression and machine learning models for acute kidney injury. *J. Am. Med. Inform. Assoc.* **2017**, *24*, 1052–1061. [CrossRef] [PubMed]

105. Cheng, P.; Waitman, L.R.; Hu, Y.; Liu, M. Predicting Inpatient Acute Kidney Injury over Different Time Horizons: How Early and Accurate? *AMIA Annu. Symp. Proc.* **2017**, *2017*, 565–574. Available online: http://www.ncbi.nlm.nih.gov/pubmed/29854121 (accessed on 20 January 2020).
106. Ibrahim, N.E.; McCarthy, C.P.; Shrestha, S.; Gaggin, H.K.; Mukai, R.; Magaret, C.A.; Rhyne, R.F.; Januzzi, J.L., Jr. A clinical, proteomics, and artificial intelligence-driven model to predict acute kidney injury in patients undergoing coronary angiography. *Clin. Cardiol.* **2019**, *42*, 292–298. [CrossRef]
107. Koola, J.D.; Davis, S.E.; Al-Nimri, O.; Parr, S.K.; Fabbri, D.; Malin, B.A.; Ho, S.B.; Matheny, M.E. Development of an automated phenotyping algorithm for hepatorenal syndrome. *J. Biomed. Inform.* **2018**, *80*, 87–95. [CrossRef]
108. Koyner, J.L.; Carey, K.A.; Edelson, D.P.; Churpek, M.M. The Development of a Machine Learning Inpatient Acute Kidney Injury Prediction Model. *Crit. Care Med.* **2018**, *46*, 1070–1077. [CrossRef]
109. Huang, C.; Murugiah, K.; Mahajan, S.; Li, S.X.; Dhruva, S.S.; Haimovich, J.S.; Wang, Y.; Schulz, W.L.; Testani, J.M.; Wilson, F.P.; et al. Enhancing the prediction of acute kidney injury risk after percutaneous coronary intervention using machine learning techniques: A retrospective cohort study. Rahimi K, ed. *PLoS Med.* **2018**, *15*, e1002703. [CrossRef]
110. Huang, C.; Li, S.-X.; Mahajan, S.; Testani, J.M.; Wilson, F.P.; Mena, C.I.; Masoudi, F.A.; Rumsfeld, J.S.; Spertus, J.A.; Mortazavi, B.J.; et al. Development and Validation of a Model for Predicting the Risk of Acute Kidney Injury Associated With Contrast Volume Levels During Percutaneous Coronary Intervention. *JAMA Netw. Open* **2019**, *2*, e1916021. [CrossRef]
111. Tomašev, N.; Glorot, X.; Rae, J.W.; Zielinski, M.; Askham, H.; Saraiva, A.; Mottram, A.; Meyer, C.; Ravuri, S.; Protsyuk, I.; et al. A clinically applicable approach to continuous prediction of future acute kidney injury. *Nature* **2019**, *572*, 116–119. [CrossRef]
112. Adhikari, L.; Ozrazgat-Baslanti, T.; Ruppert, M.; Madushani, R.W.M.A.; Paliwal, S.; Hashemighouchani, H.; Zheng, F.; Tao, M.; Lopes, J.M.; Li, X.; et al. Improved predictive models for acute kidney injury with IDEA: Intraoperative Data Embedded Analytics. *PLoS ONE* **2019**, *14*, e0214904. [CrossRef] [PubMed]
113. Flechet, M.; Falini, S.; Bonetti, C.; Güiza, F.; Schetz, M.; Van den Berghe, G.; Meyfroidt, G. Machine learning versus physicians' prediction of acute kidney injury in critically ill adults: A prospective evaluation of the AKIpredictor. *Crit. Care* **2019**, *23*, 282. [CrossRef] [PubMed]
114. Parreco, J.; Soe-Lin, H.; Parks, J.J.; Byerly, S.; Chatoor, M.; Buicko, J.L.; Namias, N.; Rattan, R. Comparing Machine Learning Algorithms for Predicting Acute Kidney Injury. *Am. Surg.* **2019**, *85*, 725–729. Available online: http://www.ncbi.nlm.nih.gov/pubmed/31405416 (accessed on 20 January 2020). [PubMed]
115. Xu, Z.; Luob, Y.; Adekkanattua, P.; Ancker, J.S.; Jiang, G.; Kiefer, R.C.; Pacheco, J.A.; Rasmussen, L.V.; Pathak, J.; Wang, F. Stratified Mortality Prediction of Patients with Acute Kidney Injury in Critical Care. *Stud. Health Technol. Inform.* **2019**, *264*, 462–466.
116. Tran, N.K.; Sen, S.; Palmieri, T.L.; Lima, K.; Falwell, S.; Wajda, J.; Rashidi, H.H. Artificial intelligence and machine learning for predicting acute kidney injury in severely burned patients: A proof of concept. *Burns* **2019**, *45*, 1350–1358. [CrossRef]
117. Zhang, Z.; Ho, K.M.; Hong, Y. Machine learning for the prediction of volume responsiveness in patients with oliguric acute kidney injury in critical care. *Crit. Care* **2019**, *23*, 112. [CrossRef]
118. Zimmerman, L.P.; Reyfman, P.A.; Smith, A.D.R.; Zeng, Z.; Kho, A.; Sanchez-Pinto, L.N.; Luo, Y. Early prediction of acute kidney injury following ICU admission using a multivariate panel of physiological measurements. *BMC Med. Inform. Decis. Mak.* **2019**, *19* (Suppl. S1), 16. [CrossRef]
119. Rashidi, H.H.; Sen, S.; Palmieri, T.L.; Blackmon, T.; Wajda, J.; Tran, N.K. Early Recognition of Burn- and Trauma-Related Acute Kidney Injury: A Pilot Comparison of Machine Learning Techniques. *Sci. Rep.* **2020**, *10*, 205. [CrossRef]

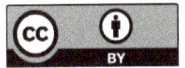

© 2020 by the authors. Licensee MDPI, Basel, Switzerland. This article is an open access article distributed under the terms and conditions of the Creative Commons Attribution (CC BY) license (http://creativecommons.org/licenses/by/4.0/).

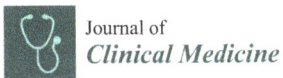

Article

Torquetenovirus Serum Load and Long-Term Outcomes in Renal Transplant Recipients

Edmund J. Gore [1,*], António W. Gomes-Neto [2], Lei Wang [3], Stephan J. L. Bakker [2], Hubert G. M. Niesters [1], Anoek A. E. de Joode [2], Erik A. M. Verschuuren [4], Johanna Westra [3] and Coretta Van Leer-Buter [1]

1. Department of Medical Microbiology, Rijksuniversiteit Groningen, University Medical Centre Groningen, 9713GZ Groningen, The Netherlands; h.g.m.niesters@umcg.nl (H.G.M.N.); c.van.leer@umcg.nl (C.V.L.-B.)
2. Department of Internal Medicine, Rijksuniversiteit Groningen, University Medical Centre Groningen, 9713GZ Groningen, The Netherlands; a.w.gomes.neto@umcg.nl (A.W.G.-N.); s.j.l.bakker@umcg.nl (S.J.L.B.); a.a.e.joode@umcg.nl (A.A.E.d.J.)
3. Department of Rheumatology and Clinical Immunology, Rijksuniversiteit Groningen, University Medical Centre Groningen, 9713GZ Groningen, The Netherlands; l.wang@umcg.nl (L.W.); johanna.westra@umcg.nl (J.W.)
4. Department of Pulmonology, Rijksuniversiteit Groningen, University Medical Centre Groningen, 9713GZ Groningen, The Netherlands; e.a.m.verschuuren@umcg.nl
* Correspondence: e.j.gore@umcg.nl; Tel.: +31-(0)-50-36-17-535

Received: 29 December 2019; Accepted: 4 February 2020; Published: 6 February 2020

Abstract: Following transplantation, patients must take immunosuppressive medication for life. Torquetenovirus (TTV) is thought to be marker for immunosuppression, and TTV–DNA levels after organ transplantation have been investigated, showing high TTV levels, associated with increased risk of infections, and low TTV levels associated with increased risk of rejection. However, this has been investigated in studies with relatively short follow-up periods. We hypothesized that TTV levels can be used to assess long term outcomes after renal transplantation. Serum samples of 666 renal transplant recipients were tested for TTV DNA. Samples were taken at least one year after renal transplantation, when TTV levels are thought to be relatively stable. Patient data was reviewed for graft failure, all-cause mortality and death due to infectious causes. Our data indicates that high TTV levels, sampled more than one year post-transplantation, are associated with all-cause mortality with a hazard ratio (HR) of 1.12 (95% CI, 1.02–1.23) per $\log_{10}$ increase in TTV viral load, ($p = 0.02$). Additionally, high TTV levels were also associated with death due to infectious causes (HR 1.20 (95% CI 1.01–1.43), $p = 0.04$). TTV levels decrease in the years following renal transplantation, but remain elevated longer than previously thought. This study shows that TTV level may aid in predicting long-term outcomes, all-cause mortality and death due to an infectious cause in renal transplant patients sampled over one year post-transplantation.

Keywords: torquetenovirus; immunosuppression; transplantation; immunosuppressed host; outcome; renal transplantation

1. Introduction

Immunosuppressive therapy is vital for organ transplantation medicine; in the last 20 years, antirejection treatment has improved enormously thanks to the increased availability of new antirejection drugs. All these drugs, however, lead to some degree of immunosuppression, and subsequently increased infection risk. Measuring trough levels of antirejection drugs is currently standard of care in determining the optimal dosing of these drugs, but is well recognized that these trough levels do not accurately reflect the risk of under-immunosuppression, potentially resulting in rejection, or over-immunosuppression, potentially resulting in increased infections [1–3]. It is, therefore, important to identify the parameters that reflect the net immune status and have predictive capacities for long-term outcomes. Torquetenovirus (TTV) is a single stranded, negative sense, non-encapsulated DNA virus; it was first discovered in 1997 by Nishizawa et al. [4–6] and is present in 46%–100% of healthy people [7]. The international commission on taxonomy (ICTV) recognizes 29 different genotypes, but their relative circulation has not been researched sufficiently [8]. Attempts to discover viable antibody assays have been hampered by the hypervariable nature of the viral capsid protein [9]. A few assays have been described by various groups; however, these assays have not proven to be scalable for large-scale clinical use [9–11]. In recent years, TTV has been studied by various research groups as a potential marker of immunosuppression following transplantation. TTV levels have been shown to increase at the start of antirejection treatment, reaching a relative plateau phase between 3 and 6 months after transplantation [12]. It is currently thought that an ideal viral loads exists for each type of organ transplantation, signifying optimal antirejection dosing. Viral loads above this ideal level have been shown to increase the chance of infections, whereas low viral loads have been shown to be associated with increased chance of rejection [13]. No formal cut-off TTV levels for optimal immunosuppression have been established, however, since these levels show great variation between different research groups, even in seemingly similar patient populations. These variations may be due to differences in circulation of TTV genotypes or due to differences in the PCR test used in these studies.

Additionally, most studies have looked at longitudinal TTV measurements relatively shortly after transplantation. The follow-up periods have also been brief, usually up to one year after solid organ transplantation (SOT). The immunosuppressed condition of these patients and the increased risk of infection nevertheless persists for a lifetime. To date, very little is known about TTV levels past the first year after transplantation, and if these TTV levels are associated with increased risk of infection or rejection in the long term. In this study, we focused on TTV measurements after the first year following renal transplantation, and hypothesized that TTV levels are associated with outcome over several years. We studied this in a cohort of 666 renal transplant recipients.

2. Materials and Methods

2.1. Study Population

This cohort study was based on a previously described set of 706 renal transplant recipients [14,15]. Included were patients (aged ≥ 18 years) who visited the outpatient clinic of the University Medical Centre Groningen (UMCG), Groningen, the Netherlands, between November 2008 and June 2011, and who had a graft that had been functioning for at least one year with no history of alcohol and/or drug addiction. Of 706 renal transplant recipients that provided written informed consent, we excluded subjects with missing biomaterial (40 cases) from further analyses, which resulted in 666 cases eligible for study. The study protocol was approved by the UMCG institutional review board (METc 2008/186); clinical trials number NCT02811835 and adhered to the Declarations of Helsinki and Istanbul.

2.2. TTV Viral Load Measurements

Serum samples were stored at −80 °C, until analysis. One serum sample per patient was used; this was collected at enrollment. DNA was extracted from thawed serum samples using the eMAG Nucleic Acid Extraction System (bioMerieux, Marcy, France). The Argene R-Gene TTV quantification kit (bioMerieux, Marcy, France) was used to perform qPCR on an Applied Biosystems 7500 (Thermo fisher, Waltham, MA, USA) according to the manufacturer's instructions. Due to limited sample volumes, 100 µL, a 1 in 4 dilution using DMEM, was performed prior to sample extraction (ThermoFisher, Waltham, MA, USA). A control experiment (data not shown) showed no significant differences in the Ct values. The R gene assay is designed to detect TTV genotypes 1, 6, 7, 8, 10, 12, 15, 16, 19, 27 and 28 [16–18].

2.3. Clinical End Points

The primary endpoint of this study was all-cause mortality, death due to infectious causes and death-censored graft failure as secondary aims. Deaths due to infectious causes were defined using the previously specified list of International Classification of Diseases, Ninth Revision, codes 1–139 [19,20]. For example, a patient meeting the criteria, which is positive culture or PCR for *Pneumocystis jiroveci* infection, would be given the code 136.3 and would therefore be classified as dying due to an infection. Graft failure was defined as return to dialysis therapy or re-transplantation. The cause of graft failure was obtained from patient records and was reviewed by a blinded nephrologist. Endpoints were recorded until the end of September 2015 and there was no loss of subjects to follow-up.

2.4. Data Analysis

Data analyses were performed using SPSS 23.0 for Windows (SPSS Inc., Chicago, IL, USA) and R (R Foundation for Statistical Computing, Vienna, Austria). As no cut-off values for low, medium and high TTV load have been established, and to avoid bias, renal transplant recipients were stratified into three equally sized groups based on serum TTV. This created four groups, named undetectable-TTV, low-TTV, medium-TTV, and high-TTV, which were further analyzed. Differences in all-cause mortality, death due to infectious causes and graft failure between the four groups were compared using Kaplan–Meier plots and log rank tests. Data are presented as mean ± SD for normally distributed data, as median [interquartile range (IQR)] for non-normally distributed data, and as number (percentage) for nominal data. *t*-Tests, or one-way ANOVA tests with Tukey post-hoc tests, were performed on normally distributed data. Each group was compared with the other three groups. Kruskal–Wallis or Mann–Whitney U tests were performed on non-normally distributed data. Chi-square tests were used on categorical data. A two-sided $p < 0.05$ was considered to indicate statistical significance in all analyses.

Prospective associations of TTV on study endpoints were explored by means of Cox regression analysis. Risk of all-cause mortality, death due to infectious causes and graft failure are presented as HR [95% confidence interval]. In these analyses, associations were adjusted in a cumulative fashion for potential confounders, including age, sex, eGFR, proteinuria (model 1), time since transplantation (model 2) and the number of immunosuppressant medications taken (model 3). Cox regression models were built in a stepwise fashion to avoid over-fitting. The proportionality of hazards for covariates was investigated by inspecting the Schoenfeld residuals. eGFR and age were included as categorical variables with equal numbers of events in each group, as eGFR and age breached the proportionality of hazards assumption as continuous variables.

The optimal cutoff values for death due to infectious causes was identified by using Youden's Index [21] in the area under receiver operating characteristics (auROC) curve. This approach was not used for all-cause mortality as the threshold was biologically unrealistic, therefore a sensitivity of 75% was set and the threshold was calculated. Sampling by replacement was used to create 1000 bootstrapped samples of equal size from within the study population, this was then used within our multivariate Cox regression models to validate the association of the TTV DNA thresholds with risk.

To assess in further detail how TTV levels change over time, and to validate our TTV test in patients with older transplants, the patients were subdivided into two groups. The first group had had a transplant 12 to 24 months prior to analysis. The 2nd group had had transplants over 24 months prior to analysis. Cox regression analysis was also performed as previously described.

3. Results

3.1. Recipient Demographics

There was a median 4.9 [IQR 3.4–5.5] years of follow-up for our study population, with 117 (18%) of renal transplant recipients having undetectable TTV, 183 (27%) having low TTV, (median 1.52 (IQR 1.00–1.85) Log_{10} copies/mL), 184 (28%) medium TTV, (median 3.00 (IQR 2.61–3.40) Log_{10} copies/mL), and 182 (27%) high TTV, (median 5.52 (IQR 4.08–5.27) Log_{10}copies/mL) (Table 1). Median time from transplant to TTV sampling was different for each group; undetectable TTV 7.1 (IQR 4.0–12.4) years, low TTV 6.4 (IQR 3.1–11.0) years, medium TTV 5.3 (IQR 2.2–14.3) years and high TTV 3.2 (1.0–9.0) years ($p < 0.001$).

Table 1. Recipient demographics.

	Undetectable TTV	Low	Medium	High	p
Number of Patients (%)	117 (18)	183 (27)	184 (28)	182 (27)	
Age (years)	49 ± 14 *a	53 ± 16	53 ± 13	55 ± 12	0.01 *
Male (%)	57 (49)	103 (56)	106 (58)	112 (62)	0.18
Weight (Kg)	77 ± 15	81 ± 16	81 ± 16	81 ± 18	0.15
BMI (Kg/m^2)	26.0 ± 4.3	26.6 ± 4.5	27.0 ± 5.1	26.8 ± 5.0	0.33
Renal Function					
Serum creatine (umol/L)	132 ± 67	135 ± 63	138 ± 57	145 ± 54	0.23
eGFR (mL/1.73 m^2)	50 ± 20 *b	47 ± 20 *b	45 ± 18	40 ± 16 *b	<0.001 *
Urinary protein excretion (g/24 h)	0.18 (0.00–0.27)	0.20 (0.00–0.41)	0.19 (0.00–0.47)	0.19 (0.00–0.47)	0.49
Proteinuria present, n (%)	21 (18)	42 (23)	46 (25)	40 (22)	0.57
Albuminuria (mg/24 h)	41 (8–144)	43 (11–189)	42 (12–235)	36 (9–202)	0.94
Transplantation					
Living Donation, n (%)	45 (39)	62 (34)	69 (38)	56 (31)	0.45
Warm Ischemic Time (minutes)	42 ± 17	43 ± 15	43 ± 16	44 ± 13	0.53
Cold Ischaemic Time (hours)	13 ± 10	14 ± 10	14 ± 11	15 ± 10	0.56
HLA I Antibodies, n (%)	9 (8)	33 (18)	26 (14)	33 (18)	0.05
HLA II Antibodies, n (%)	20 (17)	37 (20)	33 (18)	25 (14)	0.43
Transplant vintage (years)	7.1 (4.0–12.4)	6.4 (3.1–11.0)	5.3 (2.2–14.3)	3.2 (1.0–9.0)	<0.001
Acute rejection, n (%)	24 (21)	54 (30)	58 (32)	38 (21)	0.04
Medication					
Mono-therapy, n (%)	4 (3)	11 (6)	4 (2)	4 (2)	0.15
Dual-therapy, n (%)	82 (70)	107 (59)	94 (51)	78 (43)	0.01
Triple-therapy, n (%)	31 (27)	65 (36)	86 (47)	100 (55)	<0.001
Prednisolone dose (mg/day)	7.5 (7.5–10)	10 (7.5–10)	10 (7.5–10)	10 (7.5–10)	0.02
MTOR inhibitors, n (%)	3 (3)	9 (5)	3 (2)	3 (2)	0.17
Cyclosporin, n (%)	24 (21)	62 (34)	82 (45)	91 (50)	<0.001
Tacrolimus, n (%)	18 (15)	24 (13)	30 (16)	46 (25)	0.03
Azathioprine, n (%)	25 (21)	27 (15)	38 (21)	23 (13)	0.15
Mycophenolate, n (%)	79 (68)	126 (69)	117 (64)	120 (66)	0.94
End Points					
All-cause mortality	6.3 (6.1–6.5)	6.2 (6.0–6.4)	6.0 (5.7–6.2)	5.7 (5.4–6.0)	0.001
Infectious Death	6.6 (6.5–6.8)	6.6 (6.5–6.8)	6.7 (6.5–6.8)	6.4 (6.2–6.6)	0.08
Graft Failure	6.1 (5.8–6.4)	6.5 (6.3–6.6)	6.3 (6.0–6.5)	6.3 (6.0–6.5)	0.5

* a Tukey post-hoc undetectable TTV vs. TTV low, medium, high groups $p = 0.01$. * b Tukey post-hoc undetectable TTV vs. TTV low group $p < 0.001$. BMI: body mass index, eGFR: estimated glomerular filtration rate, MTOR: mammalian target of Rapamycine.

The median prednisolone dose taken by the patients was different across the groups, 7.5 mg/day for the undetectable TTV group and 10 mg/day for low, medium, high groups ($p = 0.02$). The numbers of renal transplant recipients on calcineurin inhibitors (CNIs) were different across the groups with 36%, 47%, 61% and 75% for undetectable, low, medium and high ($p < 0.001$), respectively. There were comparable numbers of renal transplant recipients on proliferation inhibitors in each group ($p = 0.13$). Twenty-three recipients were on mono-therapy, 361 on dual-therapy and 282 were on triple-therapy post-transplant. Renal transplant recipients on mono-therapy had a lower median TTV 1.67 (IQR 0.71–2.68) Log_{10}copies/mL, than recipients on dual-therapy 2.1 (IQR 0.48–3.52) Log_{10}copies/mL, or on triple-therapy 3.06 (IQR 2.57–4.22) Log_{10}copies/mL.

There were no differences between the groups in regard to the type of donation (living vs. post mortal, $p = 0.45$), warm ischemic time ($p = 0.53$), cold ischemic time ($p = 0.55$) or proteinuria ($p = 0.57$). The patient demographics are represented in Table 1.

3.2. TTV and All-Cause Mortality

Patient mortality was attributed to a variety of causes, with a total of 141 patient deaths. Fifty-eight patients (41%) died due to a cardiovascular event and 40 (28%) died due to an infection. Most infectious deaths were caused by bacteria, with 29 events, five viral illness events, two fungal infections, and finally four patients died with multiple organisms. An additional 21 patients died due to malignancy and 22 due to miscellaneous causes.

We observed differences in all-cause mortality across the four categories of TTV status (log-rank test $p < 0.001$) (Figure 1A). Fourteen (12%), 30 (16%), 44 (24%), and 53 (29%) died in the undetectable group, the low group, the medium group and the high group, respectively. Time to death was shortest for the high TTV group with 5.7 (5.4–6.0) years. This compares to 6.0 (5.7–6.2) years, 6.2 (6.0–6.4) years and 6.3 (6.1–6.5) years for the medium, low and undetectable groups, respectively. As the time between transplantation and sampling was significantly shorter in the high-TTV group, it was possible that the differences in mortality and time to death were caused by disproportionally high mortality in the early years after transplantation, a period which was not observed for the patients in the low-TTV group, who were not included in the study until a median of 6.4 years after transplantation. We therefore determined the death rate within six years after transplantation and overall in the different TTV-level groups. This did not show a significant change in death rate during the follow-up period. The death rate in the first six years after transplantation was 16% in the low-TTV group and 18% overall in the follow-up period. In the high-TTV group, the mortality was 24% in the first six years after transplantation and 33% overall. It is therefore unlikely that the high all-cause mortality in the high-TTV group was attributable to the relatively early inclusion of these patients as compared to the low-TTV group. Log TTV is significantly associated with all-cause mortality in renal transplant recipients (HR 1.12 (95%CI 1.02–1.23), $p = 0.02$ per $\log_{10}$ increase in TTV), independent of potential confounders including age, gender, eGFR, time since transplantation and number of immunosuppressant medications taken (Figure 2A). Using Youden's index, we calculated the sensitivity and specificity of a single TTV measurement, using a cut-off TTV level of 3.65 $\text{Log}_{10}\text{copies/mL}$ for identifying patients with increased chance of death; the specificity was 75% and sensitivity was 40%.

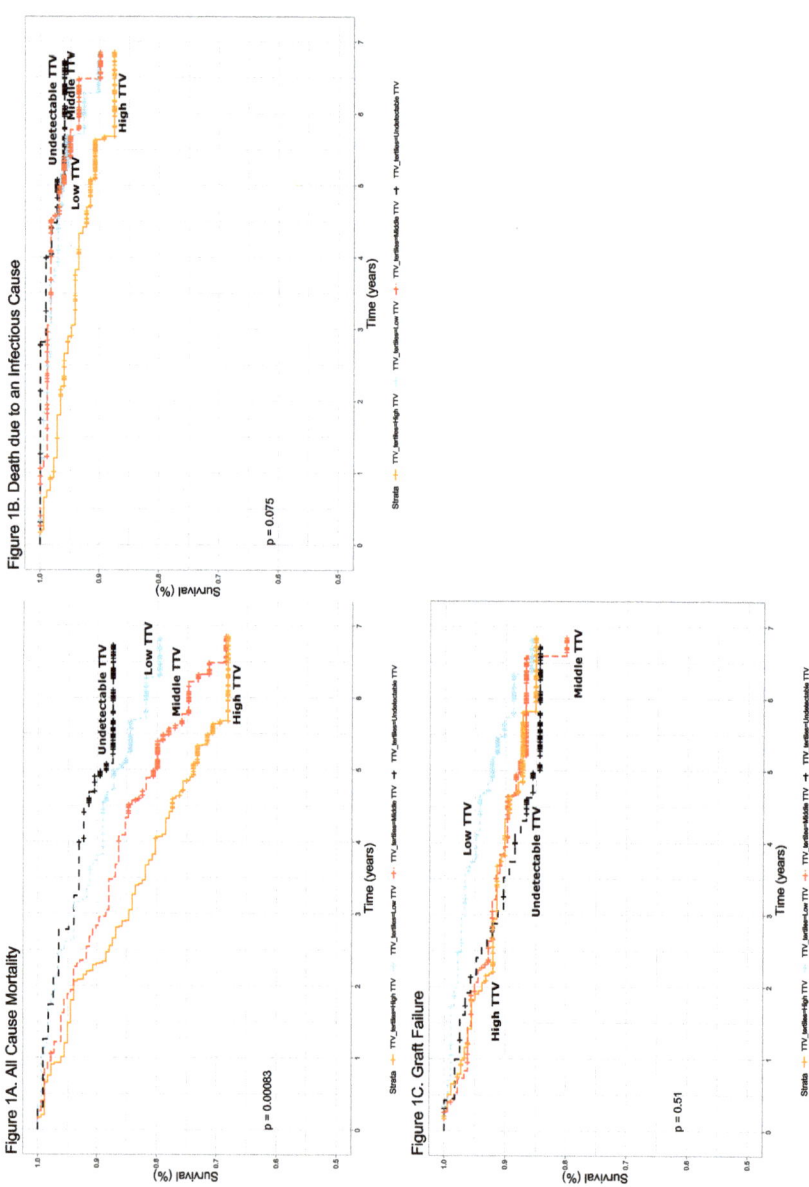

Figure 1. Kaplan–Meier plots showing differences in survival (**A**,**B**), and graft failure (**C**) over time between undetectable low torquetenovirus TTV (black), low TTV (light blue), medium TTV (red) and high TTV (orange), as measured in a serum sample tested at least 12 months after transplantation. Time from testing is displayed (**A**) All-cause mortality ($p < 0.001$, (**B**) Death due to infectious causes ($p = 0.08$), (**C**) graft survival ($p = 0.51$).

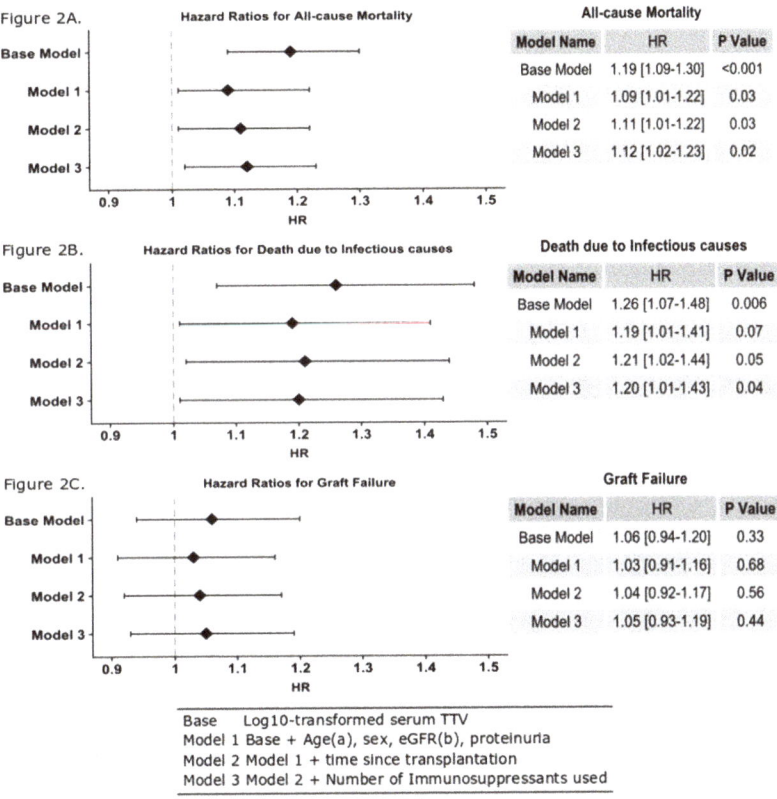

Figure 2. Hazard ratios calculated using Cox models and presented as a forest plot. (**A**) Log_{10} TTV is predictive of all-cause mortality after adjustment for age, gender, eGFR proteinuria, time since transplant and the number of immunosuppressant's used. This means that for each log increase in TTV, there is a 12% increase for a patient's risk of death (HR 1.12 (95% CI 1.0.2–1.23), $p = 0.02$). (**B**) Log_{10} TTV is predictive of death due to an infectious cause after adjustment for age, gender, eGFR proteinuria, time since transplant and the number of immunosuppressant's used. This means that for each log increase in TTV, there is a 20% increase for a patient's risk of death (HR 1.20 (95% CI 1.01–1.43), $p = 0.04$). (**C**) Log_{10} TTV is not predictive of graft failure after adjustment for age, gender, eGFR, proteinuria, time since transplant and the number of immunosuppressant's used. [a] Categorical variable used for death due to an infectious cause. [b] Categorical variable used for all-cause mortality and graft failure.

3.3. TTV and Death Due to a Cause

As over-immunosuppression is associated with risk of infection, we investigated the relationship between TTV levels and death due to infectious cause. In the TTV-undetectable group, four (3%) patients died from infections, whereas, 10 (6%), nine (5%) and 17 (9%) renal transplant recipients died in low group, the medium group and the high group, respectively (log-rank $p = 0.08$, Figure 1B) (Table 1). Mean time to death due to an infectious cause was not significantly different between the groups, i.e., for the undetectable group this was 6.6 (6.5–6.8) years, for the low-TTV group 6.6 (6.5–6.8) years, medium-TTV group 6.7 (6.5–6.8) years and high-TTV group 6.4 (6.2–6.6) years. Furthermore, we observed that log TTV is significantly associated with death due to infections (HR 1.20 (95% CI 1.01–1.43), $p = 0.04$), independent of potential confounders (Figure 2B). Using Youden's index, we determined that a single TTV measurement with a level over 3.38 Log_{10}copies/mL identified patients at risk of death due to infections with a sensitivity of 55%, and a specificity of 67%.

3.4. TTV and Graft Failure

We also observed no difference in mean graft survival across the four groups, ($p = 0.51$, Figure 1C). The numbers of patients with graft failure was not significantly different across the four groups, with 17 (15%), 17 (9%), 23 (13%) and 22 (12%) for the undetectable group, the low group, the medium group and the high group respectively ($p = 0.57$). This result is replicated when looking at the Cox model data (HR 1.01 (95% CI 0.93–1.19) $p = 0.44$, Figure 2C).

3.5. Time since Transplantation and TTV

Because there is limited data on TTV levels in renal transplant recipients beyond the first year after transplantation, we divided our transplant population into two groups. One group which were sampled 12–24 months post-transplant ($n = 164$ patients) and the other over 24 months since transplant ($n = 502$ patients). This showed that TTV levels up to 24 months from transplantation were significantly higher than TTV levels in patients 2–3 years, 3–4 years, 4–5 years and over five years from transplantation ($p < 0.05$) (Figure 3).

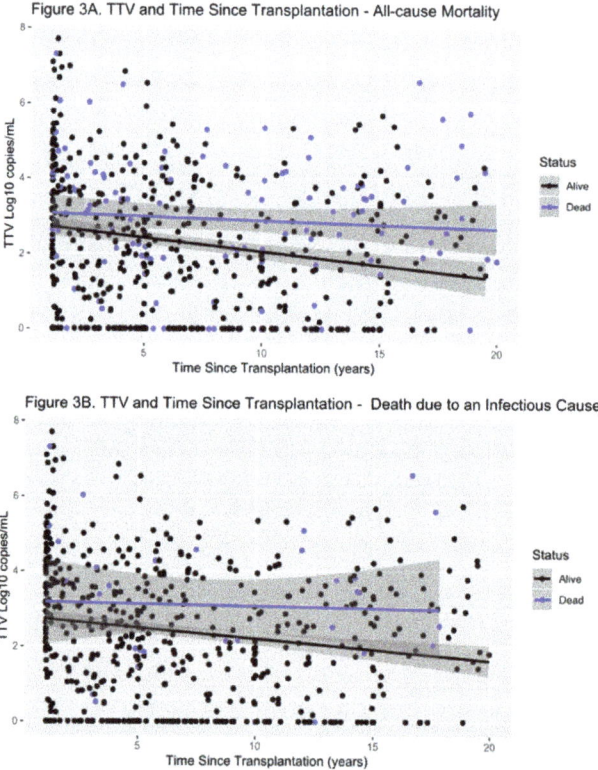

Figure 3. Scatter plot showing levels of TTV in our transplant patients and their outcomes in all-cause mortality (**A**), and death due to infectious causes (**B**). TTV levels are higher in the first years after transplantation than in later years. Patients with worse outcome show a trend of higher TTV levels over the entire follow-up period.

TTV measured within 24 months of transplantation was not associated with an increased risk of death by all causes of due to an infectious cause (Figure 4).

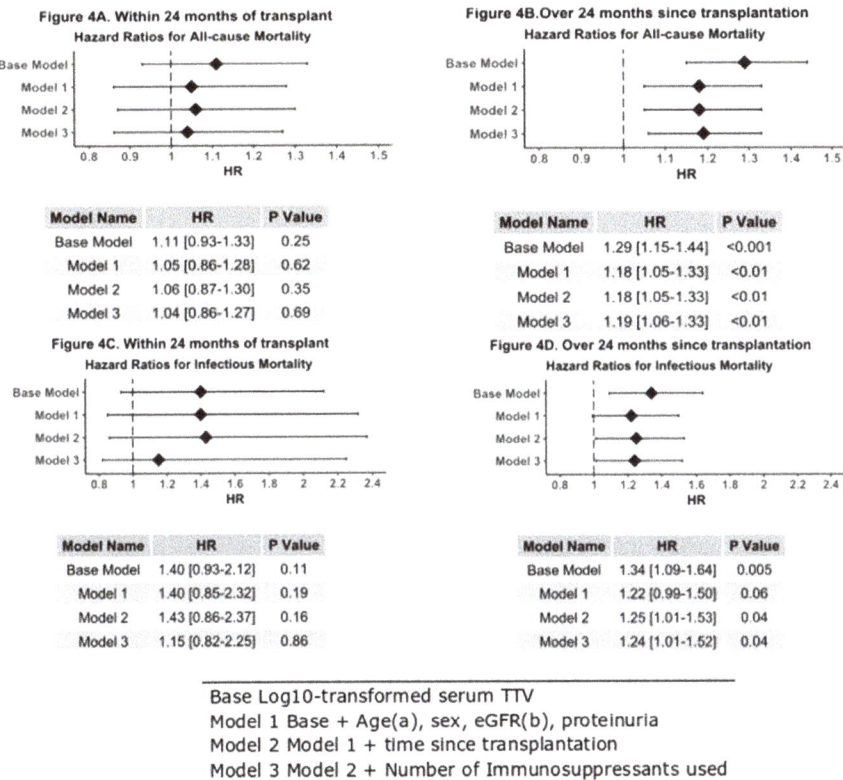

Base Log10-transformed serum TTV
Model 1 Base + Age(a), sex, eGFR(b), proteinuria
Model 2 Model 1 + time since transplantation
Model 3 Model 2 + Number of Immunosuppressants used

Figure 4. Forest plots with hazard table of Cox models after adjustment for age, gender, eGFR proteinuria, and the number of immunosuppressant's used. (**A**) All-cause mortality in patients transplanted within 24 months of TTV analysis; this includes 31 events. Log_{10} TTV cannot be used to predict risk of death transplanted within 24 months of TTV analysis. (**B**) All-cause mortality in patients tested over 24 months after transplantation, this includes 110 events. Log_{10} TTV is highly predictive of the risk of death for patients with elevated TTV (HR 1.19 (95%CI 1.06–1.33), $p < 0.01$). (**C**) Log_{10} TTV is not predictive of death due to an infectious cause in patients tested over 24 months since transplantation (HR 1.15 (95% CI 0.82–2.25), $p = 0.86$). (**D**) Log_{10} TTV is predictive of death due to an infectious cause in patients 24 months after transplantation (HR 1.24 (95%CI 1.01–1.52), $p = 0.04$). [a] Categorical variable used for death due to an infectious cause. [b] Categorical variable used for all-cause mortality.

On the contrary, TTV measured in patients over 24 months from transplantation show that there is a significant difference in survival between patients with high, medium, low or undetectable TTV ($p < 0.001$, Figure 4). Cox modeling also shows an increased all-cause mortality when adjusting for age, gender, eGFR, and number of immunosuppressant medications taken (HR 1.18 (95% CI 0.05–1.33), $p < 0.004$). Time to death due to death due infectious causes is also shorter in the high-TTV population that are over 24 months post-transplant ($p = 0.04$, Figure 4C). This conclusion is supported by Cox analysis (HR 1.24 (1.01–1.52), $p = 0.04$). Graft failure again shows no relationship with measured TTV either within 24 months after transplantation or thereafter.

4. Discussion

In recent years, the use of TTV levels as a means to gauge immunosuppression has been investigated by several groups. Most of this research has used longitudinal samples taken relatively shortly after transplantation and has been aimed to predict either infection risk, due to over-immunosuppression, or rejection, due to under-immunosuppression, during the first post-transplant year. These studies have shown mixed results, with some reporting elevated TTV in patients who subsequently died of sepsis and a higher risk of CMV reactivation in patients with high TTV levels [22–25], while others showed no connection between TTV and the overall risk of infection [26]. A reason for this apparent discrepancy may be that non-specified "risk for infection" is difficult to assess, because infections are diverse and may not be observed by the transplantation center but by referring hospitals and general practitioners instead, but may also be because TTV levels are only related to certain types of infections. Because we were interested in the relationship between TTV levels and long-term outcome after renal transplantation, we focused on all-cause mortality and death due to infectious causes, as this information can be traced reliably. We found that high TTV levels are associated with both all-cause mortality and with death due to infections. The excess mortality in the high TTV group was not attributable to other factors such as age, gender, eGFR, number of immunosuppressive medications used, proteinuria and years after transplantation. Our findings suggest that TTV-levels may be predictive of much longer-term outcomes then have been investigated thus far. Other studies have shown that a relative plateau phase in TTV levels is reached in most patients, after a first period of increasing TTV levels caused by induction immunosuppression, and subsequent tapering to maintenance therapy [17]. Our study suggests that sampling during this relative plateau phase could be useful in identifying patients at risk of adverse outcomes. However, our study also suggests the relative plateau phase is relative indeed, as the TTV-levels show a decreasing trend after this first year which continues until a final stable phase develops after 24 months, and that high TTV levels are especially predictive of long-term adverse outcome if samples are taken after 24 months.

Several papers have been published looking at the role of TTV in graft failure in different types of organ transplantation [22,27–31]. A role for TTV measurements in predicting antibody mediated rejection in renal transplantation was suggested, with lower levels of TTV found to correlate with this type of rejection [31–33]. Likewise, TTV levels were also shown to be significantly lower before the diagnosis of chronic lung allograft dysfunction in lung transplant patients [31]. These results support the theory that lower levels of TTV are a risk factor for graft failure. In our study, we did not find an association between TTV and graft failure. The main reason for this may be that we looked at patients a minimum of 12 months after transplantation, past the period which represents the highest risk for acute rejection [2,34,35]. This means we likely removed several patients with a risk of rejection, reducing our power to detect rejection. Another reason for the lack of association between TTV levels and graft failure is may be that graft failure is also caused by non-immunogenic factors such as vascular damage, which TTV is unlikely to be associated with.

Although our study investigated the use of a single TTV measurement for predicting outcome after renal transplantation, and was able to show a relationship in a large group, we do not consider this method accurate enough for use in individual patients. The sensitivity and specificity of a single measurement in identifying patients with increased risk of death is so low that no real conclusions could be drawn. The cut-off TTV level which should alert clinicians to potential over immunosuppression has not become clear from this study. Our calculated cut-offs for mortality risk and infectious mortality risk are similar to the ones calculated by Fernandez-Ruiz. et al. for increased risk of infections (i.e., 3–4 Log copies/mL) [36] but are much lower than the values suggested by other authors by several orders of magnitude [22,37]. These differences stress the need for TTV assay standardization and make it difficult to draw a consensus opinion as to clinically relevant TTV viral load measurements, which would warrant action.

Nevertheless, our study results show that time since transplantation is a consideration when attempting to evaluate TTV levels as a marker for optimal immunosuppression. What may be eventually be considered a marker for either infectious risk or rejection risk may depend on when the patient is sampled.

The group of TTV-negative renal transplant recipients in our study and their collective favorable outcome after transplantation deserves attention in future research. In all studies investigating the use of TTV after transplantation, TTV-negative recipients are found. This group logically includes patients without TTV, as well as patients whose immune systems are able to suppress TTV effectively. The fact that this group has the lowest risk of death due to infections and the lowest all-cause mortality, is not surprising. However, in studies investigating TTV levels within the first year after transplantation, this group appeared to have a higher rejection risk and more graft failure. We were not able to show a connection between graft failure and TTV level. Although the set-up of our study, with a single sample taken at least one year after renal transplantation, was not inappropriate to assess acute rejection risk, the fact that there is no association between negative TTV and graft failure stresses that more investigation is needed to determine TTV level cut-offs for optimal immunosuppression after the first year post-transplantation.

When writing it was interesting to note that many studies on TTV in transplantation medicine, including this study, have come from Central and Western Europe, while the exact geographic variation of TTV has not been fully elucidated. These are also studies that, in general, have shown a correlation between TTV and various outcomes. With the advent of a minimum of four available PCR detection methods, including one commercial kit, capable of detecting various TTV genotypes with varying levels of efficiency, it would be interesting to know exactly which TTV genotype is being detected by each kit. Several authors have noted a correlation between genogroup 4 and specifically genotype 21, which has been associated with arthritis and acute respiratory disease in children [25,38]. It may be time rethink our detection strategies by using specific PCR reactions or by using sequencing more readily.

In conclusion, our data suggest a use for TTV viral load monitoring in renal transplant recipients for long term follow-up. While cut-off values remain to be determined, high TTV levels are associated with increased all-cause mortality and increased risk of death due to infections.

Author Contributions: Conceptualization: A.A.E.d.J., S.J.L.B., E.A.M.V., J.W., C.V.L.-B.; Methodology: S.J.L.B., H.G.M.N.; Validation: H.G.M.N., C.V.L.-B., E.J.G., L.W.; Formal analyses: E.J.G., A.W.G.-N.; Investigation: E.J.G., C.V.L.-B.; Resources: H.G.M.N., S.J.L.B., J.W., E.A.M.V.; Data validation: E.J.G., A.W.G.-N.; Writing—original draft preparation: E.J.G., C.V.L.-B.; Writing—review and editing: J.W., S.J.L.B., E.A.M.V., H.G.M.N.; Supervision: C.V.L.-B., J.W., E.A.M.V. All authors have read and agreed to the published version of the manuscript.

Funding: For this project was generously provided by a Healthy Aging Research Grant (grant number HAP2017-1-299) from the University Medical Center Groningen. The authors are grateful to BioMerieux, France for providing test kits. The authors are grateful to Tim Schuurman for technical assistance in the laboratory and to Lyanne Kieneker for providing the serum samples.

Acknowledgments: The cohort on which the study was based is registered at clinicaltrials.gov as "TransplantLines Food and Nutrition Biobank and Cohort Study (TxL-FN)" with number NCT02811835.

Conflicts of Interest: The authors declare no conflict of interest.

References

1. Meier-Kriesche, H.-U.; Schold, J.D.; Srinivas, T.R.; Kaplan, B. Lack of Improvement in Renal Allograft Survival Despite a Marked Decrease in Acute Rejection Rates Over the Most Recent Era. *Am. J. Transplant.* **2004**, *4*, 378–383. [CrossRef] [PubMed]
2. Chand, S.; Atkinson, D.; Collins, C.; Briggs, D.; Ball, S.; Sharif, A.; Skordilis, K.; Vydianath, B.; Neil, D.; Borrows, R. The Spectrum of Renal Allograft Failure. *PLoS ONE* **2016**, *11*, e0162278. [CrossRef] [PubMed]
3. Morrissey, P.E.; Reinert, S.; Yango, A.; Gautam, A.; Monaco, A.; Gohh, R. Factors Contributing to Acute Rejection in Renal Transplantation: The Role of Noncompliance. *Transplant. Proc.* **2005**, *37*, 2044–2047. [CrossRef] [PubMed]
4. Maggi, F.; Bendinelli, M. Human Anelloviruses and the Central Nervous System. *Rev. Med. Virol.* **2010**, *20*, 392–407. [CrossRef] [PubMed]
5. Nishizawa, T.; Okamoto, H.; Konishi, K.; Yoshizawa, H.; Miyakawa, Y.; Mayumi, M. A Novel DNA Virus (TTV) Associated with Elevated Transaminase Levels in Posttransfusion Hepatitis of Unknown Etiology. *Biochem. Biophys. Res. Commun.* **1997**, *241*, 92–97. [CrossRef] [PubMed]

6. Okamoto, H.; Nishizawa, T.; Ukita, M. A Novel Unenveloped DNA Virus (TT Virus) Associated with Acute and Chronic Non-A to G Hepatitis. *Intervirology* **1999**, *42*, 196–204. [CrossRef]
7. Spandole, S.; Cimponeriu, D.; Berca, L.M.; Mihaescu, G. Human Anelloviruses: An Update of Molecular, Epidemiological and Clinical Aspects. *Arch. Virol.* **2015**, *160*, 893–908. [CrossRef]
8. Focosi, D.; Antonelli, G.; Pistello, M.; Maggi, F. Torquetenovirus: The Human Virome from Bench to Bedside. *Clin. Microbiol. Infect.* **2016**, *22*, 589–593. [CrossRef]
9. Ott, C.; Duret, L.; Chemin, I.; Trepo, C.; Mandrand, B.; Komurian-Pradel, F. Use of a TT Virus ORF1 Recombinant Protein to Detect Anti-TT Virus Antibodies in Human Sera. *J. Gen. Virol.* **2000**, *81*, 2949–2958. [CrossRef]
10. Mankotia, D.S.; Irshad, M. Cloning and Expression of N22 Region of Torque Teno Virus (TTV) Genome and Use of Peptide in Developing Immunoassay for TTV Antibodies. *Virol. J.* **2014**, *11*, 96. [CrossRef]
11. Nishizawa, T.; Okamoto, H.; Tsuda, F.; Aikawa, T.; Sugai, Y.; Konishi, K.; Akahane, Y.; Ukita, M.; Tanaka, T.; Miyakawa, Y.; et al. Quasispecies of TT Virus (TTV) with Sequence Divergence in Hypervariable Regions of the Capsid Protein in Chronic TTV Infection. *J. Virol.* **1999**, *73*, 9604–9608. [CrossRef] [PubMed]
12. Kulifaj, D.; Essig, M.; Meynier, F.; Pichon, N.; Munteanu, E.; Moulinas, R.; Joannes, M.; Heckel, D.; Combrissson, J.; Barranger, C.; et al. Torque Teno Virus (TTV) in Immunosuppressed Host: Performances Studies of TTV R-Gene Registered Kit and Donors and Recipients Kidney Samples Genotyping: Presentation at ESCV 2016: Poster 166. *J. Clin. Virol.* **2016**, *82*, S103–S104. [CrossRef]
13. Rezahosseini, O.; Drabe, C.H.; Sørensen, S.S.; Rasmussen, A.; Perch, M.; Ostrowski, S.R.; Nielsen, S.D. Torque-Teno Virus Viral Load as a Potential Endogenous Marker of Immune Function in Solid Organ Transplantation. *Transplant. Rev.* **2019**, *33*, 137–144. [CrossRef] [PubMed]
14. Minović, I.; Eisenga, M.F.; Riphagen, I.J.; van den Berg, E.; Kootstra-Ros, J.E.; Frenay, A.-R.S.; van Goor, H.; Rimbach, G.; Esatbeyoglu, T.; Levy, A.P.; et al. Circulating Haptoglobin and Metabolic Syndrome in Renal Transplant Recipients. *Sci. Rep.* **2017**, *7*, 14264. [CrossRef]
15. Eisenga, M.F.; Kieneker, L.M.; Soedamah-Muthu, S.S.; van den Berg, E.; Deetman, P.E.; Navis, G.J.; Gans, R.O.B.; Gaillard, C.A.J.M.; Bakker, S.J.L.; Joosten, M.M. Urinary Potassium Excretion, Renal Ammoniagenesis, and Risk of Graft Failure and Mortality in Renal Transplant Recipients. *Am. J. Clin. Nutr.* **2016**, *104*, 1703–1711. [CrossRef]
16. Kulifaj, D.; Durgueil-Lariviere, B.; Meynier, F.; Munteanu, E.; Pichon, N.; Dubé, M.; Joannes, M.; Essig, M.; Hantz, S.; Barranger, C.; et al. Development of a Standardized Real Time PCR for Torque Teno Viruses (TTV) Viral Load Detection and Quantification: A New Tool for Immune Monitoring. *J. Clin. Virol.* **2018**, *105*, 118–127. [CrossRef]
17. Solis, M.; Velay, A.; Gantner, P.; Bausson, J.; Filiputti, A.; Freitag, R.; Moulin, B.; Caillard, S.; Fafi-Kremer, S. Torquetenovirus Viremia for Early Prediction of Graft Rejection after Kidney Transplantation. *J. Infect.* **2019**, *79*, 56–60. [CrossRef]
18. Macera, L.; Spezia, P.G.; Medici, C.; Rofi, E.; Re, M.D.; Focosi, D.; Mazzetti, P.; Navarro, D.; Antonelli, G.; Danesi, R.; et al. Comparative Evaluation of Molecular Methods for the Quantitative Measure of Torquetenovirus Viremia, the New Surrogate Marker of Immune Competence. *J. Med. Virol.* **2019**. [CrossRef]
19. World Health Organisation; Centre for Disease Control; Prevention. *ICD-9-CM CDC Copy*; National Center for Health Statistics: Hyattsville, MD, USA, 2015.
20. World Health Organisation. *ICD 9 001-139*; Pan American Health Organization: Washington, DC, USA, 2012; ISBN 9241540044.
21. Youden, W.J. Index for Rating Diagnostic Tests. *Cancer* **1950**, *3*, 32. [CrossRef]
22. Görzer, I.; Haloschan, M.; Jaksch, P.; Klepetko, W.; Puchhammer-Stöckl, E. Plasma DNA Levels of Torque Teno Virus and Immunosuppression after Lung Transplantation. *J. Hear. Lung Transplant.* **2014**, *33*, 320–323. [CrossRef]
23. Walton, A.H.; Muenzer, J.T.; Rasche, D.; Boomer, J.S.; Sato, B.; Brownstein, B.H.; Pachot, A.; Brooks, T.L.; Deych, E.; Shannon, W.D.; et al. Reactivation of Multiple Viruses in Patients with Sepsis. *PLoS ONE* **2014**, *9*, e98819. [CrossRef] [PubMed]
24. Maggi, F.; Focosi, D.; Statzu, M.; Bianco, G.; Costa, C.; Macera, L.; Spezia, P.G.; Medici, C.; Albert, E.; Navarro, D.; et al. Early Post-Transplant Torquetenovirus Viremia Predicts Cytomegalovirus Reactivations In Solid Organ Transplant Recipients. *Sci. Rep.* **2018**, *8*, 15490–15498. [CrossRef] [PubMed]

25. Maggi, F.; Pifferi, M.; Fornai, C.; Andreoli, E.; Tempestini, E.; Vatteroni, M.; Presciuttini, S.; Marchi, S.; Pietrobelli, A.; Boner, A.; et al. TT Virus in the Nasal Secretions of Children with Acute Respiratory Diseases: Relations to Viremia and Disease Severity. *J. Virol.* **2003**, *77*, 2418–2425. [CrossRef] [PubMed]
26. Nordén, R.; Magnusson, J.; Lundin, A.; Tang, K.-W.; Nilsson, S.; Lindh, M.; Andersson, L.-M.; Riise, G.C.; Westin, J. Quantification of Torque Teno Virus and Epstein-Barr Virus Is of Limited Value for Predicting the Net State of Immunosuppression After Lung Transplantation. *Open Forum Infect. Dis.* **2018**, *5*, ofy050. [CrossRef] [PubMed]
27. Shang, D.; Lin, Y.H.; Rigopoulou, I.; Chen, B.; Alexander, G.J.M.; Allain, J.-P. Detection of TT Virus DNA in Patients with Liver Disease and Recipients of Liver Transplant. *J. Med. Virol.* **2000**, *61*, 455–461. [CrossRef]
28. Burra, P.; Masier, A.; Boldrin, C.; Calistri, A.; Andreoli, E.; Senzolo, M.; Zorzi, M.; Sgarabotto, D.; Guido, M.; Cillo, U.; et al. Torque Teno Virus: Any Pathological Role in Liver Transplanted Patients? *Transpl. Int.* **2008**, *21*, 972–979. [CrossRef]
29. Béland, K.; Dore-Nguyen, M.; Gagné, M.-J.; Patey, N.; Brassard, J.; Alvarez, F.; Halac, U. Torque Teno Virus in Children Who Underwent Orthotopic Liver Transplantation: New Insights About a Common Pathogen. *J. Infect. Dis.* **2014**, *209*, 247–254. [CrossRef]
30. Görzer, I.; Jaksch, P.; Kundi, M.; Seitz, T.; Klepetko, W.; Puchhammer-Stöckl, E. Pre-Transplant Plasma Torque Teno Virus Load and Increase Dynamics after Lung Transplantation. *PLoS ONE* **2015**, *10*, e0122975. [CrossRef]
31. Görzer, I.; Jaksch, P.; Strassl, R.; Klepetko, W.; Puchhammer-Stöckl, E. Association between Plasma Torque Teno Virus Level and Chronic Lung Allograft Dysfunction after Lung Transplantation. *J. Hear. Lung Transplant.* **2017**, *36*, 366–368. [CrossRef]
32. Schiemann, M.; Puchhammer-Stöckl, E.; Eskandary, F.; Kohlbeck, P.; Rasoul-Rockenschaub, S.; Heilos, A.; Kozakowski, N.; Görzer, I.; Kikić, Ž.; Herkner, H.; et al. Torque Teno Virus Load-Inverse Association with Antibody-Mediated Rejection after Kidney Transplantation. *Transplantation* **2017**, *101*, 360–367. [CrossRef]
33. Strassl, R.; Doberer, K.; Rasoul-Rockenschaub, S.; Herkner, H.; Görzer, I.; Kläger, J.P.; Schmidt, R.; Haslacher, H.; Schiemann, M.; Eskandary, F.A.; et al. Torque Teno Virus for Risk Stratification of Acute Biopsyproven Alloreactivity in Kidney Transplant Recipients. *J. Infect. Dis.* **2019**, *219*, 1934–1939. [CrossRef] [PubMed]
34. El-Zoghby, Z.M.; Stegall, M.D.; Lager, D.J.; Kremers, W.K.; Amer, H.; Gloor, J.M.; Cosio, F.G. Identifying Specific Causes of Kidney Allograft Loss. *Am. J. Transplant.* **2009**, *9*, 527–535. [CrossRef] [PubMed]
35. Sellarés, J.; De Freitas, D.G.; Mengel, M.; Reeve, J.; Einecke, G.; Sis, B.; Hidalgo, L.G.; Famulski, K.; Matas, A.; Halloran, P.F. Understanding the Causes of Kidney Transplant Failure: The Dominant Role of Antibody-Mediated Rejection and Nonadherence. *Am. J. Transplant.* **2012**, *12*, 388–399. [CrossRef] [PubMed]
36. Fernández-Ruiz, M.; Albert, E.; Giménez, E.; Ruiz-Merlo, T.; Parra, P.; López-Medrano, F.; San Juan, R.; Polanco, N.; Andrés, A.; Navarro, D.; et al. Monitoring of Alphatorquevirus DNA Levels for the Prediction of Immunosuppression-Related Complications after Kidney Transplantation. *Am. J. Transplant.* **2019**, *19*, 1139–1149. [CrossRef] [PubMed]
37. Strassl, R.; Schiemann, M.; Doberer, K.; Görzer, I.; Puchhammer-Stöckl, E.; Eskandary, F.; Kikić, Ž.; Gualdoni, G.A.; Vossen, M.G.; Rasoul-Rockenschaub, S.; et al. Quantification of Torque Teno Virus Viremia as a Prospective Biomarker for Infectious Disease in Kidney Allograft Recipients. *J. Infect. Dis.* **2018**, *218*, 1191–1199. [CrossRef]
38. Rocchi, J.; Ricci, V.; Albani, M.; Lanini, L.; Andreoli, E.; Macera, L.; Pistello, M.; Ceccherini-Nelli, L.; Bendinelli, M.; Maggi, F. Torquetenovirus DNA Drives Proinflammatory Cytokines Production and Secretion by Immune Cells via Toll-like Receptor 9. *Virology* **2009**, *394*, 235–242. [CrossRef]

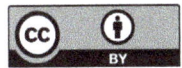

© 2020 by the authors. Licensee MDPI, Basel, Switzerland. This article is an open access article distributed under the terms and conditions of the Creative Commons Attribution (CC BY) license (http://creativecommons.org/licenses/by/4.0/).

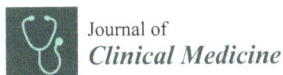

Article

Acute Kidney Injury Patterns Following Transplantation of Steatotic Liver Allografts

Caroline Jadlowiec [1,*], Maxwell Smith [2], Matthew Neville [3], Shennen Mao [4], Dina Abdelwahab [5], Kunam Reddy [1], Adyr Moss [1], Bashar Aqel [6] and Timucin Taner [7]

1. Division of Transplant Surgery, Mayo Clinic, Phoenix, AZ 85054, USA; Reddy.Kunam@mayo.edu (K.R.); Moss.Adyr@mayo.edu (A.M.)
2. Division of Anatomic Pathology, Mayo Clinic, Phoenix, AZ 85054, USA; Smith.Maxwell@mayo.edu
3. Instructor in Biostatistics, Mayo Clinic College of Medicine, Phoenix, AZ 85054, USA; Neville.Matthew@mayo.edu
4. Division of Transplant Surgery, Mayo Clinic, Jacksonville, FL 32224, USA; Mao.Shennen@mayo.edu
5. Division of Nephrology, Mayo Clinic, Phoenix, AZ 85054, USA; elhamahmi.dina@mayo.edu
6. Division of Transplant Hepatology, Mayo Clinic, Phoenix, AZ 85054, USA; Aqel.Bashar@mayo.edu
7. Division of Transplant Surgery, William J von Liebig Transplant Center, Rochester, MN 55902, USA; Taner.timucin@mayo.edu
* Correspondence: Jadlowiec.Caroline@mayo.edu; Tel.: +1-480-3421010; Fax: +1-480-3422324

Received: 29 February 2020; Accepted: 27 March 2020; Published: 30 March 2020

Abstract: Background: Steatotic grafts are increasingly being used for liver transplant (LT); however, the impact of graft steatosis on renal function has not been well described. Methods: A total of 511 allografts from Mayo Clinic Arizona and Minnesota were assessed. We evaluated post-LT acute kidney injury (AKI) patterns, perioperative variables and one-year outcomes for patients receiving moderately steatotic allografts (>30% macrovesicular steatosis, $n = 40$) and compared them to non-steatotic graft recipients. Results: Post-LT AKI occurred in 52.5% of steatotic graft recipients versus 16.7% in non-steatotic recipients ($p < 0.001$). Ten percent of steatotic graft recipients required new dialysis post-LT ($p = 0.003$). At five years, there were no differences for AKI vs. no AKI patient survival (HR 0.95, 95% CI 0.08–10.6, $p = 0.95$) or allograft survival (HR 1.73, 95% CI 0.23–13.23, $p = 0.59$) for those using steatotic grafts. Lipopeliosis on biopsy was common in those who developed AKI (61.0% vs. 31.6%, $p = 0.04$), particularly when the Model for End-Stage Liver Disease (MELD) was ≥20 (88.9%; $p = 0.04$). Lipopeliosis was a predictor of post-LT AKI (OR 6.0, 95% CI 1.1–34.6, $p = 0.04$). Conclusion: One-year outcomes for moderately steatotic grafts are satisfactory; however, a higher percentage of post-LT AKI and initiation of dialysis can be expected. Presence of lipopeliosis on biopsy appears to be predictive of post-LT AKI.

Keywords: acute kidney injury; allograft steatosis; lipopeliosis

1. Introduction

Due to the ongoing organ shortage, there has been an increased interest in utilizing moderately steatotic donor liver allografts to maximize opportunities for transplantation. Historically, the use of liver allografts with significant steatosis has been associated with increased risk of primary nonfunction, poor early graft function, and decreased patient and allograft survival [1–5]. The degree of steatosis, as well as its histological pattern, appears to impact patient and allograft survival [2,6]. While allografts with severe macrovesicular steatosis (>60%) carry a very high risk of primary non-function, those with mild macrovesicular steatosis (<30%) yield results similar to those of non-steatotic liver allografts [2]. The outcomes of liver allografts with moderate steatosis (30% to 60%) remain variable and the impact of graft steatosis on renal function has not been well described [7,8]. As such, the objectives of this study were to: (1) evaluate postoperative acute kidney injury (AKI) patterns in recipients of steatotic grafts; (2) assess biopsy-findings predictive of AKI in the use of steatotic livers; (3) examine one-year patient and allograft outcomes.

2. Materials and Methods

2.1. Study Population

This was an eight-year, two-center retrospective study of patients who underwent a liver transplant at Mayo Clinic Arizona and Mayo Clinic Minnesota between January 2009 and December 2016 ($n = 810$). This study was approved by the Mayo Clinic Institutional Review Board. Outcomes were compared between moderately steatotic (>30% macrovesicular steatosis) and non-steatotic (<30% macrovesicular steatosis) grafts. In order to assess post-liver transplant (LT) acute kidney injury (AKI) patterns, patients with pre-LT acute kidney injury (AKI) ($n = 143$) were excluded. The majority of LT were performed via piggyback technique; 2.7% ($n = 14$) were performed via caval interposition. The data that supports the findings of this study is available from the corresponding author upon reasonable request.

Pre-LT AKI was defined using the Kidney Disease Improving Global Outcomes (KDIGO) guidelines by an increase in serum creatinine > 0.3 mg/dL or 1.5–1.9 times baseline. Post-LT AKI was defined by those patients satisfying the KDIGO guidelines within 48 h post-LT and maintaining the criteria for > 48 h. Patients with pre-existing chronic kidney disease were not excluded unless they had pre-LT AKI. Mean follow-up was 4.2 years.

All liver allografts were biopsied at the time of transplant and the biopsies were reviewed by a group of designated liver pathologists. Biopsy reports were retrospectively reviewed and macrovesicular steatosis percentage was recorded (less than 30% vs. greater than 30%). Early allograft dysfunction was defined as an aspartate aminotransferase (AST) greater than 2000 U/L within the first 7 days post-LT.

Liver biopsies reported as having moderate (>30% macrovesicular) steatosis were prospectively re-reviewed by a single liver pathologist (M.S.) to specifically assess for macro- and microvesicular steatosis, the percentage of small- and large droplet macrovesicular steatosis, zonation, features of steatohepatitis, fibrosis, preservation reperfusion injury (PRI), and lipopeliosis. Percentages of steatosis were based on the percentage of hepatic parenchyma involved by fat and were estimated using previously published reference figures [9].

Operative hemodynamics were quantified using a modified operative inotrope score (inotrope score = dopamine (×1) + dobutamine (×1) + amrinone (×1) + milrinone (×15) + epinephrine (×100) + norepinephrine (×100) + phenylephrine (×1) + vasopressin (×1), with each drug dosed in µg/kg/min). The inotrope score was calculated during the pre-anhepatic, anhepatic, and post-reperfusion phases for the moderately macrovesicular steatosis cohort [10]. An average of systolic blood pressure (SBP) and mean arterial pressure (MAP) was also recorded for these operative periods.

Immunosuppression was maintained per our center's protocol. All recipients were started on mycophenolate mofetil (MMF), tacrolimus, and prednisone post-LT. MMF was withdrawn at 2–4 months; prednisone was discontinued at 4 months. Tacrolimus trough levels were set at 7–10 ng/mL for the first 2 months post-LT; at one-year post-LT, trough levels were reduced to 4–6 ng/mL. By protocol at our centers, tacrolimus is typically started immediately following transplant unless there are concerns for renal insufficiency. In the setting of post-LT renal insufficiency (defined as creatinine >2.0 mg/dL, estimated glomerular filtration rate (eGFR) <40 mL/minute or dialysis), Basiliximab 20 mg is given on post-operative days 0 and 4 to allow for a delay in tacrolimus initiation. In this setting, tacrolimus initiation is delayed until postoperative day 5.

2.2. Statistical Methods

Descriptive analysis was performed using t-tests for continuous variables and Chi-square for categorical variables. Continuous variables are shown using mean and standard deviation; categorical variables using count and percentage. Wilcoxon rank-sum tests were used for non-normally distributed continuous variables. Survival analysis was performed using Kaplan-Meier analysis. Logistic regression was applied to clinically significant variables. Statistical analysis was performed using Prism software version 7.03 (La Jolla, CA, USA) and SAS version 9.4. A p value of <0.05 was considered significant.

3. Results

3.1. Postoperative Outcomes

Of the 511 grafts that were included in this analysis, 40 were found to have moderate (>30%) macrovesicular steatosis. The average steatosis percentage was 41.1% ± 15.8% in the moderate group, compared to 3.8% ± 5.8% in the non-steatotic group ($p < 0.001$) (Table 1, Figure 1A,B). For the entire cohort, the incidence of post-LT AKI was 19.6% ($n = 100$). In assessing clinical risk factors for kidney disease, 12.5% ($n = 64$) of LT recipients were diabetic, 12.7% ($n = 65$) had hypertension, and 13.5% ($n = 69$) were both diabetic and hypertensive. The distribution of diabetes and hypertension did not vary between the steatotic and non-steatotic grafts ($p = 0.95$). There were no differences in age ($p = 0.39$), sex ($p = 0.18$), ethnicity ($p = 0.72$), race ($p = 0.57$), the biologic Model for End-Stage Liver Disease (MELD) ($p = 0.14$) or indications for liver transplant ($p = 0.16$) between the recipients receiving moderately steatotic and non-steatotic grafts (Table 1).

Table 1. Pre- and Post-Liver Transplant Recipient Demographics.

	Steatotic Grafts ($n = 40$)	Non-Steatotic Grafts ($n = 471$)	p Value
Pre-Liver Transplant			
Steatosis (%)	41.1 ± 15.8	3.8 ± 5.8	<0.0001
Recipient Age (years)	57.4 ± 9.7	56.0 ± 10.3	0.39
Biologic MELD	18.0 ± 8.3	16.1 ± 7.0	0.14
Female	9 (22.5%)	155 (32.9%)	0.18
Indication for LT			0.16
Hepatitis C (HCV)	6 (22.5%)	55 (11.6%)	
Cholestatic	5 (12.5%)	53 (11.3%)	
Hepatocellular Carcinoma (HCC)/Other MELD Exception	11 (27.5%)	223 (47.3%)	
Alcohol-Related Liver Disease (ALD)	8 (20.0%)	46 (9.8%)	
Nonalcoholic Steatohepatitis (NASH)	6 (15.0%)	49 (10.4%)	
Other	4 (10.0%)	45 (9.6%)	
Pre-LT Creatinine (mg/dL)	1.0 ± 0.3	0.9 ± 0.9	0.14
Pre-LT eGFR	57.7 ± 6.3	57.7 ± 6.6	0.97
Post-Liver Transplant			
Post-LT AKI	21 (52.5%)	79 (16.8%)	<0.0001
Post-LT Temporary Dialysis	4 (10.0%)	5 (1.1%)	0.003
ICU LOS (days)	2.0 ± 1.8	1.8 ± 2.6	0.62
Total Hospital LOS (days)	9.1 ± 10.3	9.9 ± 10.9	0.67
One-Year Post-Liver Transplant			
Creatinine (mg/dL)	1.3 ± 0.3	1.3 ± 0.7	0.97
eGFR (mL/min)	53.1 ± 7.9	53.5 ± 10.1	0.70
New Chronic Post-LT Dialysis	0 (0.0%)	2 (0.4%)	>0.99

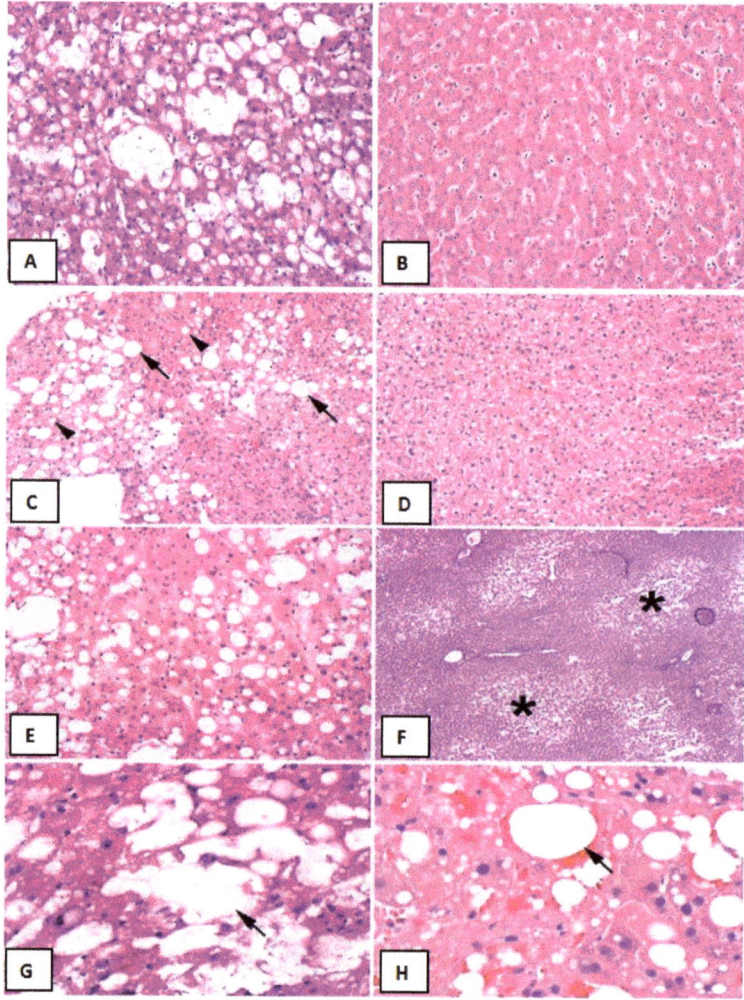

Figure 1. Liver Graft Biopsy Findings Liver Biopsy Findings. (**A**) Representative biopsy of a >30% macrovesicular steatotic allograft. (**B**) Representative biopsy of a non-steatotic allograft. (**C**) Approximately 30% macrovesicular steatosis with a mixture of large (arrows) and small (arrowheads) droplet fat (hematoxylin and eosin (H&E), 200×). (**D**) Microvesicular steatosis characterized by diffuse deposition of fat droplets in the hepatocyte cytoplasm without any macrovesicular steatosis (H&E, 200×). (**E**) Approximately 40% macrovesicular steatosis seen on a pre-implantation biopsy (H&E frozen section, 400×). (**F**) Zonal distribution of macrovesicular steatosis with fat deposition accentuated in zone three (asterisks) around the central veins (H&E, frozen section, 100×). (**G**), Lipopeliosis characterized by the rupture of hepatocytes with coalescence of fat droplets (arrow) in the sinusoidal spaces (H&E, frozen section, 600×). (**H**), Lipopeliosis (arrow) in post-reperfusion biopsy (H&E, 600×).

Post-LT AKI was observed in 52.5% of patients receiving moderately steatotic grafts versus 16.8% in the non-steatotic cohort ($p < 0.0001$). No patients in the entire cohort had liver allograft primary non-function. Patients transplanted with moderately steatotic grafts had significantly more early allograft dysfunction immediately following surgery (AST: 3212 ± 2413 U/L vs. 1118 ± 1473 U/L,

$p < 0.0001$). The rise in AST was four-fold higher for recipients of steatotic grafts that went on to develop post-LT AKI ($p < 0.0001$). There was a greater need for newly initiated temporary post-LT dialysis in the moderately steatotic group (10.0% vs. 1.1%, $p = 0.003$). There were no differences in intensive care unit (ICU) length of stay (2.0 ± 1.8 vs. 1.8 ± 2.6, $p = 0.62$) or total hospital length of stay (9.1 ± 10.3 vs. 9.9 ± 10.9, $p = 0.67$). At one-year post-LT, there were no observed differences in the need for new chronic (ongoing) post-LT dialysis ($p > 0.99$), serum creatinine (1.3 ± 0.3 vs. 1.3 ± 0.7, $p = 0.97$), or eGFR (53.1 ± 7.9 vs. 53.5 ± 10.1, $p = 0.70$) (Table 1).

3.2. Moderately Steatotic Graft Subgroup Analysis

In order to investigate postoperative outcomes in moderately steatotic livers allografts in further detail, we reviewed the characteristics of the 40 patients who were transplanted with such grafts (Table 2). In this cohort, there were no differences in age ($p = 0.61$), sex ($p = 0.43$), ethnicity ($p = 0.60$), race ($p = 0.64$), or indication for transplant ($p = 0.53$) among those who developed AKI versus those who did not (Table 2). Of those receiving steatotic grafts, 52.5% went on to develop AKI; the other 47.5% maintained normal renal function post-transplant. Recipients of steatotic grafts that went on to develop post-LT AKI had a higher biologic MELD (20.5 ± 8.9 vs. 15.3 ± 6.9, $p = 0.04$) (Table 2). There were no differences in pre-LT creatinine ($p = 0.21$) or eGFR ($p = 0.88$).

Table 2. Moderately Steatotic Graft Subgroup Analysis.

	Post-LT AKI (n = 21)	No AKI (n = 19)	p Value
Pre-Liver Transplant			
Macrovesicular Steatosis (%)	41.9 ± 15.7	40.3 ± 16.2	0.75
Recipient Age (years)	56.7 ± 8.3	58.3 ± 11.3	0.61
Biologic MELD	20.5 ± 8.9	15.3 ± 6.9	0.04
Female	3 (14.3%)	6 (31.6%)	0.43
Indication for LT			0.53
HCV	4 (19.0%)	2 (10.5%)	
Cholestatic	1 (4.8%)	4 (21.1%)	
HCC/Other MELD Exception	5 (23.8%)	6 (31.6%)	
ALD	4 (19.0%)	4 (21.1%)	
NASH	4 (19.0%)	2 (10.5%)	
Other	3 (14.3%)	1 (5.3%)	
Total Hospital LOS (median)	10.4 ± 13.5 (7.0)	7.1 ± 4.1 (6.0)	0.32
One-Year Post-LT			
Creatinine (mg/dL)	1.3 ± 0.2	1.2 ± 0.4	0.27
eGFR (mL/min)	52.7 ± 6.9	53.6 ± 9.1	0.74

Recipients of moderately steatotic grafts were all noted to have early allograft dysfunction as demonstrated through a significantly elevated AST immediately following surgery (Figure 2). This occurred regardless of whether or not they developed AKI. The rise in AST was four-fold higher for recipients of steatotic grafts that went on to develop post-LT AKI as compared to non-steatotic grafts (40001.0 ± 2471.0 U/L vs. 1118.0 ± 1473.0, $p < 0.0001$). The rise in AST was also two-fold higher when comparing steatotic grafts of recipients with and without post-LT AKI (40001.0 ± 2471.0 U/L vs. 2339.0 ± 2074.0, $p < 0.0001$). There were no differences between the post-LT AKI and no AKI groups with regards to graft type (i.e., donation after brain death, DBD, vs. donation after cardiac death, DCD) (19.0% vs. 10.5%, $p = 0.66$), sex (female: 42.9% vs. 47.4%, $p = 0.38$), or BMI (32.8 ± 5.9 kg/m^2 vs. 32.6 ± 9.4 kg/m^2, $p = 0.92$). Donor age was younger (43.2 ± 12.6 vs. 52.8 ± 14.9%, $p = 0.03$) in steatotic grafts that went on to develop AKI. In addition, there were no differences in allograft cold ischemia time (CIT) ($p = 0.28$) or estimated operative blood loss (EBL) ($p = 0.49$) (Table 3).

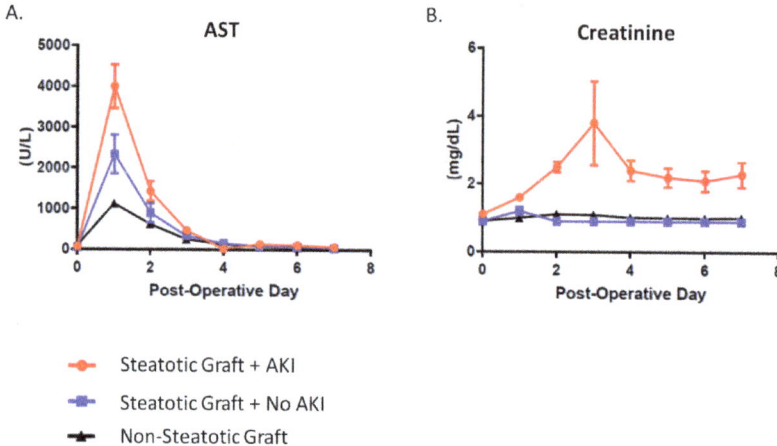

Figure 2. Post-Liver Transplant Patterns in Steatotic and Non-Steatotic Grafts. (**A**) Post-LT aspartate aminotransferase (AST) levels. Compared to non-steatotic graft, AST levels were 2-times higher in steatotic grafts without post-LT AKI and 4-times higher for steatotic grafts with AKI. (**B**) Post-LT creatinine levels.

Table 3. Steatotic Graft Recipient Operative Variables.

	Post-LT AKI (n = 21)	No AKI (n = 19)	p Value
CIT (h)	6.8 ± 2.1	6.1 ± 1.7	0.28
EBL (mL)	2157 ± 1649	1821 ± 1405	0.49
Pre-Anhepatic			
SBP (mmHg)	111.2 ± 21.8	104.2 ± 14.5	0.25
MAP	75.1 ± 13.3	73.8 ± 13.6	0.76
Inotrope Score	4.1 ± 11.9	1.7 ± 6.9	0.45
Anhepatic			
SBP (mmHg)	106.5 ± 15.4	104.4 ± 15.1	0.67
MAP	75.4 ± 11.0	76.7 ± 9.6	0.71
Inotrope Score	4.3 ± 11.9	2.6 ± 6.8	0.58
Post Reperfusion			
SBP (mmHg)	95.6 ± 13.8	96.2 ± 7.9	0.87
MAP	67.0 ± 11.8	65.5 ± 9.8	0.69
Inotrope Score	19.5 ± 20.0	3.8 ± 4.4	0.03

When operative hemodynamics of AKI and non-AKI recipients receiving moderately steatotic grafts were compared, there were no differences observed in inotrope requirements ($p = 0.45$), systolic blood pressure (SBP) ($p = 0.25$) or mean arterial pressure (MAP) ($p = 0.76$) during the pre-anhepatic phase or anhepatic phase (inotrope score $p = 0.58$; SBP $p = 0.67$; MAP $p = 0.71$) of the operation (Table 3). Post-reperfusion, SBP ($p = 0.87$) and MAP ($p = 0.69$) were similar in patients who went on to develop post-LT AKI versus those who did not suggesting appropriate perfusion parameters were able to be maintained. The post-reperfusion inotrope requirements, however, were significantly higher in the post-LT AKI group (19.5 ± 20.0 vs. 3.8 ± 4.4, $p = 0.03$). Ten percent of the patients in the steatotic post-LT AKI group ($n = 4$) required initiation of new dialysis post-LT ($p = 0.003$) (Table 2). There were no differences in ICU length of stay ($p = 0.62$) and total hospital length of stay ($p = 0.67$) between steatotic AKI and no AKI groups.

At one-year post-LT, there were no observed differences between those receiving steatotic grafts that developed AKI versus those who did not with regards to serum creatinine (1.3 ± 0.2 vs. 1.2 ± 0.4,

$p = 0.27$) and eGFR (52.7 ± 6.9 vs. 53.6 ± 9.1, $p = 0.74$) (Table 2). At five years, there were no differences for AKI vs. no AKI patient survival (HR 0.95, 95% CI 0.08–10.6, $p = 0.95$) or allograft survival (HR 1.73, 95% CI 0.23–13.23, $p = 0.59$) for those using steatotic grafts (Figure 3).

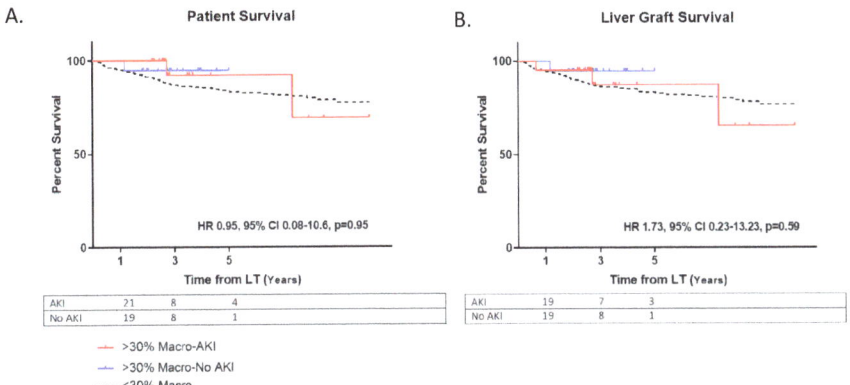

Figure 3. Survival. (**A**) Patient survival post-LT. Hazard ratio (HR); Confidence Interval (CI). (**B**) Liver allograft survival post-transplant. Moderately steatotic grafts with AKI (>30% Macro-AKI); Moderately steatotic grafts without AKI (>30% Macro-No AKI); Non-steatotic grafts (<30% Macro).

3.3. Liver Graft Biopsy Findings

In prospectively re-reviewing biopsies of all liver allografts with moderate (>30%) macrovesicular steatosis, the majority of the steatosis was found to be large droplet (Table 4) (Figure 1C,E). When comparing biopsies in patients with and without post-LT AKI, no differences were observed with regard to large droplet versus small droplet percentage composition (Figure 1C) ($p = 0.41$). Although microvesicular steatosis was minimal in both groups (Figure 1D) (0.0% vs. 21.1%), a higher frequency was observed in the no AKI group ($n = 4$, $p = 0.04$) (Table 4). No significant differences were observed in the histologic distribution of the steatosis (zonation) in the allograft ($p = 0.75$) (Figure 1F), inflammation ($p = 0.73$), ballooning ($p = 0.65$), or Mallory hyaline (Table 4). A larger percentage of biopsies in the post-LT AKI group contained lipopeliosis (61% vs. 31.6%, $p = 0.04$) (Figure 1G–H). When plotted against MELD at the time of transplant, recipients of moderately steatotic grafts with lipopeliosis with a MELD ≥ 20 were found to more likely to develop AKI (88.9%) than recipients of such grafts with MELD < 20 (40.0%; $p = 0.04$) (Figure 4). In using logistic regression, variables predictive of post-LT AKI included the finding of lipopeliosis on liver biopsy and donor age (Table 5).

Table 4. Steatotic Liver Graft Biopsy Findings.

	Post-LT AKI ($n = 21$)	No AKI ($n = 19$)	p Value
Macrovesicular Steatosis			
Large Droplet (%)	69.2 ± 16.1	64.7 ± 16.9	0.41
Small Droplet (%)	30.8 ± 16.1	35.3 ± 16.9	
Microvesicular Steatosis	0 (0.0%)	4 (21.1%)	0.04
Zonation	14 (66.7%)	11 (57.9%)	0.75
Inflammation	5 (23.8%)	6 (31.5%)	0.73
Ballooning	2 (9.5%)	3 (15.8%)	0.65
Mallory Hyaline	0 (0.0%)	0 (0.0%)	-
Lipopeliosis	13 (61.9%)	6 (31.6%)	0.03

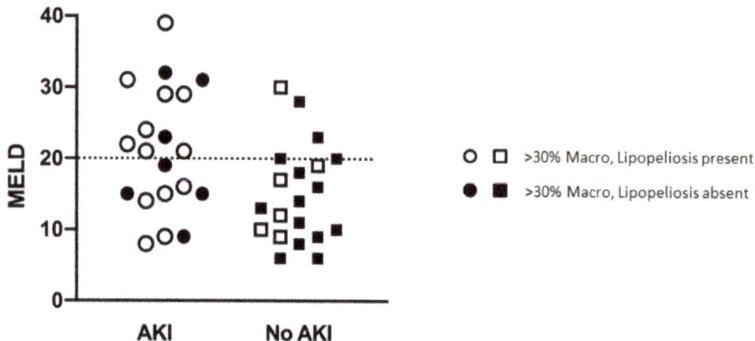

Figure 4. Relationship between MELD, Lipopeliosis and Post-LT AKI.

Table 5. Predictors of AKI in Steatotic Grafts—Logistic Regression.

Effect	Odds Ratio	95% CI		p Value
Donor Age	0.93	0.87	0.99	0.02
Lipopeliosis	6.04	1.05	34.61	0.04
Post-Reperfusion Systolic BP	1.01	0.95	1.08	0.75

4. Discussion

Primary nonfunction, poor early graft function, and decreased patient and allograft survival have all been associated with the use of steatotic liver allografts for transplantation [1–3,5]. This, combined with inaccurate and inconsistent reporting of liver allograft biopsies, has led to a high discard rate of grafts with moderate (>30%) steatosis [11]. While the risk of adverse events with severely steatotic liver allografts (>60%) remains well recognized, the use of moderately steatotic grafts (30%–60%) has been increasing [7].

It has been our experience that steatotic grafts almost universally exhibit early allograft dysfunction and require additional resource utilization postoperatively specific to the development of post-LT AKI and the need to initiate new dialysis [7,12–15]. In this study, the occurrence of AKI post-LT was noted to be markedly increased at 52.5% compared to 19.6% observed in the general liver transplant recipient pool. Although early allograft dysfunction, best demonstrated by significantly elevated transaminases, was common to all steatotic grafts, not all recipients developed post-LT AKI (Figure 2). We have clinically observed this divergent pattern; however, it remains difficult to quantify why some steatotic grafts behave in this manner while others do not. In this study, patients receiving steatotic grafts that developed post-LT AKI were noted to have higher inotrope requirements post-reperfusion. Despite having higher inotrope requirements, no differences were observed in hemodynamic parameters (systolic blood pressure and MAP) between the patients with and without post-LT AKI, suggesting that variables other than hemodynamics influence the development of AKI. Not surprisingly, a higher MELD score was associated with an increased risk of post-LT AKI. This association was particularly strong when steatotic grafts with lipopeliosis on biopsy were transplanted to patients with MELD scores of 20 or above (Tables 2 and 5) (Figure 4).

Proper classification of graft steatosis remains challenging even within the transplant community [9]. Historically, steatosis was classified as microvesicular or macrovesicular, based on hepatocyte fat droplet size and nucleus displacement. Although often reported, true microvesicular steatosis is rare and manifests histologically as diffuse deposition of small lipid droplets in the hepatocyte cytoplasm with a resulting foamy appearance (Figure 1D). Two types of fat droplets are seen in the setting of macrovesicular steatosis: small droplets and large droplets (Figure 1C). Fat droplets in small droplet steatosis are not large enough to displace the nucleus; this finding is often inaccurately reported as being microvesicular steatosis on biopsy. Although both small and large droplet steatosis contribute to overall macrovesicular steatosis, historically small droplet macrovesicular steatosis and microvesicular steatosis were used synonymously, resulting in ongoing confusion [3]. We hypothesize that some of the observed differences in post-LT AKI between otherwise similarly-appearing steatotic grafts might be related to this histological variation.

The term lipopeliosis was first identified in the early days of hepatic transplantation and describes the coalescence of fat droplets from ruptured hepatocytes into larger droplets of fat in the sinusoidal space [16]. Due to the universal finding of preservation-related injury in these biopsies, lipopeliosis was presumed to not be of clinical significance [17]. In our experience, however, the histologic finding of lipopeliosis is, by far, more common in patients who develop post-LT AKI and, in our experience, has been associated with inferior post-transplant outcomes [18].

Although the current study was not designed to elucidate the mechanisms of AKI post-LT, we have previously shown that fat droplets, through the process of lipopeliosis, embolize to the pulmonary vasculature following reperfusion with resulting respiratory failure [18]. This mechanism is likely similar to that seen after long bone traumatic injuries, where fat droplets are released into the venous system and migrate to the pulmonary capillary beds [19,20]. Microvascular lodging results in ischemia, inflammation, and release of inflammatory mediators. The breakdown of fat emboli by pneumocytes can results in release of free fatty acids that, in turn, enter systemic circulation and result in multisystem dysfunction [21]. The finding of fat droplets in the urine under these circumstances correlates with the development of AKI and a systemic process triggered by fat embolization [22]. Whether lipopeliosis in steatotic liver graft biopsies can be used to predict clinical instability and the development of post-LT AKI will need to be validated in a larger prospective study. Limitations to this study include its overall small cohort size. The results also represent the experience of only two centers. Patients with pre-LT AKI were also excluded in this study to better assess post-LT outcomes specific to AKI development. The impact of steatosis on renal function in patients with preexisting AKI remains uncertain.

In conclusion, utilization of moderately steatotic grafts is associated with a significantly higher risk for developing post-LT AKI. This risk appears to be independent of pre-reperfusion operative hemodynamics. In utilizing these grafts, laboratory abnormalities persist 2 to 3 months post-LT, but there does not appear to be an impact on long-term renal function, patient, or graft survival. The risk for AKI in this setting appears increased when the MELD score is greater than 20 and lipopeliosis is histologically present on biopsy. These outcomes are more favorable as compared to older studies, and suggest that, with lower MELD recipients, satisfactory outcomes can be achieved with the use of these grafts [5].

Author Contributions: For research articles with several authors, a short paragraph specifying their individual contributions must be provided. The following statements should be used "Conceptualization, C.J. and T.T.; methodology, C.J. and T.T.; software, C.J. and M.N.; validation, C.J., M.N and T.T.; formal analysis, C.J., M.S., M.N., S.M., D.A., K.R., A.M., B.A., T.T.; investigation, C.J., M.S., T.T.; resources, C.J.; data curation, C.J., M.S., M.N., S.M, D.A. and T.T.; writing—original draft preparation, C.J., M.S., M.N., S.M., D.A., K.R., A.M., B.A., T.T.; writing—review and editing, C.J., M.S., M.N., S.M., D.A., K.R., A.M., B.A., T.T.; visualization, C.J. and T.T.; supervision, T.T.; project administration, C.J.; funding acquisition, Not applicable. All authors have read and agreed to the published version of the manuscript.

Conflicts of Interest: The authors declare no conflict of interest.

References

1. Verran, D.; Kusyk, T.; Painter, D.; Fisher, J.; Koorey, D.; Strasser, S.; Stewart, G.; McCaughan, G. Clinical experience gained from the use of 120 steatotic donor livers for orthotopic liver transplantation. *Liver Transpl.* **2003**, *9*, 500–505. [CrossRef]
2. Selzner, M.; Clavien, P.A. Fatty liver in liver transplantation and surgery. *Semin. Liver Dis.* **2001**, *21*, 105–113. [CrossRef] [PubMed]
3. Wu, C.; Lu, C.; Xu, C. Short-term and long-term outcomes of liver transplantation using moderately and severely steatotic donor livers: A systemic review. *Medicine (Baltimore)* **2018**, *97*, e12026. [CrossRef] [PubMed]

4. Spitzer, A.L.; Lao, O.B.; Dick, A.A.; Bakthavatsalam, R.; Halldorson, J.B.; Yeh, M.M.; Upton, M.P.; Reyes, J.D.; Perkins, J.D. The biopsied donor liver: Incorporating macrosteatosis into high-risk donor assessment. *Liver Transpl.* **2010**, *16*, 874–884. [CrossRef] [PubMed]
5. Wadei, H.M.; Lee, D.D.; Croome, K.P.; Mai, M.L.; Golan, E.; Brotman, R.; Keaveny, A.P.; Taner, C.B. Early Allograft Dysfunction After Liver Transplantation Is Associated With Short- and Long-Term Kidney Function Impairment. *Am. J. Transplant.* **2016**, *16*, 850–859. [CrossRef]
6. Fishbein, T.M.; Fiel, M.I.; Emre, S.; Cubukcu, O.; Guy, S.R.; Schwartz, M.E.; Miller, C.M.; Sheiner, P.A. Use of livers with microvesicular fat safely expands the donor pool. *Transplantation* **1997**, *64*, 248–251. [CrossRef]
7. Croome, K.P.; Lee, D.D.; Croome, S.; Chadha, R.; Livingston, D.; Abader, P.; Keaveny, A.P.; Taner, C.B. The impact of postreperfusion syndrome during liver transplantation using livers with significant macrosteatosis. *Am. J. Transpl.* **2019**, *19*, 2550–2559. [CrossRef]
8. McCormack, L.; Dutkowski, P.; El-Badry, A.M.; Clavien, P.A. Liver transplantation using fatty livers: Always feasible? *J. Hepatol.* **2011**, *54*, 1055–1062. [CrossRef]
9. Hall, A.R.; Dhillon, A.P.; Green, A.C.; Ferrell, L.; Crawford, J.M.; Alves, V.; Balabaud, C.; Bhathal, P.; Bioulac-Sage, P.; Guido, M.; et al. Hepatic steatosis estimated microscopically versus digital image analysis. *Liver Int.* **2013**, *33*, 926–935. [CrossRef] [PubMed]
10. Kobashigawa, J.; Zuckermann, A.; Macdonald, P.; Leprince, P.; Esmailian, F.; Luu, M.; Mancini, D.; Patel, J.; Razi, R.; Reichenspurner, H.; et al. Report from a consensus conference on primary graft dysfunction after cardiac transplantation. *J. Heart Lung Transpl.* **2014**, *33*, 327–340. [CrossRef]
11. Doyle, M.M.; Vachharajani, N.; Wellen, J.R.; Anderson, C.D.; Lowell, J.A.; Shenoy, S.; Brunt, E.M.; Chapman, W.C. Short- and long-term outcomes after steatotic liver transplantation. *Arch Surg.* **2010**, *145*, 653–660. [CrossRef]
12. Leithead, J.A.; Rajoriya, N.; Gunson, B.K.; Muiesan, P.; Ferguson, J.W. The evolving use of higher risk grafts is associated with an increased incidence of acute kidney injury after liver transplantation. *J. Hepatol.* **2014**, *60*, 1180–1186. [CrossRef] [PubMed]
13. Cabezuelo, J.B.; Ramirez, P.; Acosta, F.; Bueno, F.S.; Robles, R.; Pons, J.A.; Miras, M.; Munitiz, V.; Fernandez, J.A.; Lujan, J.; et al. Prognostic factors of early acute renal failure in liver transplantation. *Transpl. Proc.* **2002**, *34*, 254–255. [CrossRef]
14. O'Riordan, A.; Wong, V.; McQuillan, R.; McCormick, P.A.; Hegarty, J.E.; Watson, A.J. Acute renal disease, as defined by the RIFLE criteria, post-liver transplantation. *Am. J. Transpl.* **2007**, *7*, 168–176. [CrossRef] [PubMed]
15. Leithead, J.A.; Armstrong, M.J.; Corbett, C.; Andrew, M.; Kothari, C.; Gunson, B.K.; Muiesan, P.; Ferguson, J.W. Hepatic ischemia reperfusion injury is associated with acute kidney injury following donation after brain death liver transplantation. *Transpl. Int.* **2013**, *26*, 1116–1125. [CrossRef]
16. Ferrell, L.; Bass, N.; Roberts, J.; Ascher, N. Lipopeliosis: Fat induced sinusoidal dilation in transplanted liver mimicking peliosis hepatitis. *J. Clin. Pathol.* **1992**, *45*, 1109–1110. [CrossRef] [PubMed]
17. Cha, I.; Bass, N.; Ferrell, L.D. Lipopeliosis: An Immunohistochemical and Clinicopathologic Study of Five Cases. *Am. J. Surg. Pathol.* **1994**, *18*, 789–795. [CrossRef] [PubMed]
18. Rosenfeld, D.M.; Smith, M.L.; Seamans, D.P.; Giorgakis, E.; Gaitan, B.D.; Khurmi, N.; Aqel, B.A.; Reddy, K.S. Fatal diffuse pulmonary fat microemboli following reperfusion in orthotopic liver transplantation with the use of marginal steatotic allografts. *Am. J. Transpl.* **2019**, *19*, 2640–2645. [CrossRef]
19. Shaikh, N. Emergency management of fat embolism syndrome. *J. Emergencies Trauma Shock* **2009**, *2*, 29–33. [CrossRef]
20. Glossing, H.R.; Pellegrini, V.D. Fat embolism syndrome: A review of pathology and physiological basis of treatment. *Clin. Orthop. Relat. Res.* **1982**, *165*, 68–82.
21. Baker, P.L.; Paxel, J.A.; Pettier, L.F. Free fatty acids, catecholamine and arterial hypoxia in patients with fat embolism. *J. Trauma* **1971**, *11*, 1026–1030. [CrossRef] [PubMed]
22. Evarts, C.M. Diagnosis and treatment of fat embolism. *JAMA* **1965**, *194*, 899–901. [CrossRef] [PubMed]

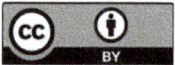

© 2020 by the authors. Licensee MDPI, Basel, Switzerland. This article is an open access article distributed under the terms and conditions of the Creative Commons Attribution (CC BY) license (http://creativecommons.org/licenses/by/4.0/).

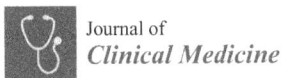

Article

Inpatient Burden and Mortality of Goodpasture's Syndrome in the United States: Nationwide Inpatient Sample 2003–2014

Wisit Kaewput [1,*], Charat Thongprayoon [2], Boonphiphop Boonpheng [3], Patompong Ungprasert [4], Tarun Bathini [5], Api Chewcharat [2], Narat Srivali [6], Saraschandra Vallabhajosyula [7] and Wisit Cheungpasitporn [8]

1. Department of Military and Community Medicine, Phramongkutklao College of Medicine, Bangkok 10400, Thailand
2. Division of Nephrology, Department of Medicine, Mayo Clinic, Rochester, MN 55905, USA; charat.thongprayoon@gmail.com (C.T.); api.che@hotmail.com (A.C.)
3. Department of Medicine, David Geffen School of Medicine, University of California, Los Angeles, Los Angeles, CA 90095, USA; boonpipop.b@gmail.com
4. Clinical Epidemiology Unit, Department of Research and Development, Faculty of Medicine, Siriraj Hospital, Mahidol University, Bangkok, 10700, Thailand; p.ungprasert@gmail.com
5. Department of Internal Medicine, University of Arizona, Tucson, AZ 85721, USA; tarunjacobb@gmail.com
6. Department of Internal Medicine, St. Agnes Hospital, Baltimore, MD 21229, USA; nsrivali@gmail.com
7. Department of Cardiovascular Medicine, Mayo Clinic, Rochester, MN 55905, USA; Vallabhajosyula.Saraschandra@mayo.edu
8. Division of Nephrology, Department of Medicine, University of Mississippi Medical Center, Jackson, MS 39216, USA; wcheungpasitporn@gmail.com
* Correspondence: wisitnephro@gmail.com; Tel.: +66-235-4760093613; Fax: +6623547733

Received: 15 January 2020; Accepted: 5 February 2020; Published: 6 February 2020

Abstract: Background: Goodpasture's syndrome is a rare, life-threatening, small vessel vasculitis. Given its rarity, data on its inpatient burden and resource utilization are lacking. We conducted this study aiming to assess inpatient prevalence, mortality, and resource utilization of Goodpasture's syndrome in the United States. **Methods:** The 2003–2014 National Inpatient Sample was used to identify patients with a principal diagnosis of Goodpasture's syndrome. The inpatient prevalence, clinical characteristics, in-hospital treatment, end-organ failure, mortality, length of hospital stay, and hospitalization cost were studied. Multivariable logistic regression was performed to identify independent factors associated with in-hospital mortality. **Results:** A total of 964 patients were admitted in hospital with Goodpasture's syndrome as the principal diagnosis, accounting for an overall inpatient prevalence of Goodpasture's syndrome among hospitalized patients in the United States of 10.3 cases per 1,000,000 admissions. The mean age of patients was 54 ± 21 years, and 47% were female; 52% required renal replacement therapy, whereas 39% received plasmapheresis during hospitalization. Furthermore, 78% had end-organ failure, with renal failure and respiratory failure being the two most common end-organ failures. The in-hospital mortality rate was 7.7 per 100 admissions. The factors associated with increased in-hospital mortality were age older than 70 years, sepsis, the development of respiratory failure, circulatory failure, renal failure, and liver failure, whereas the factors associated with decreased in-hospital mortality were more recent year of hospitalization and the use of therapeutic plasmapheresis. The median length of hospital stay was 10 days. The median hospitalization cost was $75,831. **Conclusion:** The inpatient prevalence of Goodpasture's syndrome in the United States is 10.3 cases per 1,000,000 admissions. Hospitalization of patients with Goodpasture's syndrome was associated with high hospital inpatient utilization and costs.

Keywords: Goodpasture syndrome; anti-GBM disease; epidemiology; hospitalization; outcomes

1. Introduction

Goodpasture's syndrome (GS) is a rare, life-threatening, small vessel vasculitis that is mediated by circulating anti-glomerular basement membrane (anti-GBM) autoantibodies against the NC1 domain of the alpha 3 chain of type IV collagen, targeting capillaries of the kidneys and lungs [1–4]. It is considered as one of the organ-specific autoimmune diseases that typically presents as a rapidly progressive glomerulonephritis (RPGN), accompanied by alveolar hemorrhage with pathology characterized by crescentic glomerulonephritis with classic linear polyclonal immunoglobulin (Ig) G deposits on immunofluorescence staining of the GBM on analysis of kidney biopsy samples [1,2,5–7]. Without prompt diagnosis and treatment, patients with GS can develop organ failure, resulting in significant morbidities and mortality [1–3].

Among European and Asian populations, the incidence of GS is estimated to have a frequency of 0.5 to 1.8 cases per million population per year [1–3,8,9]. A recent study from Ireland reported a nationwide disease incidence of GS of 1.64 per million population per year [10]. While it is well known that patients with GS can have both pulmonary and renal involvement requiring a mechanical ventilator and renal replacement therapy [3,4], data on its inpatient burden and resource utilization are lacking.

Thus, we conducted this study using the 2003–2014 National Inpatient Sample (NIS) database to assess inpatient prevalence, mortality, and resource utilization of GS in the United States.

2. Materials and Methods

2.1. Data Source

The 2003–2014 NIS database was used to conduct this cohort study. The NIS is the publicly available, inpatient, all-payer database in the United States. This database was developed and maintained by the Healthcare Cost and Utilization Project (HCUP) under the sponsorship of the Agency for Healthcare Research and Quality (AHRQ). The dataset contains more than 7 million hospitalizations annually, which were obtained from a 20% stratified sample of over 4000 non-federal acute care hospitals in more than 40 states of the United States. A survey procedure using discharge weights provided by the HCUP-NIS database was used to generate national estimates for 95% of hospitalizations nationwide [11]. This dataset includes codes for principal and secondary diagnosis as well as codes for procedures performed during the hospitalization.

2.2. Study Population

All patients with a principal diagnosis of GS, based on the International Classification of Diseases, Ninth Revision, Clinical Modification (ICD-9 CM) diagnosis code of 446.21 for the hospitalization were included.

2.3. Variables and Outcome of Interest

Patient characteristics included age, sex, race, year of hospitalization, smoking, hemoptysis, and the presence of anti-neutrophil cytoplasmic antibody (ANCA)-associated vasculitis, which consisted of granulomatosis polyangiitis, microscopic polyangiitis, and sepsis. Treatments included respiratory support consisting of invasive mechanical ventilation and non-invasive ventilation, renal replacement therapy, therapeutic plasmapheresis, and blood transfusion. Patient outcomes included organ failure or dysfunction, which consisted of respiratory failure, circulatory failure, renal failure, liver failure, hematologic failure, metabolic failure, and neurologic failure, as well as in-hospital mortality. Resource utilization included length of hospital stay and hospitalization cost.

2.4. Statistical Analysis

Discharge-level weights published by the HCUP were used to estimate the total number of GS patients. Continuous variables were summarized as mean ± standard deviation for normally-distributed data, and median with interquartile range for skewed data. Categorical variables were summarized as count with percentage. The annual inpatient prevalence of GS in hospitalized patients in the United States from 2003 to 2014 was calculated. Independent factors associated with in-hospital mortality were identified using multivariable logistic regression with the forward stepwise selection method. A two-tailed p-value of less than 0.05 was considered statistically significant. All analyses were performed using JMP statistical software (version 10, SAS Institute, Cary, NC).

3. Results

3.1. Patient Characteristics and In-Hospital Treatment

Of 93,377,054 hospital admissions during the study period, 964 patients were admitted to hospital with GS as the principal diagnosis. The mean age of patients was 54 ± 21 years; 47% were female, 65% were Caucasian, and 9% had a co-diagnosis of ANCA-associated vasculitis. Of patients with GS, 19% needed invasive mechanical ventilation, 5% needed non-invasive ventilation support, and 52% required renal replacement therapy. Plasmapheresis was performed in 39% of patients. Table 1 shows clinical characteristics and in-hospital treatment of GS patients in this cohort.

Table 1. Clinical characteristics, treatments, outcomes, and resource utilization of Goodpasture's syndrome patients.

	All (N = 964)
Clinical characteristics	
Age (years)	54 ± 21
≤39	260 (27)
40–49	91 (9)
50–59	141 (15)
60–69	199 (21)
≥70	273 (28)
Male sex	456 (47)
Caucasian	622 (65)
Year of hospitalization	
2003–2006	281 (29)
2007–2010	357 (37)
2011–2014	326 (34)
Smoking	95 (10)
Hemoptysis	267 (28)
ANCA vasculitis	84 (9)
Granulomatosis with polyangiitis	54 (6)
Microscopic polyangiitis	30 (3)
Sepsis	62 (6)

Table 1. Cont.

	All (N = 964)
Treatments	
Respiratory support	216 (23)
Invasive mechanical ventilation	181 (19)
Non-invasive ventilation	49 (5)
Renal replacement therapy	499 (52)
Hemodialysis	494 (51)
Peritoneal dialysis	10 (1)
Therapeutic plasmapheresis	376 (39)
Blood transfusion	391 (41)
Outcomes	
Number of organ failure	
0	230 (24)
1	369 (38)
2	242 (25)
≥3	123 (13)
Respiratory failure	283 (29)
Circulatory failure/shock	53 (6)
Renal failure	597 (62)
Liver failure	10 (1)
Hematologic failure	127 (13)
Metabolic failure	159 (17)
Neurological failure	50 (5)
In-hospital death	74 (8)
Resource utilization	
Length of stay (days), median (IQR)	10 (5–18)
<5	215 (22)
5–9	229 (24)
10–14	188 (20)
≥15	332 (34)
Hospitalization cost ($), median (IQR)	75,831.5 (31,687.3–163,201.0)

3.2. Inpatient Prevalence of GS

Table 2 shows the annual distribution and inpatient prevalence of GS in hospitalized patients. The inpatient prevalence of GS ranged from 6.7 to 12.1 per 1,000,000 admissions between the years 2003 and 2014 in the United States with an overall inpatient prevalence of GS over 12 years of 10.3 cases per 1,000,000 admissions (Figure 1).

Table 2. The distribution and inpatient prevalence of Goodpasture's syndrome from 2003 to 2014.

Year	Total Number of Goodpasture's Syndrome Patients	Total Number of Admissions	Inpatient Prevalence (per 1,000,000 Admissions)
2003	72	7,977,728	9.0
2004	54	8,004,571	6.7
2005	66	7,995,048	8.3
2006	89	8,074,825	11.0
2007	97	8,043,415	12.1
2008	84	8,158,381	10.3
2009	85	7,810,762	10.9
2010	91	7,800,441	11.7
2011	92	8,023,590	11.5
2012	75	7,296,968	10.3
2013	86	7,119,563	12.1
2014	73	7,071,762	10.3
Total	964	93,377,054	10.3

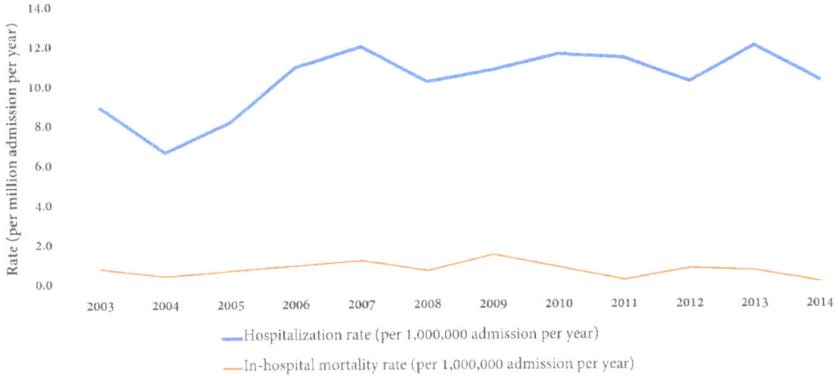

Figure 1. Rate of hospital admission and in-hospital mortality rate for Goodpasture's syndrome stratified by year.

3.3. Organ Failure and In-Hospital Mortality

Seventy-six percent of patients had at least one end-organ failure. Renal failure was the most common end-organ failure (62%), followed by respiratory failure (29%), metabolic failure (17%), hematologic failure (13%), circulatory failure (6%), neurological failure (5%), and liver failure (1%) (Table 1). The number of end-organ failures was significantly associated with increased in-hospital mortality with an adjusted OR of 2.19 (95% CI 0.45–10.58) for one end-organ failure, 7.60 (95% CI 1.67–34.56) for two end-organ failures, and 19.86 (95% CI 4.10–96.19) for ≥3 end-organ failures.

Of 964 patients with GS, 74 (8%) died in the hospital. In the multivariable logistic regression, age older than 70 years (OR 3.62; 95% CI 1.52–8.61 compared to age ≤ 39 years), sepsis (OR 5.38; 95% CI 2.53–11.45), respiratory failure (OR 7.41; 95% CI 3.85–14.26), circulatory failure (OR 7.85; 95% CI 3.37–18.26), renal failure (OR 2.55; 95% CI 1.21–5.37), and liver failure (OR 32.32; 95% CI 3.51–297.19) were associated with increased in-hospital mortality. In contrast, more recent year of hospitalization (OR 0.23; 95% CI 0.10–0.55 for year 2011–2014 compared to year 2003–2006) and the use of therapeutic plasmapheresis (OR 0.43; 95% CI 0.22–0.84) were associated with decreased in-hospital mortality (Table 3).

Table 3. Univariable and multivariable analysis assessing factors associated with in-hospital mortality in Goodpasture's syndrome patients.

Characteristics	Univariable Analysis		Multivariable Analysis	
	Crude OR (95% CI)	P-Value	Adjusted OR (95% CI)	P-Value
Age (years)				
≤39	1 (ref)		1 (ref)	
40–49	0.85 (0.23–3.17)	0.81	0.76 (0.17–3.35)	0.71
50–59	0.54 (0.15–2.01)	0.36	0.58 (0.13–2.52)	0.47
60–69	2.34 (1.05–5.22)	0.04	1.68 (0.62–4.54)	0.31
≥70	4.42 (2.16–9.02)	<0.001	3.62 (1.52–8.61)	<0.01
Male	1.34 (0.83–2.16)	0.23		
Caucasian	1.34 (0.83–2.17)	0.23		
Year of admission				
2003–2006	1 (ref)		1 (ref)	
2007–2010	1.11 (0.65–1.91)	0.70	0.92 (0.47–1.79)	0.80
2011–2014	0.46 (0.23–0.90)	0.02	0.23 (0.10–0.55)	0.001
Smoking	0.24 (0.06–0.99)	0.04		
Hemoptysis	1.99 (1.22–3.23)	<0.01		
Granulomatosis with polyangiitis	1.42 (0.59–3.43)	0.43		
Microscopic polyangiitis	0.41 (0.06–3.03)	0.38		
Sepsis	14.03 (7.85–25.10)	<0.001	5.38 (2.53–11.45)	<0.001
Respiratory failure	10.71 (6.04–19.02)	<0.001	7.41 (3.85–14.26)	<0.001
Circulatory failure/shock	11.72 (6.35–21.66)	<0.001	7.85 (3.37–18.26)	<0.001
Renal failure	3.10 (1.68–5.72)	<0.001	2.55 (1.21–5.37)	0.01
Liver failure	16.90 (3.71–76.99)	<0.001	32.32 (3.51–297.19)	<0.01
Hematologic failure	1.17 (0.60–2.28)	0.66		
Metabolic failure	1.32 (0.73–2.39)	0.36		
Neurological failure	3.32 (1.59–6.95)	0.001		
Invasive mechanical ventilation	11.26 (6.72–18.86)	<0.001		
Non-invasive ventilation	1.74 (0.71–4.23)	0.22		
Dialysis	1.40 (0.87–2.27)	0.17		
Therapeutic plasmapheresis	0.89 (0.54–1.46)	0.64	0.43 (0.22–0.84)	0.01
Blood transfusion	0.83 (0.51–1.36)	0.46		

3.4. Length of Hospital Stay and Hospitalization cost

The median length of hospital stay was 10 (IQR 5–18) days. The median hospitalization cost was $75,831 (IQR 31,687–163,201) (Table 1).

4. Discussion

To the best of our knowledge, our study is the first to evaluate inpatient prevalence, mortality, and resource utilization of GS in the United States. We demonstrated overall inpatient prevalence of GS among hospitalized patients in the United States of 10.3 cases per 1,000,000 admissions. The in-hospital mortality rate was 8%. The factors associated with increased in-hospital mortality were age older than 70 years, sepsis, the development of respiratory failure, circulatory failure, renal failure, and liver failure, whereas the factors associated with decreased in-hospital mortality were more recent year of hospitalization and the use of therapeutic plasmapheresis.

GS is often described to have an incidence of GS of 0.5 to 1.8 cases per million population per year in European and Asian populations, primarily based on single-center biopsy or serology-based series [1–3,8,9,12]. A recent nationwide study from Ireland identified all GS cases over a decade via reference immunology laboratories and a nationwide pathology database over an 11-year period, which reported a disease rate of 1.64 per million population per year [10]. In this study, we utilized the United States inpatient hospitalization data from the NIS database and demonstrated inpatient prevalence of GS among hospitalized patients in the United States of 10.3 cases per 1,000,000 admissions. Although hospitalization for GS is infrequent, we found that hospitalized patients with GS commonly had high rates of end-organ failure, including renal failure (62%) and respiratory failure (29%). While 19% of hospitalization for GS required invasive mechanical ventilation, 52% required renal replacement therapy. The median hospitalization cost for GS was as high as $75,831.

Our findings confirmed a bimodal age distribution of GS, with younger patients <39 years having a male predominance, whereas older patients >60 years old were more frequently female [2,12]. We also observed an increase in the inpatient prevalence of GS from 2004 to 2007, which subsequently stabilized (Figure 1). Although the reason remains unclear, we speculated that this is because of the increasing awareness and widespread availability of diagnostic tests around that time [4,13]. Previous studies have suggested that, in addition to genetic factors, environmental factors can also trigger the development of GS, such as cigarette smoking, inhaled hydrocarbons, or potential infectious triggers damaging the alveolar basement membrane and exposing type IV collagen epitopes [3,4,6,14–18]. Future studies are needed to assess if these factors play an important role in the trends of inpatient prevalence of GS in the United States.

Our study demonstrated that 52% of hospitalization for GS required dialysis, which was consistent with previous literature indicating that approximately half of patients with GS require hemodialysis [19]. There are limited data on how frequently artificial ventilation is required. Small series estimated that this occurred in 11% of patients with GS [20–23]. Our study demonstrated that 19% of hospitalizations for GS needed invasive mechanical ventilation, and 5% needed non-invasive ventilation support. GS is life-threatening, with irreversible kidney damage and respiratory failure. Aggressive therapy with modern treatment protocols with antibody removal by plasmapheresis, use of corticosteroids, and immunosuppressive agents, particularly cyclophosphamide, has dramatically improved patient outcomes compared to the past [4,18,24–26]. The 5-year survival rate exceeds 80% and fewer than 30% of patients require long-term dialysis [2]. In our study, we demonstrated that in-hospital mortality rate of GS in the United States between the years 2003 and 2014 was 8%. Although the data on medication were limited in the database, we found that recent year of hospitalization and the use of therapeutic plasmapheresis were associated with decreased in-hospital mortality among patients with GS. While the underlying explanations of decreased in-hospital mortality among patients with GS in the recent years of hospitalization remain unclear and require further investigations, this finding may potentially represent an improvement in patient care of GS in recent years of hospitalization.

There are several limitations of this study. Firstly, although the utilization of the NIS database allowed us to evaluate U.S. inpatient prevalence and burden of patients with GS, possible inaccuracies in ICD-9 CM coding may have confounded the results. Secondly, given the administrative nature of the dataset, the data on medication such as immunosuppression were limited in this study. Consequently, we could not assess the potential effects of immunosuppression, such as cyclophosphamide treatment on hospital outcomes of patients with GS. Thirdly, this was an analysis of an inpatient database in the United States. Sixty-five percent of patient populations with GS in NIS database were Caucasian, and this limits generalizability to the patient population in other countries. Fourthly, kidney biopsy, and laboratory data were lacking in the database. Previous studies have suggested that no patient with 100% glomerular crescents and dialysis dependence at presentation recovered kidney function, and so current guidelines do not recommend treatment in these cases [27,28]. Furthermore, studies have also demonstrated that those patients with higher serum creatinine (5.7 mg/dL or higher) and reduced proportion of normal glomeruli on kidney biopsy have poor renal outcomes [2,13]. Therefore, future studies are needed to assess the impacts of kidney biopsy findings on the treatment and outcomes during hospitalizations for GS.

5. Conclusions

In summary, we demonstrate overall inpatient prevalence among patients with GS between the years 2003 and 2014 in the United States, with 10.3 cases per 1,000,000 admissions. Although the in-hospital mortality rate was only 8%, hospitalization of patients with GS was associated with high hospital inpatient utilization and costs.

Author Contributions: Conceptualization, W.K., C.T., P.U., T.B., A.C., N.S., S.V., and W.C.; Data curation, WK and BB; Formal analysis, W.K.; Investigation, W.K., C.T., and W.C.; Methodology, W.K., C.T., S.V., and W.C.; Project administration, B.B., P.U., T.B., A.C., and N.S.; Resources, B.B.; Software, W.K.; Supervision, W.C.; Validation, W.K. and W.C.; Visualization, C.T. and T.B.; Writing—original draft, W.K.; Writing—review and editing, W.K., C.T., B.B., P.U., A.C., N.S., S.V., and W.C. All authors have read and agreed to the published version of the manuscript.

Funding: This research received no external funding.

Conflicts of Interest: We do not have any financial or non-financial potential conflict of interest.

References

1. Gulati, K.; McAdoo, S.P. Anti-Glomerular Basement Membrane Disease. *Rheum. Dis. Clin. North. Am.* **2018**, *44*, 651–673. [CrossRef]
2. Greco, A.; Rizzo, M.I.; De Virgilio, A.; Gallo, A.; Fusconi, M.; Pagliuca, G.; Martellucci, S.; Turchetta, R.; Longo, L.; De Vincentiis, M. Goodpasture's syndrome: A clinical update. *Autoimmun. Rev.* **2015**, *14*, 246–253. [CrossRef] [PubMed]
3. McAdoo, S.P.; Pusey, C.D. Anti-Glomerular Basement Membrane Disease. *Clin. J. Am. Soc. Nephrol.* **2017**, *12*, 1162–1172. [CrossRef] [PubMed]
4. Henderson, S.R.; Salama, A.D. Diagnostic and management challenges in Goodpasture's (anti-glomerular basement membrane) disease. *Nephrol. Dial. Transplant.* **2018**, *33*, 196–202. [CrossRef] [PubMed]
5. Alchi, B.; Griffiths, M.; Sivalingam, M.; Jayne, D.; Farrington, K. Predictors of renal and patient outcomes in anti-GBM disease: Clinicopathologic analysis of a two-centre cohort. *Nephrol. Dial. Transplant.* **2015**, *30*, 814–821. [CrossRef]
6. Angioi, A.; Cheungpasitporn, W.; Sethi, S.; De Vriese, A.S.; Lepori, N.; Schwab, T.R.; Fervenza, F.C. Familial antiglomerular basement membrane disease in zero human leukocyte antigen mismatch siblings. *Clin. Nephrol.* **2017**, *88*, 277–283. [CrossRef]
7. Cheungpasitporn, W.; Zacharek, C.C.; Fervenza, F.C.; Cornell, L.D.; Sethi, S.; Herrera Hernandez, L.P.; Nasr, S.H.; Alexander, M.P. Rapidly progressive glomerulonephritis due to coexistent anti-glomerular basement membrane disease and fibrillary glomerulonephritis. *Clin. Kidney J.* **2016**, *9*, 97–101. [CrossRef]
8. Tang, W.; McDonald, S.P.; Hawley, C.M.; Badve, S.V.; Boudville, N.C.; Brown, F.G.; Clayton, P.A.; Campbell, S.B.; Zoysa, J.R.; Johnson, D.W. Anti-glomerular basement membrane antibody disease is an uncommon cause of end-stage renal disease. *Kidney Int.* **2013**, *83*, 503–510. [CrossRef]
9. Kluth, D.C.; Rees, A.J. Anti-Glomerular Basement Membrane Disease. *J. Am. Soc. Nephrol.* **1999**, *10*, 2446–2453.
10. Canney, M.; O'Hara, P.V.; McEvoy, C.M.; Medani, S.; Connaughton, D.M.; Abdalla, A.A.; Doyle, R.; Stack, A.G.; O'Seaghdha, C.M.; Clarkson, M.R.; et al. Spatial and Temporal Clustering of Anti-Glomerular Basement Membrane Disease. *Clin. J. Am. Soc. Nephrol.* **2016**, *11*, 1392–1399. [CrossRef]

11. Introduction to the HCUP Nationwide Inpatient Sample (NIS) 2009. Available online: http://www.hcup-us.ahrq.gov/db/nation/nis/NIS_2009_INTRODUCTION.pdf (accessed on 1 February 2020).
12. Savage, C.O.; Pusey, C.D.; Bowman, C.; Rees, A.J.; Lockwood, C.M. Antiglomerular basement membrane antibody mediated disease in the British Isles 1980-4. *Br. Med. J. (Clin. Res. Ed.).* **1986**, *292*, 301–304. [CrossRef]
13. Moroni, G.; Ponticelli, C. Rapidly progressive crescentic glomerulonephritis: Early treatment is a must. *Autoimmun. Rev.* **2014**, *13*, 723–729. [CrossRef]
14. Donaghy, M.; Rees, A.J. CIGARETTE SMOKING AND LUNG HAEMORRHAGE IN GLOMERULONEPHRITIS CAUSED BY AUTOANTIBODIES TO GLOMERULAR BASEMENT MEMBRANE. *Lancet.* **1983**, *2*, 1390–1393. [CrossRef]
15. Huart, A.; Josse, A.G.; Chauveau, D.; Korach, J.M.; Heshmati, F.; Bauvin, E.; Cointaul, O.; Kamar, N.; Ribes, D.; Pourrat, J.; et al. Outcomes of patients with Goodpasture syndrome: A nationwide cohort-based study from the French Society of Hemapheresis. *J. Autoimmun.* **2016**, *73*, 24–29. [CrossRef]
16. Taylor, D.M.; Yehia, M.; Simpson, I.J.; Thein, H.; Chang, Y.; De Zoysa, J.R. Anti-glomerular basement membrane disease in Auckland. *Int. Med. J.* **2012**, *42*, 672–676. [CrossRef]
17. Srivastava, A.; Rao, G.K.; Segal, P.E.; Shah, M.; Geetha, D. Characteristics and outcome of crescentic glomerulonephritis in patients with both antineutrophil cytoplasmic antibody and anti-glomerular basement membrane antibody. *Clin. Rheumatol.* **2013**, *32*, 1317–1322. [CrossRef]
18. Pusey, C.D. Anti-glomerular basement membrane disease. *Kidney Int.* **2003**, *64*, 1535–1550. [CrossRef]
19. Levy, J.B.; Turner, A.N.; Rees, A.J.; Pusey, C.D. Long-Term Outcome of Anti-Glomerular Basement Membrane Antibody Disease Treated with Plasma Exchange and Immunosuppression. *Ann. Intern. Med.* **2001**, *134*, 1033–1042. [CrossRef]
20. Lazor, R.; Bigay-Game, L.; Cottin, V.; Cadranel, J.; Decaux, O.; Fellrath, J.M.; Cordier, J.F. Alveolar Hemorrhage in Anti-Basement Membrane Antibody Disease: A Series of 28 cases. *Medicine.* **2007**, *86*, 181–193. [CrossRef]
21. Herbert, D.G.; Buscher, H.; Nair, P. Prolonged venovenous extracorporeal membrane oxygenation without anticoagulation: A case of Goodpasture syndrome-related pulmonary haemorrhage. *Crit. Care Resusc.* **2014**, *16*, 69–72.
22. Balke, L.; Both, M.; Arlt, A.; Rosenberg, M.; Bewig, B. Severe Adult Respiratory Distress Syndrome from Goodpasture syndrome. Survival Using Extracorporeal Membrane Oxygenation. *Am. J. Respir. Crit. Care Med.* **2015**, *191*, 228–229. [CrossRef]
23. Legras, A.; Mordant, P.; Brechot, N.; Bel, A.; Boussaud, V.; Guillemain, R.; Cholley, B.; Gibault, L.; Le Pimpec-Barthes, F.; Combes, A. Prolonged extracorporeal membrane oxygenation and lung transplantation for isolated pulmonary anti-GBM (Goodpasture) disease. *Intensive Care Med.* **2015**, *41*, 1866–1868. [CrossRef]
24. Shah, M.K.; Hugghins, S.Y. Characteristics and outcomes of patients with Goodpasture's syndrome. *South. Med. J.* **2002**, *95*, 1411–1418. [CrossRef]
25. Johnson, J.P.; Moore, J., Jr.; Austin, H.A., 3rd; Balow, J.E.; Antonovych, T.T.; Wilson, C.B. Therapy of anti-glomerular basement membrane antibody disease: Analysis of prognostic significance of clinical, pathologic and treatment factors. *Medicine.* **1985**, *64*, 219–227. [CrossRef]
26. Cui, Z.; Zhao, J.; Jia, X.Y.; Zhu, S.N.; Jin, Q.Z.; Cheng, X.Y.; Zhao, M.H. Anti-Glomerular Basement Membrane Disease: Outcomes of Different Therapeutic Regimens in a Large Single-Center Chinese Cohort Study. *Medicine.* **2011**, *90*, 303–311. [CrossRef]
27. Booth, A.; Harper, L.; Hammad, T.; Bacon, P.; Griffith, M.; Levy, J.; Savage, C.; Pusey, C.; Jayne, D. Prospective Study of TNFα Blockade with Infliximab in Anti-Neutrophil Cytoplasmic Antibody-Associated Systemic Vasculitis. *J. Am. Soc. Nephrol.* **2004**, *15*, 717–721. [CrossRef]
28. Van Daalen, E.E.; Jennette, J.C.; McAdoo, S.P.; Pusey, C.D.; Alba, M.A.; Poulton, C.J.; Wolterbeek, R.; Nguyen, T.Q.; Goldschmeding, R.; Alchi, B.; et al. Predicting Outcome in Patients with Anti-GBM Glomerulonephritis. *Clin. J. Am. Soc. Nephrol.* **2018**, *13*, 63–72. [CrossRef]

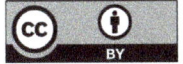

© 2020 by the authors. Licensee MDPI, Basel, Switzerland. This article is an open access article distributed under the terms and conditions of the Creative Commons Attribution (CC BY) license (http://creativecommons.org/licenses/by/4.0/).

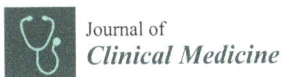

Article

Changes in Office Blood Pressure Control, Augmentation Index, and Liver Steatosis in Kidney Transplant Patients after Successful Hepatitis C Infection Treatment with Direct Antiviral Agents

Aureliusz Kolonko [1,*], Joanna Musialik [1], Jerzy Chudek [2], Magdalena Bartmańska [1], Natalia Słabiak-Błaż [1], Agata Kujawa-Szewieczek [1], Piotr Kuczera [1], Katarzyna Kwiecień-Furmańczuk [1] and Andrzej Więcek [1]

[1] Department of Nephrology, Transplantation and Internal Medicine, Medical University of Silesia, Francuska 20/24, 40-027 Katowice, Poland; jmusialik@sum.edu.pl (J.M.); bartmanska.m@gmail.com (M.B.); nataliablaz@gazeta.pl (N.S.-B.); agata.szewieczek@gmail.com (A.K.-S.); p.m.kuczera@gmail.com (P.K.); kapril@go2.pl (K.K.-F.); awiecek@spskm.katowice.pl (A.W.)
[2] Department of Internal Medicine and Oncological Chemotherapy, Medical University of Silesia, Reymonta 8, 40-035 Katowice, Poland; chj@poczta.fm
* Correspondence: uryniusz@wp.pl; Tel.: +48-322591429; Fax: +48-322553726

Received: 22 January 2020; Accepted: 27 March 2020; Published: 30 March 2020

Abstract: Hepatitis C virus (HCV) infection in kidney transplant recipients (KTRs) can be successfully treated with direct antiviral agents (DAA). The aim of our study was to analyze different measures of vascular function during and after the DAA treatment. As we have observed the improvement of blood pressure (BP) control in some individuals, we have conducted an analysis of potential explanatory mechanisms behind this finding. Twenty-eight adult KTRs were prospectively evaluated before and 15 months after start of DAA therapy. Attended office BP (OBP), augmentation index (AIx), pulse wave velocity (PWV), flow-mediated dilation (FMD), liver stiffness measurement (LSM), and liver steatosis assessment (controlled attenuation parameter (CAP)) were measured. In half of the patients, improvement of OBP control (decline of systolic BP by at least 20 mmHg or reduction of the number of antihypertensive drugs used) and parallel central aortic pressure parameters, including AIx, was observed. There was a significant decrease in CAP mean values (241 ± 54 vs. 209 ± 30 dB/m, $p < 0.05$) only in patients with OBP control improvement. Half of our KTRs cohort after successful HCV eradication noted clinically important improvement of both OBP control and central aortic pressure parameters, including AIx. The concomitant decrease of liver steatosis was observed only in the subgroup of patients with improvement of blood pressure control.

Keywords: blood pressure; eradication; interferon-free regimen; hepatitis C infection; kidney transplant

1. Introduction

Arterial hypertension is highly prevalent in kidney transplant recipients (KTRs) as a consequence of common pretransplant hypertension and as an additional effect of immunosuppressive medications [1,2]. It has been shown that blood pressure (BP) control is suboptimal (systolic BP > 140 mmHg) in 50% of KTRs [3–5]. In addition, higher BP values were associated with reduced graft and patient survival [5]. Notably, cardiovascular disease is the primary cause of mortality among kidney transplant recipients, mostly due to long-term consequences of chronic kidney disease (CKD) [6]. CKD-related systemic inflammation, calcium-phosphate abnormalities, and oxidative stress promote endothelial dysfunction, vascular calcification, and accelerated atherosclerosis in addition to the traditional risk factors [7,8]. Vascular injury caused by the uremic milieu results in an increased arterial stiffness and reduced flow-mediated dilation (FMD) [9,10].

Chronic hepatitis C virus (HCV) infection has been shown to independently worsen posttransplant survival [11]. HCV infection is a risk factor for increased aortic stiffness and cardiovascular events in dialysis patients [12], whereas advanced HCV-derived liver fibrosis is associated with increased endothelial dysfunction, independently of common cardiovascular risk factors [13]. On the other hand, patients with chronic HCV infection also demonstrate impaired autonomic nervous system function [14]. All the above disturbances caused by coexisting HCV infection may partially worsen blood pressure control in KTRs.

A few years ago a breakthrough in the treatment of chronic hepatitis C occurred. The previous interferon-based therapy, which was contraindicated for kidney transplanted patients due to increased risk of organ rejection, was replaced by new, direct acting antiviral (DAA) drug regimens. In our observation, the effectiveness of this therapy, based on sofosbuvir, reached 100% [15]. We hypothesized that the successful eradication of HCV infection may directly or indirectly improve the endothelial function. In the present study, patients were prospectively evaluated regarding different measures of their vascular function, including endothelial function, arterial stiffness measurement, and blood pressure control. Concurrently, we assessed the liver stiffness and steatosis before and after the DAA treatment. As we observed the improvement of blood pressure control in some individuals, we conducted an analysis of potential explanatory mechanisms behind this finding.

2. Material and Methods

2.1. Study Group

The study protocol was accepted by the Bioethics Committee of the Medical University of Silesia in Katowice (KNW/0022/KB1/119/16) and all participants provided written informed consent. The study was conducted in accordance with the Declaration of Helsinki. We prospectively studied all eligible adult kidney transplant recipients (KTRs) who completed treatment with DAA therapy due to HCV infection and completed both baseline and follow-up examination at least 12 months after the start of DAA therapy.

2.2. Clinical, Anthropometric, and Laboratory Measurements

Body weight and height were measured following standard procedures and body mass index (BMI) was then calculated (kg/m^2). Body surface area (BSA) was calculated according to the DuBois formula and was expressed in m^2.

Kidney graft function was measured by the estimated glomerular filtration rate (eGFR), which was calculated according to the abbreviated Modification of Diet in Renal Disease formula.

HOMA-IR (Homeostatic model assessment of insulin resistance) was calculated to assess insulin resistance.

HCV RNA was measured with COBAS® AmpliScreen HCV v.1.0, with lower limit of detection of 15 IU/mL (Roche Diagnostics, USA). HCV genotyping and viral load was performed with Linear Array Genotyping Test and COBAS®TaqMan® Quantitative test v.1.0, with lower limit of detection of 21 IU/mL (TaqMan; Roche Diagnostics, Branchburg, NJ, USA).

Concentrations of blood glycated hemoglobin (HbA$_{1C}$), serum creatinine, total cholesterol, triglycerides, and total bilirubin concentrations, as well as aspartate aminotransferase (AST), alanine aminotransferase (ALT), and gamma glutamyl transpeptidase (GGT) activity were routinely measured during standard outpatient visits. Additional blood samples were withdrawn in a closed system into tubes containing citrate and ethylenediaminetetraacetic acid (EDTA) for nonroutine analyses. The tubes were allowed to stand for 2 h at room temperature, then centrifuged (15 min, 3000 rpm), and finally plasma aliquots were preserved at −70 °C.

The plasma concentrations of high-sensitivity C-reactive protein (hsCRP) were assessed with the use of an enzyme-linked immunosorbent assay (ELISA) (Immundiagnostic AG, Bensheim, Germany), with the limit of quantification (LoQ) of 0.09 mg/L, intra-assay variation <6%, and inter-assay variation <11.6%. Plasma concentrations of interleukin-6 (IL-6) were assessed with an ELISA (R&D Systems, Minneapolis, MN, USA) with a LoQ of 0.7 pg/mL, intra-assay variation <4.2%, and inter-assay variation <6.4%. Plasma concentrations of fibroblast growth factor 21 (FGF-21) were assessed with an ELISA (Biovendor, Brno, Czech Republic) with a LoQ of 7 pg/mL, intra-assay variation <2.0%, and inter-assay variation <3.3%. Plasma concentrations of C-peptide and insulin were measured using a Cobas E411 analyzer with intermediate precision <5.0% and <2.8%, respectively.

Each study examination consisted of the measurement of office BP and central arterial pressure parameters. Echocardiography, pulse wave velocity (PWV), FMD, liver stiffness measurement (LSM), and liver steatosis assessment (controlled attenuation parameter (CAP)) were also performed at the same time points.

Attended office blood pressure measurements (OBP) were performed three times in the sitting position after more than a 5-min rest in the sitting position on the arm without arterio-venous fistula at the beginning of the study. Patients with systolic BP values ≥140 mmHg and/or diastolic BP values ≥90 mmHg or those who received antihypertensive medication were diagnosed as hypertensive. For the present post hoc analysis, the OBP control improvement was defined as the decline of attended office systolic pressure by at least 20 mmHg without pharmacotherapeutic changes or the reduction of antihypertensive treatment due to the BP decline during the follow-up period. The cut-off value (20 mmHg) was established based on doubled maximum measurement error of 10 mmHg [16,17]. Patients were divided into two study subgroups based on the BP control improvement during the follow-up period.

2.3. Echocardiography

Echocardiographic measurements were performed using Toshiba Xario 100 Diagnostic Ultrasound System (Toshiba, Toshiba Medical System Corporation, Tochigi 324-8550, Japan). M-mode and two-dimensional measurements were performed as recommended by the American Society of Echocardiography [18], including left ventricular end-diastolic and end-systolic diameters, intraventricular septum, and posterior wall end-diastolic thickness. Left ventricular mass (LVM) was calculated according to the Devereux formula [19]. LVM was indexed for BSA (LVMI).

2.4. Brachial Artery Flow-Mediated Dilation

FMD was measured in the morning, after 10 min of lying in a quiet dimmed room using the Toshiba Xario 100. During the examination, the patients rested in a seated position with their forearms and backs supported. A manual sphygmomanometer cuff was placed on the arm without arteriovenous fistula and the diameter (lumen) of the brachial artery was measured with a linear transducer. The cuff was then inflated at approximately 50 mmHg above the current systolic pressure for 5 min [20]. After the deflation of the cuff, the serial measurements during diastole were recorded and the widest dilation of the brachial artery was used for FMD calculation: FMD% = (A − B)/B × 100%, where A is the diameter of the artery during reactive hyperemia, and B is the initial diameter of the artery.

Non-endothelial dependent vasodilation (NMD) was assessed after at least a 15-min rest from the FMD acquisition. Similarly to FMD measurements, vessel diameters were assessed before and after sublingual nitroglycerin (400 μg) application (Nitromint (glyceroli trinitras), Proterapia, Poland). Of importance, as we observed unexpected reduction of NMD values in some patients, we repeated all NMD measurements using a double dose of nitroglycerin, i.e., 800 μg, after approximately 6 months from the previous follow-up series.

2.5. Central Aortic Pressure and Arterial Stiffness Measurement

Pulse waveform analysis was performed with the commercially available SphygmoCor 2000 (AtCor Medical, Sydney, Australia). Peripheral pressure waveforms were recorded from the radial artery using applanation tonometry. After the acquisition of at least 20 sequential waveforms, a validated generalized transfer function was used to generate the corresponding central aortic pressure waveform. Central blood pressure measurements, including central aortic systolic and diastolic blood pressure, central pulse pressure, and augmentation index were performed. Augmentation index was then normalized according to the heart rate (AIx@75). Only high-quality recordings, defined as an in-device quality index greater than 80% and visually acceptable curves by the investigator, were included in the analysis. The entire pulse wave analysis was performed in the sitting position under standardized conditions in the morning hours, after at least 15 min of rest in the supine position.

Arterial stiffness was also assessed using SphygmoCor 2000 placed over the carotid and femoral arteries. Pressure signals were calibrated using brachial BP and PWV was calculated as the time of the pulse wave between the diagnosed points (distance (m)/time (s)).

2.6. Liver Elastography

The controlled attenuation parameter (CAP) and liver stiffness measurement (LSM) were performed using transient elastography with a M-probe (FibroScan 502 Touch, Echosense, Paris, France). The operator was a technician certified by Echosense and unaware of patient status. The measurements were performed using a 3.5-MHz standard probe on the right hepatic lobe through the intercostal spaces with the patient lying in a supine position. As recommended by the manufacturer, 10 successful measurements were performed for each patient and only those with a success rate of at least 60% and an interquartile range/median value of less than 0.3 were considered reliable. The final CAP and liver stiffness were expressed in dB/m and kPa, respectively [21,22].

2.7. Data and Statistical Analysis

Statistical analyses were performed using the STATISTICA 13.0 PL for Windows software package (StatSoft Poland, Cracow, Poland). The values were presented as mean values with 95% confidence interval (CI) (for variables with normal distribution), medians with Q25-Q75 quartile values (for variables with not normal distribution), or frequencies. Comparisons between groups were done by using the Student t-test for quantitative variables or the χ^2 test for qualitative variables. Variables with not normal distribution were compared using the Mann–Whitney U test. The comparison of baseline and follow-up values was performed using the Student t-test, or the Wilcoxon test for variables with not normal distribution. Correlation coefficients were calculated using the Pearson test. Due to its not normal distribution, FGF-21 data were logarithmized before the correlation analyses. In all statistical tests, 'p' values below 0.05 were considered as statistically significant.

3. Results

3.1. Study Group

Out of all 73 KTRs with the presence of anti-HCV antibodies, HCV-RNA was detected in 40 patients. These patients were qualified to further HCV genotyping and viral load. Out of them, 8 patients had started DAA therapy without baseline examination planned for the present study and were not included in the final analysis. The other 32 patients were treated with the DAA anti-HCV protocol, including 8 with a 6-month regimen and 24 patients with a 3-month regimen based on sofosbuvir. The DAA regimen was shortened in the later enrolled patients as the treatment recommendations were updated during the study period. Out of this group, 4 KTRs were excluded: 2 of them were normotensive prior to HCV treatment and 2 others did not finalize the study protocol (Figure 1). Hence, the final study group consisted of 28 hypertensive patients who completed DAA therapy and both baseline and follow-up examinations. In all study patients, the diagnosis of HCV infection was established prior to kidney transplantation. In all patients, HCV viremia was not detectable after the first month of treatment and they all reached sustained virologic response at 48 weeks from DAA treatment start (SVR48) time point. The clinical characteristics of the study patients are presented in Table 1.

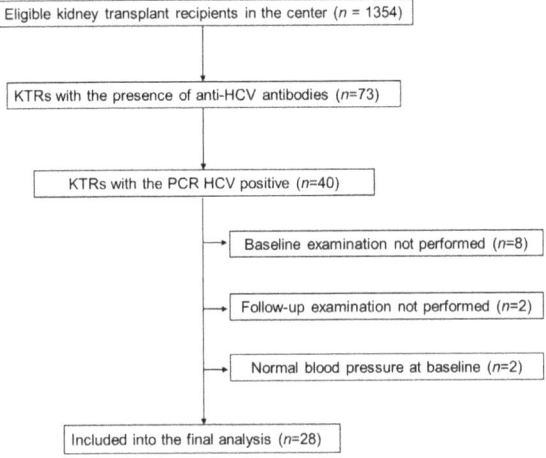

Figure 1. Study flow chart. KTRs, kidney transplant recipients; HCV, hepatitis C virus; PCR, polymerase chain reaction.

Table 1. Characteristics of direct antiviral agents-treated kidney transplant recipients stratified to subgroups based on blood pressure control improvement in the follow-up period.

	OBP Control Improvement $n = 14$	No OBP Control Improvement $n = 14$	p
Age at the start of DAA therapy (years, means and 95%CI)	49.8 (42.8–56.8)	48.5 (42.2–54.9)	0.78
Sex (M/F)	8/6	11/3	0.23
Baseline BMI (kg/m^2, means and 95%CI)	24.9 (22.8–26.9)	24.0 (22.3–25.7)	0.48
Follow-up BMI (kg/m^2, means and 95%CI)	25.6 (23.5–27.6) ##	24.4 (22.6–26.3)	0.40
Baseline eGFR (mL/min/1.73 m^2, means and 95%CI)	58.1 (45.1–71.2)	54.2 (36.3–72.1)	0.51
Follow-up eGFR (mL/min/1.73 m^2, means and 95%CI)	54.6 (39.4–69.8)	51.7 (35.0–68.5)	0.51
Diabetes (n (%))	4 (28.6)	4 (28.6)	1.0
Duration of HCV infection (years, means and 95%CI)	11.0 (6.9–15.1)	16.4 (12.6–20.1)	<0.05
Dialysis vintage (months, median and IQR)	30 (18–59)	42 (20–83)	0.37
Time after KTx (months, means and 95%CI)	121 (56–186)	125 (80–169)	0.92
Calcineurin inhibitor (CyA/Tc) (n)	8/6	7/7	0.70
Baseline HCV viremia (IU/mL, median and IQR)	340,258 (29,882–1,149,502)	78,631 (14,847–330,000)	0.40

$p < 0.01$ versus baseline. CI, confidence interval; IQR, interquartile range; OBP, attended office blood pressure; DAA, direct antiviral drug therapy; BMI, body mass index; eGFR, estimated glomerular filtration rate; KTx, kidney transplantation; CyA, cyclosporine A; Tc, tacrolimus.

3.2. Study Subgroups Based on Blood Pressure Control

In the follow-up period, half of the patients showed an improvement of OBP control (subgroup 1). Patients with OBP improvement had initially higher systolic BP (SBP) ($p = 0.02$), but similar diastolic BP (DBP) (Table 2). In addition, they received more antihypertensive medications (mean: 2.5 vs. 1.9 drugs) before the start of DAA therapy; however, this difference was not statistically significant. The observed overall SBP (Δ −20.4, 95% CI, −26.2 to −14.6 mmHg) and DBP (Δ −12.5, 95% CI, −16.5 to −8.5 mmHg) decline in subgroup 1 was obtained despite the reduction in the number of antihypertensive drugs in 9 subjects. We also observed mild reduction in SBP (Δ −5.2, 95 % CI, −9.7 to −0.8 mmHg) and DBP (Δ −4.6, 95% CI, −9.6 to 0.3 mmHg) in the second subgroup.

At baseline, the antihypertensive treatment was used in all patients: Beta-blockers in 67.9%, calcium channel blockers in 25%, angiotensin-converting enzyme inhibitor or angiotensin receptor blocker in 32.1%, alpha-blocker in 25%, and diuretics in 32.1% of study participants. The structure of antihypertensive medication classes was similar in both study subgroups (data not shown).

Both study subgroups did not differ in respect to age, gender, BMI, pretransplant dialysis vintage, time after kidney transplantation, and the occurrence of diabetes (Table 1). The time from diagnosis of HCV infection to DAA treatment was significantly longer in the subgroup 2 (Table 1), however, the percentage of patients with HCV infection lasting more than 13.7 years (mean value in the whole group) did not differ between study subgroups ($p = 0.13$). Out of whole group, only 4 patients were previously treated with interferon-based anti-HCV regimens. There were no differences in regards to baseline values of serum lipid concentrations, fasting glucose and insulin concentrations, glycated hemoglobin, and HOMA-IR values between subgroups (Supplementary Table S1).

Also, the HCV genotypes were similar in both subgroups, including 11 patients with genotype 1b in each group. The percentage of patients with advanced fibrosis, defined based on a METAVIR score >2, was comparable (28.6 vs. 38.5%, $p = 0.59$). The mean time between baseline and follow-up study examinations was also similar (15.0 ± 1.4 vs. 15.9 ± 2.1 months, $p = 0.22$).

Both study subgroups were similar in respect to calcineurin inhibitor (CNI) structure (Table 1). There were no CNI-type conversions during the whole study period. At baseline, median cyclosporine (CyA) doses were comparable (100 (100–125) mg in subgroup 1 vs. 125 (100–150) mg in subgroup 2, $p = 0.60$), whereas median tacrolimus (Tc) doses were significantly greater in subgroup 2 (4.0 (2.5–6.0) mg vs. 1.0 (1.0–2.0) mg in subgroup 1, $p < 0.05$). Notably, median CyA (97 (70–128) vs. 125 (100–146) ng/mL, respectively; $p = 0.30$) and Tc (7.1 (6.1–7.4) vs. 8.4 (6.7–8.7) ng/mL, respectively; $p = 0.22$) blood trough concentrations were similar. During and after DAA treatment, the improved liver function resulted in the reduction of calcineurin inhibitor (cyclosporine or tacrolimus) blood trough concentrations as compared with baseline values, which were similar in both study subgroups (−21.4 (−37.2 to −5.7) vs. −11.3 (−33.5 to 10.9)%, respectively; $p = 0.42$) and required individual dose adjustments in 61% of patients ($n = 17$) as soon as after one month of therapy. The consecutive CNI dose adjustments were made at physician discretion and were guided by the drug blood concentration, to prevent the CyA level decreasing below 70 ng/mL or Tc level decreasing below 5 ng/mL. Overall, the median CNI dose changes in both study subgroups were similar (13.4 (interquartile range (IQR) 0–25) vs. 25 (0–75)%, respectively; $p = 0.26$). Also, the absolute median dose changes of CyA (0 (0–75) vs. 25 (12.5–25) mg, respectively; $p = 0.73$) and Tc (0.5 (0.5–1.0) vs. 0 (−1.5–0.5) mg, respectively; $p = 0.26$) were similar.

Table 2. Office BP measurements and antihypertensive treatment before and after successful DAA therapy, divided into two subgroups based on changes in OBP control after treatment.

	OBP Control Improvement (n = 14)			p	No OBP Control Improvement (n = 14)			p
	Baseline	Follow-up	Δ		Baseline	Follow-up	Δ	
SBP (mmHg, mean and 95% CI)	145.5 (138.3–152.7)	125.1 (116.3–133.8)	−20.4 (−26.2–−14.6)	<0.001	135.6 (130.4–140.1)	130.4 (125.1–135.6)	−5.2 (−9.7–−0.8)	<0.05
DBP (mmHg, mean and 95% CI)	84.3 (78.8–89.8)	71.8 (67.0–76.6)	−12.5 (−16.5–−8.5)	<0.01	86.9 (83.6–90.1)	82.2 (79.3–85.1)	−4.6 (−9.6–−0.3)	0.07
PP (mmHg, mean and 95% CI)	61.2 (52.7–69.7)	53.3 (43.2–63.3)	−7.9 (−14.1–−1.8)	<0.05	48.7 (43.8–53.6)	48.1 (42.1–54.2)	−0.6 (−5.3–4.2)	0.86
Number of antihypertensive drugs (mean and 95% CI)	2.5 (1.3–3.7)	1.9 (0.8–2.9)	−0.6 (−1.0–−0.3)	<0.05	1.9 (1.4–2.5)	2.2 (1.5–3.0)	0.3 (0.0–0.6)	<0.07

CI, confidence interval; OBP, attended office blood pressure; DAA, direct antiviral drug therapy; SBP, systolic blood pressure; DBP, diastolic blood pressure; PP, pulse pressure.

3.3. Liver Function Tests and Liver Morphologic Assessments

At baseline, there was a numerical difference in HCV viremia between subgroups (Table 1), but neither HCV viremia nor baseline liver function tests differed significantly. In both subgroups, there was a significant reduction in aminotransferases and GGT activities after DAA treatment (Supplemental Materials Table S2). Liver elastography measurements were performed with a success rate near 100% (only 3 out of 28 patients needed 11 total measurements to obtain 10 valid results). Baseline liver stiffness measurements did not differ between subgroups and remained unchanged thereafter. On the contrary, CAP values only declined significantly in subgroup 1 (Supplementary Materials Table S2 and Figure 2).

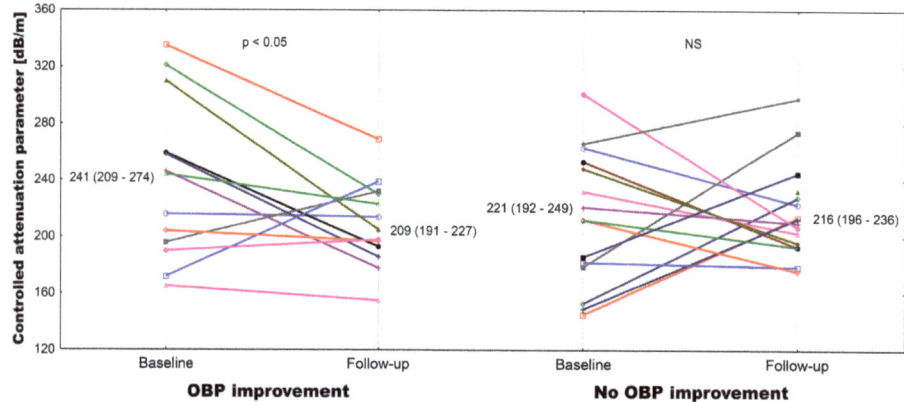

Figure 2. Individual plot of the controlled attenuation parameter at baseline and after the follow-up in patients with and without attended office blood pressure control improvement.

3.4. Central Blood Pressure Parameters

Both baseline and follow-up values of central aortic systolic pressure and central aortic pulse pressure correlated with corresponding values of OBP (baseline $r = 0.669$, $p < 0.001$, follow-up $r = 0.557$, $p < 0.01$ for SBP; and baseline $r = 0.730$, $p < 0.001$, follow-up $r = 0.502$, $p < 0.01$ for pulse pressure, respectively). There were also significant correlations between baseline augmentation index values standardized to heart rate (AIx@75) and both baseline and follow-up values of office SBP and pulse pressure (baseline $r = 0.660$, $p < 0.001$ and $r = 0.562$, $p < 0.01$, respectively; follow-up $r = 0.484$, $p < 0.01$ and $r = 0.545$, $p < 0.01$, respectively) (Table 3).

Parallel to OBP, we observed a 15.4% decline in aortic systolic pressure, a 12.1% decline in aortic diastolic pressure, and a 21.7% decline in aortic pulse pressure in subgroup 1 after successful DAA treatment (Table 3). Of note, AIx@75 values decreased significantly only in subgroup 1. On the contrary, only a mild decline of systolic aortic pressure (7.2%) was observed in subgroup 2. There was a positive correlation between the percentage change in CAP values and both the change in central aortic systolic pressure ($r = 0.438$, $p < 0.05$) and the change in AIx@75 ($r = 0.446$, $p < 0.05$). Of note, both baseline ($r = 0.479$, $p < 0.05$) and follow-up ($r = 0.431$, $p < 0.05$) CAP results correlated with corresponding BMI values.

Table 3. The central blood pressure parameters and the measurements of arterial stiffness (pulse wave velocity (PWV)) and endothelial function (flow-mediated dilation, (FMD) and nitroglycerine-mediated dilation (NMD)) measured before and after successful DAA treatment in kidney transplant recipients in both study subgroups, based on changes in OBP control after treatment.

	OBP Control Improvement (n = 14)				No OBP Control Improvement (n = 14)			
	Baseline	Follow-up	Δ	p	Baseline	Follow-up	Δ	p
Central blood pressure measurement								
AoSys (mmHg, mean and 95%CI)	136 (124–148)	114 (104–124)	−21.8 (−30.1–−13.5)	<0.01	131 (121–141)	120 (114–127)	−10.6 (−19.4–−1.9)	0.06
AoDia (mmHg, mean and 95%CI)	89 (81–96)	77 (71–83)	−11.6 (−19.2–−4.1)	<0.05	87 (81–92)	82 (76–87)	−5.0 (−12.8–−2.8)	0.19
AoPP (mmHg, mean and 95%CI)	47 (38–57)	37 (29–46)	−10.1 (−14.1–−6.2)	0.09	44 (37–51)	39 (33–44)	−5.6 (−12.3–−1.1)	0.19
AIx@75 (%, median and IQR)	20.5 (8.6–25.1)	16.9 (2.0–20.2)	−4.4 (−13.4–−1.1)	<0.05	15.5 (10.6–21.1)	16.5 (8.2–21.8)	0.0 (−8.2–7.8)	0.85
Arterial wall assessments								
PWV (m/s, mean and 95%CI)	8.5 (7.4–9.7)	8.7 (7.5–9.8)	0.1 (−0.7–0.9)	0.65	8.3 (7.1–9.5)	8.0 (6.9–9.2)	−0.3 (−1.4–0.8)	0.55
FMD (%, median and IQR)	9.2 (8.1–12.5)	9.3 (4.9–17.9)	2.1 (−6.5–3.3)	0.88	9.9 (7.5–15.0)	9.6 (5.6–12.2)	−1.6 (−2.8–0.6)	0.36
NMD (%, mean and 95%CI)	12.9 (10.3–15.6)	11.1 (8.4–13.8)	−1.8 (−5.5–−1.8)	0.30	11.8 (9.9–13.7)	6.3 (3.7–8.9)	−5.5 (−9.1–−2.0)	<0.001
NMD with double dose (%, mean and 95%CI)	12.9 (10.3–15.6)	13.4 (10.3–16.6)	0.5 (−2.2–3.2)	0.80	11.8 (9.9–13.7)	10.5 (5.7–15.3)	−1.3 (−6.0–3.5)	0.59

CI, confidence interval; IQR, interquartile range; OBP, office blood pressure; AoSys, aortic systolic pressure; AoDia, aortic diastolic pressure; AoPP, aortic pulse pressure; AIx75, aortic augmentation index normalized to heart rate of 75/min; PWV, pulse wave velocity; FMD, flow-mediated dilation; NMD, nitroglycerin-mediated dilation. For all comparisons of baseline values between two study subgroups, p values were >0.05.

3.5. Arterial Structural and Functional Measurements

At baseline and in the follow-up period, PWV values were similar in both subgroups (Table 3). FMD values were stable in both subgroups, while NMD measured using the standard (400 µg) dose of nitroglycerin did not change in subgroup 1, but showed a significant reduction in subgroup 2 (Table 3). However, in an additional repeated NMD measurement with a double dose of nitroglycerin there was no significant NMD change compared with baseline values in both study subgroups.

3.6. Cardiac Parameters

At baseline, both mean LVM (210 (169–250) vs. 211 (173–250) g, $p = 0.84$)) and mean LVMI (113 (94–131) vs. 114 (95–133) g/m^2, $p = 0.98$) were comparable in subgroups 1 and 2, respectively. Similarly, there were no differences in the follow-up LVM and LVMI values (0.70 and 0.87, respectively), and their absolute changes during the study period did not differ significantly (LVM 7.9 (−23.5 to 39.2) vs. −0.3 (−44.4 to 43.8), $p = 0.57$; LVMI 3.3 (−13.4 to 19.9) vs. −1.3 (−23.2 to 20.6) g/m^2, $p = 0.70$).

3.7. Inflammatory Markers

The baseline median of CRP concentration was slightly higher in subgroup 1 (1.7 (IQR 1.1–2.4) vs. 0.9 (0.4–1.4) mg/L in subgroup 2, with borderline significance ($p = 0.07$)). At follow-up assessment, there was a borderline increase of median hsCRP in subgroup 2 (3.6 (0.5–6.7), $p = 0.06$), whereas no difference was noted in subgroup 1 (1.8 (1.5–3.0), $p = 0.33$). There were no significant differences in IL-6 concentration median values, both at baseline (2.7 (2.2–3.2) vs. 2.2 (1.8–2.5) pg/mL, $p = 0.23$) and at the follow-up examination (2.7 (1.7–4.1) vs. 2.6 (1.7–5.7) pg/mL, $p = 0.76$). Levels did not change significantly during the study period.

3.8. Fibroblast Growth Factor 21 Levels

Median values of FGF-21 measured at follow-up increased significantly in subgroup 1 (411 (204–706) vs. 215 (120–535) pg/mL at baseline, $p < 0.01$), while they remained unchanged in subgroup 2 (189 (147–481) vs. 226 (116–267) pg/mL at baseline, $p = 0.22$). The baseline number of antihypertensive drugs was borderline associated with log values of baseline FGF-21 ($r = 0.375, p = 0.05$) and significantly associated with follow-up values of FGF-21 ($r = 0.467, p < 0.05$). However, the log values of both baseline and follow-up FGF-21 did not correlate with baseline SBP or DBP values, whereas they correlated significantly with baseline central systolic aortic pressure ($r = 0.388, p < 0.05$, and $r = 0.434$, $p < 0.05$, for baseline and follow-up FGF-21 log values, respectively) and borderline with central diastolic aortic pressure ($r = 0.357, p < 0.05$, and $r = 0.385, p < 0.05$, respectively). Moreover, the log values of follow-up FGF-21 negatively correlated with the change of central systolic and diastolic aortic pressures ($r = -0.361$ and $r = -0.367$, respectively) with both p values $= 0.06$.

4. Discussion

In the present study, we demonstrated the clinically important improvement of blood pressure control, defined as the decline of attended office systolic pressure by at least 20 mmHg without pharmacotherapeutic changes or the reduction of antihypertensive treatment due to the BP decline, in half of our cohort of HCV-infected stable kidney transplant recipients after successful HCV eradication with sofosbuvir-based DAA therapy. In this subgroup of patients, we observed the reduction of systolic BP values despite the de-escalation of antihypertensive treatment in 9 out of 14 subjects. Moreover, we also documented the parallel decline of central aortic pressure parameters, obtained with the Sphygmo-Cor device, including augmentation index, in patients with improved BP control. Finally, we noted the corresponding decrease of liver steatosis, measured by the controlled attenuation parameter, in this subgroup of patients, which may suggest the potential underlying mechanism of beneficial vascular changes.

We are aware that nowadays a majority of dialysis patients with previously diagnosed HCV infection have already been successfully treated with DAA regimen even before they get a kidney transplant. Nevertheless, the confirmation of relatively moderate BP control improvement in patients being currently on dialysis would be much more difficult due to procedural-related fluctuations in volemia. Thus, the present study findings may help to elucidate or confirm some mechanisms linking the HCV infection with BP control in CKD patients.

There are several possible pathomechanisms linking the chronic HCV infection with elevated blood pressure and increased cardiovascular risk, including increased arterial stiffness [23], endothelial dysfunction [13], and the direct effect of liver steatosis on BP regulation [24]. The virus plays an etiological and pathogenic role in the development of vasculitis and renal involvement with subsequent elevated BP and cardiovascular events. Notably, in the present study, the time from HCV diagnosis to DAA treatment was significantly shorter in the subgroup with improved BP control thereafter, which may confirm that the longer duration of HCV infection determines the degree of irreversible vascular damage and, therefore, influences the net effect of HCV eradication on BP control. Recently, an increased augmentation index following viral eradication with DAA therapy was found in patients with advanced fibrosis ($\geq$9.5 kPa) [25]. Of note, in patients with non-advanced fibrosis, the authors observed a stable augmentation index and significantly lower values of both office and central systolic pressure at the SVR12 time point [25]. In contrast, we observed a significant decrease of the normalized augmentation index in a subgroup with BP improvement, whereas any change in arterial stiffness, measured by pulse wave velocity, was found in our cohort, independently of BP changes after DAA treatment.

When considering the possible changes of endothelial function after successful HCV eradication with DAA, the reduction of endothelium-derived adhesion molecule levels at the SVR12 time point was confirmed by two small studies [26,27], but the improvement of FMD values was observed only in one group [26], and Davis et al. did not find changes in bedside microvascular reactivity, measured by peripheral arterial tonometry [27]. Of note, both studies were performed in individuals with normal renal function. In our cohort, we observed stable FMD values and significantly lower NMD values after DAA treatment; however, a repeated measurement with a double dose of nitroglycerin did not confirm the preceding finding. As we previously reported, the significant decrease of calcineurin inhibitor levels shortly after successful HCV eradication in this group [15], we may speculate that this effect was caused by an improved liver metabolic efficiency, which limited the biologic effect of a standard nitroglycerin dose used originally. Furthermore, the calcineurin inhibitor co-medication may also influence the endothelial function in our group [28], though the proportion of cyclosporine A- and tacrolimus-treated patients was similar in both study subgroups.

It is important to notice that both analyzed subgroups did not differ at baseline in terms of demographics, co-morbidity, or kidney graft function. Also, arterial stiffness and endothelial function measures, as well as liver function tests and liver stiffness measurements, were comparable. There were significantly higher baseline office systolic blood pressure and pulse pressure values, but not central blood pressure parameters, in subgroup 1. The posttreatment follow-up evaluation, along with the substantial BP control improvement, revealed a significant decrease of CAP values in these patients. Notably, in patients without known cause of chronic liver disease, increased CAP was shown to be a good indicator of fatty liver disease with metabolic abnormalities that manifest even before a sonographic fatty change appears [29].

In HCV-infected patients, an intrahepatic viral load directly enhances the liver steatosis [30], especially in the setting of multiple metabolic abnormalities (expansion of visceral adipose tissue, insulin resistance, reversible hypocholesterolemia, arterial hypertension, and hyperuricemia). On the other hand, in patients with non-alcoholic fatty liver disease (NAFLD), steatosis grade was the most important factor for endothelial dysfunction [31]. Furthermore, lower FMD values were shown in pediatric NAFLD patients, in whom systolic and diastolic blood pressures were significantly higher than in healthy controls, but also higher than obese children with normal livers [32]. Even more importantly, fatty liver was shown to be associated with 24-h systolic blood pressure and daytime diastolic blood pressure measurements [24]. Recently, Wang et al. demonstrated that NAFLD is independently associated with hypertension and blood pressure category [33]. In this study, the CAP value was the predictor of diastolic, but not systolic BP in stepwise analysis for the whole study group, not only in NAFLD participants [33]. Of note, CAP alone was not sufficient for predicting hypertension in this study.

It is well known that in the population of KTRs, the measures of vascular damage are conditioned by many factors, including the duration of chronic kidney disease, pretransplant dialysis vintage, concomitant immunosuppressive regimen, and non-optimal kidney graft function. Thus, the possibility for marked improvement of vascular elasticity and distensibility after the successful HCV treatment is much lower than in the general population. Nonetheless, overall results of our investigation may indirectly confirm the notable role of decreasing liver steatosis in the BP control improvement in the study group.

Finally, FGF-21 levels are reported to increase in acute liver injury, but decrease in chronic hepatitis B patients [34], especially those with advanced fibrosis [35]. We analyzed FGF-21 concentrations before and after the successful treatment of chronic HCV infection. Its levels significantly increased only in patients with initially more advanced steatosis as shown by CAP and improved BP control after DAA therapy and HCV elimination. The concomitant decrease of liver steatosis after DAA therapy observed in our study is in line with previously published papers [36,37] and may play a significant role in improved BP control.

The main limitation of our analyzed cohort was its small size, which limited multivariate analysis of factors independently associated with the BP control improvement. Therefore, our preliminary data should be investigated in a larger multicenter cohort. However, we included all eligible KTRs with the sustained elimination of chronic HCV infection. Of note, the structure of DAA regimen in our patients was uniform: All were treated with a sofosbuvir-based therapy. Another limitation was the method of OBP measurement used in this study, specifically the lack of unattended BP measurement, which eliminated the potential bias related to the 'white coat' effect. In addition, we did not perform the 24-h ambulatory blood pressure monitoring; however, we observed the central blood pressure values and found a strong association with OBP results. Lastly, we would like to acknowledge the lack of monitoring of the adherence to antihypertensive medication in our study.

5. Conclusions

In conclusion, we observed the clinically important improvement of both office blood pressure control and central aortic pressure parameters, including augmentation index, in half of our cohort of HCV-infected stable kidney transplant recipients after successful HCV eradication with a sofosbuvir-based DAA therapy. The concomitant decrease of liver steatosis, measured by the controlled attenuation parameter, was only observed in this subgroup of patients, which may suggest the potential underlying mechanism of beneficial hemodynamic changes. Further investigation would elucidate the pathomechanism of the observed improvement of blood pressure control, however, the increased availability of DAA therapy already resulted in pretransplant eradication of HCV infection in a majority of currently dialysis patients. We believe that patients receiving DAA therapy in the pretransplant period will benefit even more. Nevertheless, the confirmation of relatively moderate BP improvement in dialysis patients would be much more difficult due to procedural-related fluctuations in volemia.

Supplementary Materials: The following are available online at http://www.mdpi.com/2077-0383/9/4/948/s1, Table S1: Laboratory parameters before and after successful DAA therapy, divided into subgroups based on changes in OBP control after treatment, Table S2: The results of liver function tests as well as the measurements of liver stiffness (LSM) and liver steatosis (controlled attenuation parameter—CAP) in kidney transplant recipients before and after the successful DAA therapy, divided into 2 subgroups based on the changes in OBP control after treatment.

Author Contributions: Conceptualization and methodology, A.K. and J.M.; formal analysis, A.K. and J.C.; investigation, M.B., N.S.-B., A.K.-S., and P.K.; data curation, A.K. and K.K.-F.; writing—original draft preparation, A.K., J.M., and J.C.; writing—review and editing, A.W.; supervision, A.K. and A.W.; funding acquisition, A.K. All authors have read and agreed to the published version of the manuscript.

Funding: This research was funded by Medical University of Silesia in Katowice, Grant KNW-1-058/N/8/K.

Conflicts of Interest: The authors declare no conflict of interest.

References

1. Divac, N.; Naumovic, R.; Stojanovic, R.; Prostran, M. The role of immunosuppressive medications in the pathogenesis of hypertension and efficacy of antihypertensive agents in kidney transplant recipients. *Curr. Med. Chem.* **2015**, *23*, 1941–1952. [CrossRef]
2. Wadei, H.M.; Textor, S.C. Hypertension in the kidney transplant recipients. *Transplant. Rev.* **2010**, *24*, 105–120. [CrossRef]
3. Arias, M.; Fernández-Fresnedo, G.; Gago, M.; Rodrigo, E.; Gómez-Alamillo, C.; Toyos, C.; Allende, N. Clinical characteristics of resistant hypertension in renal transplant recipients. *Nephrol. Dial. Transplant.* **2012**, *27* (Suppl. 4), 36–38. [CrossRef]
4. Azancot, M.A.; Ramos, N.; Moreso, F.J.; Ibernon, M.; Espinel, E.; Torres, I.B.; Fort, J.; Seron, D. Hypertension in chronic kidney disease: The influence of renal transplantation. *Transplantation* **2014**, *98*, 537–542. [CrossRef] [PubMed]
5. Opelz, G.; Wujciak, T.; Ritz, E. Association of chronic kidney graft failure with recipient blood pressure. *Kidney Int.* **1998**, *53*, 217–222. [CrossRef] [PubMed]
6. Sarnak, M.J.; Levey, A.S.; Schoolwerth, A.C.; Coresh, J.; Culleton, B.; Hamm, L.L.; McCullough, P.A.; Kasiske, B.L.; Kelepouris, E.; Klag, M.J.; et al. Kidney disease as a risk factor for development of cardiovascular disease: A statement from the American Heart Association Councils on Kidney in Cardiovascular Disease, High Blood Pressure Research, Clinical Cardiology, and Epidemiology and Prevention. *Circulation* **2002**, *108*, 154–169.
7. Stenvinkel, P.; Carrero, J.J.; Axelsson, J.; Lindholm, B.; Heimburger, O.; Massy, Z. Emerging biomarkers for evaluating cardiovascular risk in the chronic kidney disease patient: How do new pieces fit into the uremic puzzle? *Clin. J. Am. Soc. Nephrol.* **2008**, *3*, 505–521. [CrossRef]
8. Hogas, S.M.; Voroneanu, L.; Serban, D.N.; Segall, L.; Hogas, M.M.; Serban, I.L.; Covic, A. Methods and potential biomarkers for the evaluation of endothelial dysfunction in chronic kidney disease: A critical approach. *J. Am. Soc. Hypertens.* **2010**, *4*, 116–127. [CrossRef]
9. Wang, M.C.; Tsai, W.C.; Chen, J.Y.; Huang, J.J. Stepwise increase in arterial stiffness corresponding with the stages of chronic kidney disease. *Am. J. Kidney Dis.* **2005**, *45*, 494–501. [CrossRef]
10. Recio-Mayoral, A.; Banerjee, D.; Streather, C.; Kaski, J.C. Endothelial dysfunction, inflammation and atherosclerosis in chronic kidney disease—A cross-sectional study of predialysis, dialysis and kidney-transplantation patients. *Atherosclerosis* **2011**, *216*, 446–451. [CrossRef]
11. Pedroso, S.; Martins, L.; Fonseca, I.; Dias, L.; Henriques, A.C.; Sarmento, A.M.; Cabrita, A. Impact of hepatitis C virus on renal transplantation: Association with poor survival. *Transplant. Proc.* **2006**, *38*, 1890–1894. [CrossRef] [PubMed]
12. Oyake, N.; Shimada, T.; Murakami, Y.; Ishibashi, Y.; Satoh, H.; Suzuki, K.; Matsumory, A.; Oda, T. Hepatitis C virus infection as a risk factor for increased aortic stiffness and cardiovascular events in dialysis patients. *J. Nephrol.* **2008**, *21*, 345–353. [PubMed]
13. Barone, M.; Viggiani, M.T.; Amoruso, A.; Schiraldi, S.; Zito, A.; Devito, F.; Cortese, F.; Gesualdo, M.; Brunetti, N.; Di Leo, A.; et al. Endothelial dysfunction correlates with liver fibrosis in chronic HCV infection. *Gastroenterol. Res. Pract.* **2015**, *2015*, 682174. [CrossRef] [PubMed]
14. Osztovits, J.; Horváth, T.; Abonyi, M.; Tóth, T.; Visnyei, Z.; Bekö, G.; Csák, T.; Lakatos, P.L.; Littvay, L.; Fehér, J.; et al. Chronic hepatits C virus infection associated with autonomic dysfunction. *Liver Int.* **2009**, *29*, 1473–1478. [CrossRef] [PubMed]
15. Musialik, J.; Kolonko, A.; Kwiecień, K.; Owczarek, A.J.; Więcek, A. Effectiveness and safety of sofosbuvir-based therapy against hepatitis C infection after successful kidney transplantation. *Transpl. Infect. Dis.* **2019**, *21*, e13090. [CrossRef] [PubMed]

16. Babbs, C.F. The origin of Korotkoff sounds and the accuracy of auscultatory blood pressure measurements. *J. Am. Soc. Hypertens.* **2015**, *9*, 935–950. [CrossRef] [PubMed]
17. Padwal, R.; Jalali, A.; McLean, D.; Anwar, S.; Smith, K.; Raggi, P.; Ringrose, J.S. Accuracy of oscillometric blood pressure algorithms in healthy adults and in adults with cardiovascular risk factors. *Blood Press. Monit.* **2019**, *24*, 33–37. [CrossRef]
18. Lang, R.M.; Bierig, M.; Devereux, R.B.; Flaschkampf, F.A.; Foster, E.; Pellikka, P.A.; Picard, M.H.; Roman, M.J.; Seward, J.; Shanewise, J.S.; et al. Recommendations for Chamber Quantification: A report from the American Society of Echocardiography's Guidelines and Standards Committee and the Chamber Quantification Writing group. *J. Am. Soc. Echocardiogr.* **2005**, *18*, 1440–1463. [CrossRef]
19. Devereux, R.B.; Reichek, N. Echocardiographic determination of left ventricular mass in man. Anatomic validation of the method. *Circulation* **1977**, *55*, 613–618. [CrossRef]
20. Thijssen, D.H.J.; Bruno, R.M.; van Mil, A.C.C.M.; Holder, S.M.; Faita, F.; Greyling, A.; Zock, P.L.; Taddei, S.; Deanfield, J.E.; Luscher, T.; et al. Expert consensus and evidence-based recommendations for the assessment of flow-mediated dilation in humans. *Eur. Heart J.* **2019**, *40*, 2534–2547. [CrossRef]
21. Jun, B.G.; Park, W.Y.; Park, E.J.; Jang, J.Y.; Jeong, S.W.; Lee, S.H.; Kim, S.G.; Cha, S.W.; Kim, Y.S.; Cho, Y.D.; et al. A prospective comparative assessment of the accuracy of the FibroScan in evaluating liver steatosis. *PLoS ONE* **2017**, *12*, e01827784. [CrossRef] [PubMed]
22. Sandrin, L.; Fourquet, B.; Hasquenoph, J.M.; Yon, S.; Fournier, C.; Mal, F.; Christidis, C.; Ziol, M.; Poulet, B.; Kazemi, F.; et al. Transient elastography: A new noninvasive method for assessment of hepatic fibrosis. *Ultrasound Med. Biol.* **2003**, *29*, 1705–1713. [CrossRef] [PubMed]
23. Chou, C.-H.; Ho, C.-S.; Tsai, W.-C.; Wang, M.-C.; Tsai, Y.-S.; Chen, J.-Y. Effects of chronic hepatitis C infection on arterial stiffness. *J. Am. Soc. Hypertens.* **2017**, *11*, 716–723. [CrossRef] [PubMed]
24. Vasunta, R.-L.; Kesaniemi, Y.A.; Ylitalo, A.S.; Ukkola, O.H. High ambulatory blood pressure values associated with non-alcoholic fatty liver in middle-aged adults. *J. Hypert.* **2012**, *30*, 2015–2019. [CrossRef] [PubMed]
25. Cheng, P.-N.; Chen, J.-Y.; Chiu, Y.-C.; Chiu, H.-C.; Tsai, L.-M. Augmenting central arterial stiffness following eradication of HCV by direct acting antivirals in advanced fibrosis patients. *Sci. Rep.* **2019**, *9*, 1426. [CrossRef] [PubMed]
26. Schmidt, F.P.; Zimmermann, T.; Wenz, T.; Schnorbus, B.; Ostad, M.A.; Feist, C.; Grambihler, A.; Schattenberg, J.M.; Sprinzl, M.F.; Münzel, T.; et al. Interferon- and ribavirin-free therapy with new direct acting antivirals (DAA) for chronic hepatitis C improves vascular endothelial function. *Int. J. Cardiol.* **2018**, *271*, 296–300. [CrossRef]
27. Davis, J.S.; Young, M.; Lennox, S.; Jones, T.; Piera, K.; Pickles, R.; Oakley, S. The effect of curing hepatitis C with direct-acting antiviral treatment on endothelial function. *Antivir. Ther.* **2018**, *23*, 687–694. [CrossRef]
28. Akoglu, H.; Seringec, N.; Yildirim, T.; Yilmaz, R.; Okutucu, S.; Turkmen, E.; Evranos, B.; Kaya, E.B.; Dikmenoglu, N.; Arici, M.; et al. Relationship between hemorheology and endothelial dysfunction in renal transplant patients receiving calcineurin inhibitors. *J. Nephrol.* **2013**, *26*, 931–940. [CrossRef]
29. Kwak, M.S.; Chung, G.E.; Yang, J.I.; Yim, J.Y.; Chung, S.J.; Jung, S.Y.; Kim, J.S. Clinical implications of controlled attenuation parameter in a health check-up cohort. *Liver Int.* **2017**, *38*, 915–923. [CrossRef]
30. Ramalho, F. Hepatitis C virus infection and liver steatosis. *Antivir. Res.* **2003**, *60*, 125–127. [CrossRef]
31. Sapmaz, F.; Uzman, M.; Basyigit, S.; Ozkan, S.; Yavuz, B.; Yeniova, A.; Kefeli, A.; Asilturk, Z.; Nazligül, Y. Steatosis grade is the most important risk factor for development of endothelial dysfunction in NAFLD. *Medicine* **2016**, *95*, e3280. [CrossRef] [PubMed]
32. Pacifico, L.; Anania, C.; Martino, F.; Cantisani, V.; Pascone, R.; Marcantonio, A.; Chiesa, C. Functional and morphological vascular changes in pediatric nonalcoholic fatty liver disease. *Hepatology* **2010**, *52*, 1643–1651. [CrossRef] [PubMed]
33. Wang, Y.; Zeng, Y.; Lin, C.; Chen, Z. Hypertension and non-alcoholic fatty liver disease proven by transient elastography. *Hepatol. Res.* **2016**, *46*, 1304–1310. [CrossRef] [PubMed]
34. Wu, L.; Pan, Q.; Wu, G.; Qian, L.; Zhang, J.; Zhang, L.; Fang, Q.; Zang, G.; Wang, Y.; Lau, G.; et al. Diverse changes of circulating fibroblast growth factor 21 levels in hepatitis B virus-related diseases. *Sci. Rep.* **2017**, *7*, 16482. [CrossRef] [PubMed]
35. Iwasa, M.; Mifuji-Moroka, R.; Kobayashi, Y.; Takei, Y.; D'Alessandro-Gabazza, C.; Gabazza, E.C. Comment on serum FGF21 and RBP4 levels in patients with chronic hepatits C. *Scand. J. Gastroent.* **2012**, *48*, 252–253. [CrossRef] [PubMed]

36. Tada, T.; Kumada, T.; Toyoda, H.; Sone, Y.; Takeshima, K.; Ogawa, S.; Goto, T.; Wakahata, A.; Nakashima, M.; Nakamuta, M.; et al. Viral eradication reduces both liver stiffness and steatosis in patients with chronic hepatitis C virus infection who received direct-acting anti-viral therapy. *Aliment. Pharmacol. Ther.* **2018**, *7*, 1012–1022. [CrossRef]
37. Kobayashi, N.; Iijima, H.; Tada, T.; Kumada, T.; Yoshida, M.; Aoki, T.; Nishimura, T.; Nakano, C.; Takata, R.; Yoh, K.; et al. Changes in liver stiffness and steatosis among patients with hepatitis C virus infection who received direct-acting antiviral therapy and achieved sustained virological response. *Eur. J. Gastroenterol. Hepatol.* **2018**, *5*, 546–551. [CrossRef]

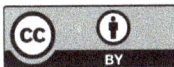 © 2020 by the authors. Licensee MDPI, Basel, Switzerland. This article is an open access article distributed under the terms and conditions of the Creative Commons Attribution (CC BY) license (http://creativecommons.org/licenses/by/4.0/).

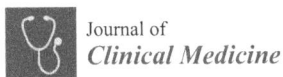

Perspective

Is There Decreasing Public Interest in Renal Transplantation? A Google Trends™ Analysis

Andreas Kronbichler [1,*], Maria Effenberger [2,*], Jae Il Shin [3,4,5], Christian Koppelstätter [1], Sara Denicolò [1], Michael Rudnicki [1], Hannes Neuwirt [1], Maria José Soler [6], Kate Stevens [7], Annette Bruchfeld [8], Herbert Tilg [2], Gert Mayer [1] and Paul Perco [1]

1. Department of Internal Medicine IV (Nephrology and Hypertension), Medical University Innsbruck, Anichstrasse 35, 6020 Innsbruck, Austria; christian.koppelstaetter@tirol-kliniken.at (C.K.); sara.denicolo@i-med.ac.at (S.D.); michael.rudnicki@i-med.ac.at (M.R.); hannes.neuwirt@i-med.ac.at (H.N.); gert.mayer@i-med.ac.at (G.M.); paul.perco@i-med.ac.at (P.P.)
2. Department of Internal Medicine I (Gastroenterology, Hepatology, Endocrinology and Metabolism), Medical University Innsbruck, Anichstrasse 35, 6020 Innsbruck, Austria; herbert.tilg@i-med.ac.at
3. Department of Pediatrics, Yonsei University College of Medicine, 03722 Seoul, Korea; shinji@yuhs.ac
4. Department of Pediatric Nephrology, Severance Children's Hospital, Seoul 03722, Korea
5. Institute of Kidney Disease Research, Yonsei University College of Medicine, Seoul 03722, Korea
6. Department of Nephrology, Hospital Universitari Vall d'Hebron, Nephrology Research Group, Vall d'Hebron Research Institute (VHIR), 08035 Barcelona, Spain; mjsoler01@gmail.com
7. Glasgow Renal and Transplant Unit, Queen Elizabeth University Hospital, Glasgow G51 4TF, UK; kate.stevens@glasgow.ac.uk
8. Department of Clinical Sciences Interventions and Technology (CLINTEC), Division of Renal Medicine, Karolinska Institutet, Karolinska University Hospital, 171 77 Stockholm, Sweden; annette.bruchfeld@ki.se
* Correspondence: andreas.kronbichler@i-med.ac.at (A.K.); Maria.effenberger@tirol-kliniken.at (M.E.)

Received: 6 March 2020; Accepted: 6 April 2020; Published: 7 April 2020

Abstract: Background and objectives: Renal transplantation is the preferred form of renal replacement therapy for the majority of patients with end stage renal disease (ESRD). The Internet is a key tool for people seeking healthcare-related information. This current work explored the interest in kidney transplantation based on Internet search queries using Google Trends™. Design, setting, participants, and measurements: We performed a Google Trends™ search with the search term "kidney transplantation" between 2004 (year of inception) and 2018. We retrieved and analyzed data on the worldwide trend as well as data from the United Network for Organ Sharing (UNOS), the Organización Nacional de Trasplantes (ONT), the Eurotransplant area, and the National Health Service (NHS) Transplant Register. Google Trends™ indices were investigated and compared to the numbers of performed kidney transplants, which were extracted from the respective official websites of UNOS, ONT, Eurotransplant, and the NHS. Results: During an investigational period of 15 years, there was a significant decrease of the worldwide Google Trends™ index from 76.3 to 25.4, corresponding to an absolute reduction of −50.9% and a relative reduction by −66.7%. The trend was even more pronounced for the UNOS area (−75.2%), while in the same time period the number of transplanted kidneys in the UNOS area increased by 21.9%. Events of public interest had an impact on the search queries in the year of occurrence, as shown by an increase in the Google Trends™ index by 39.2% in the year 2005 in Austria when a person of public interest received his second live donor kidney transplant. Conclusions: This study indicates a decreased public interest in kidney transplantation. There is a clear need to raise public awareness, since transplantation represents the best form of renal replacement therapy for patients with ESRD. Information should be provided on social media, with a special focus on readability and equitable access, as well as on web pages.

Keywords: kidney transplantation; transplant numbers; live donors; public awareness; Google Trends™

1. Introduction

Kidney transplantation is considered to be the optimal form of renal replacement therapy and has a positive impact on quality of life, survival rates of the recipients, and overall is considered cost-effective [1]. Due to organ shortage and longer waiting time, death on the waiting list is a serious concern and criteria for suitable organs have been extended. There are several advantages of live donor transplantation compared with deceased donor transplantation including lower risk of rejection, reduced waiting time for transplantation, and improved allograft and overall survival [2]. The frequency of live kidney donation is stable in the United States (US), while increasing in the Eurotransplant area and in the United Kingdom (UK) over the last 15 years. Despite these efforts there are currently 94,621 patients on the kidney waiting list in the US according to the United Network for Organ Sharing (UNOS), 10,791 (at the end of 2018) potential recipients in the Eurotransplant area and as of March 2019, approximately 5000 patients were waiting for a kidney transplant in the UK. Analysis of different surveys among the public revealed barriers towards live kidney transplantation [3], and strategies to overcome these barriers are necessary to increase the number of transplants.

Google Trends™ generates data on spatial and temporal patterns according to specified keywords. A study comparing the reliability of Google Trends™ in two settings, more common diseases with low media coverage and less common diseases with higher media coverage, found that Google Trends™ seems to be influenced by media presence rather than by true epidemiological burden of one disease [4]. Several studies using Google Trends™ data have been conducted recently. One of these investigated the influence of meteorological variables on relative search volumes for pain and found that selected local weather conditions were associated with online search volumes for specific musculoskeletal pain symptoms [5]. Analysis of Google Trends™ search volume queries not only holds great promise in medicine, but also in other areas of research. Analysis of northern Europeans' (Finland, Germany, Norway, Ireland, and the UK) web searching behavior on Mediterranean tourist destinations revealed a relationship between thermal conditions and the searching behavior, and the authors observed no time lag between the prevalence of thermal conditions and searching of the keywords [6].

In transplant medicine, public awareness is key to promote discussion around organ donation, both live and deceased. In the current study, we investigate the public interest in kidney transplantation using data on Internet search queries extracted from the Google Trends™ tool.

2. Materials and Methods

2.1. Retrieving Transplantation Numbers for UNOS, ONT, and Eurotransplant

Data were retrieved by accessing the respective websites of the transplant organizations ((https://unos.org) for the UNOS, (http://www.ont.es) for the Organización Nacional de Trasplantes (ONT), (https://www.eurotransplant.org) for the Eurotransplant countries, and (https://www.nhsbt.nhs.uk) for the UK.

Information about live and deceased donor kidney transplantation over a period of 15 years (2004–2018) for the following countries was extracted from the web pages as stated above: United States of America (UNOS), Spain (ONT), Austria, Belgium, Croatia, Germany, Hungary, Slovenia, and the Netherlands (belonging to the Eurotransplant countries), and the UK (NHS Transplant Register).

2.2. Retrieving Google Trends™ Data on Kidney Transplantation

The Google Trends™ tool (https://trends.google.com/trends/) was used to retrieve data on Internet user search activities in the context of kidney transplantation. Google Trends™ is a freely accessible tool that enables researchers to study trends and patterns of Google search queries [7]. It was implemented in 2004 and data on Internet search queries are available since then on a monthly basis. Google Trends^{TM} expresses the absolute number of searches relative to the total number of searches over the defined period of interest. The retrieved Google Trends^{TM} index ranges from 0 to 100, with 100 being the highest relative search term activity for the specified search query in any given month [7]. Thus, a search index of 50 indicates that the search activity for kidney transplantation was 50% of that seen at the time when search activity was most intense [7].

Worldwide Google Trends^{TM} indices were retrieved between January 2004 and December 2018 using the search term "kidney transplantation". We retrieved Google Trends^{TM} indices for the US, Spain, the following European countries being part of the Eurotransplant network, namely Austria, Belgium, Croatia, Germany, Hungary, Slovenia, and the Netherlands, and the UK. No Google Trends^{TM} indices could be retrieved for Luxembourg. Whereas the worldwide search was performed in English, the individual searches in the respective countries were performed in the official languages (see Table S1).

2.3. Data Analysis

Annual average Google Trends^{TM} indices were calculated based on the monthly data downloaded from the Google Trends^{TM} webpage. Time-lag correlations between transplant numbers and Google Trends^{TM} indices were calculated using the ccf function of the tseries R package using a time lag between −3 and +3. The ggplot2 R package was used to generate all graphics. R version 3.4.1 was used for all analyses.

None of the queries in the Google database for this study can be associated to a particular individual. The database retains no information about the identity, Internet protocol address or specific physical location of any user. Furthermore, any original web search logs older than nine months are anonymized in accordance with Google's privacy policy (www.google.com/privacypolicy.html).

3. Results

The worldwide search query using Google Trends^{TM} highlighted a decrease from an index of 76.3 in 2004 to 25.4 in 2018 (absolute reduction −50.9, or a relative reduction of −66.7%, see Figure 1). This trend was particularly confirmed in the US, with a decrease of the Google Trends^{TM} index from an index of 68.4 to 17.0 (absolute reduction −51.4, relative reduction of −75.2%) over time. While an initial sharp decrease in search results was observed from an index of 68.4 to 37.6 (absolute reduction −30.8, relative reduction of −45.0%) within two years, there was a further decrease by 54.8% over the following thirteen years. In the same period of time, UNOS reported an increase of deceased donor kidney transplants from 16,007 in 2004 to 21,167 in 2018 (+32.2%); within the same period the live donor kidney transplantation rate remained stable (6648 in 2004 and 6442 in 2018, −3.1%). A similar search tendency of a decreased Google Trends^{TM} index was found for the Eurotransplant area and the UK. There was a modest increase in Google Trends^{TM} search queries in Spain, with a very low number in 2004 (index of 8.3) and 10.1 in 2018 (absolute increase +1.8, or a relative increase of +21.7%). In the same time-period the number of transplanted kidneys increased from 2125 to 3313 (+55.9%). In smaller countries, it is likely that events of interest to the public lead to an increase in search queries in that particular year. This for example might explain the increase in search queries in Austria in 2005 when a person of public interest received a second live-related kidney transplant in the same year. We observed an increase of Google Trends^{TM} search queries from an index of 26.3 in 2004 to 36.6 in 2005 (absolute increase +10.3 or relative increase of +39.2%). In the following years, a decrease was found with an index of 12.9 in 2018 (absolute reduction −13.4 or a relative decrease of −51.0%). Similar curves were observed in all Eurotransplant countries, even in countries with a higher number of live-related kidney transplants, for example, the Netherlands (48.1% in 2004 and 40.0% in 2018), where more web-based information retrieval might be expected. Online searches assessed by Google Trends^{TM} decreased from 49.3 to 37.8 (−11.5, or −23.3%) over 15 years. In Germany a decrease from 52.4 to 30.7

(−21.7, or −41.4%) was found in the same period, with even more pronounced reductions observed in Belgium (from 21.5 to 8.1, corresponding to a decrease of 13.4, or −62.3%) and Hungary (from 8.3 to 2.6, absolute reduction of −5.7 or relative reduction by −68.7%). In the UK, Google Trends™ indices decreased from 33.25 to 7.58 with an absolute reduction of 25.67 and a relative reduction of −77.2%, mirroring the decrease observed in the US. An overview of Google Trends™ changes over time and number of transplants (deceased donor and live donor transplantation) in the respective countries is highlighted in Table 1, Table S2, and Figure 2.

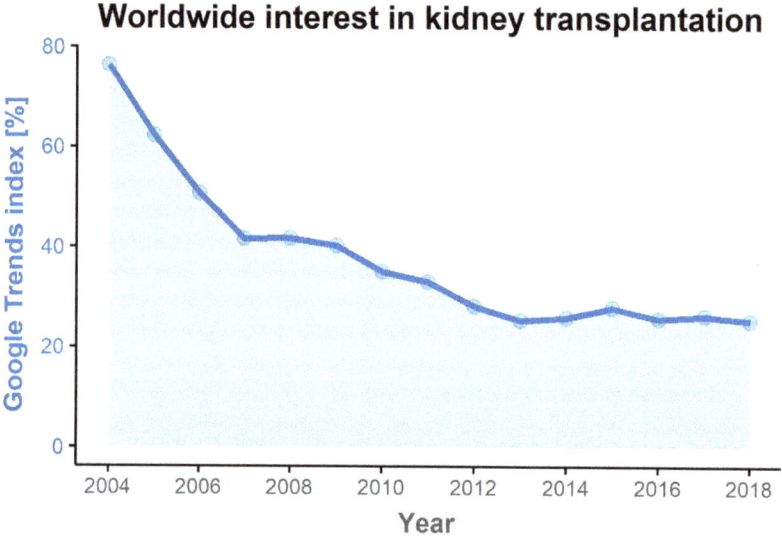

Figure 1. A worldwide decrease in the Google Trends™ indices from inception to 2018 was found. During a period of 15 years, the index decreased from 76.3 to 25.4, corresponding to a change of −66.7%.

We used correlation analysis to compare the Google Trends™ indices to the number of transplants over time and found negative correlations in particular for the UK, Belgium, and Austria, but also for Hungary, Slovenia, Germany, and the US. Spain is the only country where both transplant numbers as well as Google Trends™ indices show positive correlations above 0.5 (Figure 3).

Table 1. The respective year, number of search queries using Google Trends[TM], and the total number of kidney transplantations performed (deceased donor and living donor).

Year	World GT	US GT	US Tx	UK GT	UK Tx	ESP GT	ESP Tx	B GT	B Tx	NL GT	NL Tx	GER GT	GER Tx	AUT GT	AUT Tx	SLO GT	SLO Tx	H GT	H Tx	CRO GT	CRO Tx
2004	76.3	68.4	22,655	33.25	1836	8.3	2125	21.5	235	49.3	520	52.4	1991	26.3	253	17.4	35	8.3	0	0.0	0
2005	62.3	49.1	23,057	36.75	1783	0.0	2200	28.4	260	53.5	762	40.0	2165	36.6	255	14.8	20	5.8	0	0.0	0
2006	50.8	37.6	23,530	30.67	1915	4.0	2157	18.6	324	32.8	752	31.5	2206	30.3	303	19.5	30	8.2	0	18.8	0
2007	41.6	33.8	22,677	20.58	2130	0.0	2211	16.9	338	32.4	968	36.7	2336	26.6	299	8.5	22	8.3	0	21.0	26
2008	41.8	29.8	22,489	15.00	2282	9.3	2229	11.6	325	31.3	1012	30.8	2257	26.9	273	9.2	34	3.3	0	4.7	46
2009	40.3	32.6	23,216	16.08	2495	5.7	2328	13.3	335	31.8	1036	28.4	2317	22.8	331	9.0	31	7.4	0	10.2	57
2010	35.1	24.1	23,178	14.00	2694	5.3	2225	12.4	313	31.8	1151	28.7	2512	17.8	300	8.2	38	2.8	0	11.2	70
2011	33.1	25.7	22,589	11.83	2686	10.3	2498	10.1	338	33.3	1091	32.6	2660	13.2	293	9.0	29	3.7	0	8.3	47
2012	28.2	21.9	22,106	10.50	2799	9.8	2551	10.6	373	37.5	1215	30.0	2471	17.2	307	8.8	39	3.8	13	9.6	57
2013	25.4	19.6	22,629	8.67	3001	8.0	2552	8.9	361	33.9	1273	30.8	2241	17.7	321	8.5	40	3.8	120	7.5	46
2014	25.9	16.2	22,646	9.58	3259	8.9	2678	8.0	353	35.1	1321	33.5	2021	15.0	336	8.3	37	3.9	276	8.7	57
2015	27.9	20.2	23,506	7.50	3121	9.3	2905	10.5	374	28.2	1280	30.0	2089	12.3	305	10.7	43	3.1	242	8.3	53
2016	25.8	17.6	24,689	8.50	3268	8.9	2997	6.1	380	28.8	1348	29.5	1957	14.3	324	11.5	35	3.9	238	6.8	52
2017	26.3	15.1	25,660	9.75	3351	11.0	3269	8.7	386	30.5	1329	34.2	1814	12.7	330	10.8	32	2.8	218	8.0	50
2018	25.4	17.0	27,609	7.58	3608	10.1	3313	8.1	373	37.8	1274	30.7	2130	12.9	320	11.2	37	2.6	244	8.8	43
Change (%).	−66.7	−75.1	+21.9	−77.2	+196.5	+21.7	+55.9	−62.3	+58.7	−23.3	+245.0	−41.4	+7.0	−51.0	+26.5	−35.6	+5.7	−68.7	-	-	-

Abbreviations: GT (Google Trends[TM]), US (United States of America), UK (United Kingdom), ESP (Spain), B (Belgium), NL (the Netherlands), GER (Germany), AUT (Austria), SLO (Slovenia), H (Hungary), CRO (Croatia), Tx. (transplants).

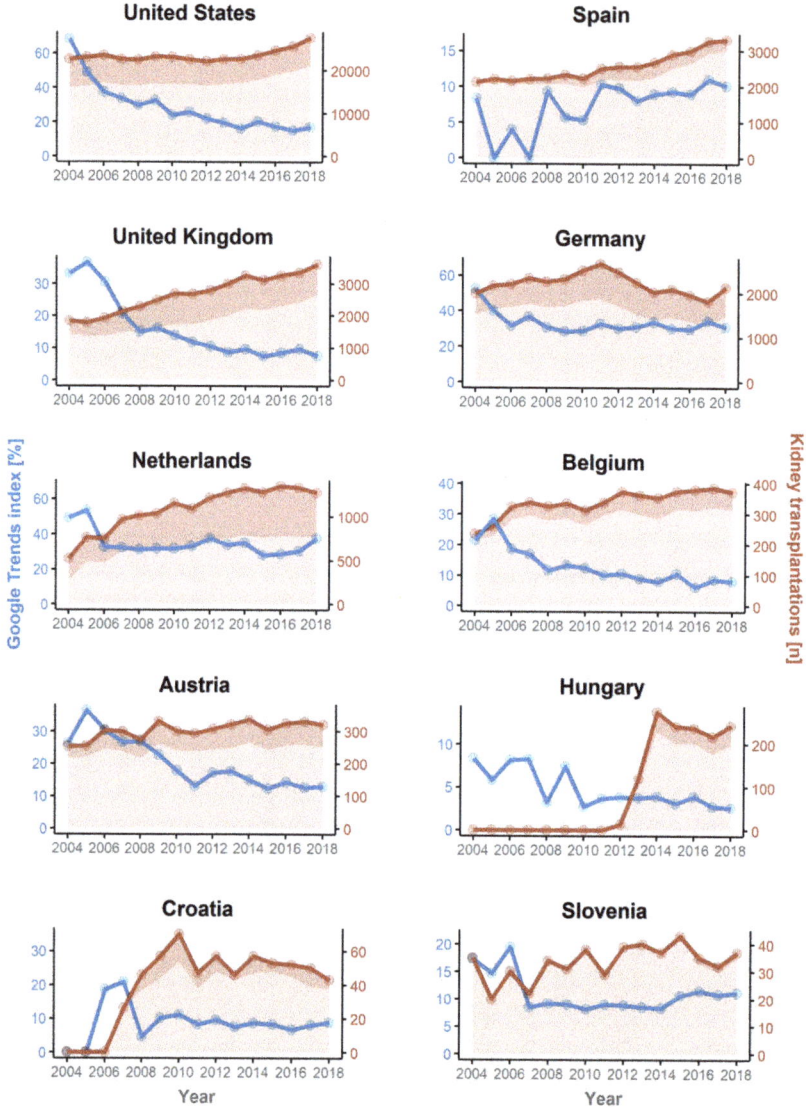

Figure 2. The respective numbers of renal transplants (red line) and the Google Trends™ indices (blue line) are given for the United Nations of Organ Sharing (UNOS), the Organización Nacional de Trasplantes (ONT), the Eurotransplant areas, and the UK National Register. Numbers of deceased and living donor transplants are indicated by light and dark red areas. While there was a marginal increase in the Google Trends™ index observed in Spain, the curves obtained from the UNOS, Eurotransplant areas, and the UK National Register mirror the worldwide trend.

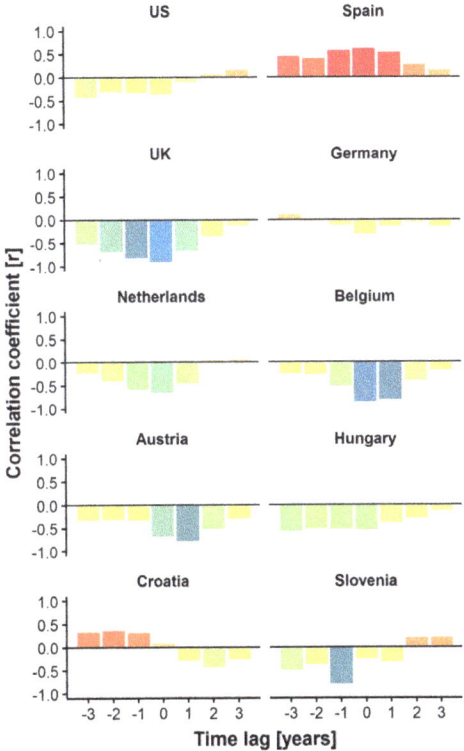

Figure 3. Time-lag correlations of Google Trends™ indices and number of performed transplants for the countries under study. Negative correlations between Google Trends™ indices and number of transplants are highlighted in green to blue whereas positive correlations are given in orange to red.

4. Discussion

To our knowledge, this is the first study investigating the trend of search queries for kidney transplantation. We observed a global decrease in public interest regarding kidney transplant, in particular in the UNOS, the Eurotransplant areas, and the UK. There is a global increase in transplanted kidneys, however, an increase in waiting time and a shortage of kidney donors highlight the demand [8]. Kidney transplant is the optimal form of renal replacement therapy for patients with end stage renal disease, improving both quality and quantity of life. Whilst this is true for both live and deceased organ donation, recipients of a live donor kidney transplant demonstrate better outcomes at both, one and five-years post transplantation [9]. Thus, raising and maintaining awareness about kidney transplants is imperative. How can we achieve this essential goal? Along with strategies discussed below, supra-national alliances such as the European Kidney Health Alliance (EKHA) are essential.

Efforts should be made to increase the number of live kidney donor transplants which are performed [9]. To help overcome hurdles like lack of awareness, particularly in populations with lower rates of live donor kidney transplants, namely ethnic minority populations and in groups who suffer from socioeconomic deprivation [10,11], successful campaigns have been orchestrated using both traditional media as well as online media, and community-based venues. By using Google Analytics™, the authors found an eight-fold increase in traffic to the Infórmate website, a website developed by the Northwestern University faculty in partnership with the National Kidney Foundation, compared to the pre-campaign period [12]. Website exposure was associated with a significant knowledge score increase between pretest and posttest assessments, which was maintained at a follow-up assessment at three weeks [13]. Readability and accessibility of online living donor and deceased donor recipient material is essential. An analysis of the top ten websites for both revealed that the reading level for the living donor materials was 12.54, while it was 12.87 for the deceased donor materials, corresponding to a university level. Overall, the readability of online material remains too high for the corresponding health literacy rates among potential kidney transplant recipients [14]. Whilst the readability must be increased, Information Score (IS) assessment also revealed a poor quality of many websites and that more input from transplant physicians is needed. Information should be freely available in multiple languages, as well as in Braille format and as audio text. Generally, websites belonging to academic institutions have higher IS than professional, or commercial websites [15]. Among 46 Italian YouTube® videos analyzed for usefulness to inform about live donor kidney transplantation, only a minority (15.2%) were categorized to contain useful information for the general population [16].

Kidney transplant knowledge should be improved in potential recipients. The Knowledge Assessment of Renal Transplantation (KART) contains 15 items including basic information about the procedure, prognosis, and insurance issues, and has an acceptable evidenced reliability. The KART distinguished patients who spent more or less than one hour receiving different types of education, including communication between doctors and medical staff, reading brochures, browsing the Internet, and watching videos [17]. Limited knowledge is not only present among patients but is also evident amongst medical students. In total, 96% were aware of the possibility of live donor kidney transplantation, but only 8% of the surveyed students were registered as potential donors in this South African study [18]. Similarly, a study from Leeds found that students had a basic understanding of organ donation and transplantation but lack detailed knowledge, such as understanding the criteria which are commonly used for brain death testing [19]. A study from India reporting on 200 interviews found that awareness will promote organ donation and there is a need for effective campaigns that educate people with relevant information, since a majority (59%) believed that donated organs might be misused, abused, or misappropriated [20].

Potential kidney transplant donors and recipients and those who have donated or received a transplant should be invited to share their experience online, in person, and on social media platforms. A survey involving 199 patients revealed that half use social media (52.3%, not further specified which channels were used) and most reported to be willing to post information about live kidney donation on their social networks (51%) [21]. Renal patients' organizations must also be supported and encouraged to provide information via social media.

Transplant physicians, surgeons, and nursing staff may also use social media to increase awareness of kidney transplantation. A survey among members of the American Society of Transplant Surgeons indicated that among 299 physicians who completed the survey, 59% use social media to communicate with surgeons, 57% with transplant professionals, 21% with transplant recipients, 16% with living donors, and 15% with waitlisted candidates. Younger age and fewer years of experience in transplantation were significantly associated with a stronger belief that social media may be influential in living organ donation [22].

Religious differences in mixed communities may play a role. In a Dutch study, the impact of religion on live donor kidney transplantation was assessed. The authors reported that religion is not perceived as an obstacle to live donation in the Netherlands. However, there is a necessity for increased clarity and awareness for different religions with respect to live donation [23]. While most of the patients seemed to favor live donor kidney transplantation, a variety of potentially modifiable barriers were identified, including inadequate patient education, emotional factors, restrictive social influences, and suboptimal communication [24].

Altruistic live donation will play an increasing role in the future. Social media is used to facilitate transplantation (i.e., through websites such as MatchingDonors.com), which was implemented as early as 1994. An organ registration fee is one of the ethical concerns of such strategies. Facebook and

Twitter are freely available platforms to communicate with others within groups and via hashtags and offer the opportunity to connect with potential live donors [25]. Moorlock et al. critically assessed the so-called "identifiable victim effect" and proposed that institutionally organized personal case-based campaigns aimed at promoting specific recipients for directed donation, despite its ethical concerns, should be preferred to facilitate altruistic live donation [26]. Building a framework for social media and organ donation is necessary and recommendations for transplant hospitals have been issued [27]. Programs such as the Kidney Coach Program (KCP) need to be implemented in the clinical practice to equip individuals (candidates and advocates for candidates) with tools to identify potential donors, which enables individuals to discuss donation with people in their social network [28].

Amongst countries participating in the Eurotransplant program, different legal strategies are employed; for instance, in Germany a potential donor needs to declare willingness to be registered as a deceased donor or 'opt in' [29]. This can increase the time it takes to ascertain suitability and thus delay transplant surgery. It also means that there are likely to be many willing donors, who simply do not register but if the system were 'opt out' would be very willing to be organ donors. Furthermore, 'opt in' systems for deceased donor donation lead to ongoing political debate which one might anticipate would help to raise awareness. When this was assessed via a Google Trends™ search, the decrease in the Google Trends™ index mirrored the changes observed in other Eurotransplant countries and thus this ongoing debate did not influence the public interest as assessed by Google Trends™. By the end of 2020, the organ donation laws in the UK will have moved from an 'opt in' system for deceased donor organ donation to an 'opt out' system (i.e., a deemed authorization system, applicable to the vast majority of the population with some notable exceptions). Northern Ireland is excepted from this change and the donation system there remains 'opt in' [30]. A significant factor in this change in legislation is the result of campaigning and lobbying from a nine-year old boy, Max Johnson, and his family. Max was awaiting a heart transplant which he ultimately received from Keira Ball, a nine-year old girl whose parents selflessly agreed to donate her organs. The legislation is to be commonly referred to as Max and Keira's Law [31].

Whilst this study shows a decreasing interest in web-based information over time in most areas, the number of live kidney donations increased in the ONT, the Eurotransplant areas, and the UK, while it was almost stable over time in the UNOS area (−3.1% from 2004 to 2018). This highlights that in most countries information from the treating physicians is more important than from the World Wide Web. A scoping review addressed strategies to increase live kidney donation and found that recipient-based education that reaches friends and family has the best evidence of being effective [32]. In contrast to the global trend, the Google Trends™ search highlighted an increase in search queries in Spain. In the same time period, the number of live and deceased kidney transplantation increased by 480.3% and 46.3%. It is tempting to speculate that either a sharp increase in transplant numbers or the implementation of non-heart-beating donation increased public interest [33].

This study has a few limitations. While Google Trends™ captures Google search queries and might act as a surrogate for public interest, Google is not the only available search engine next to other social media networks being used to search for information on the Internet. Previous work by others however indicates that Google Trends™ is a very valid measure of public interest. Additionally, the results obtained from Google Trends™ represent only relative numbers with no information on the absolute interest being available. We restricted our analysis to countries with an excellent documentation of transplant numbers and excluded countries from Asia and Africa, although they were included in the worldwide Google Trends™ analysis.

In conclusion, our Google Trends™ analysis found a decreasing public interest in renal transplantation. Strategies to inform the general population about unmet needs in the transplant setting (i.e., reduction of the waiting list time and live kidney donation) need to be utilized by all involved in the care of patients with kidney disease, by the patients themselves, and by national societies and academic institutions. Easily accessible information must be provided which is coherent and available in multiple languages including Braille and audio text. The message conveyed should be consistent and the information should be made available on multiple platforms including webpages, social media, and paper format. This may help reduce barriers in accessing information for different groups and improve outcomes according to the principles of patient-centered care.

Supplementary Materials: The following are available online at http://www.mdpi.com/2077-0383/9/4/1048/s1, Table S1: Search terms for the respective countries and languages are given, Table S2: The numbers of deceased donor and living donor kidney transplantations over time are given.

Author Contributions: Conceptualization, A.K., M.E., and P.P. Data curation, A.K., M.E., and P.P. Formal analysis, P.P. Investigation, P.P. Supervision, A.K., M.E., and P.P., Validation, A.K., M.E., J.I.S., C.K., S.D., M.R., H.N., M.J.S., K.S., A.B., H.T., G.M., and P.P. Visualization, P.P. Writing—original draft A.K., M.E., J.I.S., C.K., S.D., M.R., H.N., M.J.S., K.S., A.B., H.T., G.M., and P.P. Writing—review & editing, A.K., M.E., J.I.S., C.K., S.D., M.R., H.N., M.J.S., K.S., A.B., H.T., G.M., and P.P. All authors have read and agreed to the published version of the manuscript.

Funding: This research received no external funding.

Conflicts of Interest: The authors declare no conflicts of interest.

References

1. Shrestha:, B.; Haylor, J.; Raftery, A. Historical perspectives in kidney transplantation: An updated review. *Prog. Transplant.* **2015**, *25*, 64–76. [CrossRef]
2. Reese, P.P.; Boudville, N.; Garg, A.X. Living kidney donation: Outcomes, ethics, and uncertainty. *Lancet* **2015**, *385*, 2003–2013. [CrossRef]
3. Tong, A.; Chapman, J.R.; Wong, G.; Josephson, M.A.; Craig, J.C. Public awareness and attitudes to living organ donation: Systematic review and integrative synthesis. *Transplantation* **2013**, *96*, 429–437. [CrossRef] [PubMed]
4. Cervellin, G.; Comelli, I.; Lippi, G. Is Google Trends a reliable tool for digital epidemiology? Insights from different clinical settings. *J. Epidemiol. Glob. Health* **2017**, *7*, 185–189. [CrossRef]
5. Telfer, S.; Obradovich, N. Local weather is associated with rates of online searches for musculoskeletal pain symptoms. *PLoS ONE* **2017**, *12*, e0181266. [CrossRef] [PubMed]
6. Charalampopoulos, I.; Nastos, P.T.; Didaskalou, E. Human Thermal Conditions and North Europeans' Web Searching Behavior (Google Trends) on Mediterranean Touristic Destinations. *Urban Sci.* **2017**, *1*, 8. [CrossRef]
7. Arora, V.S.; McKee, M.; Stuckler, D. Google Trends: Opportunities and limitations in health and health policy research. *Health Policy* **2019**, *123*, 338–341. [CrossRef]
8. Andre, M.; Huang, E.; Everly, M.; Bunnapradist, S. The UNOS Renal Transplant Registry: Review of the Last Decade. *Clin. Transpl.* **2014**, 1–12.
9. Terasaki, P.I.; Cecka, J.M.; Gjertson, D.W.; Takemoto, S. High survival rates of kidney transplants from spousal and living unrelated donors. *N. Engl. J. Med.* **1995**, *333*, 333–336. [CrossRef] [PubMed]
10. Bratton, C.; Chavin, K.; Baliga, P. Racial disparities in organ donation and why. *Curr. Opin. Organ. Transpl.* **2011**, *16*, 243–249. [CrossRef]
11. Reed, R.D.; Sawinski, D.; Shelton, B.A.; MacLennan, P.A.; Hanaway, M.; Kumar, V.; Long, D.; Gaston, R.S.; Kilgore, M.L.; Julian, B.A.; et al. Population Health, Ethnicity, and Rate of Living Donor Kidney Transplantation. *Transplantation* **2018**, *102*, 2080–2087. [CrossRef] [PubMed]
12. Gordon, E.J.; Shand, J.; Black, A. Google analytics of a pilot mass and social media campaign targeting Hispanics about living kidney donation. *Internet Interv.* **2016**, *6*, 40–49. [CrossRef]
13. Gordon, E.J.; Feinglass, J.; Carney, P.; Vera, K.; Olivero, M.; Black, A.; O'Connor, K.; MacLean, J.; Nichols, S.; Sageshima, J.; et al. A Culturally Targeted Website for Hispanics/Latinos About Living Kidney Donation and Transplantation: A Randomized Controlled Trial of Increased Knowledge. *Transplantation* **2016**, *100*, 1149–1160. [CrossRef]
14. Zhou, E.P.; Kiwanuka, E.; Morrissey, P.E. Online patient resources for deceased donor and live donor kidney recipients: A comparative analysis of readability. *Clin. Kidney J.* **2018**, *11*, 559–563. [CrossRef] [PubMed]
15. Hanif, F.; Abayasekara, K.; Willcocks, L.; Jolly, E.C.; Jamieson, N.V.; Praseedom, R.K.; Goodacre, J.A.; Read, J.C.; Chaudhry, A.; Gibbs, P. The quality of information about kidney transplantation on the World Wide Web. *Clin. Transpl.* **2007**, *21*, 371–376. [CrossRef]

16. Bert, F.; Gualano, M.R.; Scozzari, G.; Alesina, M.; Amoroso, A.; Siliquini, R. YouTube((R)): An ally or an enemy in the promotion of living donor kidney transplantation? *Health Inform. J.* **2018**, *24*, 103–110. [CrossRef] [PubMed]
17. Peipert, J.D.; Hays, R.D.; Kawakita, S.; Beaumont, J.L.; Waterman, A.D. Measurement Characteristics of the Knowledge Assessment of Renal Transplantation. *Transplantation* **2019**, *103*, 565–572. [CrossRef]
18. Sobnach, S.; Borkum, M.; Hoffman, R.; Muller, E.; McCurdie, F.; Millar, A.; Numanoglu, A.; Kahn, D. Medical students' knowledge about organ transplantation: A South African perspective. *Transpl. Proc.* **2010**, *42*, 3368–3371. [CrossRef] [PubMed]
19. Bedi, K.K.; Hakeem, A.R.; Dave, R.; Lewington, A.; Sanfey, H.; Ahmad, N. Survey of the knowledge, perception, and attitude of medical students at the University of Leeds toward organ donation and transplantation. *Transpl. Proc.* **2015**, *47*, 247–260. [CrossRef]
20. Balwani, M.R.; Gumber, M.R.; Shah, P.R.; Kute, V.B.; Patel, H.V.; Engineer, D.P.; Gera, D.N.; Godhani, U.; Shah, M.; Trivedi, H.L. Attitude and awareness towards organ donation in western India. *Ren. Fail.* **2015**, *37*, 582–588. [CrossRef]
21. Kazley, A.S.; Hamidi, B.; Balliet, W.; Baliga, P. Social Media Use Among Living Kidney Donors and Recipients: Survey on Current Practice and Potential. *J. Med. Internet Res.* **2016**, *18*, e328. [CrossRef]
22. Henderson, M.L.; Adler, J.T.; Van Pilsum Rasmussen, S.E.; Thomas, A.G.; Herron, P.D.; Waldram, M.M.; Ruck, J.M.; Purnell, T.S.; DiBrito, S.R.; Holscher, C.M.; et al. How Should Social Media Be Used in Transplantation? A Survey of the American Society of Transplant Surgeons. *Transplantation* **2019**, *103*, 573–580. [CrossRef]
23. Ismail, S.Y.; Massey, E.K.; Luchtenburg, A.E.; Claassens, L.; Zuidema, W.C.; Busschbach, J.J.; Weimar, W. Religious attitudes towards living kidney donation among Dutch renal patients. *Med. Health Care Philos.* **2012**, *15*, 221–227. [CrossRef]
24. Ismail, S.Y.; Claassens, L.; Luchtenburg, A.E.; Roodnat, J.I.; Zuidema, W.C.; Weimar, W.; Busschbach, J.J.; Massey, E.K. Living donor kidney transplantation among ethnic minorities in the Netherlands: A model for breaking the hurdles. *Patient Educ. Couns.* **2013**, *90*, 118–124. [CrossRef] [PubMed]
25. Henderson, M.L. Social Media in the Identification of Living Kidney Donors: Platforms, Tools, and Strategies. *Curr. Transpl. Rep.* **2018**, *5*, 19–26. [CrossRef] [PubMed]
26. Moorlock, G.; Draper, H. Empathy, social media, and directed altruistic living organ donation. *Bioethics* **2018**, *32*, 289–297. [CrossRef] [PubMed]
27. Henderson, M.L.; Clayville, K.A.; Fisher, J.S.; Kuntz, K.K.; Mysel, H.; Purnell, T.S.; Schaffer, R.L.; Sherman, L.A.; Willock, E.P.; Gordon, E.J. Social media and organ donation: Ethically navigating the next frontier. *Am. J. Transpl.* **2017**, *17*, 2803–2809. [CrossRef] [PubMed]
28. LaPointe Rudow, D.; Geatrakas, S.; Armenti, J.; Tomback, A.; Khaim, R.; Porcello, L.; Pan, S.; Arvelakis, A.; Shapiro, R. Increasing living donation by implementing the Kidney Coach Program. *Clin. Transpl.* **2019**, *33*, e13471. [CrossRef] [PubMed]
29. Metz, C.; Hoppe, N. Organ transplantation in Germany: Regulating scandals and scandalous regulation. *Eur. J. Health Law* **2013**, *20*, 113–116. [CrossRef]
30. Organ Donation Laws. Available online: https://www.organdonation.nhs.uk/uk-laws/ (accessed on 7 April 2020).
31. Max, Heart Transplant Recipient and Campaigner. Available online: https://www.organdonation.nhs.uk/helping-you-to-decide/real-life-stories/people-who-have-benefitted-from-receiving-a-transplant/max-heart-transplant-recipient-and-campaigner/ (accessed on 7 April 2020).
32. Barnieh, L.; Collister, D.; Manns, B.; Lam, N.N.; Shojai, S.; Lorenzetti, D.; Gill, J.S.; Klarenbach, S. A Scoping Review for Strategies to Increase Living Kidney Donation. *Clin. J. Am. Soc. Nephrol.* **2017**, *12*, 1518–1527. [CrossRef]
33. Gentil, M.A.; Castro de la Nuez, P.; Gonzalez-Corvillo, C.; de Gracia, M.C.; Cabello, M.; Mazuecos, M.A.; Rodriguez-Benot, A.; Ballesteros, L.; Osuna, A.; Alonso, M. Non-Heart-Beating Donor Kidney Transplantation Survival Is Similar to Donation After Brain Death: Comparative Study With Controls in a Regional Program. *Transpl. Proc.* **2016**, *48*, 2867–2870. [CrossRef] [PubMed]

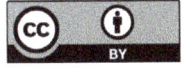

© 2020 by the authors. Licensee MDPI, Basel, Switzerland. This article is an open access article distributed under the terms and conditions of the Creative Commons Attribution (CC BY) license (http://creativecommons.org/licenses/by/4.0/).

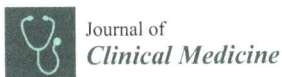

Article

Prognostic Value of Neutrophil-To-Lymphocyte Ratio and Platelet-To-Lymphocyte Ratio for Renal Outcomes in Patients with Rapidly Progressive Glomerulonephritis

Yukari Mae, Tomoaki Takata *, Ayami Ida, Masaya Ogawa, Sosuke Taniguchi, Marie Yamamoto, Takuji Iyama, Satoko Fukuda and Hajime Isomoto

Division of Medicine and Clinical Science, Faculty of Medicine, Tottori University, Yonago, Tottori 683-8504, Japan
* Correspondence: t-takata@tottori-u.ac.jp; Tel.:+81-859-38-6527

Received: 26 March 2020; Accepted: 12 April 2020; Published: 15 April 2020

Abstract: Background: Rapidly progressive glomerulonephritis (RPGN) is a syndrome characterized by a rapid decline in renal function that often causes end-stage renal disease. Although it is important to predict renal outcome in RPGN before initiating immunosuppressive therapies, no simple prognostic indicator has been reported. The aim of this study was to investigate the associations of neutrophil-to-lymphocyte ratio (NLR) and platelet-to-lymphocyte ratio (PLR) to renal outcomes in patients with RPGN. Methods: Forty-four patients with a clinical diagnosis of RPGN who underwent renal biopsy were enrolled. The relationships between NLR and PLR and renal outcome after 1 year were investigated. Results: NLR and PLR were significantly higher in patients with preserved renal function in comparison to patients who required maintenance hemodialysis ($p < 0.05$ and $p < 0.01$, respectively). An NLR of 4.0 and a PLR of 137.7 were the cutoff values for renal outcome (area under the curve, 0.782 and 0.819; sensitivity, 78.4% and 89.2%; specificity, 71.4% and 71.4%, respectively). Furthermore, an NLR of 5.0 could predict recovery from renal injury in patients requiring hemodialysis (area under the curve, 0.929; sensitivity, 83.3%; specificity, 85.7%). Conclusion: NLR and PLR could be candidates for predicting renal outcomes in patients with RPGN.

Keywords: NLR; PLR; RPGN; predictive value; hemodialysis; withdrawal; cellular crescent; global sclerosis

---

1. Introduction

Rapidly progressive glomerulonephritis (RPGN) is a syndrome characterized by hematuria, proteinuria, anemia, and a rapid decline in renal function [1]. The diagnosis of RPGN is made when renal dysfunction occurs within a short period of time and is complicated with proteinuria or hematuria [2]. The etiology of RPGN is divided into three classifications: immune complex crescentic glomerulonephritis, pauci-immune crescentic glomerulonephritis, and anti-glomerular basement membrane (GBM) crescentic glomerulonephritis. In Japan, the number of end-stage renal disease (ESRD) cases caused by RPGN has increased approximately 3.1 times between 1994 and 2018, which represents the fifth most common etiology of ESRD [2,3]. Since RPGN causes a progressive decline in renal function, patients with RPGN require aggressive treatment with steroids and immunosuppressive agents [4]. However, these treatments are not always effective and, in such cases, RPGN is refractory and requires maintenance hemodialysis (HD). Considering that steroids and immunosuppressive agents can cause life-threatening infections, conservative treatment is also considered for patients with RPGN. Although it is critically important to predict renal outcomes in the early stages of RPGN [5], a simple prognostic marker for RPGN is yet to be established.

In recent years, neutrophil-to-lymphocyte ratio (NLR) and platelet-to-lymphocyte ratio (PLR) have received attention as potential new markers of systemic inflammation. In previous studies, NLR and PLR have been reported to be useful in systemic inflammatory diseases such as aortitis syndrome [6], Behçet's disease [7], Kawasaki disease [8], Henoch–Schönlein purpura [9], systemic lupus erythematosus [10], and anti-neutrophil cytoplasmic antibody (ANCA)-associated vasculitis (AAV) [11,12]. Furthermore, NLR and PLR have been proposed as markers of inflammation in patients with ESRD [13,14]. Therefore, we speculated that NLR and PLR could be simple predictors of renal decline in RPGN. The purpose of this study was to investigate the associations of NLR and PLR to renal outcome in patients with RPGN.

2. Materials and Methods

2.1. Study Population

In this study, we enrolled 501 patients who underwent renal biopsy at the Tottori University Hospital between 2009 and 2019. Renal biopsies were performed according to the indications of the guidelines from the Japanese Society of Nephrology [15]; persistent hematuria and/or proteinuria, proteinuria more than 0.5 g/day, a rapid decline in renal function, or gross hematuria. Among the 501 patients enrolled, 47 patients were clinically diagnosed with RPGN based on the guidelines from the Japanese Society of Nephrology [16]. Excluding 2 cases with an active bacterial infection and 1 case with a relapse of the glomerulonephritis, 44 patients were included in the analyses (Figure 1). None of the patients included had a history of cancer or prescribed corticosteroids. Immunosuppressive therapies were determined according to the guidelines [16]. This study was conducted in accordance with the Declaration of Helsinki and approved by the Ethics Committee of Tottori University Hospital (approval number: 19A138).

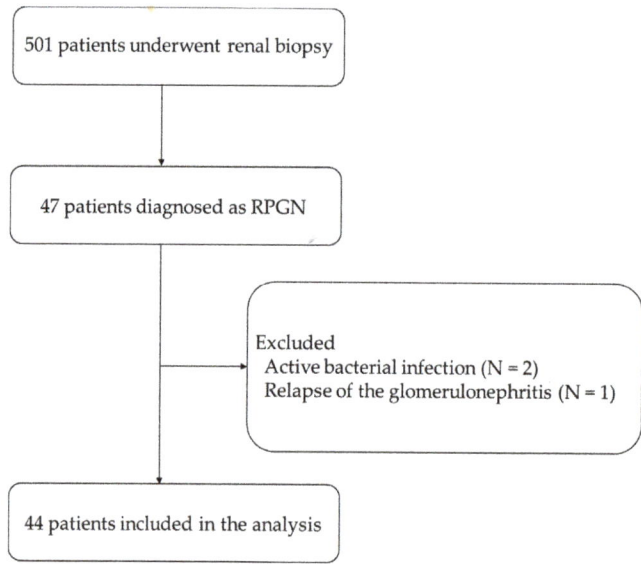

Figure 1. Study design. Of the 501 patients who underwent renal biopsy, 44 patients were included in the analysis.

2.2. Clinical and Laboratory Findings

The patient's characteristics and laboratory findings on admission, including white blood cell count (WBC), neutrophil count (Neu), lymphocyte count (Lym), platelet count (Plt), creatinine (Cr), estimated glomerular filtration rate (eGFR) [17], C-reactive protein (CRP), erythrocyte sedimentation rate (ESR), myeloperoxidase (MPO)-ANCA, proteinase 3 (PR3)-ANCA, and the anti-GBM antibody, were acquired retrospectively. NLR was calculated as the ratio of neutrophil count to lymphocyte count (NLR = Neu/Lym), and PLR was calculated as the ratio of platelet count to lymphocyte count (PLR = Plt/Lym). Renal outcomes 1 year from diagnosis were also recorded.

2.3. Histological Findings

Ultrasound-guided renal biopsy was performed as previously described [18]. In brief, renal tissue was obtained using a 16-gauge biopsy gun (Acecut; TSK Laboratory, Tochigi, Japan). The specimen was fixed in 10% formalin and embedded in paraffin. Sections (4 μm thickness) were stained with periodic acid-Schiff (PAS). Pathological changes in glomeruli were defined as global sclerosis, cellular crescent, fibrocellular crescent, fibrous crescent, and others. Pathological analyses were performed by an experienced nephrologist (S.F.), who was independent of the acquisition and analysis of the clinical information.

2.4. Statistical Analyses

Continuous variables were expressed as the mean ± standard deviation or the median (range) according to the distribution. The Kolmogorov–Smirnov test was used to assess normal distribution. Differences between groups were analyzed using the Student's t test for normally distributed variables, the Mann–Whitney U test for non-normally distributed variables, or the chi-square test for categorical variables. In addition, receiver operating characteristic (ROC) curve analysis was performed to determine the optimal cutoff values for NLR and PLR. The optimal cutoff point was determined by minimizing the square of the distance between the point (sensitivity of 1, 1-specificity of 0) and any point on the ROC curve. Multivariate regression analysis was carried out, in which age, eGFR, CRP, and NLR or PLR were selected, with the stepwise forward selection method, to investigate independent predictors of renal outcomes in the 44 patients. StatFlex Ver7 for Windows (Artec, Osaka, Japan) was used for the statistical analyses. A two-tailed p-value of < 0.05 was considered statistically significant.

3. Results

3.1. Differences between Patients with Preserved Renal Function and Renal Failure

All patients enrolled in this study were ethnically homogenous. The etiology of the 44 patients was as follows: ANCA-associated vasculitis ($n = 34$), ANCA-negative vasculitis ($n = 6$), and anti-GBM disease ($n = 4$). We first divided the patients into two groups according to their renal outcomes at 1 year post diagnosis. The characteristics of the 37 cases with preserved renal function (pre-dialysis group) and 7 cases with renal failure (maintenance HD group) are shown in Table 1 and Figure 2. WBC, Neu, Plt, Cr, eGFR and the anti-GBM antibody all showed significant differences between the groups. We also observed significant differences in NLR (8.2 (2.0–32.0) vs. 3.9 (2.8–8.4), $p = 0.019$) and PLR (265.7 (82.9–2255.0) vs. 126.0 (107.1–269.0), $p = 0.008$) between the pre-dialysis and maintenance HD groups, respectively. Multivariate regression analysis revealed that renal function was the strongest influencing factor for renal outcome (stdβ = 0.363, $p = 0.012$). There was also a trend suggesting the significance of NLR as a predictive value (stdβ = 0.276, $p = 0.052$); PLR, however, did not display this significance (stdβ = 0.207, $p = 0.148$).

Table 1. Patient's characteristics between the pre-dialysis and maintenance hemodialysis (HD) groups.

	Pre-dialysis ($n = 37$)	Maintenance HD ($n = 7$)	p Value
Sex (Male/Female)	22/15	5/2	0.132
Age (years)	71.4 ± 11.6	65.7 ± 7.8	0.222
Classifications of RPGN			
Immune complex CGN	33 (89.2%)	1 (14.3%)	
Pauci-immune CGN	4 (10.8%)	2 (28.6%)	
Anti-GBM CGN	0 (0%)	4 (57.1%)	
Immunosuppressive therapy			
Pulse corticosteroids	29/8	6/1	0.557
Cyclophosphamide	13/24	0/7	0.069
Plasma exchange	0/37	3/4	0.003
White blood cell count ($10^3/\mu L$)	10.2 (4.9–23.5)	6.2 (4.7–12.4)	0.037
Neutrophil count ($10^3/\mu L$)	8.5 (3.6–22.1)	4.6 (3.3–8.4)	0.012
Lymphocyte count ($10^3/\mu L$)	1.17 ± 0.59	1.31 ± 0.43	0.550
Platelet count ($10^3/\mu L$)	327 (98–808)	189 (117–269)	0.015
Creatinine (mg/dL)	2.80 ± 2.01	8.74 ± 1.80	<0.001
eGFR (mL/min/1.73 m^2)	27.3 ± 21.2	5.4 ± 2.0	<0.001
CRP (mg/dL)	5.0 (0–24.8)	4.0 (0.4–26.9)	0.987
ESR (mm/h)	99 (10–140)	111 (62–134)	0.771
MPO-ANCA (U/mL)	166 (0–860)	0 (0–2440)	0.109
PR3-ANCA (U/mL)	0 (0–35.8)	0 (0–0)	0.308
anti-GBM antibody (U/mL)	0 (0–0)	42.3 (0–858.0)	<0.001
NLR	8.2 (2.0–32.0)	3.9 (2.8–8.4)	0.019
PLR	265.7 (82.9–2255.0)	126.0 (107.1–269.0)	0.008

Data are presented as the mean ± standard deviation, median (range), or number (%). HD—hemodialysis; RPGN—rapidly progressing glomerulonephritis; CGN—crescentic glomerulonephritis; eGFR—estimated glomerular filtration rate; CRP—C-reactive protein; ESR—erythrocyte sedimentation rate; MPO—myeloperoxidase; ANCA—anti-neutrophil cytoplasmic antibody; PR3—proteinase 3; GBM—glomerular basement membrane; NLR—neutrophil-to-lymphocyte ratio; PLR—platelet-to-lymphocyte ratio.

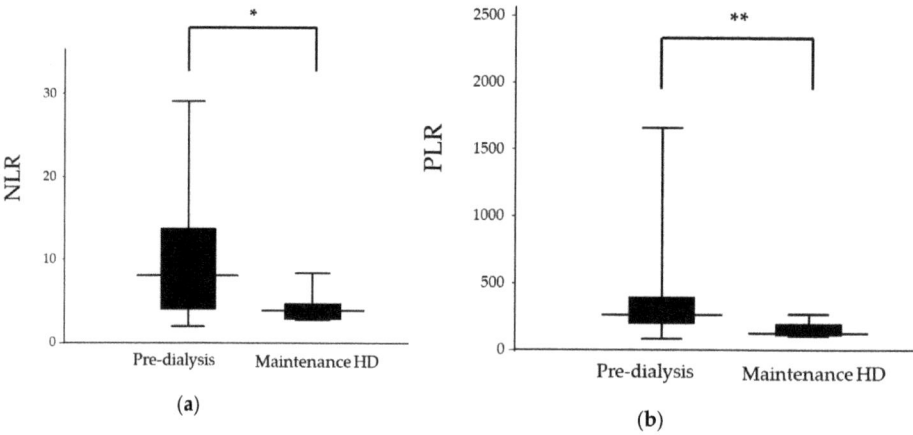

Figure 2. Neutrophil-to-lymphocyte ratios (NLR) and platelet-to-lymphocyte ratios (PLR) in the pre-dialysis and maintenance hemodialysis (HD) groups. (**a**) NLR in the pre-dialysis and maintenance HD groups. (**b**) PLR in the pre-dialysis and maintenance HD groups. The top and the bottom of the boxes are the first and third quartile, respectively. The length of the box represents the interquartile range. The line through the middle of each box represents the median. The error bars show the minimum and maximum values (range). *, $p < 0.05$; **, $p < 0.01$. NLR—neutrophil-to-lymphocyte ratio; PLR—platelet-to-lymphocyte ratio; HD—hemodialysis.

The ROC curves analyses were performed to define the cutoff value of PLR and NLR for predicting renal outcomes after 1 year (Figure 3). Both NLR and PLR were accurate predictors of renal outcomes, with an area under the curve (AUC) of 0.782 in NLR and 0.819 in PLR. The cutoff values defined were 4.0 in NLR, with a sensitivity of 78.4% and specificity of 71.4%, and 137.7 in PLR, with a sensitivity of 89.2% and specificity of 71.4%.

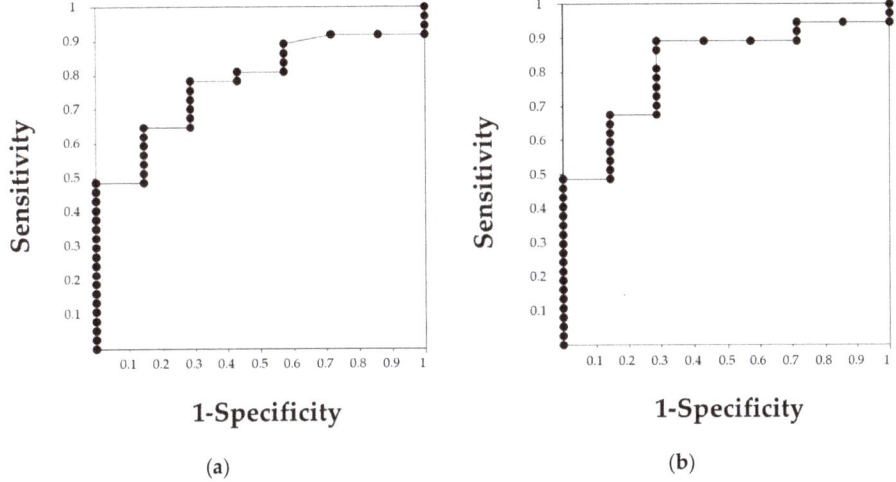

Figure 3. The receiver operating characteristic (ROC) curve of neutrophil-to-lymphocyte ratio (NLR) and platelet-to-lymphocyte ratio (PLR) for predicting renal outcome. (**a**) The ROC curve of NLR showing an area under the curve (AUC) of 0.782. An NLR of 4.0 was the cutoff value with a sensitivity of 78.4% and a specificity of 71.4%. (**b**) The ROC curve of PLR showing an AUC of 0.819. The cutoff value of 137.7 was determined with a sensitivity of 89.2% and a specificity of 71.4%.

3.2. Differences between Patients with Temporary Hemodialysis and Maintenance Hemodialysis

Since renal function on admission was a strong predicting factor for renal outcome, we divided the 13 patients who required HD into two groups as follows: 6 patients with recovery of renal function (temporary HD group) and 7 patients with persistent renal failure (maintenance HD group). Sex, WBC and Neu showed significant differences between the groups (Table 2). NLR was significantly higher in the temporary HD group compared to the maintenance HD group (12.4 (4.1–21.4) vs. 3.9 (2.8–8.4), $p = 0.008$, respectively, Figure 4). However, no significant difference was observed in PLR between the temporary HD group and the maintenance HD group (341.7 ± 217.7 vs. 156.1 ± 62.6, $p = 0.053$, respectively). The ROC curve analysis showed that an NLR of 5.0 could predict withdrawal from HD with a sensitivity of 83.3% and a specificity of 85.7%, with an AUC of 0.929 (Figure 5).

Table 2. Patient's characteristics between temporary the HD and maintenance HD groups.

	Temporary HD (n = 6)	Maintenance HD (n = 7)	p Value
Sex (Male/Female)	1/5	5/2	0.048
Age (years)	72.7 ± 18.4	65.7 ± 7.8	0.381
Classifications of RPGN			
Immune complex CGN	0 (0%)	1 (14.3%)	
Pauci-immune CGN	6 (100%)	2 (28.6%)	
Anti-GBM CGN	0 (0%)	4 (57.1%)	
Immunosuppressive therapy			
Pulse corticosteroids	6/0	6/1	0.538
Cyclophosphamide	1/5	0/7	0.462
Plasma exchange	6/0	3/4	0.049
White blood cell count ($10^3/\mu L$)	12.6 ± 5.1	7.6 ± 2.9	0.048
Neutrophil count ($10^3/\mu L$)	11.0 ± 5.0	5.3 ± 2.1	0.018
Lymphocyte count ($10^3/\mu L$)	1.10 ± 0.58	1.31 ± 0.43	0.470
Platelet count ($10^3/\mu L$)	289.7 ± 112.7	191.4 ± 55.6	0.066
CRP (mg/dL)	11.2 ± 7.0	8.1 ± 10.3	0.554
ESR (mm/h)	104 ± 32	103 ± 27	0.985
MPO-ANCA (U/mL)	160 (17.0–469.0)	0 (0–2440)	0.138
anti-GBM antibody (U/mL)	0 (0–0)	42.3 (0–858.0)	0.065
NLR	12.4 (4.1–21.4)	3.9 (2.8–8.4)	0.008
PLR	341.7 ± 217.7	156.1 ± 62.6	0.053

Data are presented as the mean ± standard deviation, median (range), or number (%). HD—hemodialysis; RPGN—rapidly progressing glomerulonephritis; CGN—crescentic glomerulonephritis; eGFR—estimated glomerular filtration rate; CRP—C-reactive protein; ESR—erythrocyte sedimentation rate; MPO—myeloperoxidase; ANCA—anti-neutrophil cytoplasmic antibody; PR3—proteinase 3; GBM—glomerular basement membrane; NLR—neutrophil-to-lymphocyte ratio; PLR—platelet-to-lymphocyte ratio.

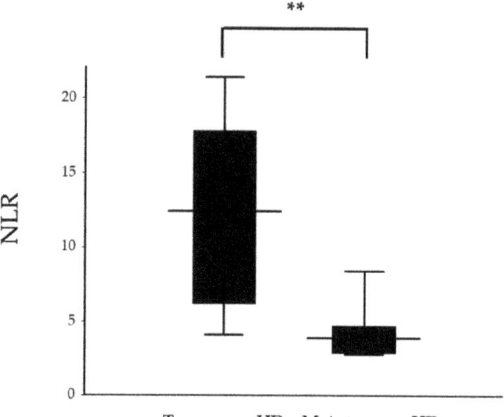

Figure 4. Neutrophil-to-lymphocyte ratios (NLR) of the temporary and maintenance hemodialysis (HD) groups. The top and the bottom of the boxes are the first and third quartile, respectively. The length of the box represents the interquartile range. The line through the middle of each box represents the median. The error bars show the minimum and maximum values (range). ** $p < 0.01$. NLR—neutrophil-to-lymphocyte ratio; HD—hemodialysis.

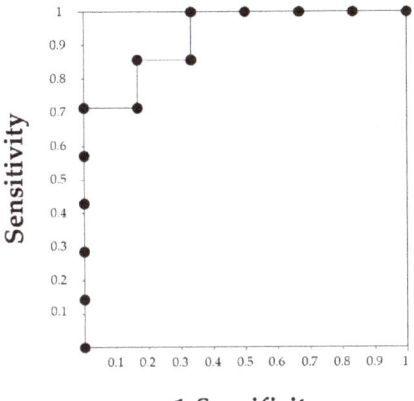

Figure 5. The receiver operating characteristic (ROC) curve for neutrophil-to-lymphocyte ratio (NLR) for recovery from renal failure. The NLR of 5.0 was determined to be a cutoff value with a sensitivity of 83.3% and a specificity of 85.7%, and the area under the curve was 0.929.

We further investigated histological changes in the temporary HD group and maintenance HD group (Table 3, Figures 6 and 7). The number of globally sclerotic glomeruli was significantly lower in the temporary HD group (9.0% ± 10.1% vs. 53.0% ± 9.7%, $p < 0.001$), whereas the number of glomeruli with cellular crescent was significantly higher in the temporary HD group (27.9 (0–73.3) vs. 0 (0–13.3), $p = 0.022$).

Table 3. Histological changes in the temporary hemodialysis (HD) and maintenance HD groups.

	Temporary HD (n = 6)	Maintenance HD (n = 7)	p Value
Cellular crescent (%)	30.4 ± 24.1	4.4 ± 5.7	0.022
Fibrocellular crescent (%)	11.9 ± 14.1	10.2 ± 9.4	0.945
Fibrous crescent (%)	19.0 ± 22.9	20.1 ± 16.3	0.921
Global sclerosis (%)	9.0 ± 10.1	53.0 ± 9.7	<0.001

Data are presented as the mean ± standard deviation. HD—hemodialysis.

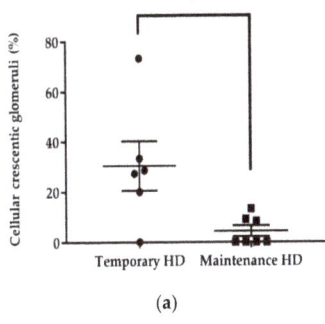

(a)

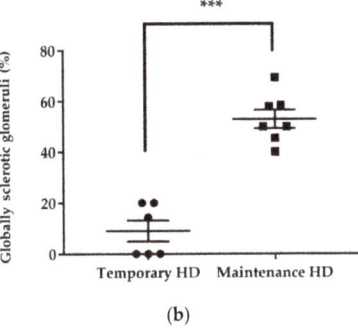

(b)

Figure 6. Quantification of histological findings in the temporary and maintenance hemodialysis (HD) groups. (a) Comparison of the percentage of glomeruli with cellular crescent between the temporary and maintenance HD groups. (b) Comparison of the percentage of globally sclerotic glomeruli between the temporary and maintenance HD groups. Bars indicate mean ± SEM. *, $p < 0.05$; *** $p < 0.001$. HD—hemodialysis.

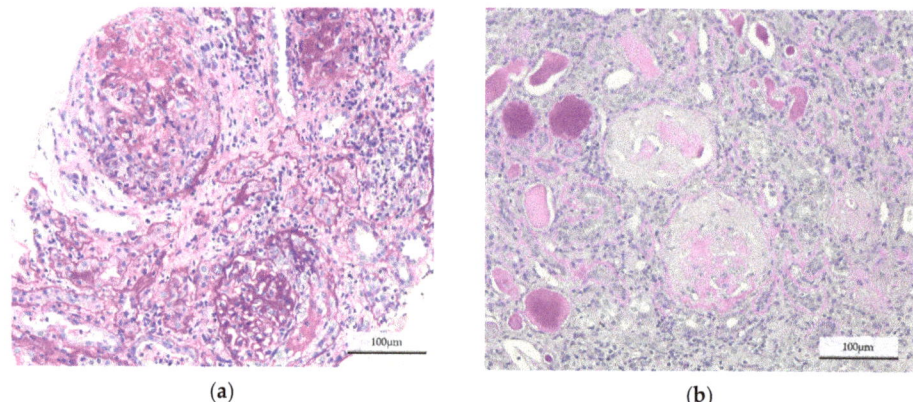

Figure 7. Histological findings in each group. Representative images of Periodic acid-Schiff staining on paraffin-embedded kidney sections, from patients in (**a**) the temporary hemodialysis (HD) group, and (**b**) the maintenance HD group. Cellular crescentic glomeruli were dominant in the temporary HD group, whereas most of the glomeruli were globally sclerotic in the maintenance HD group.

4. Discussion

In this study, we found that NLR and PLR at the point of diagnosis of RPGN are associated with renal outcome. In particular, NLR was considered to be a useful prognostic indicator for the recovery from HD in patients with RPGN.

RPGN often causes a progressive decline in renal function that leads to ESRD at a high rate. In this study, we observed that around 16% of the cases resulted in ESRD. Several renal prognostic indicators of RPGN, such as the degree of decline in renal function on admission, histological classification, and the level of the anti-GBM antibody, have been suggested in previous reports [4,19]. However, it is difficult to accurately predict renal outcome without a renal biopsy or in patients who require HD. Therefore, it is important to establish a simple renal prognostic indicator other than renal function or histological assessment.

NLR and PLR are simple and cost-effective markers, that represent the ratio of the number of cells with two different hemocytes. Neu and Plt increase with inflammation [11,20], while Lym may decrease with inflammation in autoimmune diseases [21]. Since the majority of the patients included in this study had an etiology of autoimmune vasculitis, it was expected that the increase in Neu and Plt, and the decrease in Lym, would be proportionate to the degree of inflammation. Therefore, we considered that NLR and PLR could be more reliable than a single hemocyte number. Infection, cancers, ischemic heart disease and peripheral vascular disease affect NLR and PLR [22]. In addition, steroids increase Neu, while immunosuppressive agents may reduce Neu by myelosuppression. Thus, in this study, we excluded patients who had infectious diseases and who were already administered steroids or immunosuppressive drugs at diagnosis, and confirmed no patient had a history of malignancy, ischemic heart disease or peripheral vascular disease.

NLR and PLR have been reported to be associated with AAV disease activity; high NLR and PLR indicate a higher disease activity [11,12,20,22]. On the other hand, several studies have mentioned that the application of NLR and PLR is limited. It has been demonstrated that NLR is a good predictor of the relapse rate, but not of death in patients with AAV [22]. PLR is also able to predict the disease activity but cannot predict relapse in AAV patients [20]. In this study, both NLR and PLR at diagnosis were significantly higher in patients with preserved renal function than in patients with maintenance HD. We speculate that a higher NLR and PLR indicate acute disease and an active phase, sustaining the possibility of a positive response to immunosuppressive therapy, whereas a lower NLR and PLR may suggest a chronic phase with irreversible renal injury. This was confirmed by the histological analysis, which revealed significant differences in glomerular changes. The majority of the glomeruli in the maintenance HD group were globally sclerosing, indicating irreversible renal injury. Cellular crescent presence, suggesting a possibility of improvement, was highly observed in the temporary HD group. We demonstrated that an NLR < 4.0 or PLR < 137.7 at diagnosis were associated with negative renal outcomes, especially in patients requiring HD. An NLR < 5.0 at diagnosis could predict irreversible renal failure.

Since the patients in the pre-dialysis group showed variable renal function, and the multivariate analysis revealed that renal function was the strongest influencing factor, we investigated the predictive abilities of NLR and PLR in patients requiring HD. Among the 13 patients, NLR at diagnosis was significantly higher in the temporary HD group than in the maintenance HD group. Although PLR showed an increased presence in the temporary HD group, the difference was not significant. The half-life of Neu and Plt could affect this result. Neu can survive for less than 24 h, while Plt survives for 10 days, and their lifespans are controlled by endogenous apoptosis [23,24]. Plt, which is increased by inflammation, circulates for a longer period than Neu. In predicting the course of patients requiring HD, it would be desirable to evaluate the acute phase of inflammation and disease activity. Therefore, NLR would be a better predictor than PLR for withdrawal of HD.

There are some limitations to our study. First, all the patients were treated based on the clinical guidelines for the ANCA-associated RPGN [25]; thus, the treatment strategy differed in each patient. Since all four patients with an anti-GBM disease required maintenance HD, this may affect the result of our study. However, we observed a significant difference in NLR between the temporary and maintenance HD groups when these patients were eliminated. In addition to the variations in NLR and PLR, this study was a retrospective study, with a small number of subjects. Therefore, the results of the present study should be carefully interpreted, and a prospective study with a larger number of patients is required to confirm the suitability of NLR and PLR as predicative factors in renal outcomes.

5. Conclusions

In conclusion, we revealed that the NLR and PLR at diagnosis could predict renal outcomes in patients with RPGN, and that NLR could predict withdrawal from HD in patients requiring HD. Treatment strategies could be modified according to the NLR and PLR, especially in patients whose renal function is unlikely to recover, which may reduce the risk of treatment-related complications.

Author Contributions: Conceptualization, Y.M. and T.T.; Methodology, Y.M. and T.T.; Formal analysis, Y.M.; Investigation, Y.M.; Data Curation, Y.M., A.I., M.O., S.T., M.Y., T.I., and S.F.; Writing—Original Draft Preparation, Y.M.; Writing—Review & Editing, T.T.; Supervision, T.T. and H.I. All authors have read and agreed to the published version of the manuscript.

Funding: This research received no external funding.

Conflicts of Interest: The authors declare no conflict of interest.

References

1. Nachman, P.H.; Jennette, J.C.; Falk, R.J. Primary glomerular disease. In *Brenner and Rector's The Kidney*, 9th ed.; Taal, M.W., Chertow, G.M., Marsden, P.A., Skorecki, K., Yu, A.S.L., Brenner, B.M., Eds.; Elsevier Inc.: Philadelphia, PA, USA, 2012; Volume 1, pp. 1153–1154.
2. Usui, J.; Yamagata, K. Progressive renal diseases: Recent advances in diagnosis and treatments. Topics: II. Pathophysiology and treatments; 4. Crescentic glomerulonephritis. *J. Jpn. Soc. Int. Med.* **2013**, *102*, 1128–1135. (In Japanese) [CrossRef] [PubMed]
3. Nitta, K.; Masakane, I.; Hanafusa, N.; Goto, S.; Abe, M.; Nakai, S.; Taniguchi, M.; Hasegawa, T.; Wada, A.; Hamano, T.; et al. 2018 annual dialysis data report, JSDT renal data registry. *J. Jpn. Soc. Dial. Ther.* **2018**, *52*, 679–754. (In Japanese) [CrossRef]
4. Toraman, A.; Neşe, N.; Özyurt, B.C.; Kürşat, S. Association between neutrophil-lymphocyte & platelet lymphocyte ratios with prognosis & mortality in rapidly progressive glomerulonephritis. *Indian J. Med. Res.* **2019**, *150*, 399–406. [PubMed]

5. Xu, P.C.; Chen, T.; Wu, S.J.; Yang, X.; Gao, S.; Hu, S.Y.; Wei, L.; Yan, T.K. Pathological severity determines the renal recovery for anti-myeloperoxidase antibody-associated vasculitis requiring dialysis at disease onset: A retrospective study. *BMC Nephrol.* **2019**, *20*, 287. [CrossRef] [PubMed]
6. Pan, L.; Du, J.; Li, T.; Liao, H. Platelet-to-lymphocyte ratio and neutrophil-to-lymphocyte ratio associated with disease activity in patients with Takayasu's arteritis: A case-control study. *BMJ Open* **2017**, *7*, e014451. [CrossRef]
7. Yuksel, M.; Yildiz, A.; Oylumlu, M.; Turkcu, F.M.; Bilik, M.Z.; Ekinci, A.; Elbey, B.; Tekbas, E.; Alan, S. Novel markers of endothelial dysfunction and inflammation in Behçet's disease patients with ocular involvement: Epicardial fat thickness, carotid intima media thickness, serum ADMA level, and neutrophil-to-lymphocyte ratio. *Clin. Rheumatol.* **2016**, *35*, 701–708. [CrossRef]
8. Chantasiriwan, N.; Silvilairat, S.; Makonkawkeyoon, K.; Pongprot, Y.; Sittiwangkul, R. Predictors of intravenous immunoglobulin resistance and coronary artery aneurysm in patients with Kawasaki Disease. *Paediatr. Int. Child. Health* **2018**, *38*, 209–212. [CrossRef]
9. Park, C.H.; Han, D.S.; Jeong, J.Y.; Eun, C.S.; Yoo, K.S.; Jeon, Y.C.; Sohn, J.H. The optimal cut-off value of neutrophil-to-lymphocyte ratio for predicting prognosis in adult patients with Henoch-Schönlein purpura. *PLoS ONE* **2016**, *11*, e0153238. [CrossRef]
10. Wu, Y.; Chen, Y.; Yang, X.; Chen, L.; Yang, Y. Neutrophil-to-lymphocyte ratio (NLR) and platelet-to-lymphocyte ratio (PLR) were associated with disease activity in patients with systemic lupus erythematosus. *Int. Immunopharmacol.* **2016**, *36*, 94–99. [CrossRef]
11. Küçük, H.; Göker, B.; Varan, Ö.; Dumludag, B.; Haznedaroğlu, Ş.; Öztürk, M.A.; Tufan, A.; Emiroglu, T.; Erten, Y. Predictive value of neutrophil/lymphocyte ratio in renal prognosis of patients with granulomatosis with polyangiitis. *Ren. Fail.* **2017**, *39*, 273–276. [CrossRef]
12. Abaza, N.M.; El-Latif, E.M.; Gheita, T.A. Clinical significance of neutrophil/lymphocyte ratio in patients with granulomatosis with polyangiitis. *Reumatol. Clin.* **2019**, *15*, 363–367. [CrossRef] [PubMed]
13. Turkmen, K.; Guney, I.; Yerlikaya, F.H.; Tonbul, H.Z. The relationship between neutrophil-to-lymphocyte ratio and inflammation in end-stage renal disease patients. *Ren. Fail.* **2012**, *34*, 155–159. [CrossRef] [PubMed]
14. Turkmen, K.; Erdur, F.M.; Ozcicek, F.; Ozcicek, A.; Akbas, E.M.; Ozbicer, A.; Demirtas, L.; Turk, S.; Tonbul, H.Z. Platelet-to-lymphocyte ratio better predicts inflammation than neutrophil-to-lymphocyte ratio in end-stage renal disease patients. *Hemodial. Int.* **2013**, *17*, 391–396. [CrossRef] [PubMed]
15. Sakai, H.; Kurokawa, K.; Koyama, A.; Arimura, Y.; Kida, H.; Shigematsu, H.; Suzuki, S.; Nihei, H.; Makino, H.; Ueda, N.; et al. Guidelines for the management of rapidly progressive glomerulonephritis. *Nihon Jinzo Gakkai Shi* **2002**, *44*, 55–82. (In Japanese) [PubMed]
16. Japanese Society of Nephrology. Clinical practice guidebook for diagnosis and treatment of chronic kidney disease 2012. *Nihon Jinzo Gakkai Shi* **2012**, *54*, 1034–1191.
17. Matsuo, S.; Imai, E.; Horio, M.; Yasuda, Y.; Tomita, K.; Nitta, K.; Yamagata, K.; Tomino, Y.; Yokoyama, H.; Hishida, A. Revised equations for estimated GFR from serum creatinine in Japan. *Am. J. kidney. Dis.* **2009**, *53*, 982–992. [CrossRef]
18. Iyama, T.; Takata, T.; Koda, M.; Fukuda, S.; Hoi, S.; Mae, Y.; Fukui, T.; Munemura, C.; Isomoto, H. Renal shear wave elastography for the assessment of nephron hypertrophy: A cross-sectional study in chronic kidney disease. *J. Med. Ultrason.* **2018**, *45*, 571–576. [CrossRef]
19. Jennette, J.C. Rapidly progressive crescentic glomerulonephritis. *Kidney Int.* **2003**, *63*, 1164–1177. [CrossRef]
20. Park, H.J.; Jung, S.M.; Song, J.J.; Park, Y.B.; Lee, S.W. Platelet to lymphocyte ratio is associated with the current activity of ANCA-associated vasculitis at diagnosis: A retrospective monocentric study. *Rheumatol. Int.* **2018**, *38*, 1865–1871. [CrossRef]
21. Schulze-Koops, H. Lymphopenia and autoimmune diseases. *Arthritis Res. Ther.* **2004**, *6*, 178–180. [CrossRef]
22. Ahn, S.S.; Jung, S.M.; Song, J.J.; Park, Y.B.; Lee, S.W. Neutrophil to lymphocyte ratio at diagnosis can estimate vasculitis activity and poor prognosis in patients with ANCA-associated vasculitis: A retrospective study. *BMC Nephrol.* **2018**, *19*, 187. [CrossRef] [PubMed]
23. McCracken, J.M.; Allen, L.A. Regulation of human neutrophil apoptosis and lifespan in health and disease. *J. Cell Death* **2014**, *7*, 15–23. [CrossRef] [PubMed]

24. Lebois, M.; Josefsson, E.C. Regulation of platelet lifespan by apoptosis. *Platelets* **2016**, *27*, 497–504. [CrossRef] [PubMed]
25. Matsuo, S.; Kimura, K.; Muso, E.; Fujimoto, S.; Hasegawa, M.; Kaname, S.; Usui, J.; Inohara, T.; Kobayashi, M.; Itabashi, M.; et al. Clinical guideline for rapidly progressive glomerulonephritis in Japan 2014. *Jpn. J. Nephrol.* **2015**, *57*, 139–232. (In Japanese)

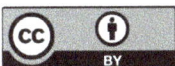

© 2020 by the authors. Licensee MDPI, Basel, Switzerland. This article is an open access article distributed under the terms and conditions of the Creative Commons Attribution (CC BY) license (http://creativecommons.org/licenses/by/4.0/).

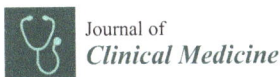

Article

Clusterin as a New Marker of Kidney Injury in Children Undergoing Allogeneic Hematopoietic Stem Cell Transplantation—A Pilot Study [†]

Kinga Musiał [1,*], Monika Augustynowicz [1], Izabella Miśkiewicz-Migoń [2], Krzysztof Kałwak [2], Marek Ussowicz [2] and Danuta Zwolińska [1]

[1] Department of Pediatric Nephrology, Wrocław Medical University, 50-556 Wrocław, Poland; monika.augustynowicz@umed.wroc.pl (M.A.); danuta.zwolinska@umed.wroc.pl (D.Z.)
[2] Department of Bone Marrow Transplantation, Oncology and Pediatric Hematology, Wrocław Medical University, 50-556 Wrocław, Poland; imiskiewicz@usk.wroc.pl (I.M.-M.); krzysztof.kalwak@umed.wroc.pl (K.K.); marek.ussowicz@umed.wroc.pl (M.U.)
* Correspondence: kinga.musial@umed.wroc.pl
† Short title: Clusterin in children after alloHSCT.

Received: 18 July 2020; Accepted: 9 August 2020; Published: 11 August 2020

Abstract: Background and aims: The markers of renal damage defining subclinical AKI are not widely used in children undergoing allogeneic hematopoietic stem cell transplantation (alloHSCT). The aim of the study was to evaluate serum and urinary clusterin as indices of kidney injury after alloHSCT in relation to damage (kidney injury molecule (KIM)-1) and functional (cystatin C) markers. Material and methods: Serum and urinary clusterin, KIM-1 and cystatin C concentrations were assessed by ELISA in 27 children before alloHSCT, 24 h, 1, 2, 3 and 4 weeks after alloHSCT and in controls. Results: All parameters were significantly higher in HSCT patients compared to controls even before the transplantation. The serum concentrations increased after HSCT and this rising trend was kept until the third (clusterin) or 4th (KIM-1, cystatin C) week. Urinary clusterin and KIM-1 were elevated until the third week and then decreased yet remained higher than before HSCT. Urinary cystatin C has risen from the second week after HSCT and decreased after the third week but was still higher than before alloHSCT. Conclusions: The features of kidney injury are present even before alloHSCT. Clusterin seems useful in the assessment of subclinical AKI and may become a new early marker of sublethal kidney injury in children.

Keywords: acute kidney injury; cystatin C; hyperfiltration; kidney injury molecule (KIM)-1; tubular damage

---

1. Introduction

Renal tubular epithelial cells are prone to hypoxia and metabolic stress, thus they become first target cells in the course of kidney injury. Contrast-induced nephropathy is a classic example of reversible acute kidney injury (AKI) with tubular involvement [1]. Animal and human studies showed that contrast administration triggers both systemic and renal cytotoxic effects [2,3]. However, if the conditions are unfavorable, further irreversible changes may lead to progression to chronic kidney disease [4].

Acute kidney injury is a well-documented phenomenon characteristic for HSCT [5–8]. However, most studies on AKI take into account the KDIGO classifications, focusing on the serum creatinine values and diuresis [9]. Such criteria do not ease the AKI diagnosis. In order to secure the patient with positive fluid balance and prevent oliguria, additional hydration and forced diuresis are implemented. These conditions may bias the values of estimated glomerular filtration rate (eGFR) and urine output.

Recent classifications have expanded the definition of AKI beyond the functional criteria. They distinguish four options, based on the combined evaluation of function and damage markers [10]. This new approach defines normal renal function as an absence of any index alteration, subclinical AKI as an isolated increase of any damage marker, functional AKI when solely function markers are modified and combined AKI with both function and damage markers altered [10,11].

The search for new markers was conditioned by the failure of serum creatinine as an early marker of renal function decrement. The indices of cellular damage—especially of tubular injury—are of particular interest as new markers of the so-called "subclinical AKI" [10]. The preliminary studies concerning children after cardiosurgery or hematopoietic stem cell transplantation (HSCT) proved that combination of the biomarkers of renal function and tubular damage may be of added value in the early diagnosis of AKI [12,13].

Indeed, the risk of AKI is increased in children undergoing hematopoietic stem cell transplantation (HSCT), mainly due to the nephrotoxicity of drugs. Additionally, renal hypoperfusion, infections and immune complications (including graft versus host disease) count. Moreover, patients with allogeneic HSCT suffer from AKI more often than those undergoing the autologous transplantation [14,15]. The assessment of renal function in the early (up to 28 days) post-transplantation period seems of paramount importance, because it may reveal the potential direction of future changes into either full renal recovery or acute kidney disease or chronic kidney disease [16,17]. First promising results in the population of children undergoing HSCT should urge further search for reliable early markers of kidney injury [13].

2. Aim of Study

Therefore, the objective of the study was to assess the usefulness of serum and urinary clusterin as new indices of kidney injury in the early post-HSCT period in relation to other renal damage (KIM-1) and functional (cystatin C) markers and to estimate their potential value as factors differentiating between children transplanted because of oncological and non-oncological reasons.

3. Material and Methods

3.1. Study Design and Settings

This observational pilot study concerned 27 children (15 girls, 12 boys) undergoing first alloHSCT in the Department of Bone Marrow Transplantation, Pediatric Oncology and Hematology, in 2019 (patient flow is shown in Figure 1). The observation period started before introducing conditioning therapy, then parameter examinations were performed 24 h, 1, 2, 3 and 4 weeks after HSCT.

The exclusion criteria for the patients were the age below 2 years and over 18 years, autologous HSCT and retransplantation. The whole alloHSCT group contained 27 patients (median age 4.5 years, interquartile range 3.1–8.0 years). The subdivision into two groups was carried out depending on the indications for allotransplantation. Seventeen patients (median age 6.6 years, interquartile range 4.0–9.8 years) were qualified for transplantation due to oncological reasons, 10 (median age 4.5 years, interquartile range 3.1–7.0 years) underwent HSCT due to non-oncological indications (mainly severe aplastic anemia). In 79% of cases the donor was unrelated, in 18%-related and in 3%-haploidentical.

The conditioning therapy concerned myeloablative (busulfan, cyclophosphamide and fludarabine or fludarabine, treosulfan, thiotepa) or non-myeloablative (cyclophosphamide, fludarabine) regimens. In most patients graft versus host disease (GvHD) protocol contained pre-HSCT ATG, cyclosporine A since 1 day before HSCT and methotrexate given in the 1st, 3rd and 6th day after transplantation. Nineteen out of 27 patients developed GvHD. None of the patients died in the observation period.

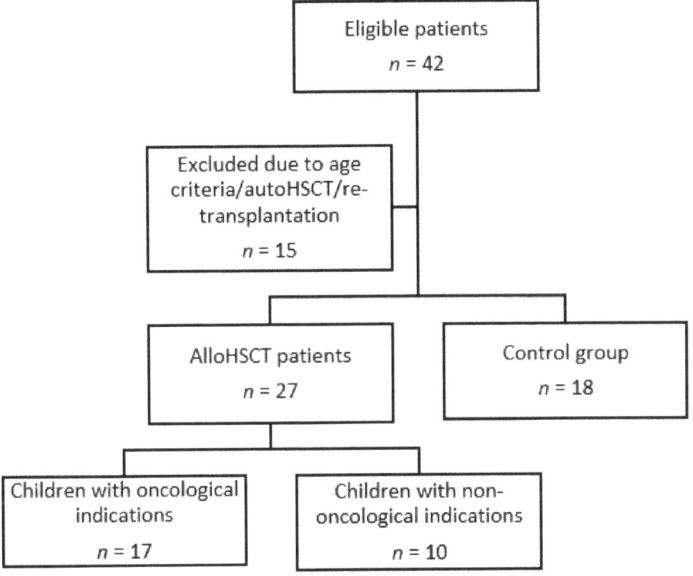

Figure 1. Patient flow.

The control group contained 18 age-matched children (9 girls, 9 boys; median age 7.8 years, interquartile range 7.0–9.8 years) with monosymptomatic nocturnal enuresis and normal kidney function.

Informed consent was obtained from the patients over 16 and their parents, if necessary.

3.2. Methods

Blood samples were drawn from peripheral veins after an overnight fast. Samples were clotted for 30 min, centrifuged at room temperature, 1000 g for 15 min, then serum was stored at −80 °C until assayed. Urine was collected aseptically from the first morning sample, centrifuged at room temperature, 1000 g for 15 min and then stored at −80 °C until assayed.

The serum and urine concentrations of clusterin, cystatin C and KIM-1 were evaluated by commercially available ELISA kits (clusterin EIAab, reagent kit E1180h; cystatin C R & D Systems, reagent kit DSCTC0; KIM-1 EIAab, reagent kit E0785 h). Standards, serum and urine samples were transferred to 96-well microplates precoated with recombinant antibodies to human clusterin, cystatin C, KIM-1 and creatinine. Captured proteins were then detected using monoclonal antibodies against clusterin, cystatin C and KIM-1 conjugated to horseradish peroxidase. Next, the assay was developed with tetramethylbenzidine substrate and blue color was developed proportionately to the amount of captured protein. The addition of acid stop solution ended the color development and converted it to the endpoint yellow. The intensity of the latter was measured in a microplate reader at 450 nm, with the correction wavelength at 550/650 nm. Each sample was tested in duplicate and the arithmetical mean was considered a final result. Measurements were performed according to the manufacturer's instructions; results were calculated by reference to standard curves. Detection limits were as follows: clusterin 1.56 ng/mL; cystatin C 3.13 ng/mL; KIM-1 0.15 ng/mL. The intra-assay and inter-assay coefficients of variation (% CV) for examined parameters did not exceed 8.5% and 9.4%, respectively.

The assessment of kidney function relied on hematological protocols assessing serum creatinine in fixed time points. Serum and urine chemistry parameters were measured using automated routine diagnostic tests on the Beckman Coulter AU2700 analyzer. The serum creatinine was assessed with the use of enzymatic method (creatinine OSR61204 reagent, creatininase–sarcosine oxidase reactions). Serum and urine concentrations of all parameters was measured before conditioning, 24 h after allotransplantation and then 1 week, 2, 3, 4 weeks after alloHSCT. eGFR was calculated in all time points, based on the Schwarz formula [18]. The eGFR changes were confronted with the pre-transplantation values.

All urinary concentrations of evaluated parameters were normalized to urinary creatinine values.

AKI was diagnosed based on the pRIFLE criteria [9]. Hyperfiltration was defined as eGFR ≥ 140 mL/min/1.73 m^2, according to recent meta-analysis and pediatric experience [19,20].

3.3. Statistical Analysis

Results were expressed as median values and interquartile ranges. The null hypothesis of normality of distribution of analyzed variables was rejected by Shapiro–Wilk test. Thus, the comparisons between paired and unpaired data were evaluated by using nonparametric tests (Friedman, Wilcoxon, Kruskal–Wallis, Mann–Whitney U). The correlations between parameters were assessed with the use of Spearman's correlation coefficient R. Statistical analysis was performed using the package Statistica ver. 13.3 (StatSoft). A p-value < 0.05 was considered significant.

4. Results

None of the patients presented with eGFR < 60 mL/min/1.73 m^2 and median eGFR values in both groups were above 90 mL/min/1.73 m^2 at any time point (Table 1) Most oncological patients demonstrated hyperfiltration until the 3rd week after transplantation (with peak incidence in the first week after HSCT). Non-oncological children with eGFR > 140 mL/min/1.73 m^2 were in minority. The median eGFR values in non-oncological children were comparable to those of the controls during the whole study except for the early (24 h after HSCT) measurement, when they became significantly higher (Table 1). Contrarily, the eGFR records in oncological patients remained significantly elevated compared to controls from point zero until the 3rd week after alloHSCT. They were increased throughout the whole study period compared to the non-oncological patients (Table 1).

Table 1. eGFR values in examined groups.

eGFR (mL/min/1.73 m^2) Median Value (Interquartile Range)	Before alloHSCT	24 h after alloHSCT	1 Week after alloHSCT	2 Weeks after alloHSCT	3 Weeks after alloHSCT	4 Weeks after alloHSCT
Oncological patients	142 (112–149) [a]	183 (153–216) [a,b]	172 (155–205) [a,b]	188 (166–195) [a,b]	149 (140–174) [a,b,c]	134 (123–149) [a,c]
Non-oncological patients	107 (96–129)	140 (126–176) [b]	131 (118–149) [b]	130 (114–136) [b]	129 (100–145) [b]	126 (92–134)

[a] $p < 0.05$ oncological pts vs. non-oncological pts; [b] $p < 0.05$ any time point vs. before alloHSCT; [c] $p < 0.05$ 2 weeks after vs. 3 weeks after; eGFR estimated glomerular filtration rate; alloHSCT allogeneic hematopoietic stem cell transplantation.

The urinary clusterin, KIM-1 and cystatin C concentrations were significantly elevated in all patients compared to controls, irrespective of the indication for transplantation (oncological or non-oncological), even before alloHSCT. Normalization of the urinary concentrations of clusterin, KIM-1 and cystatin C for urinary creatinine maintained these differences (Figures 2–4). In the case of clusterin, the urinary values have increased nearly 3-fold 24 h after transplantation, then kept the plateau phase until the second week and rose again in the 3rd week. Finally, they decreased in the 4th week after HSCT, yet remained higher than before HSCT (Figure 2). The urinary KIM-1 values rose by 50% 24 h after HSCT, then kept growing until the 3rd week and finally decreased (Figure 3). Urinary cystatin C demonstrated the delayed elevation from the 2nd week after transplantation, lasting only until the 3rd week and followed by a significant decrease 1 week later (Figure 4). After 4 weeks of observation, all urinary biomarkers were still significantly elevated compared to the pre-transplantation values.

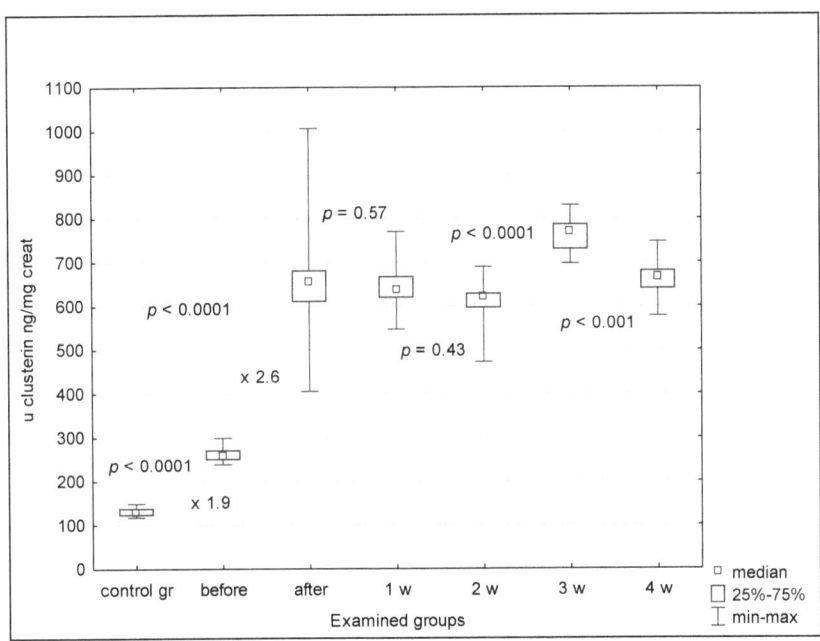

Figure 2. Urinary clusterin values in examined groups. before—before alloHSCT; after—24 h after alloHSCT; 1 w (2 w, 3 w, 4 w)—1 week (2, 3, 4 weeks) after alloHSCT.

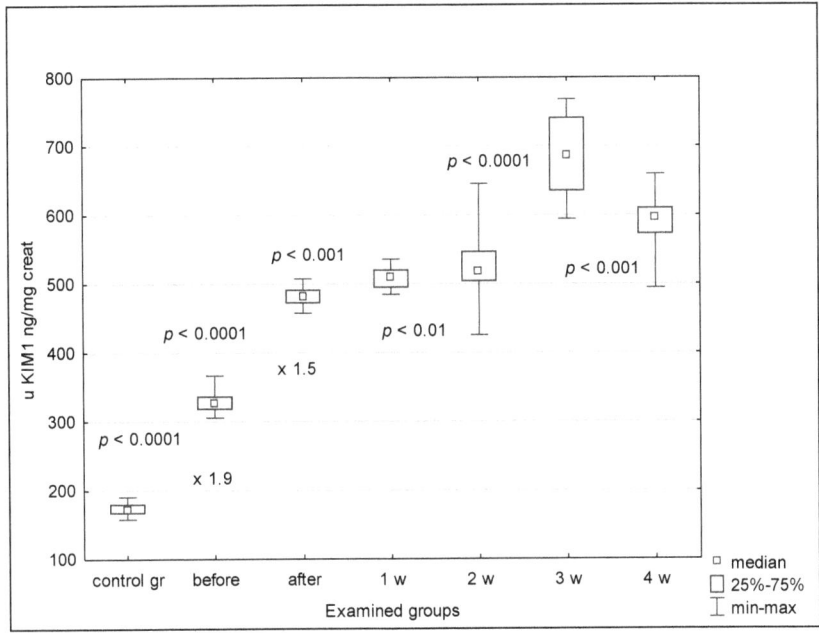

Figure 3. Urinary KIM-1 values in examined groups. before—before alloHSCT; after—24 h after alloHSCT; 1 w (2 w, 3 w, 4 w)—1 week (2, 3, 4 weeks) after alloHSCT.

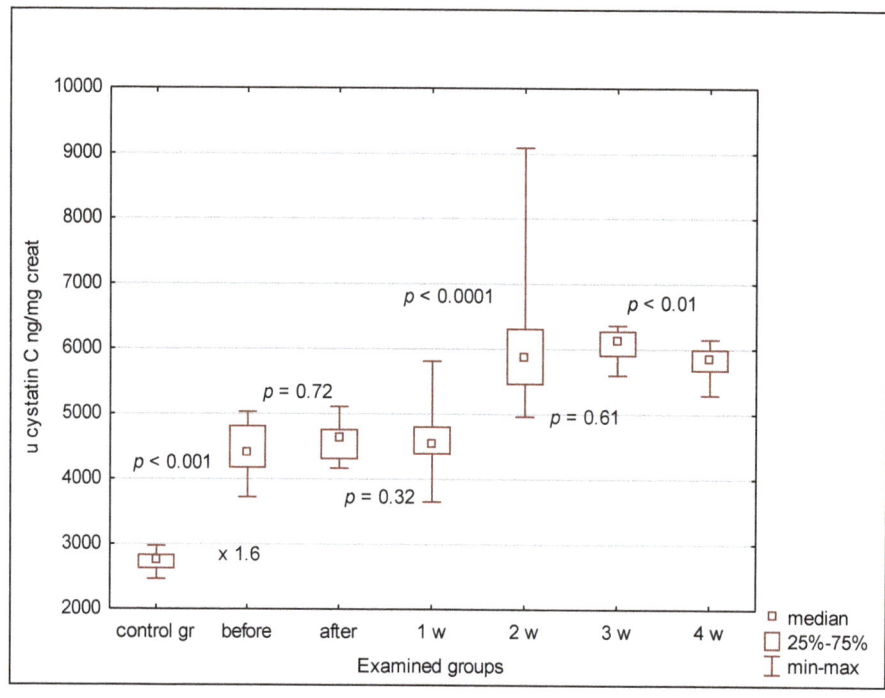

Figure 4. Urinary cystatin C values in examined groups. before—before alloHSCT; after—24 h after alloHSCT; 1 w (2 w, 3 w, 4 w)—1 week (2, 3, 4 weeks) after alloHSCT.

The serum concentrations of clusterin, KIM-1 and cystatin C in children before transplantation were significantly higher than in controls (Table 2). The serum values further increased 24 h after HSCT and the rise was most spectacular in the case of clusterin (over 2-fold) compared to 50%–60% elevation of other markers. Then the concentrations rose systematically until the 3rd week (clusterin) or 4th week (KIM-1, cystatin C) after alloHSCT. There was no significant difference in the urinary or serum marker values between oncological and non-oncological patients at any time point (Table 2).

Table 2. Serum parameter values in examined groups.

Serum Parameter Median Value (Interquartile Range)	s Clusterin (ng/mL)	s KIM1 (ng/mL)	s Cystatin C (ng/mL)
Control group	1.3 (1.2–1.4)	2.3 (2.2–2.4)	148 (141.7–164.3)
Before alloHSCT	3.1 (3.0–3.1) [a]	4.2 (4.1–4.3) [a]	408 (387.6–433) [a]
24 h after alloHSCT	7.9 (7.2–8.4) [a,b]	6.7 (6.3–6.8) [a,b]	634.8 (604.6–689.1) [a,b]
1 week after alloHSCT	8.9 (8.8–9.1) [a,c]	6.7 (6.0–6.8) [a]	905.6 (879–961.6) [a,c]
2 weeks after alloHSCT	9.5 (9.3–10) [a,d]	8 (7.8–8.2) [a,d]	898 (878.7–926.3) [a]
3 weeks after alloHSCT	13.3 (12.8–13.6) [a,e]	8.9 (8.8–8.9) [a,e]	1106 (1053–1157) [a,e]
4 weeks after alloHSCT	13.3 (12.8–13.6) [a]	9.2 (9.1–9.2) [a,f]	1262 (1222–1288) [a,f]

[a] $p < 0.05$ any time point vs. control group; [b] $p < 0.05$ 24 h after alloHSCT vs. before alloHSCT; [c] $p < 0.05$ 1 week after alloHSCT vs. 24 h after alloHSCT; [d] $p < 0.05$ 2 weeks after alloHSCT vs. 1 week after alloHSCT; [e] $p < 0.05$ 3 weeks after alloHSCT vs. 2 weeks after alloHSCT; [f] $p < 0.05$ 4 weeks after alloHSCT vs. 3 weeks after alloHSCT. No significant correlations were detected between the analyzed parameters.

AKI was diagnosed in 4 patients (3 oncological and 1 non-oncological), according to the pRIFLE criteria. Risk stage was diagnosed in 3 of them, 1 developed Injury stage. None of the patients required renal replacement therapy.

5. Discussion

Although AKI is a common finding in the patients undergoing alloHSCT, most of the classifications assessing the degree of renal impairment concentrate on the functional indices. However, damage markers seem a promising and objective alternative in the assessment of kidney injury. The fact that the number of potential AKI markers is increasing proves that the problem is emerging. Thus, our aim was to confront the known indices of tubular injury (KIM-1) and glomerular function (cystatin C, eGFR) with a new marker of cellular stress and damage. Clusterin has not been analyzed in a specific population of patients undergoing HSCT so far.

Every patient in this study group, irrespective of the indication for HSCT, demonstrated the features of cellular damage seen even before the procedure of transplantation. The interpretation of this unexpected result was quite challenging, because up-to-date studies on the populations undergoing HSCT have never compared their records to those of age-matched controls with normal renal function and no history of kidney injury. The pre-transplantation therapies, including chemotherapeutics and nephrotoxic drugs, seem of paramount importance as an explanation for this phenomenon. Indeed, all patients transplanted due to oncological reasons have undergone series of chemotherapies, whereas many of the non-oncological children were treated with potentially nephrotoxic antibiotics prior to alloHSCT. All these interventions were related to their primary diagnoses and could trigger the pre-transplantation subclinical kidney damage. Irrespective of the underlying cause, such observation would suggest that subclinical background is a common finding and, thus, the key player in the HSCT-related AKI.

The post-transplantation aggravation of cellular damage was rather predictable, taking into account the nephrotoxic and cytotoxic potentials of conditioning regimens, anti-GvHD prophylaxis and treatment of infections. The essential finding was that these signs of injury concerned both serum and urine, depicting not only renal, but also systemic cell damage after HSCT.

Among all analyzed parameters, the serum and urinary clusterin values have shown the most spectacular changes in children before HSCT compared to controls and before HSCT compared to 24 h after HSCT. The serum and urinary values before transplantation were at least two times higher than in controls and rose over 2.5-fold after transplantation. In the meantime, the other serum markers increased by no more than 60%, whereas the urinary values became 14% higher (KIM-1) or remained unchanged (cystatin C). Only in the case of clusterin the post-HSCT response was more spectacular than the difference between control group and pre-HSCT values.

Clusterin is a 75–80 kDa heat shock protein secreted by both epithelial and secretory cells in response to stress. Its protective and anti-apoptotic roles against renal ischemia-reperfusion injury have been demonstrated in murine kidneys [21]. Interestingly, clusterin was detected in both renal tubular epithelial and mesangial cells. Its decreased expression aggravated postischemic renal injury, as well as proteinuria in the course of glomerulopathy. Clusterin knockout mice suffered from the progression of renal inflammation and fibrosis after ischemia–reperfusion injury [22]. Investigation concerning humans is restricted to single reports on the urinary clusterin in patients with diabetes mellitus and promising results of a diagnostic multi-biomarker kit including urine clusterin in the scope of indices of chronic kidney injury [23,24].

Taking into account the experimental data, the above mentioned reports and our results, we could put forward the hypothesis about the protective role of clusterin in the kidney injury due to HSCT. Such presumption would provide the explanation for increasing levels in both serum and urine as a response to systemic and kidney stress conditions. Moreover, clusterin has turned out the most accurate marker predicting drug-induced AKI in adults, better than cystatin C or KIM-1 [25]. Interestingly, all three markers became higher compared to non-AKI controls already 1–3 days before the onset of AKI.

This may suggest the reason for the early pre-transplant elevation of all indices compared to healthy controls. It also shows the added value of all tested markers in diagnosing nephrotoxicity. Moreover, yet, testing big cohorts may give unequivocal results in the pediatric population, questioning for example the accuracy of KIM-1 as a predictor of AKI in children [26].

In our study group, urinary KIM-1 behaved similarly to urinary clusterin, although the elevation after HSCT did not reach 50%. However, the rising trend persisted until the third week and then a significant decrease was noticed. Yet, the values remained higher than before transplantation. Such scheme would talk into the tubular damage aggravating since the HSCT procedure. The serum KIM-1 concentrations kept the systematic growth throughout the whole observation period, except for the plateau phase between 24 h and one week after HSCT. These results have suggested the ongoing tubular damage in the course of HSCT procedure, triggered most probably by nephrotoxic drugs. Increased serum KIM-1 could point at its release by the cells damaged in the course of conditioning therapy, anti-GvHD prophylaxis or current infection treatment, as well as the accumulation of a molecule that cannot be filtered freely through glomeruli due to its molecular mass of 90–110 kDa. The possible long-term consequence has been discovered in experimental studies, when chronic KIM-1 elevation in mice promoted fibrosis, thus linking AKI to CKD [27].

However, both abovementioned markers seemed similar in the mode of early reaction to kidney injury. The usefulness of clusterin and KIM-1 could be strengthened by the fact that their elevated serum and urine values were noticed even before transplantation, both in oncological and non-oncological patients, whereas pre-transplantation eGFR changes concerned only oncological children. In detail, their eGFR values were significantly higher compared to controls and most of the patients demonstrated hyperfiltration. This finding was confirmed by other authors, who put the main stress on hypermetabolic states and previous chemotherapy as causative factors of hyperfiltration [28]. The eGFR discrepancies could also be the consequence of many transplant-related covariates like catabolism, inflammation or weight loss, directly influencing serum creatinine [29].

Whether this hyperfiltration could be the early sign of progression into chronic kidney injury, remains unexplained, because the longer time of observation would be needed. However, the elevation of both damage parameters and eGFR could be the proof for the pre-transplantation kidney injury in oncological patients. This finding justifies the current attempts to prevent renal injury or at least to minimize the impact of potential nephrotoxins on the kidney. The reduction of nephrotoxic exposure is one of the effective tools already used in oncological patients [30]. The animal models suggest the possibility to prevent AKI with the use of phosphodiesterase-5 inhibitors prior to potentially nephrotoxic treatment [31,32]. Independent of the chosen strategy, the threat of renal injury should urge careful follow-up of the patient in order to avoid additional insults triggering irreversible damage to the kidney.

Cystatin C is an established marker of glomerular function and a good predictor of AKI in children, so it seemed a good candidate to verify the abovementioned discrepant eGFR results. However, it did not confirm differences between oncological and non-oncological patients [33]. Out of the three examined markers, cystatin C was the only one with low molecular weight (13 kDa) freely filtered through glomeruli. Therefore, the fact that the elevation of cystatin C in serum has outrun the increase of the urinary value was the direct proof of the serum origin of cystatin C found in the urine. Having said that, the increased values of urinary clusterin and KIM-1, both of higher molecular weight than cystatin C, must have been of tubular cell origin. Therefore, their elevation was probably proportionate to the degree of cell damage and, in case of clusterin, to the intensity of protective mechanisms against kidney injury.

Summarizing, in our study clusterin has outperformed the targeted glomerular (cystatin C) and tubular (KIM-1) indices of kidney function. Therefore, it seems a promising early marker of the sublethal kidney injury, covering both tubular and glomerular spectrum of renal damage. Whether clusterin may become a duplex renal functional and damage marker, is yet to be established in the studies performed on a larger group of patients.

We also must acknowledge the limitations of our study. First, the clinical data were collected according to the hematological protocols, not taking into account all nephrological aspects. Thus, the full information about urine output is missing. This is the first report on the clusterin serum and urinary values in children, so it is impossible to confront them with the age-related reference values. We are also aware of the low number of patients and the heterogeneity of examined groups, which limits the power of conclusions and urges the continuation of the study throughout a longer period on a larger group of patients.

6. Conclusions

All children demonstrated the features of cell damage already before alloHSCT; thus, the subclinical AKI is a common finding in this population. Clusterin seems more useful in the assessment of subclinical AKI than the classical indices of tubular (KIM-1) and glomerular (cystatin C) damage analyzed separately. It may become a new early marker of sublethal kidney injury in this group of patients.

Author Contributions: Conceptualization: K.M., M.A., D.Z.; investigation: K.M., M.A., I.M.-M., M.U.; resources: I.M.-M., K.K., M.U.; formal analysis: K.M.; writing—original draft: K.M. writing—review and editing: K.M., D.Z.; visualization: K.M.; funding acquisition: K.K., D.Z. All authors have read and agreed to the published version of the manuscript.

Funding: The project was financed by the Foundation "Na Ratunek Dzieciom z Chorobą Nowotworową" (FNRD.C210.19.002).

Conflicts of Interest: The authors declare no conflict of interest regarding the publication of this manuscript.

Ethical Standards: All procedures were performed in accordance with the 1964 Helsinki declaration and its further amendments. The research project was approved by the Wroclaw Medical University ethics committee (decision no. KB-786/2018).

References

1. Mamoulakis, C.; Tsarouhas, K.; Fragkiadoulaki, I.; Heretis, I.; Wilks, M.; Spandidos, D.; Tsitsimpikou, C.; Tsatsakis, A. Contrast-induced nephropathy: Basic concepts, pathophysiological implications and prevention strategies. *Pharmacol. Ther.* **2017**, *180*, 99–112. [CrossRef] [PubMed]
2. Mamoulakis, C.; Fragkiadoulaki, I.; Karkala, P.; Georgiadis, G.; Zisis, I.E.; Stivaktakis, P.; Kalogeraki, A.; Tsiaoussis, T.; Burykina, T.; Lazopoulos, G.; et al. Contrast-indiced nephropathy in an animal model: Evaluation of novel biomarkers in blood and tissue samples. *Toxicol. Rep.* **2019**, *6*, 395–400. [CrossRef] [PubMed]
3. Tsarouhas, K.; Tsitsimpikou, C.; Papantoni, X.; Lazaridou, D.; Koutouzis, M.; Mazzaris, S.; Rezaee, R.; Mamoulakis, C.; Georgoulias, P.; Nepka, C.; et al. Oxidative stress and kidney injury in trans-radial catheterization. *Biomed. Rep.* **2018**, *8*, 417–425. [CrossRef] [PubMed]
4. Chevalier, R.L. The proximal tubule is the primary target of injury and progression of kidney disease: Role of the glomerulotubular junction. *Am. J. Physiol. Renal Physiol.* **2016**, *311*, F145–F161. [CrossRef]
5. Koh, K.N.; Sunkara, A.; Kang, G. Acute Kidney Injury in Pediatric Patients Receiving Allogeneic Hematopoietic Cell Transplantation: Incidence, Risk Factors, and Outcomes. *Biol. Blood Marrow Transplant.* **2018**, *24*, 758–764. [CrossRef]
6. Raina, R.; Herrera, N.; Krishnappa, V.; Sethi, S.K.; Deep, A.; Kao, W.; Bunchman, T.; Abu-Arja, R. Hematopoietic stem cell transplantation and acute kidney injury in children: A comprehensive review. *Pediatr. Transplant.* **2017**, *21*, e12935. [CrossRef]
7. Didsbury, M.S.; Mackie, F.E.; Kennedy, S.E. A systematic review of acute kidney injury in pediatric allogeneic hematopoietic stem cell recipients. *Pediatr. Transplant.* **2015**, *19*, 460–470. [CrossRef]
8. Kizilbash, S.J.; Kashtan, C.E.; Chavers, B.M.; Cao, Q.; Smith, A.R. Acute kidney injury and the risk of mortality in children undergoing hematopoietic stem cell transplantation. *Biol. Blood Marrow Transplant.* **2016**, *22*, 1264–1270. [CrossRef]

9. Sutherland, S.M.; Byrnes, J.J.; Kothari, M.; Longhurst, C.A.; Dutta, S.; Garcia, P.; Goldstein, S.L. AKI in hospitalized children: Comparing the pRIFLE, AKIN, and KDIGO definitions. *Clin. J. Am. Soc. Nephrol.* **2015**, *10*, 554–561. [CrossRef]
10. Haase, M.; Kellum, J.A.; Ronco, C. Subclinical AKI—An emerging syndrome with important consequences. *Nat. Rev. Nephrol.* **2012**, *8*, 735–739. [CrossRef]
11. Ronco, C.; Kellum, J.A.; Haase, M. Subclinical AKI is still AKI. *Crit. Care* **2012**, *16*, 313. [CrossRef] [PubMed]
12. Basu, R.K.; Wong, H.R.; Krawczeski, C.D.; Wheeler, D.S.; Manning, P.B.; Chawla, L.S.; Devarajan, P.; Goldstein, S.L. Combining functional and tubular damage biomarkers improves diagnostic precision for acute kidney injury after cardiac surgery. *J. Am. Coll. Cardiol.* **2014**, *64*, 2753–2762. [CrossRef] [PubMed]
13. Benoit, S.W.; Dixon, B.P.; Goldstein, S.L.; Bennett, M.R.; Lane, A.; Lounder, D.T.; Rotz, S.J.; Gloude, N.J.; Lake, K.E.; Litts, B.; et al. A novel strategy for identifying early acute kidney injury in pediatric hematopoietic stem cell transplantation. *Bone Marrow Transplant.* **2019**, *54*, 1453–1461. [CrossRef] [PubMed]
14. Kanduri, S.R.; Cheungpasitporn, W.; Thongprayoon, C.; Bathini, T.; Kovvuru, K.; Garla, V.; Medaura, J.; Vaitla, P.; Kashani, K.B. Incidence and mortality of acute kidney injury in patients undergoing hematopoietic stem cell transplantation: A systematic review and meta-analysis. *QJM* **2020**. [CrossRef] [PubMed]
15. Caliskan, Y.; Besisik, S.K.; Sargin, D.; Ecder, T. Early renal injury after myeloablative allogeneic and autologous hematopoietic cell transplantation. *Bone Marrow Transplant.* **2006**, *38*, 141–147. [CrossRef]
16. Basu, R.K. Targeting acute kidney injury: Can an innovative approach to existing and novel biomarkers shift the paradigm? *Nephron* **2019**, *143*, 207–210. [CrossRef]
17. Chawla, L.S.; Bellomo, R.; Bihorac, A.; Goldstein, S.L.; Siew, E.D.; Bagshaw, S.M.; Bittleman, D.; Cruz, D.; Endre, Z.H.; Fitzgerald, R.L.; et al. Acute kidney disease and renal recovery: Consensus report of the Acute Disease Quality Initiative (ADQI) 16 workgroup. *Nat. Rev. Nephrol.* **2017**, *13*, 241–257. [CrossRef]
18. Schwartz, G.J.; Muñoz, A.; Schneider, M.F.; Mak, R.H.; Kaskel, F.; Warady, B.A.; Furth, S.L. New equations to estimate GFR in children with CKD. *J. Am. Soc. Nephrol.* **2009**, *20*, 629–637. [CrossRef]
19. Cachat, F.; Combescure, C.; Cauderay, M.; Girardin, E.; Chehade, H. A systematic review of glomerular hyperfiltration assessment and definition in the medical literature. *Clin. J. Am. Soc. Nephrol.* **2015**, *10*, 382–389. [CrossRef]
20. Iduoriyekemwen, N.J.; Ibadin, M.O.; Aikhionbare, H.A.; Idogun, S.E.; Abiodun, M.T. Glomerular hyperfiltration in excess weight adolescents. *Niger. J. Clin. Pract.* **2019**, *22*, 842–848. [CrossRef]
21. Zhou, W.; Guan, Q.; Kwan, C.C.H.; Chen, H.; Gleave, M.E.; Nguan, C.Y.C.; Du, C. Loss of clusterin expression worsens renal ischemia-reperfusion injury. *Am. J. Physiol. Renal Physiol.* **2010**, *298*, F568–F578. [CrossRef] [PubMed]
22. Guo, J.; Guan, Q.; Liu, X.; Wang, H.; Gleave, M.E.; Nguan, C.Y.C.; Du, C. Relationship of clusterin with renal inflammation and fibrosis after the recovery phase of ischemia-reperfusion injury. *BMC Nephrol.* **2016**, *17*, 133. [CrossRef] [PubMed]
23. Kim, S.S.; Song, S.H.; Kim, J.H.; Jeon, Y.K.; Kim, B.H.; Kang, M.-C.; Chun, S.W.; Hong, S.H.; Chung, M.; Kim, Y.K.; et al. Urine clusterin/apolipoprotein J is linked to tubular damage and renal outcomes in patients with type 2 diabetes mellitus. *Clin. Endocrinol.* **2017**, *87*, 156–164. [CrossRef] [PubMed]
24. Watson, D.; Yang, J.; Sarwal, R.D.; Sigdel, T.K.; Liberto, J.; Damm, I.; Louie, V.; Sigdel, S.; Livingstone, D.; Soh, K.; et al. A novel multi-biomarker assay for non-invasive quantitative monitoring of kidney injury. *J. Clin. Med.* **2019**, *8*, 499. [CrossRef] [PubMed]
25. Da, Y.; Akalya, K.; Murali, T.; Vathsala, A.; Tan, C.-S.; Low, S.; Lim, H.-N.; Teo, B.-W.; Lau, T.; Ong, L.; et al. Serial quantification of urinary protein biomarkers to predict drug-induced acute kidney injury. *Curr. Drug Metab.* **2019**, *20*, 656–664. [CrossRef] [PubMed]
26. Fazel, M.; Sarveazad, A.; Ali, K.M.; Yousefifard, M.; Hosseini, M. Accuracy of urine kidney injury molecule-1 in predicting acute kidney injury in children; a systematic review and meta-analysis. *Arch. Acad. Emerg. Med.* **2020**, *8*, e44. [PubMed]
27. Humphreys, B.D.; Xu, F.; Sabbisetti, V.; Grgic, I.; Naini, S.M.; Wang, N.; Chen, G.; Xiao, S.; Patel, D.; Henderson, J.M.; et al. Chronic epithelial kidney injury molecule-1 expression causes murine kidney fibrosis. *J. Clin. Investig.* **2013**, *123*, 4023–4035. [CrossRef]
28. Kwatra, N.S.; Meany, H.J.; Ghelani, S.J.; Zahavi, D.; Pandya, N.; Majd, M. Glomerular hyperfiltration in children with cancer: Prevalence and a hypothesis. *Pediatr. Radiol.* **2017**, *47*, 221–226. [CrossRef]

29. Filler, G.; Lee, M. Educational review: Measurement of GFR in special populations. *Pediatr. Nephrol.* **2018**, *33*, 2037–2046. [CrossRef]
30. Young, J.; Dahale, D.; Demmel, K.; O'Brien, M.; Geller, J.I.; Courter, J.; Haslam, D.B.; Danziger-Isakov, L.; Goldstein, S.L. Reducing acute kidney injury in pediatric oncology patients: An improvement project targeting nephrotoxic medications. *Pediatr. Blood Cancer* **2020**, *67*, e28396. [CrossRef]
31. Georgiadis, G.; Zisis, I.-E.; Docea, A.O.; Tsarouhas, K.; Fragkiadoulaki, I.; Mavridis, C.; Karavitakis, M.; Stratakis, S.; Stylianou, K.; Tsitsimpikou, C.; et al. Current concepts on the reno-protective effects of phosphodiesterase 5 inhibitors in acute kidney injury: Systematic search and review. *J. Clin. Med.* **2020**, *9*, 1284. [CrossRef] [PubMed]
32. Iordache, A.M.; Buga, A.M.; Albulescu, D.; Vasile, R.C.; Mitrut, R.; Georgiadis, G.; Zisis, I.-E.; Mamoulakis, C.; Tsatsakis, A.; Docea, A.O.; et al. Phosphodiesterase-5 inhibitors ameliorate structural kidney damage in a rat model of contrast-induced nephropathy. *Food Chem. Toxicol.* **2020**, *143*, 111535. [CrossRef] [PubMed]
33. Nakhjavan-Shahraki, B.; Yousefifard, M.; Ataei, N.; Baikpour, M.; Ataei, F.; Bazargani, B.; Abbasi, A.; Ghelichkhani, P.; Javidilarijani, F.; Hosseini, M. Accuracy of cystatin C in prediction of acute kidney injury in children; serum or urine levels: Which one works better? A systematic review and meta-analysis. *BMC Nephrol.* **2017**, *18*, 120. [CrossRef] [PubMed]

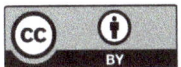

© 2020 by the authors. Licensee MDPI, Basel, Switzerland. This article is an open access article distributed under the terms and conditions of the Creative Commons Attribution (CC BY) license (http://creativecommons.org/licenses/by/4.0/).

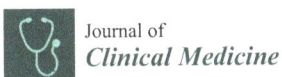

Article

Changes in Serum Creatinine Levels and Natural Evolution of Acute Kidney Injury with Conservative Management of Hemodynamically Significant Patent Ductus Arteriosus in Extremely Preterm Infants at 23–26 Weeks of Gestation

Eun Seop Seo [†], Se In Sung [†], So Yoon Ahn, Yun Sil Chang and Won Soon Park [*]

Department of Pediatrics, Samsung Medical Center, Sungkyunkwan University School of Medicine, 06351 Seoul, Korea; eunseop720@gmail.com (E.S.S.); sein.sung@samsung.com (S.I.S.); soyoon.ahn@samsung.com (S.Y.A.); yschang@skku.edu (Y.S.C.)
* Correspondence: wonspark@skku.edu; Tel.: +82-2-3410-3523; Fax: +82-2-3410-0043
† These authors equally contributed to the manuscript.

Received: 8 February 2020; Accepted: 29 February 2020; Published: 4 March 2020

Abstract: Changes in kidney function in extremely preterm infants (EPT) with conservatively managed hemodynamically significant (HS) patent ductus arteriosus (PDA) are not known well. We aimed to present the postnatal course in serum creatinine levels (sCr), prevalence of acute kidney injury (AKI), then relevance between AKI and adverse outcomes in EPT with conservatively managed HS PDA. By review of medical records, we analyzed the postnatal course of sCr and prevalence of stage 3 AKI defined by the modified Kidney Disease Improving Global Outcome (KDIGO) in EPT at gestational age of 23 to 26 weeks with conservatively treated HS PDA. We investigated if the presence and/or prolonged duration of stage 3 AKI elevated the risk of adverse outcomes. The results showed that, neither factor was associated with adverse outcomes. While the average PDA closure date was at postnatal day (P) 41 and 53, sCr peaked at P 10 and 14 and the cumulative prevalence of stage 3 AKI was 57% and 72% in the EPT of 25–26 and 23–24 weeks' gestation, respectively. The high prevalence of stage 3 AKI without adverse outcomes in EPT with conservatively managed HS PDA suggests that it might reflect renal immaturity rather than pathologic conditions.

Keywords: acute kidney injury; patent ductus arteriosus; conservative management

1. Introduction

Assessing kidney function is crucial for meticulous fluid, electrolyte, and nutritional support, and the adjustment of medication dosage in extremely preterm infants (EPT) [1–4]. Serum creatinine level (sCr) is a commonly used in evaluating renal function and could also be applied in assessment of glomerular filtration rate (GFR) in neonates and infants [4–7]. However, the use of sCr for renal function assessment in preterm infants is problematic as their sCr at birth reflects maternal levels [8,9], and sCr is quite variable according to gestational age (GA), birth weight, and chronological age [4,7,10,11]. Limited data are available on how sCr is affected by gestational age and birth weight and how this value changes over time, especially in the peri-viable EPT [5,7,10,12–14]. Despite these limitations, all the three current available acute kidney injury (AKI) definitions use change in sCr to classify the stage of AKI in the newborn infants [5,15,16].

AKI in premature infants are known to be related to increased mortality [11,17–21] and morbidities, which includes bronchopulmonary dysplasia (BPD) [2,22,23] and intraventricular hemorrhage (IVH) [24]. However, these associations have not been well reported and elucidated in EPT, although

EPT are at high risk for acute AKI because of low GFR resulting from under-developed kidney systems, exhibiting incomplete nephrogenesis and low nephron number [25,26]. Meanwhile, hemodynamically significant (HS) patent ductus arteriosus (PDA) could promote developing AKI by decreasing renal perfusion in the preterm infants in recent studies [16,17,27–29]. However, growing evidences support that the conservative management of HS PDA could be safe and feasible without increased mortality and/or morbidities [30–33]. Furthermore, the risks of developing AKI and the ensuing adverse outcomes with the conservative management of HS PDA have not yet been delineated. Therefore, we conducted this investigation to provide the natural postnatal course of changes in sCr, and the prevalence of AKI in EPT at gestation of 23–26 weeks with HS PDA exclusively managed with a conservative approach [31,32]. We also examined if the presence or persistence of AKI stage 3 adversely affected the risk of adverse events by comparing mortality and morbidities between EPT with and without AKI stage 3.

2. Experimental Section

2.1. Study Sample

The Samsung Medical Center (SMC) Institutional Review Board approved our investigation and waived the need for consent on October 10, 2019 (No. SMC 2015-10-156). We reviewed medical charts of 97 EPT at gestation of 23–26 weeks admitted to our Neonatal Intensive Care Unit (NICU) from January 2011 to June 2014 presenting with HS PDA, and treated exclusively by a conservative approach [31,32]. We stratified the extremely preterm infants into 23–24 ($n = 50$) and 25–26 ($n = 47$) weeks' gestation, and analyzed rates of mortality and morbidities, such as necrotizing enterocolitis (NEC), BPD, and intraventricular hemorrhage (IVH) in accordance with the presence/absence of and duration of AKI stage 3 [5,16,18].

2.2. AKI

AKI events occurring during the 6-week postnatal period were detected by the neonatal modified KIDGO sCr criteria [5,16,18] (Table 1). Measuring a chemistry panel including sCr q 1–3 days is usual at our NICU if the infant's condition is critical during the first few weeks of life, and increasing the interval up to q 1–2 weeks, if the infant's condition has become stabilized. Although we did not adopt urine amount criteria to classify stage, we calculated urine output from flow sheets, and reported the incidence of oliguria (<0.5 mL/kg/day) at each stage of AKI.

Table 1. The maximum AKI stage within a first month after birth according to neonatal acute kidney injury KDIGO classification.

Stage	Serum Creatinine	GA 23–24 Weeks $n = 50$	GA 25–26 Weeks $n = 47$	Total $n = 97$	Total with Oliguria (<0.5 mL/kg/day) $n = 97$
0	No change in SCr or rise < 0.3 mg/DL	4 (8%)	3 (6%)	7(7%)	1(1%)
1	SCr rise ≥ 0.3 mg/dL within 48 h or SCr rise ≥ 1.5–1.9 × reference SCr [a] within 7 days	2 (4%)	5 (11%)	7(7%)	1(1%)
2	SCr rise ≥ 2.0–2.9 × reference SCr [a]	7 (14%)	11 (23%)	18(19%)	1(1%)
3	SCr rise ≥ 3 × reference SCr [a] or SCr ≥ 2.5 mg/dL [b] or receipt of dialysis	36 (72%)	27 (57%)	63(66%)	18(19%)

[a] Reference SCr will be considered as the lowest prior SCr value. [b] SCr value of 2.5 mg/dL corresponds to GFR less than 10 mL/min/1.73 m^2. AKI, acute kidney injury; SCr, serum creatinine; KDIGO, Kidney Disease Improving Global Outcomes.

2.3. HS PDA

We defined HS PDA as more than 2 mm in ductal diameter plus predominant left to right flow on echocardiography initially performed at average postnatal day 7; requiring ventilator support accompanying signs and symptoms consistent with symptomatic PDA, such as hypotension with mean airway pressure below GA; grade ≥ 2 cardiac murmur; pulse pressure widening (>30 mmHg); or need for increased respiratory support [31,32]. We deferred until postnatal day 7 as spontaneous ductal closures could occur even in EPT for the first postnatal week [17,34]. Follow-up echocardiography was conducted regularly at 2–4 weeks intervals until PDA closure. During the study period, 50/54 (93%) and 47/74 (64%) in the EPT of 23–26 weeks of gestation were diagnosed with HS PDA, respectively.

2.4. Fluid Therapy

We managed all EPT with HS PDA with non-interventional conservative management without any pharmacologic and/or surgical intervention. We judiciously restricted the fluid intake starting with the first-day mean fluid volume around 67 mL/kg/day, and maintaining mean fluid intake around 107–115 mL/kg/day from days 7 to 28 for the first two months of life [31,32]. We individualized and adjusted the target fluid volume for each EPT q 24 h after assessment of volume status by body weight, serum sodium level, urine output and specific gravity, or cardiomegaly. In this present study, we could obtain judicious fluid restriction in EPT through meticulous NICU care including better room care delivery, minimal handling, and high humidification [35,36].

2.5. Data Collection and Definition

We analyzed clinical characteristics, which included sex, birth weight, GA, Apgar score at 1-min and 5-min, mode of delivery, chorioamnionitis, use of inotropic drugs, antenatal steroid use, and oliguria. We determined GA using the last menstrual period of mother and modified Ballard score. We confirmed chorioamnionitis using placental pathology. We reported oliguria when urine amount is less than 0.5 mL/kg for a day.

We analyzed adverse outcomes including ≥ moderate BPD [37], cystic periventricular leukomalacia, IVH (grade ≥ 3) [38], NEC (Bell's stage ≥ 2b) [39], retinopathy of prematurity (ROP) (stage ≥ 3) [40], and mortality.

To present the time course of sCr and AKI by gestational age, cumulative incidence rates of AKI in EPT at gestational age of 23–24 and 25–26 weeks were evaluated. We measured the adjusted odds ratios (ORs) of mortality and morbidities by the presence and/or persistence (per increase of week) of AKI stage 3 using multivariate regression analyses.

2.6. Statistical Analyses

We analyzed the categorical variables by χ^2 tests and Fisher's exact test. For continuous variables, we analyzed data through Student's t-tests and Mann–Whitney U tests. We also did multivariable analyses by binary logistic regression to measure adjusted ORs and 95% CI of the association between the duration of stage 3 AKI and adverse outcomes including mortality within the entire cohort. We considered a p value less than 0.05 as statistically significant. We used SPSS version 21 (SPSS Inc., Chicago, IL, USA) in all data analyses.

3. Results

3.1. Natural Course of sCr

For the time course of sCr, the initial increase in sCr peaked at postnatal day (P) 10 and postnatal week 2 in EPT at 25–26 and 23–24 weeks of gestation, respectively (Figure 1A). The peak sCr showed a higher tendency without statistical significance in EPT at gestation of 23–24 weeks than in those at 25–26 weeks. After this, sCr gradually declined until postnatal week 9 in both subgroups and reached sCr at birth at postnatal week 6 and 7 in EPT at 25–26 and 23–24 weeks' gestation, respectively. In EPT of 25–26 weeks' gestation without HS PDA, sCr showed a similar time course without statistical significance with the EPT of 25–26 weeks' gestation with HS PDA (Supplementary Figure S1).

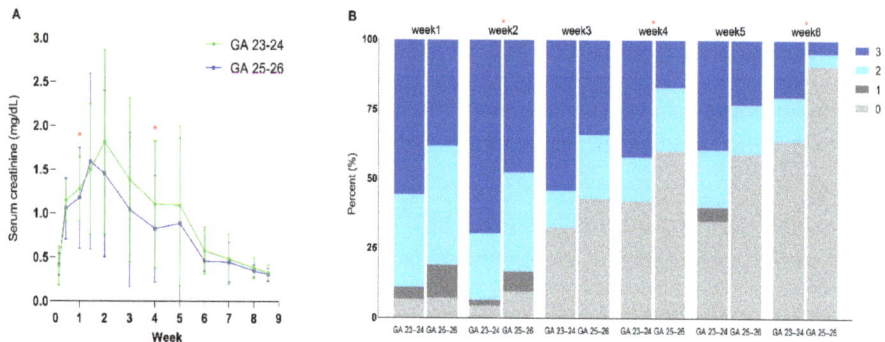

Figure 1. Time course of the mean serum creatinine levels within different gestational groups and prevalence of acute kidney injury (AKI) by stage in a week interval. (**A**) Serum creatinine profile for the 6 weeks of life in accordance to different gestational age groups; (**B**) Prevalence of AKI by stage in a week interval. * $p < 0.05$ in comparison between infants at 23–24 and those at 25–26 weeks of gestation.

3.2. AKI Prevalence

Table 1 demonstrates the cumulative AKI stage within the first six postnatal weeks according to neonatal KDIGO classification stratified by gestational age group. While only 6% and 8% were at AKI stage 0 in EPT at 25–26 and 23–24 weeks of gestation, respectively, the prevalence of AKI stage 3 tended to be higher (72%) in EPT at gestation of 23–24 weeks than in EPT of 25–26 weeks (57%) without statistical significance.

For the time course of the prevalence of AKI by stage in a week interval, postnatal increase in the prevalence of AKI stage 3 peaked at postnatal week 2 in both groups, and afterwards prevalence gradually declined till postnatal week 6 (Figure 1B). The prevalence of AKI stage 3 at postnatal week 2 and 6 in EPT at gestation of 23–24 weeks was higher significantly than that in EPT at gestation of 25–26 weeks.

3.3. Clinical Characteristics According to AKI Stage

Demographic and clinical characteristics in each study group in accordance with AKI stages are described in Table 2. In EPT with AKI stage 3, total GA was significantly lower, and male gender in EPT at gestation of 25–26 weeks had higher GA than in EPT with AKI 0–2. While total oliguria and oliguria in EPT at 25–26 weeks of gestation with AKI stage 3 were higher compared with those with AKI stage 0–2 significantly, no differences were observed in other clinical variables between AKI stage 3 and stage 0–2 groups.

3.4. Adverse Outcomes According to AKI Stage

While sepsis in EPT at 25–26 weeks of gestation with AKI stage 3 was slightly higher than infants with AKI stage 0–2, no significant differences were found in other adverse outcomes, including mortality and BPD, between the AKI stage 3 and stage 0–2 groups (Table 3).

Table 2. Demographics and clinical characteristics of EPT in period II: Stage 0–2 AKI vs. stage 3 AKI.

Clinical Characteristics	Total (n = 97)					
	GA 23–24 Weeks (n = 50)		GA 25–26 Weeks (n = 47)		Total (n = 97)	
	AKI 0–2 (n = 13)	AKI 3 (n = 36)	AKI 0–2 (n = 18)	AKI 3 (n = 27)	AKI 0–2 (n = 31)	AKI 3 (n = 63)
Gestational age (weeks)	23.9 ± 0.4	23.6 ± 0.5	25.6 ± 0.5 †	25.3 ± 0.4 †	24.8 ± 1.0	24.3 ± 1.0 *
Birth weight, mean (SD), g	684 ± 90	636 ± 79	743 ± 145	829 ± 140 †	718 ± 127	719 ± 145
Male, n (%)	6(46)	19(53)	7(39)	19(70) *	13(42)	38(60)
Apgar score at 1-min	3.9 ± 0.7	4.2 ± 1.3	4.4 ± 1.8	4.7 ± 1.4	4.2 ± 1.4	4.4 ± 1.4
Apgar score at 5-min	6.9 ± 1.1	6.5 ± 1.4	6.8 ± 1.4	6.9 ± 1.5	6.8 ± 1.3	6.7 ± 1.5
Cesarean delivery, n (%)	8 (62)	26(72)	16 (89)	24 (89)	24 (78)	50 (79)
Hypertension in pregnancy, n (%)	0	0	1 (6)	0	1 (3)	0
Chorioamnionitis, n (%)	6 (46)	25 (69)	9 (50)	15 (56)	15 (48)	40 (62)
Use of inotropic drugs, n (%)	3 (23)	8 (22)	4 (22)	1 (4)	7 (44)	9 (56)
Antenatal steroid use, n (%)	12 (92)	27 (75)	13 (72)	24 (89)	25 (81)	51 (81)
Oliguria, n (%)	1 (8)	9 (25)	1 (6)	9 (33) *	2 (7)	18 (29) *

* $p < 0.05$ compared with Stage 0–2 AKI. † $p < 0.05$ compared with infants at 23–24 weeks of gestation.

Table 3. Adverse outcomes of infants in period II: stage 0–2 AKI vs. stage 3 AKI.

Adverse Outcomes	Total (n = 97)					
	GA 23–24 Weeks (n = 50)		GA 25–26 Weeks (n = 47)		Total (n = 97)	
	AKI 0–2 (n = 13)	AKI 3 (n = 36)	AKI 0–2 (n = 18)	AKI 3 (n = 27)	AKI 0–2 (n = 31)	AKI 3 (n = 63)
Mortality, n (%)	1 (8)	7 (19)	1 (6)	1 (4)	2 (7)	8 (13)
Length of stay	111 ± 14	120 ± 64	130 ± 68	110 ± 59	122 ± 53	116 ± 62
NEC (Stage ≥ 2b), n (%)	0	5 (14)	2 (11)	3 (11)	2 (7)	8 (13)
ROP (requiring laser operation), n (%)	3 (23)	10 (28)	5 (28)	7 (26)	8 (26)	17 (27)
Blood culture-proven sepsis, n (%)	3 (23)	13 (36)	1 (6)	10 (37) *	4 (13)	23 (37) *
Cystic PVL, n (%)	3 (23)	7 (20)	3 (17)	2 (7)	6 (19)	9 (15)
IVH (Grade ≥ 3), n (%)	1 (8)	8 (22)	1 (6)	2 (7)	2 (7)	10 (16)
BPD (≥moderate BPD), n (%)	5 (39)	15 (47)	6 (33)	8 (30)	11 (36)	23 (39)
Survival without BPD, n (%)	1 (0)	0	1 (6)	3 (11)	2 (7)	3 (5)

* $p < 0.05$ compared with Stage 0–2 AKI.

3.5. Adjusted ORs for Risk of Adverse Outcomes by AKI Stage 3

The adjusted ORs for the risk of unfavorable outcomes were not increased in AKI stage 3 in multivariate analyses (Table 4). In addition, the adjusted ORs for outcomes were not elevated by prolonged duration (per week) of AKI stage 3 (Table 5).

Table 4. Adjusted ORs * for risk of adverse outcomes by presence of Stage 3 AKI.

Outcomes	Adjusted OR (95% CI)	p Value
Mortality	0.965 (0.140–6.661)	0.971
BPD (more than moderate BPD)	1.441 (0.507–4.095)	0.493
Survival without BPD	0.314 (0.018–5.559)	0.430
IVH (Grade ≥ 3), n (%)	1.923 (0.360–10.269)	0.444
Cystic PVL	0.460 (0.116–1.819)	0.268
ROP (requiring laser operation), n (%)	1.538 (0.480–4.926)	0.469
NEC (Stage ≥ 2b), n (%)	3.610 (0.439–29.654)	0.232
Blood culture-proven sepsis	3.556 (0.965–13.101)	0.057

OR, odds ratio; AKI, acute kidney injury; CI, confidence interval; BPD, bronchopulmonary dysplasia; IVH, intraventricular hemorrhage; PVL, periventricular. leukomalacia; ROP, retinopathy of prematurity; NEC, necrotizing enterocolitis. * adjusted for birth weight, gestational age, small for gestational age, antenatal steroid use, 1-min and 5-min Apgar scores, hypertension in pregnancy, chorioamnionitis.

Table 5. Adjusted ORs * for risk of adverse outcomes by duration (per week) of stage 3 AKI.

Outcomes	Adjusted OR (95% CI)	p Value
Mortality	1.040 (0.602–1.797)	0.887
BPD (more than moderate BPD)	1.043 (0.745–1.459)	0.808
Survival without BPD	0.332 (0.083–1.329)	0.119
IVH (Grade ≥ 3), n (%)	1.164 (0.074–1.823)	0.508
Cystic PVL	0.709 (0.437–1.150)	0.163
ROP (requiring laser operation), n (%)	1.000 (0.693–1.441)	0.998
NEC (Stage ≥ 2b), n (%)	1.325 (0.748–2.346)	0.335
Blood culture-proven sepsis	1.170 (0.820–1.665)	0.382

OR, odds ratio; AKI, acute kidney injury; CI, confidence interval; BPD, bronchopulmonary dysplasia; IVH, intraventricular hemorrhage; PVL, periventricular. leukomalacia; ROP, retinopathy of prematurity; NEC, necrotizing enterocolitis. * adjusted for birth weight, gestational age, small for gestational age, antenatal steroid use, 1-min and 5-min Apgar scores, hypertension in pregnancy, chorioamnionitis.

4. Discussion

This present study is the first human study demonstrating the natural postnatal evolution of sCr and the prevalence of AKI in the peri-viable EPT at gestation of 23–26 weeks with HS PDA who received exclusive conservative management. In this present study, while sCr at birth was about the same between the study groups, representing maternal levels [8,9], the peak sCr and the peak prevalence of AKI stage 3 during the first two postnatal weeks were higher in EPT at gestation of 23–24 weeks than in EPT of 25–26 weeks. These findings suggest that very low initial GFR and tubular immaturity, and its slow improvement, might be inversely related to GA in these peri-viable EPT [7,11,14,27,41]. Furthermore, as HS PDA closed averagely at postnatal day 41 and 53 in EPT of 25–26 and 23–24 weeks' gestation, respectively [31,32], our data suggests that renal immaturity inversely related to GA, rather than HS PDA induced renal hypo-perfusion [17,27–29], are primarily responsible for the initial postnatal rise in sCr and the peak prevalence of AKI stage 3 during the first two postnatal weeks [42].

sCr after peak declined rapidly, and reached a birth sCr at postnatal week 6 and 7, compatible with corrected GA of 31–32 weeks in EPT at 25–26 and 23–24 weeks of gestation, respectively, and after then, sCr approached a stable plateau in both GA subgroups, indicating a steady state between endogenous Cr production and excretion [13,27,41]. In the preterm infant, the GFR is lower until the full nephrogenesis is finished by 34–35 weeks of gestation [43–46]. Overall, our data suggest that despite its inverse relationship with GA, the postnatal renal maturation and the ensuing logarithmic increase in GFR are accelerated by 2–3 weeks in these peri-viable EPT [47].

Although AKI in premature infants has been known to be related to raised mortality [11,17–21] and morbidity rates, including BPD [2,22,23] and IVH [24], evidence supporting their direct causal relationships are lacking. In contrast, while sepsis rate was more elevated in AKI stage 3 than in stage 0–2, only in EPT at gestation of 25–26 but not of 23–24 weeks, neither the presence nor the prolonged duration of AKI stage 3 was associated with elevated mortality or any morbidities rates including BPD and IVH. The reasons for our results, which are contradictory to other studies showing increased mortality and/or morbidities [2,11,17–24], are difficult to explain. Few data are available for the peri-viable EPT of 23–24 week's gestation, and actively treated with pharmacologic agents for HS PDA could be cofounders in other studies. A further controlled study with a homogeneous patient population and same clinical management policy might be necessary to clarify these contradictory findings.

Fluid therapy and drug dosing in premature infants need to be adjusted according to renal function, i.e., GFR [3,4,45,46]. Considering our results, which showed greater and delayed peak of sCr and very high prevalence of AKI stage 3 at the first two postnatal weeks in these peri-viable EPT with HS PDA, judicious fluid restriction might be prerequisite for the success of non-interventional treatment for HS PDA [2,48,49]. In our prior studies [31,32], fluid volume of 67 mL/kg/day at day of birth, and raising up to ≤115 mL/kg/day for the first month was accomplished without restricting caloric support or elevating the risk of renal dysfunctions and electrolyte imbalance. Acute fluid overload in the newborn infants was associated with adverse outcomes, including mortality [50] and morbidities [2,48]. Furthermore, the extent of volume overload in critical adult patients also correlated with worse clinical course [51–53]. In contrast, fluid restriction was associated with reduced mortality [54] and morbidities, such as PDA and NEC [55]. Overall, these findings suggest that judicious fluid restriction might be essential for the success of the non-interventional conservative treatment of HS PDA in EPT [45].

Heterogeneous time intervals and variable number of follow-up sCr measurements for review could be limitations of this retrospective uncontrolled observational single center study. The absence of long-term outcome assessments including growth and neurodevelopment might be another limitation of this study. However, a relatively large sample size ($n = 50$) of the peri-viable EPT at gestation of 23–24 weeks with HS PDA exclusively managed with a conservative treatment, as well as less variation in clinical management policies, might be a strength of this single-center study.

5. Conclusions

In conclusion, the study findings suggest that AKI observed in EPT with conservatively managed HS PDA is not a pathological entity and might reflect a physiological postnatal developmental process of the immature renal system.

Supplementary Materials: The following are available online at http://www.mdpi.com/2077-0383/9/3/699/s1, Figure S1: Time course of the mean serum creatinine levels between infants with HS (hemodynamically significant) PDA (patent ductus arteriosus) and those with Non HS PDA for 60 days of life.

Author Contributions: Conceptualization, E.S.S., S.I.S. and W.S.P.; methodology, Y.S.C. and W.S.P.; software, E.S.S.; validation, S.Y.A.; formal analysis, E.S.S. and S.I.S.; resources, S.I.S. and W.S.P, data curation, E.S.S. and S.Y.A.; writing—original draft preparation, E.S.S. and S.I.S.; writing—review and editing, Y.S.C. and W.S.S.; visualization, E.S.S.; supervision, Y.S.C. and W.S.P.; project administration, E.S.S. and S.I.S. All authors have read and agree to the published version of the manuscript.

Funding: This research was funded by grants of the 20 by 20 Project (Best #3, GFO1150091) from Samsung Medical Center.

Conflicts of Interest: The authors declare no conflict of interest.

References

1. Aviles, D.H.; Fildes, R.D.; Jose, P.A. Evaluation of renal function. *Clin. Perinatol.* **1992**, *19*, 69–84. [CrossRef]
2. Rocha, G.; Ribeiro, O.; Guimaraes, H. Fluid and electrolyte balance during the first week of life and risk of bronchopulmonary dysplasia in the preterm neonate. *Clinics* **2010**, *65*, 663–674. [CrossRef] [PubMed]
3. Aperia, A.; Broberger, O.; Elinder, G.; Herin, P.; Zetterstrom, R. Postnatal development of renal function in pre-term and full-term infants. *Acta Paediatr. Scand.* **1981**, *70*, 183–187. [CrossRef] [PubMed]
4. Falcao, M.C.; Okay, Y.; Ramos, J.L. Relationship between plasma creatinine concentration and glomerular filtration in preterm newborn infants. *Rev. Hosp. Clin. Fac. Med. Sao Paulo* **1999**, *54*, 121–126. [CrossRef] [PubMed]
5. Chowdhary, V.; Vajpeyajula, R.; Jain, M.; Maqsood, S.; Raina, R.; Kumar, D.; Mhanna, M.J. Comparison of different definitions of acute kidney injury in extremely low birth weight infants. *Clin. Exp. Nephrol.* **2018**, *22*, 117–125. [CrossRef] [PubMed]
6. Raaijmakers, A.; Ortibus, E.; van Tienoven, T.P.; Vanhole, C.; Levtchenko, E.; Allegaert, K. Neonatal creatinemia trends as biomarker of subsequent cognitive outcome in extremely low birth weight neonates. *Early Hum. Dev.* **2015**, *91*, 367–372. [CrossRef]
7. Gallini, F.; Maggio, L.; Romagnoli, C.; Marrocco, G.; Tortorolo, G. Progression of renal function in preterm neonates with gestational age < or = 32 weeks. *Pediatr. Nephrol.* **2000**, *15*, 119–124. [CrossRef]
8. Lao, T.T.; Loong, E.P.; Chin, R.K.; Lam, Y.M. Renal function in the newborn. Newborn creatinine related to birth weight, maturity and maternal creatinine. *Gynecol. Obstet. Invest.* **1989**, *28*, 70–72. [CrossRef]
9. Gordjani, N.; Burghard, R.; Leititis, J.U.; Brandis, M. Serum creatinine and creatinine clearance in healthy neonates and prematures during the first 10 days of life. *Eur. J. Pediatr.* **1988**, *148*, 143–145. [CrossRef]

10. Walker, M.W.; Clark, R.H.; Spitzer, A.R. Elevation in plasma creatinine and renal failure in premature neonates without major anomalies: Terminology, occurrence and factors associated with increased risk. *J. Perinatol.* **2011**, *31*, 199–205. [CrossRef]
11. Lee, C.C.; Chan, O.W.; Lai, M.Y.; Hsu, K.H.; Wu, T.W.; Lim, W.H.; Wang, Y.C.; Lien, R. Incidence and outcomes of acute kidney injury in extremely-low-birth-weight infants. *PLoS ONE* **2017**, *12*, e0187764. [CrossRef] [PubMed]
12. Gilarska, M.; Raaijmakers, A.; Zhang, Z.Y.; Staessen, J.A.; Levtchenko, E.; Klimek, M.; Grudzien, A.; Starzec, K.; Allegaert, K.; Kwinta, P. Extremely Low Birth Weight Predisposes to Impaired Renal Health: A Pooled Analysis. *Kidney Blood Press. Res.* **2019**, *44*, 897–906. [CrossRef] [PubMed]
13. Thayyil, S.; Sheik, S.; Kempley, S.T.; Sinha, A. A gestation- and postnatal age-based reference chart for assessing renal function in extremely premature infants. *J. Perinatol.* **2008**, *28*, 226–229. [CrossRef] [PubMed]
14. Miall, L.S.; Henderson, M.J.; Turner, A.J.; Brownlee, K.G.; Brocklebank, J.T.; Newell, S.J.; Allgar, V.L. Plasma creatinine rises dramatically in the first 48 hours of life in preterm infants. *Pediatrics* **1999**, *104*, e76. [CrossRef]
15. Askenazi, D.; Abitbol, C.; Boohaker, L.; Griffin, R.; Raina, R.; Dower, J.; Davis, T.K.; Ray, P.E.; Perazzo, S.; DeFreitas, M.; et al. Optimizing the AKI definition during first postnatal week using Assessment of Worldwide Acute Kidney Injury Epidemiology in Neonates (AWAKEN) cohort. *Pediatr. Res.* **2019**, *85*, 329–338. [CrossRef]
16. Majed, B.; Bateman, D.A.; Uy, N.; Lin, F. Patent ductus arteriosus is associated with acute kidney injury in the preterm infant. *Pediatr. Nephrol.* **2019**, *34*, 1129–1139. [CrossRef]
17. Stojanovic, V.; Barisic, N.; Milanovic, B.; Doronjski, A. Acute kidney injury in preterm infants admitted to a neonatal intensive care unit. *Pediatr. Nephrol.* **2014**, *29*, 2213–2220. [CrossRef]
18. Jetton, J.G.; Boohaker, L.J.; Sethi, S.K.; Wazir, S.; Rohatgi, S.; Soranno, D.E.; Chishti, A.S.; Woroniecki, R.; Mammen, C.; Swanson, J.R.; et al. Incidence and outcomes of neonatal acute kidney injury (AWAKEN): A multicentre, multinational, observational cohort study. *Lancet Child Adolesc. Health* **2017**, *1*, 184–194. [CrossRef]
19. Shalaby, M.A.; Sawan, Z.A.; Nawawi, E.; Alsaedi, S.; Al-Wassia, H.; Kari, J.A. Incidence, risk factors, and outcome of neonatal acute kidney injury: A prospective cohort study. *Pediatr. Nephrol.* **2018**, *33*, 1617–1624. [CrossRef]
20. Viswanathan, S.; Manyam, B.; Azhibekov, T.; Mhanna, M.J. Risk factors associated with acute kidney injury in extremely low birth weight (ELBW) infants. *Pediatr. Nephrol.* **2012**, *27*, 303–311. [CrossRef]
21. Jetton, J.G.; Askenazi, D.J. Update on acute kidney injury in the neonate. *Curr. Opin. Pediatr.* **2012**, *24*, 191–196. [CrossRef] [PubMed]
22. Starr, M.C.; Boohaker, L.; Eldredge, L.C.; Menon, S.; Griffin, R.; Mayock, D.E.; Li, L.; Askenazi, D.; Hingorani, S.; Neonatal Kidney, C. Acute Kidney Injury and Bronchopulmonary Dysplasia in Premature Neonates Born Less than 32 Weeks' Gestation. *Am. J. Perinatol.* **2019**. [CrossRef] [PubMed]
23. Askenazi, D.; Patil, N.R.; Ambalavanan, N.; Balena-Borneman, J.; Lozano, D.J.; Ramani, M.; Collins, M.; Griffin, R.L. Acute kidney injury is associated with bronchopulmonary dysplasia/mortality in premature infants. *Pediatr. Nephrol.* **2015**, *30*, 1511–1518. [CrossRef]
24. Stoops, C.; Boohaker, L.; Sims, B.; Griffin, R.; Selewski, D.T.; Askenazi, D. The Association of Intraventricular Hemorrhage and Acute Kidney Injury in Premature Infants from the Assessment of the Worldwide Acute Kidney Injury Epidemiology in Neonates (AWAKEN) Study. *Neonatology* **2019**, *116*, 321–330. [CrossRef] [PubMed]
25. Rodriguez-Soriano, J.; Aguirre, M.; Oliveros, R.; Vallo, A. Long-term renal follow-up of extremely low birth weight infants. *Pediatr. Nephrol.* **2005**, *20*, 579–584. [CrossRef] [PubMed]
26. Hentschel, R.; Lodige, B.; Bulla, M. Renal insufficiency in the neonatal period. *Clin. Nephrol.* **1996**, *46*, 54–58. [PubMed]
27. Iacobelli, S.; Bonsante, F.; Ferdinus, C.; Labenne, M.; Gouyon, J.B. Factors affecting postnatal changes in serum creatinine in preterm infants with gestational age <32 weeks. *J. Perinatol.* **2009**, *29*, 232–236. [CrossRef]
28. Vanpee, M.; Ergander, U.; Herin, P.; Aperia, A. Renal function in sick, very low-birth-weight infants. *Acta Paediatr.* **1993**, *82*, 714–718. [CrossRef]
29. Weintraub, A.S.; Connors, J.; Carey, A.; Blanco, V.; Green, R.S. The spectrum of onset of acute kidney injury in premature infants less than 30 weeks gestation. *J. Perinatol.* **2016**, *36*, 474–480. [CrossRef]
30. Letshwiti, J.B.; Semberova, J.; Pichova, K.; Dempsey, E.M.; Franklin, O.M.; Miletin, J. A conservative treatment of patent ductus arteriosus in very low birth weight infants. *Early Hum. Dev.* **2017**, *104*, 45–49. [CrossRef]
31. Sung, S.I.; Chang, Y.S.; Chun, J.Y.; Yoon, S.A.; Yoo, H.S.; Ahn, S.Y.; Park, W.S. Mandatory closure versus nonintervention for patent ductus arteriosus in very preterm infants. *J. Pediatr.* **2016**, *177*, 66–71. [CrossRef] [PubMed]

32. Sung, S.I.; Chang, Y.S.; Kim, J.; Choi, J.H.; Ahn, S.Y.; Park, W.S. Natural evolution of ductus arteriosus with noninterventional conservative management in extremely preterm infants born at 23–28 weeks of gestation. *PLoS ONE* **2019**, *14*, e0212256. [CrossRef] [PubMed]
33. Kaempf, J.W.; Wu, Y.X.; Kaempf, A.J.; Kaempf, A.M.; Wang, L.; Grunkemeier, G. What happens when the patent ductus arteriosus is treated less aggressively in very low birth weight infants? *J. Perinatol.* **2012**, *32*, 344–348. [CrossRef] [PubMed]
34. Nemerofsky, S.L.; Parravicini, E.; Bateman, D.; Kleinman, C.; Polin, R.A.; Lorenz, J.M. The ductus arteriosus rarely requires treatment in infants >1000 grams. *Am. J. Perinatol.* **2008**, *25*, 661–666. [CrossRef]
35. Sung, S.I.; Ahn, S.Y.; Seo, H.J.; Yoo, H.S.; Han, Y.M.; Lee, M.S.; Chang, Y.S.; Park, W.S. Insensible water loss during the first week of life of extremely low birth weight infants less than 25 gestational weeks under high humidification. *Neonatal Med.* **2013**, *20*, 51–57. [CrossRef]
36. Park, J.H.; Chang, Y.S.; Sung, S.; Ahn, S.Y.; Park, W.S. Trends in overall mortality, and timing and cause of death among extremely preterm infants near the limit of viability. *PLoS ONE* **2017**, *12*, e0170220. [CrossRef]
37. Jobe, A.H.; Bancalari, E. Bronchopulmonary dysplasia. *Am. J. Respir. Crit. Care Med.* **2001**, *163*, 1723–1729. [CrossRef]
38. Papile, L.A.; Burstein, J.; Burstein, R.; Koffler, H. Incidence and evolution of subependymal and intraventricular hemorrhage: A study of infants with birth weights less than 1500 gm. *J. Pediatr.* **1978**, *92*, 529–534. [CrossRef]
39. Walsh, M.C.; Kliegman, R.M. Necrotizing enterocolitis: Treatment based on staging criteria. *Pediatr. Clin. N. Am.* **1986**, *33*, 179–201. [CrossRef]
40. International Committee for the Classification of Retinopathy of Prematurity. The International Classification of Retinopathy of Prematurity revisited. *Arch. Ophthalmol.* **2005**, *123*, 991–999. [CrossRef]
41. Bateman, D.A.; Thomas, W.; Parravicini, E.; Polesana, E.; Locatelli, C.; Lorenz, J.M. Serum creatinine concentration in very-low-birth-weight infants from birth to 34-36 wk postmenstrual age. *Pediatr. Res.* **2015**, *77*, 696–702. [CrossRef] [PubMed]
42. Velazquez, D.M.; Reidy, K.J.; Sharma, M.; Kim, M.; Vega, M.; Havranek, T. The effect of hemodynamically significant patent ductus arteriosus on acute kidney injury and systemic hypertension in extremely low gestational age newborns. *J. Matern. Fetal Neonatal Med.* **2019**, *32*, 3209–3214. [CrossRef] [PubMed]
43. Evans, N. Volume expansion during neonatal intensive care: Do we know what we are doing? *Semin. Neonatol.* **2003**, *8*, 315–323. [CrossRef]
44. Gawlowski, Z.; Aladangady, N.; Coen, P.G. Hypernatraemia in preterm infants born at less than 27 weeks gestation. *J. Paediatr. Child Health* **2006**, *42*, 771–774. [CrossRef]
45. Chow, J.M.; Douglas, D. Fluid and electrolyte management in the premature infant. *Neonatal Netw.* **2008**, *27*, 379–386. [CrossRef]
46. Awad, H.; el-Safty, I.; el-Barbary, M.; Imam, S. Evaluation of renal glomerular and tubular functional and structural integrity in neonates. *Am. J. Med. Sci.* **2002**, *324*, 261–266. [CrossRef]
47. Sutherland, M.R.; Gubhaju, L.; Moore, L.; Kent, A.L.; Dahlstrom, J.E.; Horne, R.S.; Hoy, W.E.; Bertram, J.F.; Black, M.J. Accelerated maturation and abnormal morphology in the preterm neonatal kidney. *J. Am. Soc. Nephrol.* **2011**, *22*, 1365–1374. [CrossRef]
48. Abbas, S.; Keir, A.K. In preterm infants, does fluid restriction, as opposed to liberal fluid prescription, reduce the risk of important morbidities and mortality? *J. Paediatr. Child Health* **2019**, *55*, 860–866. [CrossRef]
49. Cuzzolin, L.; Fanos, V.; Pinna, B.; di Marzio, M.; Perin, M.; Tramontozzi, P.; Tonetto, P.; Cataldi, L. Postnatal renal function in preterm newborns: A role of diseases, drugs and therapeutic interventions. *Pediatr. Nephrol.* **2006**, *21*, 931–938. [CrossRef]
50. Askenazi, D.J.; Koralkar, R.; Hundley, H.E.; Montesanti, A.; Patil, N.; Ambalavanan, N. Fluid overload and mortality are associated with acute kidney injury in sick near-term/term neonate. *Pediatr. Nephrol.* **2013**, *28*, 661–666. [CrossRef]
51. Foland, J.A.; Fortenberry, J.D.; Warshaw, B.L.; Pettignano, R.; Merritt, R.K.; Heard, M.L.; Rogers, K.; Reid, C.; Tanner, A.J.; Easley, K.A. Fluid overload before continuous hemofiltration and survival in critically ill children: A retrospective analysis. *Crit. Care Med.* **2004**, *32*, 1771–1776. [CrossRef] [PubMed]
52. Goldstein, S.L.; Currier, H.; Graf, C.; Cosio, C.C.; Brewer, E.D.; Sachdeva, R. Outcome in children receiving continuous venovenous hemofiltration. *Pediatrics* **2001**, *107*, 1309–1312. [CrossRef] [PubMed]

53. Goldstein, S.L.; Somers, M.J.; Baum, M.A.; Symons, J.M.; Brophy, P.D.; Blowey, D.; Bunchman, T.E.; Baker, C.; Mottes, T.; McAfee, N.; et al. Pediatric patients with multi-organ dysfunction syndrome receiving continuous renal replacement therapy. *Kidney Int.* **2005**, *67*, 653–658. [CrossRef] [PubMed]
54. Tammela, O.K.; Koivisto, M.E. Fluid restriction for preventing bronchopulmonary dysplasia? Reduced fluid intake during the first weeks of life improves the outcome of low-birth-weight infants. *Acta Paediatr.* **1992**, *81*, 207–212. [CrossRef] [PubMed]
55. Bell, E.F.; Acarregui, M.J. Restricted versus liberal water intake for preventing morbidity and mortality in preterm infants. *Cochrane Database Syst. Rev.* **2014**, *12*. [CrossRef] [PubMed]

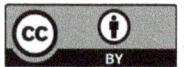

© 2020 by the authors. Licensee MDPI, Basel, Switzerland. This article is an open access article distributed under the terms and conditions of the Creative Commons Attribution (CC BY) license (http://creativecommons.org/licenses/by/4.0/).

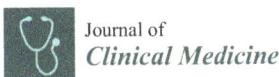

Article

Targeted Urine Metabolomics for Monitoring Renal Allograft Injury and Immunosuppression in Pediatric Patients

Tara K. Sigdel, Andrew W. Schroeder [†], Joshua Y. C. Yang [†], Reuben D. Sarwal, Juliane M. Liberto and Minnie M. Sarwal *

Division of Transplant Surgery, Department of Surgery, University of California San Francisco, San Francisco, CA 94143, USA; tara.sigdel@ucsf.edu (T.K.S.); andrew.schroeder@ucsf.edu (A.W.S.); joshua.yang@alumni.ucsf.edu (J.Y.C.Y.); reuben.sarwal@ucsf.edu (R.D.S.); jlibert7@jhmi.edu (J.M.L.)
* Correspondence: minnie.sarwal@ucsf.edu
† Authors contributed equally.

Received: 4 May 2020; Accepted: 21 July 2020; Published: 22 July 2020

Abstract: Despite new advancements in surgical tools and therapies, exposure to immunosuppressive drugs related to non-immune and immune injuries can cause slow deterioration and premature failure of organ transplants. Diagnosis of these injuries by non-invasive urine monitoring would be a significant clinical advancement for patient management, especially in pediatric cohorts. We investigated the metabolomic profiles of biopsy matched urine samples from 310 unique kidney transplant recipients using gas chromatography–mass spectrometry (GC-MS). Focused metabolite panels were identified that could detect biopsy confirmed acute rejection with 92.9% sensitivity and 96.3% specificity (11 metabolites) and could differentiate BK viral nephritis (BKVN) from acute rejection with 88.9% sensitivity and 94.8% specificity (4 metabolites). Overall, targeted metabolomic analyses of biopsy-matched urine samples enabled the generation of refined metabolite panels that non-invasively detect graft injury phenotypes with high confidence. These urine biomarkers can be rapidly assessed for non-invasive diagnosis of specific transplant injuries, opening the window for precision transplant medicine.

Keywords: kidney transplantation; metabolomics; immunosuppression; urine; acute rejection; immunosuppression; allograft

1. Introduction

Kidney transplantation (KTx) is the preferred method of treatment for end-stage kidney failure [1]. Increasing the longevity of transplanted kidneys is critical because of the shortage of available kidneys and kidney donors [2]. While improved short-term survival of the transplanted kidney has been attributed to better immunosuppressive drugs and sophistication in organ procurement and surgical methods [3], long-term survival outcomes have largely remained limited and unchanged [4]. Currently used methods of KTx monitoring, such as patient serum creatinine and proteinuria, are neither sufficiently sensitive nor specific to detect early-stage injury and only detect advanced and often irreversible tissue injury [5]. Additionally, kidney biopsies cannot easily be used to predict injury [6,7]. Over recent years, the application of high throughput technologies towards a more discovery-based approach for correlative biomarkers of graft injury have utilized sequencing [8] gene expression, proteomic [9–14], and metabolomic methods [15,16]. Many of these approaches show background signals of other clinical confounders, such as immunosuppression exposure [17], and thus require the application of more customized and robust analytical techniques for improving the diagnostic accuracy of biomarkers in blood and urine to reflect different transplant (Tx) injury phenotypes [18–20].

In this study, we hypothesized that the recipient's immune response towards the graft induces immunological and downstream metabolic changes at the time of specific injuries, such as acute rejection (AR), which result in perturbations in specific urine metabolite concentrations. We also hypothesized that specific metabolic pathways are injury-specific such that a panel of metabolites can be used as a surrogate biomarker to monitor KTx injuries. In this report, we present our findings from a comprehensive targeted metabolomics analysis of urine collected from pediatric KTx patients. These samples have been biopsy matched, providing an accurate phenotype characterization, and enabling exploration of metabolic pathways associated with KTx dysfunction.

2. Experimental Section

2.1. Patients and Samples

Biobanked urine samples available in the Sarwal lab from previously funded studies were screened for matching biopsy data on the day of urine collection. Out of a total of 2016 biobanked urine samples collected between 2006 and 2009, 770 were biopsy-matched, of which 326 unique and clinically annotated urine samples were included in the first part of this study. These patients were on calcineurin inhibitor (CNI) based immunosuppression (IS). All urine samples were stored at −80 °C with urine processing techniques, procedures, and conditions in which we have previously shown negligible degradation of urine components [11].

All samples from our biobank were matched with transplant biopsies; all biopsies were read by a central pathologist and scored by the Banff and Chronic Allograft Damage Index (CADI) [21–23] as acute cellular or humoral rejection with clinical graft dysfunction, and tubulitis and/or vasculitis on histology (AR; $n = 106$) [24], stable with no histological or clinical graft injury (stable graft function (STA); $n = 111$), interstitial fibrosis and tubular atrophy (IFTA; $n = 71$) [25], and BK viral nephritis with SV40 staining on histology, with/without clinical graft dysfunction (BK viral nephritis (BKVN); $n = 22$). Intragraft C4d stains were performed to assess for antibody-mediated rejection (ABMR). AR was defined, at minimum, by the following criteria: (i) TCMR consisting of either a tubulitis (t) score > 2 accompanied by an interstitial inflammation score > 2 or vascular changes (v) score > 0; (ii) C4d-positive ABMR consisting of positive donor-specific antibodies (DSAs) with a glomerulitis (g) score > 0 or peritubular capillaritis score (ptc) > 0 or v > 0 with unexplained acute tubular necrosis/thrombotic microangiopathy (ATN/TMA) with C4d = 2; or (iii) C4d-negative ABMR consisting of positive DSA with unexplained ATN/TMA with g + ptc ≥ 2 and C4d = 0 or 1. Stable allografts were defined by an absence of substantial injury on the matched biopsy pathology and definitions of the inflammation or i score and the tubulitis or t score. IFTA used standard pathology definitions as described by the Banff schema on the paired biopsies from each individual urine sample.

This study was conducted in accordance with the relevant guidelines and regulations as approved by the University of California San Francisco (UCSF) Human Research Protection Program Institutional Review Board (IRB) under IRB #14-13573. All patients provided written informed consent. In cases of pediatric and young adult patients, written informed consent was obtained from a parent and/or legal guardian to participate in the research, in full adherence to the Declaration of Helsinki. The clinical and research activities being reported are consistent with the Principles of the Declaration of Istanbul as outlined in the 'Declaration of Istanbul on Organ Trafficking and Transplantation Tourism'. As such, no organs or tissues were procured from prisoners. All organs or tissues were procured from the Departments of Surgery at either UCSF or Stanford University.

2.2. Urine Collection, Initial Processing, Storage, and GC/MS-TOF Analysis

Second morning void mid-stream urine (50–100 mL) was collected in sterile containers and was centrifuged at 2000× g for 20 min at room temperature within 1 h of collection. Specifically, the urine specimens were collected in sterile polypropylene collection tubes that are leak-resistant with a sterility seal. Processing of the urine was done all in one bath with sterile polypropylene plastic tubes. The supernatant was separated from the pellet containing any particulate matter including cells and cell debris. The pH of the supernatant was adjusted to 7.0 with Tris-HCL and stored at −80 °C in polypropylene plastic tubes until further analysis. The identification of metabolites followed the well-established FiehnLib protocol [26]. In brief, all metabolite reference standards underwent a two-step derivatization procedure following the previously published protocol [27]. The derivatization of urine metabolites procedure has been described previously [27]. Briefly, neat urine samples were lyophilized without further pretreatment after our initial finding of severe alterations using urease treatments. To the dried samples, 20 µL of 40 mg/mL methoxylamine hydrochloride in pyridine was added, and samples were agitated at 30 °C for 30 min. Subsequently, 180 µL of trimethylsilylating agent N-methyl-N-trimethylsilyltrifluoroacetamide (MSTFA) was added, and samples were agitated at 37 °C for 30 min. GC–MS analysis was performed using an Agilent 6890 N gas chromatograph (Atlanta, GA, USA) interfaced to a time-of-flight (TOF) Pegasus III mass spectrometer (Leco, St. Joseph, MI, USA) [27]. Automated injections were performed with a programmable robotic Gerstel MPS2 multipurpose sampler (Mülheim an der Ruhr, Germany). The GC was fitted with both an Agilent injector and a Gerstel temperature-programmed injector, cooled injection system (model CIS 4), with a Peltier cooling source. An automated liner exchange (ALEX) designed by Gerstel was used to eliminate cross-contamination from sample matrix occurring between sample runs. Multiple baffled liners for the GC inlet were deactivated with 1 µL injections of MSTFA. The Agilent injector temperature was held constant at 250 °C while the Gerstel injector was programmed (initial temperature 50 °C, hold 0.1 min, and increased at a rate of 10 °C/s to a final temperature of 330 °C, hold time 10 min). Injections of 1 µL were made in split (1:5) mode (purge time 120 s, purge flow 40 mL/min). Chromatography was performed on a Rtx-5Sil MS column (30 m × 0.25 mm inner diameter (i.d.), 0.25 µm film thickness) with an Integra-Guard column (Restek, Bellefonte, PA, USA). Helium carrier gas was used at a constant flow of 1 mL/min. The GC oven temperature program was initially 50 °C with a 1-min hold time and ramping at 20 °C/min to a final temperature of 330 °C with a 5-min hold time before cool-down for a 20 min run time. MS parameters were based on Autotune using FC43 (Perfluorotributylamine) with manufacturer-specific tune settings. Transfer line temperature was 250 °C and electron impact ionization was set at 70 eV. Filament source temperature was at 250 °C and TOF at room temperature. After a solvent delay of 350 s, mass spectra were acquired at 20 scans/s with a mass range of 50 to 500 m/z. Initial peak detection and mass spectrum deconvolution were performed with Leco Chroma-TOF software (version 2.25, Leco) and samples were exported to the netCDF format for further data evaluation with MZmine [28] and XCMS [29].

2.3. Raw Data Processing and Statistics

All chromatograms were assessed in the same manner by software packages MZmine [28] and XCMS [29]. These packages performed peak finding in an automated and unbiased way using the common MS netCDF file format that enables a unique way of data export irrespective of different instrument platforms. For the raw GC–MS data, the netCDF export function from the Leco ChromaTOF software was used. For MZmine, the m/z bin size was set to 0.01, the chromatographic threshold level was set to 0.5, the absolute intensity threshold was set to 2500, the tolerance in m/z values was set to 0.5, the tolerance in intensity was set to 1.0, and the minimum peak length was set to 2 s.

The raw data was normalized using urine creatinine, as an internal control, measured as a part of urine metabolome assessment and quantile normalization for batch correction. Moreover, 310 biopsy-matched urine samples, with resulting panels of 266 metabolites, were used for the analyses of both post-transplant injury classification and significant metabolite selection. Non-parametric imputation was applied to these samples via the missForest algorithm [30]. If more there was missing data on more than one-third of the metabolites, these samples were excluded. Sixteen samples met this criterion.

Clustering was performed and visualized with Morpheus (Broad Institute) using average linkage hierarchical clustering. The log-transformed data was median centered, per metabolite, prior to clustering for better visualization. One minus Pearson's correlation was used for the similarity metric. A fire color scheme was used in heat maps of the metabolites. Z-score analysis scaled each metabolite according to a reference distribution.

To evaluate the performance of the classification models, these 310 samples were randomly assigned to training (75%) and test (25%) sets. To avoid overfitting, 10-fold cross-validation was performed for models on the training set. The primary statistical learning method used for allograft outcome classification was Random Forests [31] via the randomForest package in R. Significant metabolites were selected from the Random Forests model using the VSURF package in R [32]. Additionally, for visualization of significant metabolites, volcano plots were produced using variable importance values derived from Random Forests models as a significance measure. Metabolite selection was done by Bonferroni-corrected p-value in addition to VSURF to display a traditional volcano plot and directly compare VSURF to traditional t-testing methods and their resulting metabolite lists. These variable importance scores are defined as the mean percentage decrease in classification accuracy of the model if the metabolite data were to be randomly permuted rather than taken as quantified (a higher score denotes a higher variable importance). Comparison of classification models was done by computing and plotting area under the curve (AUC) from the receiver operating characteristic (ROC) using the pROC package in R. Statistical comparison between full and abbreviated metabolite models to assess diagnostic accuracy similarity was carried out using the DeLong's test [33]. Given that certain clinical data variables were significantly different between groups, these variables were reviewed for any association with particular variable differences within or between groups and their impact on metabolite signatures of different transplant phenotypes. Analysis was performed using the R statistical software version 3.4.3. MetaboAnalyst (www.metaboanalyst.ca) was used to perform targeted pathway and enrichment analysis [34].

2.4. Data Availability

The datasets generated during and analyzed during the current study are not publicly available due to legacy IRB consent restrictions on public sharing of data from these patient populations but are available from the corresponding author on reasonable request.

3. Results

3.1. Metabolites in Urine Are Perturbed in Different Transplant Injuries in Kidney Transplantation

We processed 326 urine samples for a targeted metabolomics assay that identified 266 metabolites. Figure 1 summarizes the study. Sixteen samples had missing data on more than one third of total metabolites identified following a tool called MissForest on non-parametric missing value imputation for mixed-type data [30]. Metabolomics data on the remaining 310 biopsy-matched urine samples was used for the analyses of both post-Tx injury detection and associated metabolic pathways and their enrichment. Baseline characteristics of the study subjects is provided in Table 1.

The data was used for supervised clustering to generate a heat map (Figure 2A) and z-score plot (Figure 2B). The heatmap shows heterogeneity in overall metabolome data across urine samples from different phenotypes. In the z-score plot, stable-based z-scores were plotted for each of the 266 metabolites. The plots revealed robust metabolic alterations in AR (z-score range: −4.2 to 800.5) and IFTA (z-score range: −3.8 to 265.4) compared to fewer changes in BKVN samples (z-score range: −3.4 to 116.9).

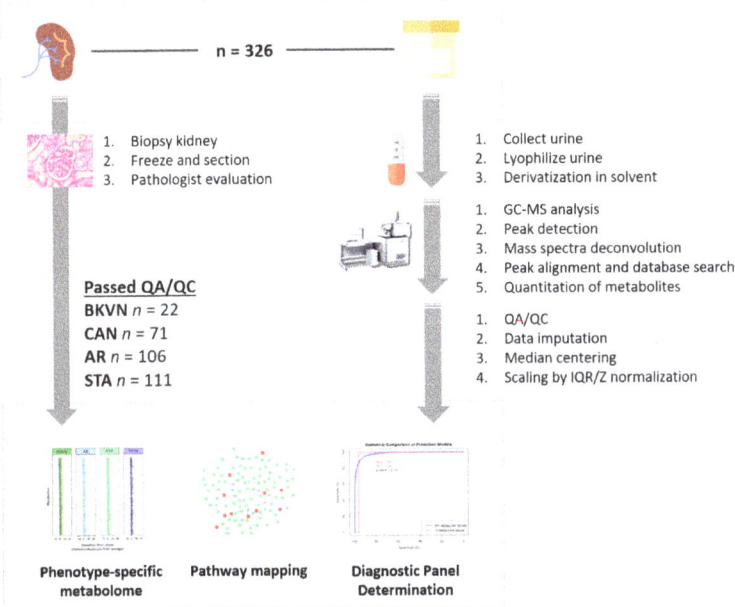

Figure 1. Sample selection and study schematic of the study. Summary outlining study samples, assay platform, study phenotypes, analysis, and results.

Table 1. Patient demographic data for the discovery cohort.

Phenotype	AR	STA	IFTA	BKVN	p-Value
Number of Patients	106	111	71	22	
Maintenance (% Steroid-free)	63.2%	50.5%	56.3%	36.4%	0.078
Recipient Gender (% M)	64.2%	58.6%	67.6%	59.1%	0.002
Recipient Age * (years)	13 ± 5 (14; 2–21)	14 ± 5 (15; 1–21)	10 ± 6 (10; 1–20)	14 ± 5 (17; 1–18)	0.003
Donor Gender (% M)	46.2%	52.3%	52.1%	72.7%	0.123
Donor Age * (years)	29 ± 11 (29; 4–50)	30 ± 10 (28; 14–51)	30 ± 10 (32; 12–50)	28 ± 10 (29; 16–49)	0.353
Month post-Tx (mean ± SD)	71 ± 32	15 ± 24	23 ± 32	8 ± 7	0.311
Donor Source (%): 1 = Living Related 2 = Living Unrelated 3 = Deceased	1 = 24.5% 2 = 40.6% 3 = 34.0%	1 = 37.8% 2 = 8.1% 3 = 44.1%	1 = 43.7% 2 = 8.5% 3 = 47.9%	1 = 9.1% 2 = 31.8% 3 = 54.5%	
Recipient Race (%): 1 = Caucasian 2 = Asian 3 = African American 4 = Hispanic 5 = Mixed and Others	1 = 42.5% 2 = 5.7% 3 = 16.0% 4 = 7.5% 5 = 12.3%	1 = 43.2% 2 = 4.5% 3 = 18.0% 4 = 2.7% 5 = 16.2%	1 = 50.7% 2 = 7.0% 3 = 18.3% 4 = 5.6% 5 = 9.9%	1 = 27.3% 2 = 0.0% 3 = 13.6% 4 = 18.2% 5 = 0.0%	
HLA Mismatch	4.64 ± 1.41	4.15 ± 1.35	3.62 ± 1.67	4.80 ± 1.15	0.245
eGFR	75.3 ± 42.3	95.4 ± 28.5	104.1 ± 36.7	N/A [#]	0.171

* Age in years: mean ± SD (median; range). AR, acute rejection; STA, stable graft function; IFTA, interstitial fibrosis and tubular atrophy; BKVN, BK virus nephropathy. [#] Estimated glomerular filtration rate (eGFR) data were unavailable for BKVN samples. Immunosuppression consisted of Tacrolimus and Mycophenolate Mofetil for all patients, with maintenance steroids for those on steroid-based immunosuppression. All patients received IL2R monoclonal antibody (Daclizumab) induction; steroid-based patients received this for 2 months and steroid-free patients received this for 6 months. Most patients were unsensitized and recipients for first allografts, with 4 repeat transplants. Of the 106 AR, 29 were ABMR. The clinical data variables that were significantly different between groups were assessed for any statistical association with their impact on metabolite signatures of different transplant phenotypes and were not found to be significant.

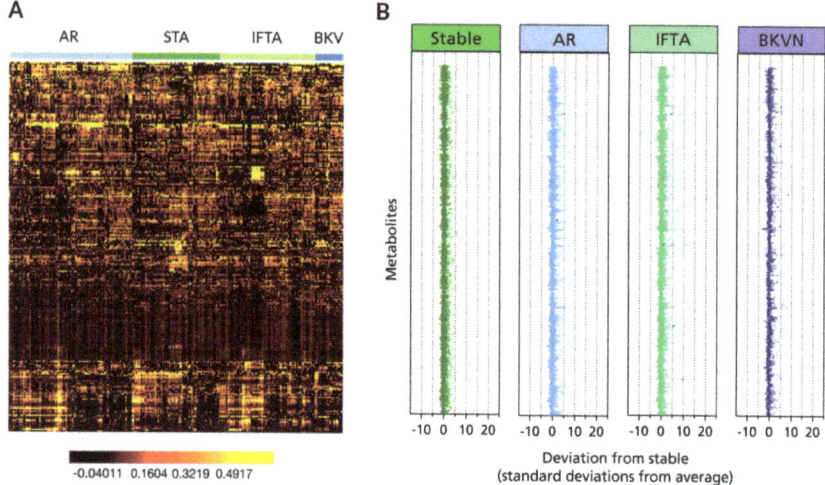

Figure 2. Metabolomic profiling of renal transplant outcomes. (**A**) Heat map representation of unsupervised hierarchical clustering by metabolite (rows) grouped by transplant phenotype (columns). Shades of black to red to orange to yellow represent continuous increases of a metabolite relative to the median metabolite levels (see color scale). (**B**) z-score plots for the data in a normalized to the mean of the stable phenotype urine samples (truncated at 25 s.d. for clarity).

3.2. Metabolite Marker Panel for Alloimmune Injury

Applying the VSURF method, a panel of 9 metabolites (Table 2) were selected out of 266 to accurately classify post-Tx alloimmune injury, combining the output from samples with either acute or chronic alloimmune injury (AR/IFTA) versus stable (STA) samples. The resulting model had a 95% accuracy of correctly discriminating between the two outcome groups (AUC = 0.950, sensitivity = 95.3%, specificity = 75.9%). This lower specificity is likely due to within group heterogeneity between AR and IFTA phenotypes. The 9 metabolite VSURF model was nearly identical in accuracy to the full 266-metabolite model, which had an AUC of 0.954. This difference in AUC values was not significant using DeLong's test ($p = 0.731$), meaning there is no significant change in classification accuracy between the full and abbreviated metabolite models (Figure 3A). This suggests that no diagnostic accuracy is lost in using the abbreviated metabolite model.

Table 2. Transplant phenotype-specific metabolite markers.

Injury-Specific (n = 9)	AR (n = 11)	BKVN (n = 5)
Glycine	Glycine	Arabinose
N-methylalanine	Glutaric acid	2-hydroxy-2-methylbutanoic acid
Adipic acid	Adipic acid	Hypoxanthine
Glutaric acid	Inulobiose	Benzyl alcohol
Inulobiose	Threose	N-acetyl-D-mannosamine
Threitol	Sulfuric acid	
Isothreitol	Taurine	
Sorbitol	N-methylalanine	
Isothreonic acid	Asparagine	
	5-aminovaleric acid lactam	
	Myo-inositol	

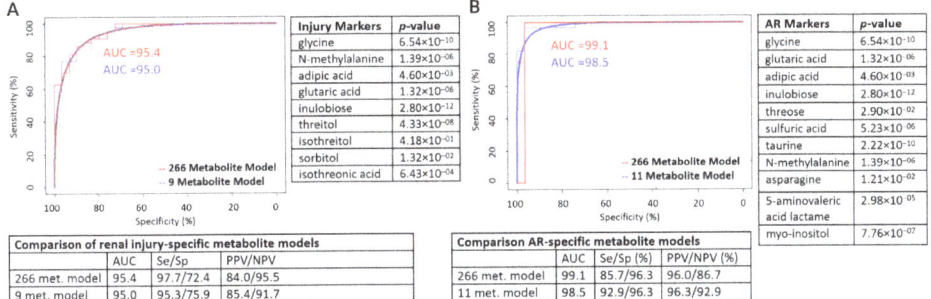

Figure 3. Identification of potential biomarker panel of metabolites for KTx alloimmune injury and acute rejection using VSURF method. (**A**) Two receiver operating characteristic (ROC) curves representing classification accuracies and a statistical comparison of the full and sparse RF models for alloimmune injury and the table displaying classification accuracy on the test set. The metabolites in the panel are listed on the right-hand side (**B**) Two ROC curves representing classification accuracies and a statistical comparison of the full and sparse Random Forests (RF) models for acute rejection (AR) injury and the bottom table displaying classification accuracy on the test set. The metabolites in the panel are listed on the right-hand side.

3.3. Metabolite Marker Panel for Acute Rejection

In order to identify a metabolite marker panel specific to acute rejection of KTx, we applied VSURF exclusively to the AR and STA urine metabolome datasets ($n = 217$). The resulting model contained 11 metabolites (Table 2) for AR detection. The ROC analysis resulted with an AUC of 0.985 with 92.9% sensitivity and 96.3% specificity (Figure 3B). Individual distributions for the three most significant metabolites, glycine, N-methylalanine, and inulobiose, are presented in the form of bean plots (Figure 4).

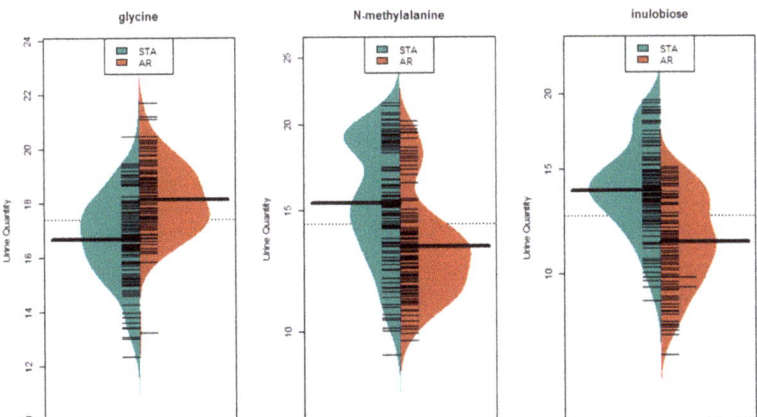

Figure 4. Significantly altered metabolites in AR versus STA. Bean plots demonstrating distribution of the 3 most significant metabolites in AR comparing to STA. The bold horizontal line represents mean value for each group.

3.4. Metabolite Marker Panel for BK Virus Nephritis

In order to identify BKVN-specific metabolites, we used VSURF on 22 BKVN urine and 288 non-BKVN urine that included AR, IFTA, and STA urine. The resulting VSURF panel contained 5 metabolites, Arabinose, 2-hydroxy-2-methylbutanoic acid, hypoxanthine, benzyl alcohol, and N-acetyl-D-mannosamine (Table 2) for BKVN classification with 72.7% sensitivity and 96.2% specificity (Table S1). When we confined our analysis to only BKVN vs. STA, VSURF resulted in a panel of 4 metabolites, arabinose, 2-hydroxy-2-methylbutanoic acid, octadecanol, and phosphate. For this panel, BKVN classification was 88.9% sensitive and 94.8% specific (Table S2). The 4-metabolite VSURF model had accuracy comparable to that of the full 266-metabolite model, which had a sensitivity of 87.5% and specificity of 93.2% (Table S3).

3.5. Metabolic Pathways Associated with Graft Injury

To explore metabolite significance by both statistical significance and magnitude of fold change in the injury group, a volcano plot with Random Forests (RF) importance score was generated (Figure 5A) that shows the relative importance of the metabolite in terms of RF score for AR-specific panel. Additionally, a volcano plot with fold changes (increased or decreased) and corresponding p-values displayed the significance of the various metabolites in AR (Figure S1). The plot reveals metabolites of increasing significance relative to the Random Forests classification model. Some metabolites from the 9-metabolite marker panel for alloimmune injury and the 11-metabolite marker panel for AR are among the very highly perturbed metabolites. The metabolites significantly perturbed in KTx injury with p-value < 0.001 (n = 42) were analyzed for metabolic pathway enrichment with MetaboAnalyst. Pathway analysis for enrichment identified nitrogen metabolism, ascorbate, and aldarate metabolism, and amino sugar and nucleotide sugar metabolism as the three most significantly enriched pathways (Figure 5B).

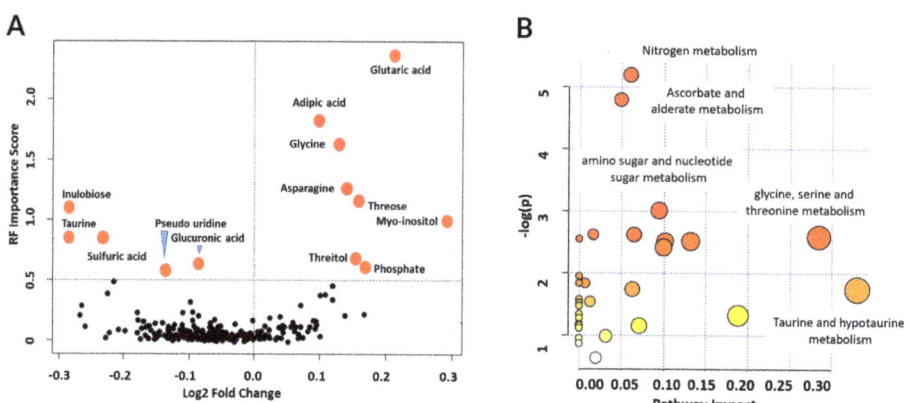

Figure 5. Metabolites and pathways significantly perturbed in KTx alloimmune injury. (**A**) Volcano plot displaying fold change and significance of metabolites. Red dots denote metabolites significant at a Random Forests importance score greater than 0.5. The right half displays metabolites in the injury group with a higher signature relative to the stable group. Some metabolites from the 9-metabolite marker panel for alloimmune injury and the 11-metabolite marker panel for AR are among the very highly perturbed metabolites labeled in red dots. (**B**) Enrichment analysis of metabolic pathways using significantly altered metabolites showed enrichment in nitrogen metabolism (p = 0.0055), ascorbate and aldarate metabolism (p = 0.0083), and amino sugar and nucleotide sugar metabolism (p = 0.05) as significantly enriched pathways. The y-axis represents the p-values as the negative of their natural logarithm.

4. Discussion

Sophisticated interrogation of urine through advanced technologies for kidney diseases is important as urine provides an attractive alternative biospecimen [35] and unlike invasive biopsies, urine metabolite changes can be diagnostic of advanced tissue injury. Additionally, our data suggest that these urine panels can have much greater sensitivity and specificity over measured serum creatinine [35–39]. Molecular perturbations in the kidney have been previously shown to occur much earlier than both histological changes and clinical alterations in kidney function, and previously published studies confirm that urine is an excellent mirror of these intra-graft molecular changes [11,35,40–49]. In this comprehensive study, we had access to a unique resource of over 300 biopsy matched urine samples archived from kidney transplant patients transplanted at multiple transplant centers, mapped with detailed clinical demographics, which enhanced the results obtained from the urine metabolomic studies conducted in this study.

Prior studies, using different assay platforms, have evaluated the urine metabolome for assessing kidney transplant injury [43,50–52]. Wang et al. [50] applied matrix-assisted laser desorption/ionization Fourier transform mass spectrometry (MALDI-FTMS) for studying acute tubular injury, Blydt-Hanson et al. [51] used liquid chromatography tandem mass spectrometry for studying transplant rejection, Dieme et al. [52] used GC-MS to study the metabolic effects of calcineurin inhibitor drugs in kidney transplant patients, Ho et al. [53] used LC-MS for analysis of alloimmune injury, and Suhre et al. [43] applied LC-MS and GC-MS. Most of these studies have larger metabolite diagnostic panels and only few studies have urine samples that are all biopsy-matched, resulting in little overlap across the identified panels to date. Using all biopsy-matched urine samples matched with pathologist blinded biopsy evaluations, GC-MS, and custom informatics analyses using nonlinear, nonparametric machine learning model development, we were able to greatly refine, as well as cross-validate the performance of small panels of urine metabolites for AR and BKVN. These clinical phenotypes are often difficult to distinguish even by biopsy, and pose a clinical challenge for patient management, specifically concerning the decision between immunosuppression augmentation (in AR) or minimization (in BKVN). In addition to selecting the most informative metabolites to provide discriminant diagnostic models for biopsy matched transplant injury categories, we have also tried to better understand the biological mechanisms that some of the metabolites suggest are dysregulated in transplant injury, using panels in this study and other published studies on the urine metabolome.

Many of the metabolites that we identified as correlated with transplant injury have previously been associated with changes in renal physiology. Taurine is a key metabolite that was included in our AR specific panel and was found to have significantly reduced levels in urine during rejection. Taurine plays a role in different physiologic and biologic processes in the kidney as reflected in urinary excretion patterns. Taurine participates in several physiological functions in the kidney [54–56], such as its role in the renal cell cycle and apoptosis. It also functions as an osmolyte during the stress response. Therefore, the changes in urinary taurine levels seen in this study may relate to the higher burden of tissue injury in AR, and its lower levels in the kidney may reflect a failure in protecting the kidney during immune-mediated damage [57]. The low level of taurine in urine during rejection may reflect a combination of decreased production in the kidney and perturbed osmolar reabsorption of taurine in the medulla [58].

Myo-inositol was found to be a significant biomarker in our model and had been previously shown by Dieme et al. [52] and Suhre et al. [43] to be relevant to and increased in transplant rejection. Urinary myo-inositol was the most important metabolite for discriminating between AR, STA, and IFTA phenotypes in our models. Myo-inositol is an osmolyte of the renal medulla that plays an important role in protecting renal cells from hyperosmotic stress [59]. It is enriched under hyperosmotic conditions via the sodium/myo-inositol cotransporter in the thick ascending limb of the loop of Henle [60]. The kidney is the most important organ for myo-inositol metabolism given that there is high expression of its associated enzymes, L-myo-inositol-1-phosphate synthetase, and myo-inositol oxygenase, in the renal parenchyma [61]. Inhibition of myo-inositol transport has been shown to cause acute renal failure in rats [62]. Furthermore, it has recently been shown through urine metabolomics profiling of humans that increased levels of myo-inositol are significantly associated with kidney disease and inversely proportional to eGFR [63]. It has also been shown to be elevated in the plasma metabolomic profiles of patients with end-stage renal disease [50,61]. These studies suggest an essential role of myo-inositol in renal physiology. Thus, its higher levels in AR may relate to the severity or progression of rejection. In looking at known perturbations in gene expression levels in AR [14] we observed that the sodium-myo-inositol transporter (SMIT), encoded by *SLC5A3*, is located in the thick ascending limb and functions to reabsorb myo-inositol into the renal medullary cells under conditions of hypertonicity [64]. Thus, perturbations of this transporter may be a key mechanism for acute rejection related tissue injury, mediated by hyperosmolar stress [63]. Given that patients with AR may have preserved kidney graft function and stable serum creatinine levels, the utility of this biomarker may be confounded given its correlation with eGFR. Further studies are needed to further validate role of myo-inositol in the progression of rejection.

These are first observations, should be consolidated with more integrative analysis of multi-omic datasets, and could be further aided by spatial metabolomics. Use of metabolomics for kidney disease outcomes generally could complement diagnostics made using other modalities, including gene expression, cell-free DNA, and proteomics [65–69].

This study benefits from the evaluation of the human urine metabolome in different geographic and demographic cohorts, as the samples came from enrolled patients at Stanford and UCSF. The diversity of patient samples supports the robustness and clinical utility of the described metabolite panels. Translation of these biomarker panels to clinical practice can be done by GC-MS/TOF based assays that are readily available in most commercial labs. Despite the fact that we have analyzed urine from a diverse population and using two different immunosuppressive drugs, additional independent validation studies that allow for prospective clinical testing and application of these metabolite panels will be required to validate the performance of these biomarker panels for diagnostic transplant monitoring. This is important because the diversity of the cohort also introduces many factors that are known to affect the metabolic profiles of patients, such as age, gender, BMI, diet, exercise, comorbidities, and even the time of day as a function of the circadian rhythm [70]. In our cohorts, age and gender were significantly different and as would be expected from a pediatric population, they had few comorbidities. A future study consisting of a larger cohort size that collected these additional details would help to delineate the effects of these parameters on the metabolic profiles. Furthermore, we note that storage length is known to affect the metabolites present and detected in urine studies. While our urine samples were stored at −80 °C, this may have influenced the distribution of the metabolites in the samples. Future work should be done to compare biobanked samples versus freshly collected samples to delineate any potential differences in the metabolomic profile.

There are a number of additional limitations to this study. We note that certain patient subsets, such as the BKVN arm had a relatively smaller number of patients ($n = 22$), and this warrants further investigation with a larger number of samples to validate the results. We also note that all samples AR samples used were collected at the time of the rejection, rather than before, and thus we could not assess the predictive value of metabolite alterations in transplant rejection. We believe this would be a useful area of future study, as predictive signatures of rejection prior to clinical AR (e.g., picking up subclinical AR) would be valuable to prevent further decline of kidney function [71].

Nevertheless, urinary metabolite profiles provide an exciting opportunity for rapid bedside–to-bench screening for risk assessment, improved immunosuppression titration, and rejection prevention to ultimately improve transplant and patient outcomes. With the increasing number of studies in this space [43,72], a comprehensive metabolomics picture of allograft outcomes can be created and further contribute to the care management of transplant patients.

Supplementary Materials: The following are available online at http://www.mdpi.com/2077-0383/9/8/2341/s1, Table S1: Metabolite selection by VSURF to discriminate BKVN from all other phenotypes, Table S2: Metabolite selection by VSURF to discriminate BKVN from STA, Table S3: Use of all 266 metabolites in VSURF to discriminate BKVN from STA, Figure S1: Volcano plot displaying fold change and significance of metabolites in the urine of acute rejection patients compared to the patients with stable grafts.

Author Contributions: Conceptualization, project administration, funding acquisition, supervision, and resources, T.K.S. and M.M.S.; visualization, T.K.S., A.W.S., and J.Y.C.Y.; methodology, software, validation, formal analysis, investigation, data curation, writing—original draft preparation, and writing—review and editing by all authors. All authors have read and agreed to the published version of the manuscript.

Funding: This research was funded by Sarwal Lab startup funds.

Acknowledgments: We are grateful for the help from physicians, clinical coordinators, research personnel, patients, and patient families. We are grateful to Maggie Kerwin for proofreading while revising the manuscript.

Conflicts of Interest: The authors declare no conflict of interest. The funders had no role in the design of the study; in the collection, analyses, or interpretation of data; in the writing of the manuscript, or in the decision to publish the results.

References

1. Abecassis, M.; Bartlett, S.T.; Collins, A.J.; Davis, C.L.; Delmonico, F.L.; Friedewald, J.J.; Hays, R.; Howard, A.; Jones, E.; Leichtam, A.B.; et al. Kidney transplantation as primary therapy for end-stage renal disease: A National Kidney Foundation/Kidney Disease Outcomes Quality Initiative (NKF/KDOQITM) conference. *Clin. J. Am. Soc. Nephrol. CJASN* **2008**, *3*, 471–480. [CrossRef] [PubMed]
2. Pomfret, E.A.; Sung, R.S.; Allan, J.; Kinkhabwala, M.; Melancon, J.K.; Roberts, J.P. Solving the organ shortage crisis: The 7th annual American Society of Transplant Surgeons' State-of-the-Art Winter Symposium. *Am. J. Transplant.* **2008**, *8*, 745–752. [CrossRef] [PubMed]
3. Meier-Kriesche, H.U.; Schold, J.D.; Srinivas, T.R.; Kaplan, B. Lack of improvement in renal allograft survival despite a marked decrease in acute rejection rates over the most recent era. *Am. J. Transplant.* **2004**, *4*, 378–383. [CrossRef] [PubMed]
4. Gaston, R.S. Improving Long-Term Outcomes in Kidney Transplantation: Towards a New Paradigm of Post-Transplant Care in the United States. *Trans. Am. Clin. Climatol. Assoc.* **2016**, *127*, 350–361. [PubMed]
5. Nasr, M.; Sigdel, T.; Sarwal, M. Advances in diagnostics for transplant rejection. *Expert Rev. Mol. Diagn.* **2016**, *16*, 1121–1132. [CrossRef]
6. Loupy, A.; Haas, M.; Solez, K.; Racusen, L.; Glotz, D.; Seron, D.; Nankivell, B.J.; Colvin, R.B.; Afrouzian, M.; Akalin, E.; et al. The Banff 2015 Kidney Meeting Report: Current Challenges in Rejection Classification and Prospects for Adopting Molecular Pathology. *Am. J. Transplant.* **2017**, *17*, 28–41. [CrossRef]
7. Filler, G.; Bendrick-Peart, J.; Christians, U. Pharmacokinetics of mycophenolate mofetil and sirolimus in children. *Ther. Drug Monit.* **2008**, *30*, 138–142. [CrossRef]
8. Yang, J.Y.; Sarwal, M.M. Transplant genetics and genomics. *Nat. Rev. Genet.* **2017**, *18*, 309–326. [CrossRef]
9. Reeve, J.; Bohmig, G.A.; Eskandary, F.; Einecke, G.; Lefaucheur, C.; Loupy, A.; Halloran, P.F. The MMDx-Kidney Study Group. Assessing rejection-related disease in kidney transplant biopsies based on archetypal analysis of molecular phenotypes. *JCI Insight* **2017**, *2*, 1–14. [CrossRef]
10. Roedder, S.; Sigdel, T.; Salomonis, N.; Hsieh, S.; Dai, H.; Bestard, O.; Metes, D.; Zeevi, A.; Gritsh, A.; Cheeseman, J.; et al. The kSORT assay to detect renal transplant patients at high risk for acute rejection: Results of the multicenter AART study. *PLoS Med.* **2014**, *11*, e1001759. [CrossRef]
11. Sigdel, T.K.; Salomonis, N.; Nicora, C.D.; Ryu, S.; He, J.; Dinh, V.; Orton, D.J.; Moore, R.J.; Hsieh, S.C.; Dai, H.; et al. The identification of novel potential injury mechanisms and candidate biomarkers in renal allograft rejection by quantitative proteomics. *Mol. Cell. Proteom. MCP* **2014**, *13*, 621–631. [CrossRef] [PubMed]
12. Khatri, P.; Roedder, S.; Kimura, N.; De Vusser, K.; Morgan, A.A.; Gong, Y.; Fischbein, M.P.; Robbins, R.C.; Naesens, M.; Bute, A.J.; et al. A common rejection module (CRM) for acute rejection across multiple organs identifies novel therapeutics for organ transplantation. *J. Exp. Med.* **2013**, *210*, 2205–2221. [CrossRef] [PubMed]
13. Yang, J.Y.; Sigdel, T.K.; Sarwal, M.M. Self-antigens and rejection: A proteomic analysis. *Curr. Opin. Organ Transplant.* **2016**, *21*, 362–367. [CrossRef] [PubMed]

14. Sarwal, M.; Chua, M.S.; Kambham, N.; Hsieh, S.C.; Satterwhite, T.; Masek, M.; Salvatierra, O., Jr. Molecular heterogeneity in acute renal allograft rejection identified by DNA microarray profiling. *N. Engl. J. Med.* **2003**, *349*, 125–138. [CrossRef] [PubMed]
15. Erpicum, P.; Hanssen, O.; Weekers, L.; Lovinfosse, P.; Meunier, P.; Tshibanda, L.; Ktzesinski, J.M.; Hustinx, R.; Jouret, F. Non-invasive approaches in the diagnosis of acute rejection in kidney transplant recipients, part II: Omics analyses of urine and blood samples. *Clin. Kidney J.* **2017**, *10*, 106–115. [CrossRef]
16. Wishart, D.S. Metabolomics: A complementary tool in renal transplantation. *Contrib. Nephrol.* **2008**, *160*, 76–87.
17. Klawitter, J.; Klawitter, J.; Kushner, E.; Jonscher, K.; Bendrick-Peart, J.; Leibfritz, D.; Christians, U.; Schmitz, V. Association of immunosuppressant-induced protein changes in the rat kidney with changes in urine metabolite patterns: A proteo-metabonomic study. *J. Proteome Res.* **2010**, *9*, 865–875. [CrossRef]
18. Bouatra, S.; Aziat, F.; Mandal, R.; Guo, A.C.; Wilson, M.R.; Knox, C.; Bjorndahl, T.C.; Krishamurthy, R.; Saleem, F.; Liu, P.; et al. The human urine metabolome. *PLoS ONE* **2013**, *8*, e73076. [CrossRef]
19. Bohra, R.; Klepacki, J.; Klawitter, J.; Klawitter, J.; Thurman, J.; Christians, U. Proteomics and metabolomics in renal transplantation-quo vadis? *Transpl. Int.* **2013**, *26*, 225–241. [CrossRef]
20. Gromski, P.S.; Muhamadali, H.; Ellis, D.I.; Xu, Y.; Correa, E.; Turner, M.L.; Goodacre, R. A tutorial review: Metabolomics and partial least squares-discriminant analysis-a marriage of convenience or a shotgun wedding. *Anal. Chim. Acta* **2015**, *879*, 10–23. [CrossRef]
21. Racusen, L.C.; Halloran, P.F.; Solez, K. Banff 2003 meeting report: New diagnostic insights and standards. *Am. J. Transplant.* **2004**, *4*, 1562–1566. [CrossRef] [PubMed]
22. Racusen, L.C.; Solez, K.; Colvin, R.B.; Bonsib, S.M.; Castro, M.C.; Cavallo, T.; Croker, B.P.; Demetris, A.J.; Drachenberg, C.B.; Fogo, A.B.; et al. The Banff 97 working classification of renal allograft pathology. *Kidney Int.* **1999**, *55*, 713–723. [CrossRef] [PubMed]
23. Solez, K.; Colvin, R.B.; Racusen, L.C.; Haas, M.; Sis, B.; Mengel, M.; Halloran, P.F.; Baldwin, W.; Banfi, G.; Collins, A.B.; et al. Banff 07 classification of renal allograft pathology: Updates and future directions. *Am. J. Transplant.* **2008**, *8*, 753–760. [CrossRef] [PubMed]
24. Nankivell, B.J.; Alexander, S.I. Rejection of the kidney allograft. *N. Engl. J. Med.* **2010**, *363*, 1451–1462. [CrossRef]
25. Fletcher, J.T.; Nankivell, B.J.; Alexander, S.I. Chronic allograft nephropathy. *Pediatric Nephrol.* **2009**, *24*, 1465–1471. [CrossRef]
26. Kind, T.; Wohlgemuth, G.; Lee, D.Y.; Lu, Y.; Palazoglu, M.; Shahbaz, S.; Fiehn, O. FiehnLib: Mass spectral and retention index libraries for metabolomics based on quadrupole and time-of-flight gas chromatography/mass spectrometry. *Anal. Chem.* **2009**, *81*, 10038–10048. [CrossRef] [PubMed]
27. Kind, T.; Tolstikov, V.; Fiehn, O.; Weiss, R.H. A comprehensive urinary metabolomic approach for identifying kidney cancerr. *Anal. Biochem.* **2007**, *363*, 185–195. [CrossRef] [PubMed]
28. Katajamaa, M.; Miettinen, J.; Oresic, M. MZmine: Toolbox for processing and visualization of mass spectrometry based molecular profile data. *Bioinformatics* **2006**, *22*, 634–636. [CrossRef]
29. Smith, C.A.; Want, E.J.; O'Maille, G.; Abagyan, R.; Siuzdak, G. XCMS: Processing mass spectrometry data for metabolite profiling using nonlinear peak alignment, matching, and identification. *Anal. Chem.* **2006**, *78*, 779–787. [CrossRef]
30. Stekhoven, D.J.; Buhlmann, P. MissForest-non-parametric missing value imputation for mixed-type data. *Bioinformatics* **2012**, *28*, 112–118. [CrossRef]
31. Breiman, L. Random forests. *Mach. Learn.* **2001**, *45*, 5–32. [CrossRef]
32. Genuer, R.; Poggi, J.M.; Tuleau-Malot, C. VSURF: An R Package for Variable Selection Using Random Forests. *R. J.* **2015**, *7*, 19–33. [CrossRef]
33. Delong, E.R.; Delong, D.M.; Clarkepearson, D.I. Comparing the Areas under 2 or More Correlated Receiver Operating Characteristic Curves-a Nonparametric Approach. *Biometrics* **1988**, *44*, 837–845. [CrossRef] [PubMed]
34. Chong, J.; Soufan, O.; Li, C.; Caraus, I.; Li, S.; Bourque, G.; Wishart, D.S.; Xia, J. MetaboAnalyst 4.0: Towards more transparent and integrative metabolomics analysis. *Nucleic Acids Res.* **2018**, *46*, W486–W494. [CrossRef]
35. Nissaisorakarn, V.; Lee, J.R.; Lubetzky, M.; Suthanthiran, M. Urine biomarkers informative of human kidney allograft rejection and tolerance. *Hum. Immunol.* **2018**, *79*, 343–355. [CrossRef] [PubMed]

36. Sigdel, T.K.; Kaushal, A.; Gritsenko, M.; Norbeck, A.D.; Qian, W.J.; Xiao, W.; Camp, D.G.; Smith, R.D.; Sarwal, M.M. Shotgun proteomics identifies proteins specific for acute renal transplant rejection. *Proteom. Clin. Appl.* **2010**, *4*, 32–47. [CrossRef]
37. Sigdel, T.K.; Lee, S.; Sarwal, M.M. Profiling the proteome in renal transplantation. *Proteom. Clin. Appl.* **2011**, *5*, 269–280. [CrossRef]
38. Sigdel, T.K.; Sarwal, M.M. The proteogenomic path towards biomarker discovery. *Pediatric Transplant.* **2008**, *12*, 737–747. [CrossRef]
39. Sigdel, T.K.; Sarwal, M.M. Recent advances in biomarker discovery in solid organ transplant by proteomics. *Expert Rev. Proteom.* **2011**, *8*, 705–715. [CrossRef]
40. Sigdel, T.K.; Gao, Y.; He, J.; Wang, A.; Nicora, C.D.; Fillmore, T.L.; Shi, T.; Webb-Robertson, B.J.; Smith, R.D.; Qian, W.J.; et al. Mining the human urine proteome for monitoring renal transplant injury. *Kidney Int.* **2016**, *89*, 1244–1252. [CrossRef] [PubMed]
41. Sigdel, T.K.; Ng, Y.W.; Lee, S.; Nicora, C.D.; Qian, W.J.; Smith, R.D.; Qian, W.J.; Salvatierra, O.; Camp, D.G.; Sarwal, M.M. Perturbations in the urinary exosome in transplant rejection. *Front. Med.* **2014**, *1*, 57. [CrossRef] [PubMed]
42. Sigdel, T.K.; Vitalone, M.J.; Tran, T.Q.; Dai, H.; Hsieh, S.C.; Salvatierra, O.; Sarwal, M.M. A rapid noninvasive assay for the detection of renal transplant injury. *Transplantation* **2013**, *96*, 97–101. [CrossRef] [PubMed]
43. Suhre, K.; Schwartz, J.E.; Sharma, V.K.; Chen, Q.; Lee, J.R.; Muthukumar, T.; Dadhania, D.M.; Ding, R.; Ikle, D.H.; Bridges, N.D.; et al. Urine Metabolite Profiles Predictive of Human Kidney Allograft Status. *J. Am. Soc. Nephrol. JASN* **2016**, *27*, 626–636. [CrossRef]
44. Fairchild, R.L.; Suthanthiran, M. Urine CXCL10/IP-10 Fingers Ongoing Antibody-Mediated Kidney Graft Rejection. *J. Am. Soc. Nephrol. JASN* **2015**, *26*, 2607–2609. [CrossRef]
45. Li, B.; Hartono, C.; Ding, R.; Sharma, V.K.; Ramaswamy, R.; Qian, B.; Serur, D.; Mouradian, J.; Schwartz, J.E.; Suthanthiran, M. Noninvasive diagnosis of renal-allograft rejection by measurement of messenger RNA for perforin and granzyme B in urine. *N. Engl. J. Med.* **2001**, *344*, 947–954. [CrossRef] [PubMed]
46. Li, R.; Guo, L.X.; Li, Y.; Chang, W.Q.; Liu, J.Q.; Liu, L.F.; Xin, G.Z. Dose-response characteristics of Clematis triterpenoid saponins and clematichinenoside AR in rheumatoid arthritis rats by liquid chromatography/mass spectrometry-based serum and urine metabolomics. *J. Pharm. Biomed. Anal.* **2017**, *136*, 81–91. [CrossRef] [PubMed]
47. Schaub, S.; Mayr, M.; Honger, G.; Bestland, J.; Steiger, J.; Regeniter, A.; Mihatsch, M.J.; Wilkins, J.A.; Rush, D.; Nickerson, P. Detection of subclinical tubular injury after renal transplantation: Comparison of urine protein analysis with allograft histopathology. *Transplantation* **2007**, *84*, 104–112. [CrossRef]
48. Schaub, S.; Rush, D.; Wilkins, J.; Gibson, I.W.; Weiler, T.; Sangster, K.; Nicolle, L.; Karpinski, M.; Jeffery, J.; Nickerson, P. Proteomic-based detection of urine proteins associated with acute renal allograft rejection. *J. Am. Soc. Nephrol. JASN* **2004**, *15*, 219–227. [CrossRef]
49. Torng, S.; Rigatto, C.; Rush, D.N.; Nickerson, P.; Jeffery, J.R. The urine protein to creatinine ratio (P/C) as a predictor of 24-hour urine protein excretion in renal transplant patients. *Transplantation* **2001**, *72*, 1453–1456. [CrossRef]
50. Choi, J.Y.; Yoon, Y.J.; Choi, H.J.; Park, S.H.; Kim, C.D.; Kim, I.S.; Kwon, T.H.; Do, J.Y.; Kim, S.H.; Ryu, D.H.; et al. Dialysis modality-dependent changes in serum metabolites: Accumulation of inosine and hypoxanthine in patients on haemodialysis. *Nephrol. Dial. Transpl.* **2011**, *26*, 1304–1313. [CrossRef]
51. Blydt-Hansen, T.D.; Sharma, A.; Gibson, I.W.; Mandal, R.; Wishart, D.S. Urinary metabolomics for noninvasive detection of borderline and acute T cell-mediated rejection in children after kidney transplantation. *Am. J. Transplant.* **2014**, *14*, 2339–2349. [CrossRef]
52. Dieme, B.; Halimi, J.M.; Emond, P.; Buchler, M.; Nadal-Desbarat, L.; Blasco, H.; Guellec, C.L. Assessing the metabolic effects of calcineurin inhibitors in renal transplant recipients by urine metabolic profiling. *Transplantation* **2014**, *98*, 195–201. [CrossRef] [PubMed]
53. Ho, J.; Sharma, A.; Mandal, R.; Wishart, D.S.; Wiebe, C.; Storsley, L.; Karpinski, M.; Gibson, I.M.; Nickerson, P.W.; Rush, D.N. Detecting Renal Allograft Inflammation Using Quantitative Urine Metabolomics and CXCL10. *Transplant. Direct* **2016**, *2*, e78. [CrossRef] [PubMed]
54. Hoffman, N.E.; Iser, J.H.; Smallwood, R.A. Hepatic bile acid transport: Effect of conjugation and position of hydroxyl groups. *Am. J. Physiol* **1975**, *229*, 298–302. [CrossRef]

55. Chesney, R.W.; Han, X.; Patters, A.B. Taurine and the renal system. *J. Biomed. Sci.* **2010**, *17* (Suppl. 1):S4, 1–10. [CrossRef] [PubMed]
56. Trachtman, H.; Sturman, J.A. Taurine: A therapeutic agent in experimental kidney disease. *Amino Acids* **1996**, *11*, 1–13. [CrossRef] [PubMed]
57. Trachtman, H.; Futterweit, S.; Prenner, J.; Hanon, S. Antioxidants reverse the antiproliferative effect of high glucose and advanced glycosylation end products in cultured rat mesangial cells. *Biochem. Biophys. Res. Commun.* **1994**, *199*, 346–352. [CrossRef]
58. Dantzler, W.H.; Silbernagl, S. Renal tubular reabsorption of taurine, gamma-aminobutyric acid (GABA) and beta-alanine studied by continuous microperfusion. *Pflug. Arch.* **1976**, *367*, 123–128. [CrossRef]
59. Brocker, C.; Thompson, D.C.; Vasiliou, V. The role of hyperosmotic stress in inflammation and disease. *Biomol. Concepts* **2012**, *3*, 345–364. [CrossRef]
60. Yorek, M.A.; Dunlap, J.A.; Lowe, W.L., Jr. Osmotic regulation of the Na+/myo-inositol cotransporter and postinduction normalization. *Kidney Int.* **1999**, *55*, 215–224. [CrossRef]
61. Niewczas, M.A.; Sirich, T.L.; Mathew, A.V.; Skupien, J.; Mohney, R.P.; Warram, J.H.; Smiles, A.; Huang, X.; Walker, W.; Byun, J.; et al. Uremic solutes and risk of end-stage renal disease in type 2 diabetes: Metabolomic study. *Kidney Int.* **2014**, *85*, 1214–1224. [CrossRef] [PubMed]
62. Kitamura, H.; Yamauchi, A.; Sugiura, T.; Matsuoka, Y.; Horio, M.; Tohyama, M.; Shimada, S.; Imai, E.; Hori, M. Inhibition of myo-inositol transport causes acute renal failure with selective medullary injury in the rat. *Kidney Int.* **1998**, *53*, 146–153. [CrossRef] [PubMed]
63. Gil, R.B.; Ortiz, A.; Sanchez-Nino, M.D.; Markoska, K.; Schepers, E.; Vanholder, R.; Glorieux, G.; Schmitt-Kopplin, P.; Heinzmann, S.S. Increased urinary osmolyte excretion indicates chronic kidney disease severity and progression rate. *Nephrol. Dial. Transplant.* **2018**, *33*, 2156–2164. [CrossRef] [PubMed]
64. Burg, M.B.; Ferraris, J.D. Intracellular organic osmolytes: Function and regulation. *J. Biol. Chem.* **2008**, *283*, 7309–7313. [CrossRef] [PubMed]
65. Yang, J.Y.C.; Sarwal, R.; Ky, K.; Dong, V.; Stoller, M.; Sarwal, M.; Chi, T. Non-Radiologic Assessment of Kidney Stones by KIT, a Spot Urine Assay. *Br. J. Urol. Int.* **2020**, *125*, 732–738. [CrossRef]
66. Yang, J.Y.C.; Sarwal, R.D.; Fervenza, F.C.; Sarwal, M.M.; Lafayette, R.A. Noninvasive Urinary Monitoring of Progression in IgA Nephropathy. *Int. J. Mol. Sci.* **2019**, *20*, 4463. [CrossRef]
67. Sigdel, T.K.; Yang, J.Y.C.; Bestard, O.; Schroeder, A.; Hsieh, S.-C.; Liberto, J.M.; Qamm, I.; Geraedts, A.C.M.; Sarwal, M.M. A urinary Common Rejection Module (uCRM) score for non-invasive kidney transplant monitoring. *PLoS ONE* **2019**, *7*, 1–15. [CrossRef]
68. Sigdel, T.; Yang, J.; Bestard, O.; Hsieh, S.; Roedder, S.; Damm, I.; Liberto, J.; Nandoe, S.; Sarwal, M. A Non-Invasive Urinary Common Rejection Module (uCRM) Gene Expression Score Quantifies and Differentiates Kidney Transplant Injury. *Am. J. Transplant.* **2017**. [CrossRef]
69. Yang, J.Y.C.; Sarwal, R.D.; Sigdel, T.K.; Damm, I.; Rosenbaum, B.; Liberto, J.M.; Chan-on, C.; Arreola-Guerra, J.M.; Alberu, J.M.; Vincenti, F.; et al. A urine score for noninvasive accurate diagnosis and prediction of kidney transplant rejection. *Sci. Transl. Med.* **2020**, *12*, 1–11. [CrossRef]
70. Bi, H.; Guo, Z.; Jia, X.; Liu, H.; Ma, L.; Xue, L. The key points in the pre-analytical procedures of blood and urine samples in metabolomics studies. *Metabolomics* **2020**, *16*, 1–15. [CrossRef]
71. Moreso, F.; Carrera, M.; Goma, M.; Hueso, M.; Sellares, J.; Martorell, J.; Grinyó, J.M.; Serón, D. Early subclinical rejection as a risk factor for late chronic humoral rejection. *Transplantation* **2012**, *93*, 41–46. [CrossRef] [PubMed]
72. Bassi, R.; Niewczas, M.A.; Biancone, L.; Bussolino, S.; Merugumala, S.; Tezza, S.; D'Addio, F.; Nasr, M.B.; Valderrama-Vasquez, A.; Usuelli, V. Metabolomic profiling in individuals with a failing kidney allograft. *PLoS ONE* **2017**, *12*, 1–14. [CrossRef] [PubMed]

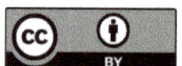

© 2020 by the authors. Licensee MDPI, Basel, Switzerland. This article is an open access article distributed under the terms and conditions of the Creative Commons Attribution (CC BY) license (http://creativecommons.org/licenses/by/4.0/).

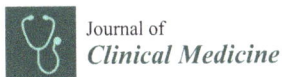

Concept Paper

Lifestyle, Inflammation, and Vascular Calcification in Kidney Transplant Recipients: Perspectives on Long-Term Outcomes

Camilo G. Sotomayor *, Charlotte A. te Velde-Keyzer, Martin H. de Borst, Gerjan J. Navis and Stephan J.L. Bakker

Department of Internal Medicine, University Medical Center Groningen, University of Groningen, 9700 RB Groningen, The Netherlands; c.a.keyzer@umcg.nl (C.A.t.V.-K.); m.h.de.borst@umcg.nl (M.H.d.B.); g.j.navis@umcg.nl (G.J.N.); s.j.l.bakker@umcg.nl (S.J.L.B.)
* Correspondence: c.g.sotomayor.campos@umcg.nl; Tel.: +31-50-361-0881

Received: 18 May 2020; Accepted: 26 May 2020; Published: 18 June 2020

Abstract: After decades of pioneering and improvement, kidney transplantation is now the renal replacement therapy of choice for most patients with end-stage kidney disease (ESKD). Where focus has traditionally been on surgical techniques and immunosuppressive treatment with prevention of rejection and infection in relation to short-term outcomes, nowadays, so many people are long-living with a transplanted kidney that lifestyle, including diet and exposure to toxic contaminants, also becomes of importance for the kidney transplantation field. Beyond hazards of immunological nature, a systematic assessment of potentially modifiable—yet rather overlooked—risk factors for late graft failure and excess cardiovascular risk may reveal novel targets for clinical intervention to optimize long-term health and downturn current rates of premature death of kidney transplant recipients (KTR). It should also be realized that while kidney transplantation aims to restore kidney function, it incompletely mitigates mechanisms of disease such as chronic low-grade inflammation with persistent redox imbalance and deregulated mineral and bone metabolism. While the vicious circle between inflammation and oxidative stress as common final pathway of a multitude of insults plays an established pathological role in native chronic kidney disease, its characterization post-kidney transplant remains less than satisfactory. Next to chronic inflammatory status, markedly accelerated vascular calcification persists after kidney transplantation and is likewise suggested a major independent mechanism, whose mitigation may counterbalance the excess risk of cardiovascular disease post-kidney transplant. Hereby, we first discuss modifiable dietary elements and toxic environmental contaminants that may explain increased risk of cardiovascular mortality and late graft failure in KTR. Next, we specify laboratory and clinical readouts, with a postulated role within persisting mechanisms of disease post-kidney transplantation (i.e., inflammation and redox imbalance and vascular calcification), as potential non-traditional risk factors for adverse long-term outcomes in KTR. Reflection on these current research opportunities is warranted among the research and clinical kidney transplantation community.

Keywords: nephrology; kidney transplant; kidney transplant recipients; long-term outcomes; graft failure; cardiovascular mortality; lifestyle; inflammation; vascular calcification; bone mineral density; dual-energy X-ray absorptiometry

1. Introduction

Chronic kidney disease (CKD) is a major public health problem, with a current worldwide prevalence of approximately 843 million individuals [1]. Global mean prevalence was recently reported at 13.4% for all CKD stages together (1–5) and at 10.6% if only the more severe CKD stages (3–5)

are considered [2]. Whereas the prevalence of all stages of CKD rises with age, older patients with similar levels of eGFR are less likely than their younger counterparts to progress to the need of renal replacement therapy, which has raised the question of whether all older patients who meet criteria for CKD actually have CKD [3].

The prevalence of CKD, its detection, treatment, and impact on health have been mainly studied in economically developed countries [1]. Nevertheless, even in these circumstances, it usually remains a silent, smoldering health threat, with, e.g., rates of awareness of being afflicted with kidney disease of approximately 10% among patients with CKD in an economically developed country like the United States [4]. Along the same line, in 2016, approximately 35% of patients diagnosed with incident end-stage kidney disease (ESKD) received little or no nephrology care prior to actually being diagnosed with ESKD [4]. Regrettably, prevalence of ESKD and prevalence of renal replacement therapy continue to increase (Figures 1 and 2) [4].

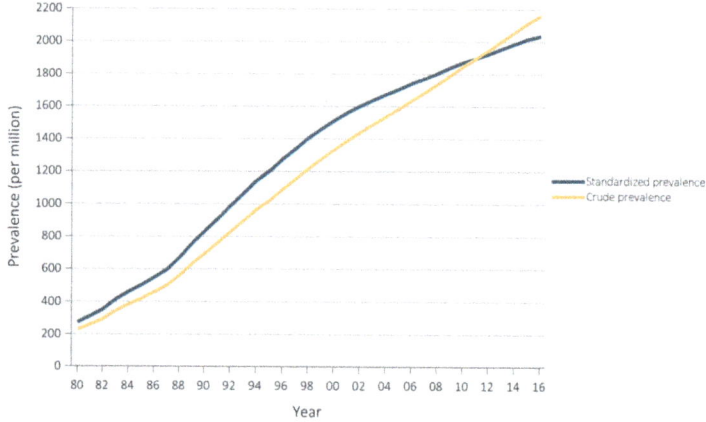

Figure 1. Prevalence of end-stage kidney disease (ESKD) in the United States (US) population, 1980–2016. This figure shows a steady increase in ESKD prevalence over recent ~35 years in the US. Standardized for age, sex, and race. Data Source: USRDS 2018 Annual Data Report [4].

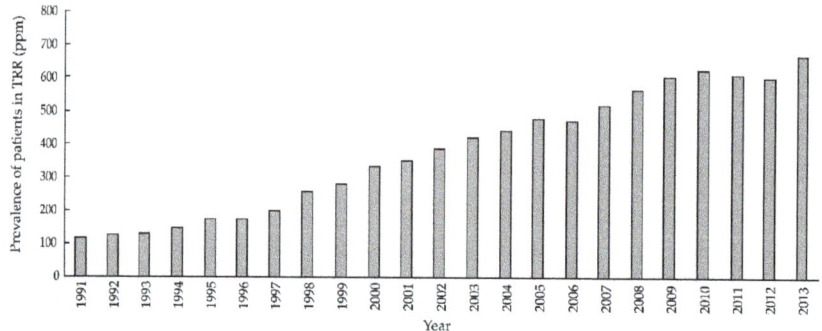

Figure 2. Prevalence of renal replacement therapy in Latin America, 1991–2013. This figure shows a steady increase in prevalence of renal replacement therapy over recent ~25 years in Latin America. Reprinted from "Latin American Dialysis and Transplant Registry: Experience and contributions to end-stage kidney disease epidemiology" [5].

Compared to chronic dialysis treatment, kidney transplantation is considered the renal replacement therapy of choice and the gold-standard treatment for most ESKD patients because it offers superior cost-effectiveness, quality of life, and life expectancy [6–10]. However, the latter has largely been due to significant improvements of short-term outcomes [11]. Advances in immunosuppression, tissue typing, treatment of infections, and surgical techniques led rates of 1-year graft survival at a pinnacle, whereas improvement of long-term outcomes post-transplant remains a major challenge in the kidney transplantation field [11].

On the one hand, the life-saving benefit of a kidney transplant remains largely hampered by cumulative injury of a multitude of hazards through immune and non-immune mechanisms of kidney damage. Over time, these mechanisms lead to chronic interstitial fibrosis and tubular atrophy as histopathological consequence and end-stage kidney allograft failure as functional repercussion, eventually requiring restart of dialysis or re-transplantation as final adverse clinical event (i.e., graft failure) [11–15].

On the other hand, kidney transplant recipients (KTR) are at particularly high risk of premature death, depicting overall mortality rates considerably higher than that of age-matched controls in the general population [16,17].

Indeed, approximately half of all kidney allograft losses are due to premature death with a functioning graft, a long-standing pattern that has remained largely unchanged over recent years [17,18].

Next, under the general understanding that cardiovascular disease is the leading cause of premature death post-kidney transplant (Figure 3) and thereby importantly challenging the improvement of longevity of KTR, great efforts have focused on the improvement of long-term cardiovascular outcomes [19–21].

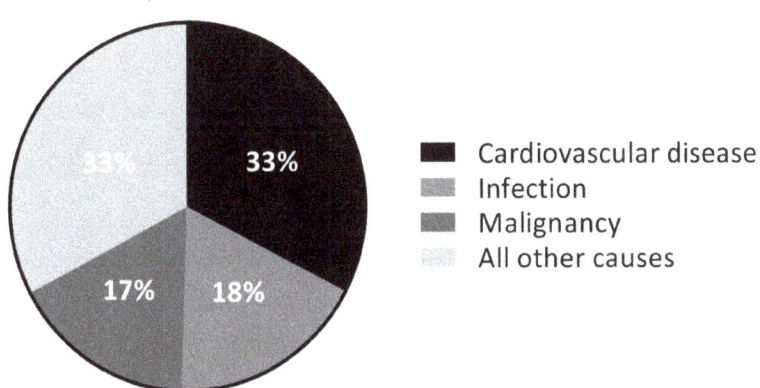

Figure 3. Mortality by causes of death with graft function in US KTR in 2015. This figure shows that cardiovascular disease was the leading cause of mortality among US KTR in 2015. Cardiovascular disease included acute myocardial infarction, atherosclerotic heart disease, congestive heart failure, cerebrovascular accident, and arrhythmia/cardiac arrest. Adapted from USRDS 2018 Annual Data Report [4].

In the clinical setting of KTR after the first-year post-transplant, beyond hazards of immunological nature, there is a pressing need to systematically study and characterize the clinical impact of potentially modifiable risk factors, such as lifestyle, diet, and exposure to toxic contaminants, which are underexplored areas in the kidney transplantation field [22–26]. This evidence is needed to guide decision making by clinicians and policy-makers in post-transplantation care. Furthermore, because kidney transplantation aims to restore kidney function but it incompletely mitigates collateral mechanisms of disease, such as chronic low-grade inflammation with persistent redox imbalance and deregulated mineral and bone metabolism, further research investigating specific clinical and laboratory readouts with a proposed involvement in such pathological pathways may point towards non-traditional risk factors and reveal novel targets for clinical intervention [27–32].

In the kidney transplantation field, future advances are expected from amelioration of adverse long-term outcomes by increasing recognition and developing novel, early, and cost-effective risk-management strategies focused on the non-immune aspects of post-kidney transplantation care and thus optimize long-term health and downturn current rates of premature death in stable KTR [11].

2. Lifestyle: Healthy Diet and Toxic Contaminants

One area with great potential for improvement is lifestyle, in particular diet and exposure to toxic contaminants. Systematic investigation of traditional and potentially modifiable risks factors in the post-kidney transplant setting may point towards otherwise overlooked early risk-management opportunities and thus provide the basis for the development of cost-effective interventional approaches to increase the lifespan of KTR. Healthy diet is a cornerstone element of cardio-metabolic health in the general population [33–38]. In general, a healthy diet is recommended as essential for cardiovascular disease prevention in all individuals. Surprisingly, however, little is known about the potential impact of a healthy diet on cardiovascular health and survival benefit in kidney patients across the continuum of CKD stages, in patients undergoing kidney replacement therapy, and remarkably limited evidence is available in the post-kidney transplantation clinical setting [39–42]. Moreover, native CKD and pre-transplant ESKD patients are generally advised to follow seemingly conflicting and challenging dietary recommendations with the aim of restricting individual nutrients such as potassium, salt, phosphorus, and protein [43]. It should be realized that there is scant evidence to support such restrictive dietary recommendations [44–46]. Finally, there is a notorious lack of studies aimed to aid on the development of evidence-based recommendations to appropriately adjust any pre-transplant dietary advice to the patient after kidney transplantation has been performed [26,43,44,47,48]. Below, we provide several examples of where opportunities may lie (Box 1).

Box 1. Characteristics of a healthy diet [49].

- ≥200 g of fruit per day (2–3 servings).
- ≥200 g of vegetables per day (2–3 servings).
- Fish 1–2 times per week, one of which to be oily fish.
- Saturated fatty acids to account for <10% of total energy intake through replacement by polyunsaturated fatty acids.
- Trans unsaturated fatty acids: as little as possible, preferably no intake from processed food and <1% of total energy intake from natural origin.
- 30 g unsalted nuts per day.
- <5 g of salt per day.
- Consumption of alcoholic beverages should be limited to 2 glasses per day (20 g/d of alcohol) for men and 1 glass per day (10 g/d of alcohol) for women.
- Sugar-sweetened soft drinks and alcoholic beverages consumption must be discouraged.

2.1. Fruit and Vegetable Consumption Post-Kidney Transplantation

With the aim of limiting potassium intake, for example, pre-transplant ESKD patients have largely been discouraged from a high consumption of fruits and vegetables, which are, however, well-known essential components of a healthy diet [50–54]. Beyond being rich in potassium, fruits and vegetables are rich in fibers, polyunsaturated and monounsaturated fatty acids, magnesium, iron, and generate less acid and contain smaller amounts of saturated fatty acids, protein, and absorbable phosphorus in comparison to meat [39,55]. At least four servings of fruit and vegetables per day are widely recommended for the prevention of major chronic diseases in the general population [49]. Indeed, increased consumption of fruits and vegetables has consistently shown to confer superior cardiovascular prognosis in the general population [52–54,56].

Recent studies show that KTR consume less fruits and vegetables than the general population, which has been associated with higher risk of cardiovascular mortality and posttransplant diabetes [57,58]. At present, however, post-kidney transplant, there is no clear incentive by transplant healthcare providers to prescribe restoration of the consumption of these basic items of a healthy diet. This attitude may respond to the fact that it remains relatively unexplored whether an increase of fruits and vegetables consumption post-kidney transplantation positively impacts outcomes of KTR, which would be hypothetically expected mainly by decreasing the excess cardiovascular burden and premature cardiovascular death. Epidemiological studies aimed to estimate a theoretical benefit of a relative increase of these specific food items are warranted as first step to, thereafter, investigate potential interventional strategies promoting novel, cost-effective, and patient-centered approaches to the nutritional management of KTR, adequately informing clinical practice and policy.

2.2. Fish Intake Post-Kidney Transplantation and Mercury Exposure

Similarly, fish are rich in the omega-3 polyunsaturated fatty acids (n-3 PUFA) EPA (eicosapentaenoic acid) and DHA (docosahexaenoic acid), which are suggested to yield several beneficial effects for cardiovascular health [59–62]. Circulating levels of EPA and DHA have been associated with reduced cardiovascular risk in both healthy populations and in patients with pre-existing cardiovascular disease [59–62]. Proposed beneficial health effects of marine-derived n-3 PUFA are wide-ranging, favorably impacting inflammation, fibrosis, lipid modulation, plaque stabilization, blood pressure, artery calcification processes, and endothelial function [63–66]. These properties render EPA and DHA as of encompassing therapeutic potential in the management of cardiovascular risk of KTR. Indeed, in this particular setting, recent observational studies showed that plasma levels of marine-derived n-3 PUFA are inversely associated with cardiovascular mortality risk [67,68].

It should be realized, however, that the results of randomized control trials using supplementation of these individual nutrients are not yet sufficiently powered to draw definitive conclusions and recommendations for KTR [69,70]. Moreover, no study has been devoted to evaluating the potential beneficial effect of a relatively high dietary fish intake, as mostly shown in the general population [71–75]. Indeed, fish is the main dietary source of n-3 PUFA, and its inclusion in diet seems reasonable because it is a good source of protein without potentially adverse effects of accompanying intake of high saturated fat as present in fatty meat products. Not exempt of drawbacks, however, fish is also the major source of human exposure to organic mercury (with the exception of industrial accidents or particular occupational exposures) [76–78]. Therefore, alongside the study of the potential health benefits of marine-derived n-3 PUFA, weighted investigation of a relatively higher fish intake has been performed as necessary step towards developing cautious evidence-based dietary guidelines for clinical uptake [79], suggesting that beneficial effects of a higher dietary intake of n-3 PUFA by increasing fish consumption post-kidney transplantation may not be mitigated by postulated increased cardiovascular risk due to concomitant exposure to mercury [79].

2.3. Cadmium Exposure and Nephrotoxicity in the Post-Kidney Transplant Setting

Cadmium is another heavy metal of environmental and lifestyle-related concern, with tobacco and diet as primary sources of exposure. Previous studies have demonstrated that cadmium may induce hypertension, which in turn is associated with accelerated kidney function decline and particularly demonstrated in KTR, by shortened allograft survival [80–84]. Most importantly, a strong body of evidence shows that the kidney is the most sensitive target organ of cadmium-induced body burden, through postulated direct mechanisms of cadmium-induced injury in this organ, wherein it accumulates with a half-life of up to 45 years [85–89]. It is important to note that, particularly in settings of long-term oxidative stress such as that of KTR, cadmium-induced nephrotoxicity may be associated with impaired kidney function at concentrations that are otherwise considered non-toxic [90–92]. Taking also into account that the most effective way to reduce cardiovascular disease in KTR may indeed be preservation of graft function, the aforementioned constellation of factors turn the investigation of cadmium-associated risk of encompassing relevance within the study of long-term outcomes of kidney allograft function [21,84]. Furthermore, bodily cadmium is susceptible to therapeutic interventions [93].

Thus, cadmium-targeted interventional strategies may offer novel opportunities to decrease the long-standing high burden of late kidney graft failure; however, whether the nephrotoxic exposure to cadmium represents an overlooked hazard for preserved graft functioning remains unknown.

3. Inflammation and Oxidative Stress and Vascular Calcification

Another area of great opportunities for further improvement may lie in a better evaluation of disease mechanisms long-term after transplantation. Traditional risk factors such as diabetes mellitus, smoking, and hypertension, among others, do not suffice to account for the excess burden of premature cardiovascular death of, otherwise, stable KTR [94–97]. Indeed, cardiovascular disease has an atypical nature in KTR when compared with the general population [20,21]. Unexplained cardiovascular risk subsidizes current efforts to provide cutting-edge evidence on the potential independent hazard of novel (non-traditional) cardiovascular risk factors post-kidney transplantation [98–102].

It should be taken into account that while kidney transplantation aims to restore kidney function, it incompletely abrogates mechanisms of disease. Moreover, an aggregate of factors specific to the transplant milieu such as a chronic low-grade immunologic response to the kidney allograft, long-term toxicity of maintenance immunosuppressive, as well as various degrees of progressive uremia, contribute to perpetuate chronic inflammation, redox imbalance, and deregulated mineral and bone metabolism, which have to be proposed as major independent and evolving pathophysiological mechanisms, whose mitigation may counterbalance—at least to a considerable extent—the excess risk of cardiovascular disease and graft failure post-kidney transplantation [30,32,101,103,104]. Below, we provide several examples of where opportunities may lie.

3.1. Inflammation and Oxidative Stress Post-Kidney Transplantation

Indeed, while the vicious circle between inflammation and oxidative stress as final common pathway of a multitude of insults plays an established pathological role in native chronic kidney disease (CKD), its characterization post-kidney transplant has been less than satisfactory [105–109]. This is relevant because, at a physiological level, the cornerstone role of the complex interplay between inflammation and oxidative stress (Box 2) provides a theoretical and conceptual framework upon which upcoming research may deepen the understanding of the pathophysiological status of KTR once they reach a seemingly stable clinical stage [105].

Box 2. Oxidative stress.

> Oxidative stress is defined as an imbalance between the generation and removal of oxidant species. The most representative biological oxidant agents are reactive oxygen species (ROS) and reactive nitrogen species (RNS). The former group includes hydrogen peroxide, superoxide anion, and hydroxyl radical, whereas within the latter group relevant species are peroxynitrite anion, nitric oxide, and nitrogen dioxide radicals. Oxidative stress occurs when ROS and/or RNS production overwhelms the endogenous antioxidant defense system, either by excess production and/or inadequate removal. The antioxidant defense system is constituted by enzymatic antioxidant agents, including catalase, glutathione peroxidase, and superoxide dismutase. Non-enzymatic antioxidant components include a diversity of biological molecules, such as ascorbic acid (vitamin C), α-tocopherol (vitamin E), reduced glutathione, carotenoids, flavonoids, polyphenols, and several other exogenous antioxidants [110].

3.1.1. Vitamin C as Anti-Inflammatory and Antioxidant Agent and Its Depletion Post-Kidney Transplant

Inflammation, specifically the established inflammatory biomarker high-sensitivity C-reactive protein (hs-CRP)—which is also an indirect marker of increased oxidant production—has been previously shown to be independently associated with increased mortality risk in KTR [98,100]. Supported by data consistently showing an inverse correlation with hs-CRP in different settings, vitamin C is well-known by its anti-inflammatory effects [111–114]. Moreover, vitamin C is a physiological antioxidant agent, with radical-scavenger and reducing activities, of paramount importance for protection against diseases and degenerative processes caused by oxidant stress [115]. This particular composite of biochemical properties renders vitamin C as compelling research candidate to broaden the understanding of the interaction of inflammation and oxidative stress in the mechanisms leading to excess risk of premature death post-kidney transplantation. It should be realized, moreover, that pre-transplant ESKD patients often have an imbalance of several critical trace elements and vitamins [39]. Vitamin C, particularly, has been shown to be removed by conventional hemodialysis membranes, leading to drastic vitamin C depletion and oxidative stress [116–118]. Through an inverse mediating effect on inflammatory signaling biomarkers, sub-physiological levels of vitamin C (depletion) may be hypothesized to be implicated in mechanisms that associate with increased risk of adverse long-term outcomes [119–123]. To date, however, relatively little is known regarding the prevalence of abnormal vitamin C status post-kidney transplantation, yet recent studies have shown that low plasma vitamin C contributes to excess risk for premature death post-kidney transplantation [124,125].

3.1.2. Advanced Glycation End products as Amplifiers of Oxidative Stress and Inflammatory Responses

Inflammation is referred to as a redox-sensitive mechanism on the basis that reactive oxygen species may activate transcription factors such as nuclear factor kappa B (NF-kB), which regulates inflammatory mediator genes expression [126]. In this regard, advanced glycation end products (AGE) are particularly interesting oxidative stress biomarkers because it has been demonstrated that, upon binding to AGE-specific receptors, AGE activate intracellular pathways that amplify inflammatory and oxidative stress responses and regulate the transcription of adhesion molecules through NF-kB activation [127]. In agreement, data derived from clinical studies in pre-transplant ESKD patients support the implication of AGE in the complex feedback loop between oxidative stress and inflammation leading to endothelial dysfunction and adverse cardiovascular effects [128–130].

Several studies have observed accumulation of AGE in native and transplant CKD patients, and a strong body of evidence on the general theory of AGE pathophysiology supports its pivotal role in the initiation and progression of mechanisms underlying cardiovascular disease. However, few attempts have been made to investigate the association of AGE with cardiovascular risk post-kidney transplantation [99,131]. Through a mediating effect on up-regulation of inflammatory, oxidative stress and endothelial dysfunction biomarkers, a relative increase of AGE may be hypothesized to actively contribute to the intracellular signaling pathways that ultimately yield excess risk of premature cardiovascular death in KTR. It remains unknown whether a hypothetical association with risk of cardiovascular mortality is independent of estimates of kidney function and traditional cardiovascular risk factors such as body mass index, diabetes, blood pressure, and smoking status.

3.1.3. Inflammation, Galectin-3, and Fibrosis

Inflammation is also referred to as a unifying mechanism of injury because—through a cornerstone signaling link with interstitial fibrosis and tubular atrophy—it may hold observations that connect hazards of several natures with structural damage and detrimental function of the kidney [12–15,132,133]. Of note, the concept that chronic rejection is responsible for all progressive long-term kidney graft failure has long ago been reformulated to a hypothesis of cumulative damage [12–15]. Thus, repeated insults of both immune and non-immune nature damage the graft by leading to interstitial fibrosis and tubular atrophy, which represents a final common pathway of injury with adverse functional consequences [13]. Galectin-3 is a β-galactoside-binding lectin with a postulated key mediating role on kidney tissue fibrosis [134–138]. In different models, it has been shown that whether a variety of insults incur on irreversible kidney fibrosis or not depends on the expression and secretion of galectin-3 [135–138]. In the general population, moreover, an increasing body of prospective evidence has related plasma galectin-3 with incident CKD [139–141]. Because galectin-3 is both a biomarker of systemic inflammation and kidney fibrosis, it may broaden our understanding and provide data to further support a unifying link between repeated inflammatory and pro-oxidant insults and increased risk of graft failure beyond the first-year post-kidney transplantation. Finally, it should be realized that the dependent role of galectin-3 on kidney fibrosis has been specifically shown in the particular post-kidney transplant setting in a murine model [138]. Within the clinical kidney transplantation field, however, a number of crucial questions remain unanswered. Especially with galectin-3, targeted pharmacological therapies are increasingly becoming available, and evidence of a hypothetical association between galectin-3 levels and risk of long-term graft survival may point towards novel interventional avenues to potentially decrease the long-standing burden of late graft failure.

3.2. Bone Disease and Vascular Calcification

Chronic kidney disease-mineral and bone disorders (CKD-MBD) is the clinical entity or syndrome that KDIGO (Kidney Disease: Improving Global Outcomes) more than a decade ago has coined to embody the disruption of the complex systems biology enclosed by the kidney, skeleton, and cardiovascular system [142]. In line with previous evidence, the results of a recent elegant study by Yilmaz et al. support the hypothesis that decline in cardiovascular risk post-kidney transplantation depends on partial resolution of inflammation but also on resolution of the CKD-MBD [143,144]. The findings of the aforementioned research group support the notion that beyond restoration of organ function post-kidney transplant, amelioration of inflammation and correction of CKD-MBD may attenuate excess cardiovascular disease through separate biological pathways. In agreement, Cozzolino et al. recently depicted inflammation and oxidative stress, on one hand, and CKD-MBD, on the other hand, as major mechanisms underlying a feedback loop that exacerbates cardiovascular disease in CKD patients (Figure 4) [145].

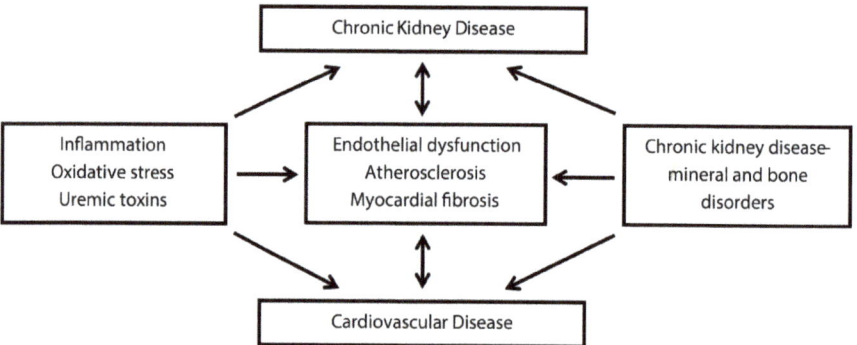

Figure 4. Cardiovascular disease in chronic kidney disease. This figure shows inflammation, oxidative stress, and uremic toxins on one side and chronic kidney disease-mineral and bone disorders on the other side of independent mechanisms linking chronic kidney and cardiovascular disease. Adapted from: "Cardiovascular disease in dialysis patients" by M. Cozzolino et al., 2019, Nephrol Dial Transplant, 33: iii28–34 [145].

Within the context of CKD-MBD, vascular calcification—a currently established cardiovascular risk factor in KTR, as shown by previous studies of our group and others [146–151]—is linked with bone disease through inter-related pathophysiological mechanisms that comprise the bone-vascular axis hypothesis, which contributes to the exceedingly high cardiovascular risk in native CKD [152–156]. Post-kidney transplant bone disease is certainly a topic of epidemiological relevance due to its high prevalence and its association with fragility fractures and reduced mobility [157–162]. Previous studies remarked that existing research had failed to explore a hypothetical contributing role of post-kidney transplant bone disease to increased risk of vascular calcification in KTR [154,158,163]. Recent evidence, however, has come to support the existence of a bone-vascular axis post-kidney transplantation, providing data to evaluate its epidemiological relevance post-kidney transplant and pointing towards an otherwise overlooked therapeutic opportunity to at least partially decrease the markedly high cardiovascular burden post-kidney transplant [164].

It has also been proposed that mediators of inflammation (e.g., interleukin 6 and tumor necrosis factor) contribute to fibroblast growth factor (FGF)-23 elevation and that, in turn, FGF-23 increases cytokine production, thus linking systemic inflammation with dysregulated phosphate metabolism in a vicious cycle [165,166]. It has been proposed that inflammatory mediators function as drug targets to decrease the burden of FGF23-associated injury in various tissues, thus offering a novel therapeutic opportunity to decrease the burden of cardiovascular diseases including vascular calcification in kidney disease patients [165,167]. Nevertheless, even in CKD patients within normal range of serum phosphate levels, vascular calcification is often observed. Calciprotein particles are calcium-phosphate nanoparticles that increase with CKD progression, which have been associated with inflammatory responses, endothelial damage, vascular stiffness, and calcification [168]. Calciprotein particles may play a pathophysiological role in the link between chronic inflammation and vascular calcification. Further research is warranted to evaluate its contribution to overall cardiovascular burden in KTR and to develop novel pharmacological strategies targeting calciprotein particles to encourage protection against the risk of vascular calcification post-kidney transplantation [169].

3.3. Immunosuppressive Therapy and Traditional Risk Factors of Vascular Calcification

The contribution of several traditional risk factors of vascular calcification may be particularly relevant in the post-kidney transplantation setting due to the effect of maintenance immunosuppressive therapy on diabetes, dyslipidemia, and vitamin D metabolism [170]. Previous studies have shown that low vitamin D along with low vitamin K may synergistically associate with higher risk of hypertension [171] and thereby contribute to higher risk of vascular calcification [172]. In KTR, particularly, we have recently shown that combined vitamin D and K deficiency is highly prevalent and is associated with increased mortality and graft failure [173]. Further research is needed to investigate both the direct and indirect role of immunosuppressive drugs in the progression of vascular calcification. There may, however, be opposing effects, because it has been described that steroids and calcineurin inhibitors inhibit inducible nitric oxide and may thereby lead to progression of vascular calcification through endothelial dysfunction [170], while mycophenolate mofetil inhibits vascular smooth muscle cell proliferation and may be protective against vascular calcification [174,175]. Similarly, we recently reported that use of cyclosporine rather than tacrolimus correlated with prevalence of osteopenia, while osteopenia was associated with higher risk of vascular calcification after kidney transplantation [164]. Future studies are warranted to assess the association between immunosuppressive agents and risk of vascular calcification, which may provide new cardiovascular risk management opportunities post-kidney transplantation.

4. Conclusions

Further research on lifestyle-related factors including diet and exposure to toxic contaminants, as well as persisting mechanisms of disease post-kidney transplantation (i.e., inflammation and redox imbalance and vascular calcification) is needed as it may bring about powerful opportunities to improve long-term outcomes post-kidney transplantation. Reflection on these current research opportunities is warranted among the research and clinical kidney transplantation community. Forthcoming analyses of the data to be generated by the long-lasting Transplant Lines Prospective Cohort Study and Biobank of Solid Organ Transplant Recipients [176] may shed light on these questions.

Author Contributions: Conceptualization, C.G.S. and S.J.L.B.; methodology, C.G.S., M.H.d.B., G.J.N., and S.J.L.B.; investigation, C.G.S. and S.J.L.B.; resources, C.G.S., M.H.d.B., and S.J.L.B.; writing—original draft preparation, C.G.S.; writing—review and editing, C.G.S., M.H.d.B., C.A.t.V.-K., G.J.N., and S.J.L.B.; supervision, M.H.d.B., G.J.N., and S.J.L.B.; project administration, C.G.S. and S.J.L.B.; funding acquisition, C.G.S. and S.J.L.B. All authors have read and agreed to the published version of the manuscript.

Funding: Camilo G. Sotomayor is supported by a personal grant from CONICYT (F 72190118).

Conflicts of Interest: The authors declare no conflict of interest. The funders had no role in the design of the study; in the collection, analyses, or interpretation of data; in the writing of the manuscript, or in the decision to publish the results.

Disclaimer: The data reported in Figure 1 have been supplied by the United States Renal Data System. The interpretation and reporting of these data are the responsibility of the author(s) of this manuscript and in no way should be seen as an official policy or interpretation of the U.S. government.

References

1. Jager, K.J.; Kovesdy, C.; Langham, R.; Rosenberg, M.; Jha, V.; Zoccali, C. A single number for advocacy and communication-worldwide more than 850 million individuals have kidney diseases. *Nephrol. Dial. Transpl.* **2019**, *34*, 1803–1805. [CrossRef] [PubMed]
2. Hill, N.R.; Fatoba, S.T.; Oke, J.L.; Hirst, J.A.; O'callaghan, C.A.; Lasserson, D.S.; Hobbs, F.D.R. Global Prevalence of Chronic Kidney Disease-A Systematic Review and Meta-Analysis. *PLoS ONE* **2016**, *11*, e0158765. [CrossRef] [PubMed]
3. Eriksen, B.O.; Ingebretsen, O.C. The progression of chronic kidney disease: A 10-year population-based study of the effects of gender and age. *Kidney Int.* **2006**, *69*, 375–382. [CrossRef] [PubMed]
4. United States Renal Data System. *USRDS 2018 Annual Data Report: Atlas of Chronic Kidney Disease and End-Stage Renal Disease in the United States*; Bethesda, M., Ed.; National Institutes of Health; National Institute of Diabetes and Digestive and Kidney Diseases: Bethesda, MD, USA, 2018. Available online: https://www.usrds.org/Default.aspx (accessed on 8 September 2019).
5. Cusumano, A.M.; Rosa-Diez, G.J.; Gonzalez-Bedat, M.C. Latin American Dialysis and Transplant Registry: Experience and contributions to end-stage renal disease epidemiology. *World J. Nephrol.* **2016**, *5*, 389. [CrossRef] [PubMed]
6. Mohnen, S.M.; Van Oosten, M.J.M.; Los, J.; Leegte, M.J.H.; Jager, K.J.; Hemmelder, M.H.; Logtenberg, S.J.J.; Stel, V.S.; Hakkaart-Van Roijen, L.; De Wit, G.A. Healthcare costs of patients on different renal replacement modalities – Analysis of Dutch health insurance claims data. *PLoS ONE* **2019**, *14*, e0220800. [CrossRef]
7. Suthanthiran, M.; Strom, T.B. Renal Transplantation. *N. Engl. J. Med.* **1994**, *331*, 365–376. [CrossRef]
8. Wolfe, R.A.; Ashby, V.B.; Milford, E.L.; Ojo, A.O.; Ettenger, R.E.; Agodoa, L.Y.C.; Held, P.J.; Port, F.K. Comparison of Mortality in All Patients on Dialysis, Patients on Dialysis Awaiting Transplantation, and Recipients of a First Cadaveric Transplant. *N. Engl. J. Med.* **1999**, *341*, 1725–1730. [CrossRef]
9. Oniscu, G.C.; Brown, H.; Forsythe, J.L.R. Impact of Cadaveric Renal Transplantation on Survival in Patients Listed for Transplantation. *J. Am. Soc. Nephrol.* **2005**, *16*, 1859–1865. [CrossRef] [PubMed]
10. Tonelli, M.; Wiebe, N.; Knoll, G.; Bello, A.; Browne, S.; Jadhav, D.; Klarenbach, S.; Gill, J. Systematic Review: Kidney Transplantation Compared With Dialysis in Clinically Relevant Outcomes. *Am. J. Transpl.* **2011**, *11*, 2093–2109. [CrossRef]
11. Lamb, K.E.; Lodhi, S.; Meier-Kriesche, H.U. Long-term renal allograft survival in the United States: A critical reappraisal. *Am. J. Transpl.* **2011**, *11*, 450–462. [CrossRef]
12. Nankivell, B.J.; Borrows, R.J.; Fung, C.L.-S.; O'Connell, P.J.; Allen, R.D.M.; Chapman, J.R. The natural history of chronic allograft nephropathy. *N. Engl. J. Med.* **2003**, *349*, 2326–2333. [CrossRef] [PubMed]
13. Nankivell, B.J.; Chapman, J.R. Chronic allograft nephropathy: Current concepts and future directions. *Transplantation* **2006**, *81*, 643–654. [CrossRef] [PubMed]
14. Nankivell, B.J.; Kuypers, D.R.J. Diagnosis and prevention of chronic kidney allograft loss. *Lancet* **2011**, *378*, 1428–1437. [CrossRef]
15. Nankivell, B.J.; Borrows, R.J.; Fung, C.L.-S.; O'Connell, P.J.; Allen, R.D.M.; Chapman, J.R. Natural history, risk factors, and impact of subclinical rejection in kidney transplantation. *Transplantation* **2004**, *78*, 242–249. [CrossRef]

16. Arend, S.M.; Mallat, M.J.K.; Westendorp, R.J.W.; Van Der Woude, F.J.; Van Es, L.A. Patient survival after renal transplantation; more than 25 years follow-up. *Nephrol. Dial. Transpl.* **1997**, *12*, 1672–1679.
17. Oterdoom, L.H.; de Vries, A.P.J.; van Ree, R.M.; Gansevoort, R.T.; van Son, W.J.; van der Heide, J.J.H.; Navis, G.; de Jong, P.E.; Gans, R.O.B.; Bakker, S.J.L. N-Terminal Pro-B-Type Natriuretic Peptide and Mortality in Renal Transplant Recipients Versus the General Population. *Transplantation* **2009**, *87*, 1562–1570. [CrossRef]
18. U.S. Renal Data System. *USRDS 2010 Annual Data Report: Atlas of Chronic Kidney Disease and End-Stage Renal Disease in the United States, National Institutes of Health*; National Institute of Diabetes and Digestive and Kidney Diseases: Bethesda, MD, USA, 2010.
19. Ojo, A.O.; Hanson, J.A.; Wolfe, R.A.; Leichtman, A.B.; Agodoa, L.Y.; Port, F.K. Long-term survival in renal transplant recipients with graft function. *Kidney Int.* **2000**, *57*, 307–313. [CrossRef]
20. Shirali, A.C.; Bia, M.J. Management of cardiovascular disease in renal transplant recipients. *Clin. J. Am. Soc. Nephrol.* **2008**, *3*, 491–504. [CrossRef]
21. Jardine, A.G.; Gaston, R.S.; Fellstrom, B.C.; Holdaas, H. Prevention of cardiovascular disease in adult recipients of kidney transplants. *Lancet* **2011**, *378*, 1419–1427. [CrossRef]
22. Fry, K.; Patwardhan, A.; Ryan, C.; Trevillian, P.; Chadban, S.; Westgarth, F.; Chan, M. Development of Evidence-Based Guidelines for the Nutritional Management of Adult Kidney Transplant Recipients. *J. Ren. Nutr.* **2009**, *19*, 101–104. [CrossRef]
23. Zelle, D.M.; Kok, T.; Dontje, M.L.; Danchell, E.I.; Navis, G.; van Son, W.J.; Bakker, S.J.L.; Corpeleijn, E. The role of diet and physical activity in post-transplant weight gain after renal transplantation. *Clin. Transpl.* **2013**, *27*, E484–E490. [CrossRef] [PubMed]
24. Nolte Fong, J.V.; Moore, L.W. Nutrition Trends in Kidney Transplant Recipients: The Importance of Dietary Monitoring and Need for Evidence-Based Recommendations. *Front. Med.* **2018**, *5*, 302. [CrossRef] [PubMed]
25. Klaassen, G.; Zelle, D.M.; Navis, G.J.; Dijkema, D.; Bemelman, F.J.; Bakker, S.J.L.; Corpeleijn, E. Lifestyle intervention to improve quality of life and prevent weight gain after renal transplantation: Design of the Active Care after Transplantation (ACT) randomized controlled trial. *BMC Nephrol.* **2017**, *18*, 296. [CrossRef] [PubMed]
26. Sabbatini, M.; Ferreri, L.; Pisani, A.; Capuano, I.; Morgillo, M.; Memoli, A.; Riccio, E.; Guida, B. Nutritional management in renal transplant recipients: A transplant team opportunity to improve graft survival. *Nutr. Metab. Cardiovasc. Dis.* **2019**, *29*, 319–324. [CrossRef] [PubMed]
27. Monier-Faugere, M.-C.; Mawad, H.; Qi, Q.; Friedler, R.M.; Malluche, H.H. High Prevalence of Low Bone Turnover and Occurrence of Osteomalacia after Kidney Transplantation. *J. Am. Soc. Nephrol.* **2000**, *11*, 1093–1099. [PubMed]
28. Sprague, S.M.; Belozeroff, V.; Danese, M.D.; Martin, L.P.; Olgaard, K. Abnormal bone and mineral metabolism in kidney transplant patients—A review. *Am. J. Nephrol.* **2008**, *28*, 246–253. [CrossRef]
29. Evenepoel, P.; Lerut, E.; Naesens, M.; Bammens, B.; Claes, K.; Kuypers, D.; Vermeersch, P.; Meijers, B.; Van Damme, B.; Vanrenterghem, Y. Localization, etiology and impact of calcium phosphate deposits in renal allografts. *Am. J. Transpl.* **2009**, *9*, 2470–2478. [CrossRef]
30. Kalantar-Zadeh, K.; Molnar, M.Z.; Kovesdy, C.P.; Mucsi, I.; Bunnapradist, S. Management of mineral and bone disorder after kidney transplantation. *Curr. Opin. Nephrol. Hypertens.* **2012**, *21*, 389–403. [CrossRef]
31. Lou, I.; Foley, D.; Odorico, S.K.; Leverson, G.; Schneider, D.F.; Sippel, R.; Chen, H. How Well Does Renal Transplantation Cure Hyperparathyroidism? *Ann. Surg.* **2015**, *262*, 653–659. [CrossRef]
32. Wolf, M.; Weir, M.R.; Kopyt, N.; Mannon, R.B.; Von Visger, J.; Deng, H.; Yue, S.; Vincenti, F. A Prospective Cohort Study of Mineral Metabolism After Kidney Transplantation. *Transplantation* **2016**, *100*, 184–193. [CrossRef]
33. Willett, W. Diet and health: What should we eat? *Science* **1994**, *264*, 532–537. [CrossRef] [PubMed]
34. Stampfer, M.J.; Hu, F.B.; Manson, J.E.; Rimm, E.B.; Willett, W.C. Primary Prevention of Coronary Heart Disease in Women through Diet and Lifestyle. *N. Engl. J. Med.* **2000**, *343*, 16–22. [CrossRef] [PubMed]
35. Hu, F.B.; Manson, J.E.; Stampfer, M.J.; Colditz, G.; Liu, S.; Solomon, C.G.; Willett, W.C. Diet, lifestyle, and the risk of type 2 diabetes mellitus in women. *N. Engl. J. Med.* **2001**, *345*, 790–797. [CrossRef]
36. Chiuve, S.E.; McCullough, M.L.; Sacks, F.M.; Rimm, E.B. Healthy Lifestyle Factors in the Primary Prevention of Coronary Heart Disease Among Men. *Circulation* **2006**, *114*, 160–167. [CrossRef]
37. Chiuve, S.E.; Rexrode, K.M.; Spiegelman, D.; Logroscino, G.; Manson, J.E.; Rimm, E.B. Primary prevention of stroke by healthy lifestyle. *Circulation* **2008**, *118*, 947–954. [CrossRef] [PubMed]

38. Chiuve, S.E.; Fung, T.T.; Rexrode, K.M.; Spiegelman, D.; Manson, J.E.; Stampfer, M.J.; Albert, C.M. Adherence to a low-risk, healthy lifestyle and risk of sudden cardiac death among women. *JAMA* **2011**, *306*, 62–69. [CrossRef]
39. Kalantar-Zadeh, K.; Fouque, D. Nutritional Management of Chronic Kidney Disease. *N. Engl. J. Med.* **2017**, *377*, 1765–1776. [CrossRef]
40. Kelly, J.T.; Palmer, S.C.; Wai, S.N.; Ruospo, M.; Carrero, J.-J.; Campbell, K.L.; Strippoli, G.F.M. Healthy Dietary Patterns and Risk of Mortality and ESRD in CKD: A Meta-Analysis of Cohort Studies. *Clin. J. Am. Soc. Nephrol.* **2017**, *12*, 272–279. [CrossRef]
41. Chauveau, P. Nutrition in chronic kidney disease: Nephrology dialysis transplantation notable advances in 2018. *Nephrol. Dial. Transpl.* **2019**, *34*, 893–896. [CrossRef]
42. Saglimbene, V.M.; Wong, G.; Ruospo, M.; Palmer, S.C.; Garcia-Larsen, V.; Natale, P.; Teixeira-Pinto, A.; Campbell, K.L.; Carrero, J.-J.; Stenvinkel, P.; et al. Article Fruit and Vegetable Intake and Mortality in Adults undergoing Maintenance Hemodialysis. *Clin. J. Am. Soc. Nephrol.* **2019**, *14*, 250–260. [CrossRef]
43. Levin, A.; Stevens, P.E.; Bilous, R.W.; Coresh, J.; De Francisco, A.L.M.; De Jong, P.E.; Griffith, K.E.; Hemmelgarn, B.R.; Iseki, K.; Lamb, E.J.; et al. Notice. *Kidney Int. Suppl.* **2013**, *3*, 1. [CrossRef]
44. Palmer, S.C.; Hanson, C.S.; Craig, J.C.; Strippoli, G.F.M.; Ruospo, M.; Campbell, K.; Johnson, D.W.; Tong, A. Dietary and fluid restrictions in CKD: A thematic synthesis of patient views from qualitative studies. *Am. J. Kidney Dis.* **2015**, *65*, 559–573. [CrossRef] [PubMed]
45. Mcmahon, E.J.; Campbell, K.L.; Bauer, J.D.; Mudge, D.W. Altered dietary salt intake for people with chronic kidney disease. *Cochrane Database Syst. Rev.* **2015**, *18*, CD010070. [CrossRef]
46. Liu, Z.; Su, G.; Guo, X.; Wu, Y.; Liu, X.; Zou, C.; Zhang, L.; Yang, Q.; Xu, Y.; Ma, W. Dietary interventions for mineral and bone disorder in people with chronic kidney disease. *Cochrane Database Syst. Rev.* **2015**, *16*, CD010350. [CrossRef] [PubMed]
47. Gordon, E.J.; Prohaska, T.R.; Gallant, M.; Siminoff, L.A. Self-care strategies and barriers among kidney transplant recipients: A qualitative study. *Chronic Illn.* **2009**, *5*, 75–91. [CrossRef]
48. Stanfill, A.; Bloodworth, R.; Cashion, A. Lessons learned: Experiences of gaining weight by kidney transplant recipients. *Prog. Transpl.* **2012**, *22*, 71–78. [CrossRef]
49. Piepoli, M.F.; Hoes, A.W.; Agewall, S.; Albus, C.; Brotons, C.; Catapano, A.L.; Cooney, M.-T.; Corrà, U.; Cosyns, B.; Deaton, C.; et al. European Guidelines on cardiovascular disease prevention in clinical practice. *Eur. Heart J.* **2016**, *37*, 2315–2381. [CrossRef]
50. Lloyd-Jones, D.M.; Hong, Y.; Labarthe, D.; Mozaffarian, D.; Appel, L.J.; Van Horn, L.; Greenlund, K.; Daniels, S.; Nichol, G.; Tomaselli, G.F.; et al. Defining and setting national goals for cardiovascular health promotion and disease reduction: The american heart association's strategic impact goal through 2020 and beyond. *Circulation* **2010**, *121*, 586–613. [CrossRef]
51. Crowe, F.L.; Roddam, A.W.; Key, T.J.; Appleby, P.N.; Overvad, K.; Jakobsen, M.U.; Tjonneland, A.; Hansen, L.; Boeing, H.; Weikert, C.; et al. Fruit and vegetable intake and mortality from ischaemic heart disease: Results from the European Prospective Investigation into Cancer and Nutrition (EPIC)-Heart study. *Eur. Heart J.* **2011**, *32*, 1235–1243. [CrossRef]
52. Lim, S.S.; Vos, T.; Flaxman, A.D.; Danaei, G.; Shibuya, K.; Adair-Rohani, H.; AlMazroa, M.A.; Amann, M.; Anderson, H.R.; Andrews, K.G.; et al. A comparative risk assessment of burden of disease and injury attributable to 67 risk factors and risk factor clusters in 21 regions, 1990–2010: A systematic analysis for the Global Burden of Disease Study 2010. *Lancet* **2012**, *380*, 2224–2260. [CrossRef]
53. Larsson, S.C.; Virtamo, J.; Wolk, A. Total and specific fruit and vegetable consumption and risk of stroke: A prospective study. *Atherosclerosis* **2013**, *227*, 147–152. [CrossRef] [PubMed]
54. Zhang, X.; Shu, X.-O.; Xiang, Y.-B.; Yang, G.; Li, H.; Gao, J.; Cai, H.; Gao, Y.-T.; Zheng, W. Cruciferous vegetable consumption is associated with a reduced risk of total and cardiovascular disease mortality. *Am. J. Clin. Nutr.* **2011**, *94*, 240–246. [CrossRef] [PubMed]
55. Cases, A.; Cigarrán-Guldrís, S.; Mas, S.; Gonzalez-Parra, E. Vegetable-Based Diets for Chronic Kidney Disease? It Is Time to Reconsider. *Nutrients* **2019**, *11*, 1263. [CrossRef] [PubMed]

56. Forouzanfar, M.H.; Alexander, L.; Anderson, H.R.; Bachman, V.F.; Biryukov, S.; Brauer, M.; Burnett, R.; Casey, D.; Coates, M.M.; Cohen, A.; et al. Global, regional, and national comparative risk assessment of 79 behavioural, environmental and occupational, and metabolic risks or clusters of risks in 188 countries, 1990–2013: A systematic analysis for the Global Burden of Disease Study 2013. *Lancet* **2015**, *386*, 2287–2323. [CrossRef]
57. Sotomayor, C.G.; Gomes-Neto, A.W.; Eisenga, M.F.; Nolte, I.M.; Anderson, J.L.; de Borst, M.H.; Osté, M.C.; Rodrigo, R.; Gans, R.O.; Berger, S.P.; et al. Consumption of fruits and vegetables and cardiovascular mortality in renal transplant recipients: A prospective cohort study. *Nephrol. Dial. Transpl.* **2020**, *35*, 357–365. [CrossRef] [PubMed]
58. Gomes-Neto, A.W.; Osté, M.C.; Sotomayor, C.; Berg, E.V.D.; Geleijnse, J.M.; Gans, R.O.; Navis, G.J.; Bakker, S.J. Fruit and Vegetable Intake and Risk of Posttransplantation Diabetes in Renal Transplant Recipients. *Diabetes Care* **2019**, *42*, 1644–1652. [CrossRef]
59. Mozaffarian, D.; Gottdiener, J.S.; Siscovick, D.S. Intake of tuna or other broiled or baked fish versus fried fish and cardiac structure, function, and hemodynamics. *Am. J. Cardiol.* **2006**, *97*, 216–222. [CrossRef]
60. Chin, J.P.; Gust, A.P.; Nestel, P.J.; Dart, A.M. Marine oils dose-dependently inhibit vasoconstriction of forearm resistance vessels in humans. *Hypertension* **1993**, *21*, 22–28. [CrossRef]
61. Nestel, P.J. Fish oil and cardiovascular disease: Lipids and arterial function. *Am. J. Clin. Nutr.* **2000**, *71*, 228S–231S. [CrossRef]
62. Kristensen, S.D.; Bach Iversen, A.M.; Schmidt, E.B. n-3 polyunsaturated fatty acids and coronary thrombosis. *Lipids* **2001**, *36*, S79–S82. [CrossRef]
63. Bar-Or, A.; Bashinskaya, V.V.; Kulakova, O.G.; Boyko, A.N.; Favorov, A.V.; Favorova, O.O.; Medicina, F.D.E.; Bos, S.D.; Berge, T.; Celius, E.G.; et al. The genetics of multiple sclerosis: SNPs to pathways to pathogenesis. *PLoS ONE* **2012**, *7*, 457. [CrossRef]
64. Christensen, J.H. Omega-3 polyunsaturated Fatty acids and heart rate variability. *Front. Med.* **2011**, *2*, 84. [CrossRef] [PubMed]
65. Masson, S.; Marchioli, R.; Mozaffarian, D.; Bernasconi, R.; Milani, V.; Dragani, L.; Tacconi, M.; Marfisi, R.M.; Borgese, L.; Cirrincione, V.; et al. Plasma n-3 polyunsaturated fatty acids in chronic heart failure in the GISSI-heart failure trial: Relation with fish intake, circulating biomarkers, and mortality. *Am. Heart J.* **2013**, *165*, 208–215. [CrossRef] [PubMed]
66. Calder, P.C. Omega-3 fatty acids and inflammatory processes. *Nutrients* **2010**, *2*, 355–374. [CrossRef] [PubMed]
67. Eide, I.A.; Jenssen, T.; Hartmann, A.; Diep, L.M.; Dahle, D.O.; Reisæter, A.V.; Bjerve, K.S.; Christensen, J.H.; Schmidt, E.B.; Svensson, M. The association between marine n-3 polyunsaturated fatty acid levels and survival after renal transplantation. *Clin. J. Am. Soc. Nephrol.* **2015**, *10*, 1246–1256. [CrossRef] [PubMed]
68. Gomes-Neto, A.W.; Sotomayor, C.G.; Pranger, I.; van den Berg, E.; Gans, R.O.; Soedamah-Muthu, S.; Navis, G.J.; Bakker, S.J. Intake of Marine-Derived Omega-3 Polyunsaturated Fatty Acids and Mortality in Renal Transplant Recipients. *Nutrients* **2017**, *9*, 363. [CrossRef]
69. Tatsioni, A.; Chung, M.; Sun, Y.; Kupelnick, B.; Lichtenstein, A.H.; Perrone, R.; Chew, P.; Lau, J.; Bonis, P.A. Effects of fish oil supplementation on kidney transplantation: A systematic review and meta-analysis of randomized, controlled trials. *J. Am. Soc. Nephrol.* **2005**, *16*, 2462–2670. [CrossRef]
70. Lim, A.K.; Manley, K.J.; Roberts, M.A.; Fraenkel, M.B. Fish oil for kidney transplant recipients. *Cochrane Database Syst. Rev.* **2016**, *8*, CD005282. [CrossRef]
71. Kromhout, D.; Feskens, E.J.; Bowles, C.H. The protective effect of a small amount of fish on coronary heart disease mortality in an elderly population. *Int. J. Epidemiol.* **1995**, *24*, 340–345. [CrossRef]
72. Stone, N.J. Fish consumption, fish oil, lipids, and coronary heart disease. *Circulation* **1996**, *94*, 2337–2340. [CrossRef]
73. Krauss, R.M.; Eckel, R.H.; Howard, B.; Appel, L.J.; Daniels, S.R.; Deckelbaum, R.J.; Erdman, J.W.; Kris-Etherton, P.; Goldberg, I.J.; Kotchen, T.A.; et al. AHA Dietary Guidelines: revision 2000: A statement for healthcare professionals from the Nutrition Committee of the American Heart Association. *Circulation* **2000**, *102*, 2284–2299. [CrossRef] [PubMed]
74. Psota, T.L.; Gebauer, S.K.; Kris-Etherton, P. Dietary Omega-3 Fatty Acid Intake and Cardiovascular Risk. *Am. J. Cardiol.* **2006**, *98*, 3–18. [CrossRef] [PubMed]

75. Wang, C.; Harris, W.S.; Chung, M.; Lichtenstein, A.H.; Balk, E.M.; Kupelnick, B.; Jordan, H.S.; Lau, J. n-3 Fatty acids from fish or fish-oil supplements, but not α-linolenic acid, benefit cardiovascular disease outcomes in primary- and secondary-prevention studies: A systematic review. *Am. J. Clin. Nutr.* **2006**, *84*, 5–17. [CrossRef] [PubMed]
76. World Health Organization. *Preventing Disease through Healthy Environment—Exposure to Mercury: A Major Public Health Concern*; WHO: Geneva, Switzerland, 2010.
77. Hightower, J.M.; Moore, D. Mercury levels in high-end consumers of fish. *Environ. Health Perspect.* **2003**, *111*, 604–608. [CrossRef] [PubMed]
78. Joshi, A.; Douglass, C.W.; Kim, H.D.; Joshipura, K.J.; Park, M.C.; Rimm, E.B.; Carino, M.J.; Garcia, R.I.; Morris, J.S.; Willett, W.C. The relationship between amalgam restorations and mercury levels in male dentists and nondental health professionals. *J. Public Health Dent.* **2003**, *63*, 52–60. [CrossRef]
79. Sotomayor, C.G.; Gomes-Neto, A.W.; Gans, R.O.; de Borst, M.; Berger, S.P.; Rodrigo, R.; Navis, G.J.; Touw, D.J.; Bakker, S.J.; Sotomayor, C.G.; et al. Fish Intake, Circulating Mercury and Mortality in Renal Transplant Recipients. *Nutrients* **2018**, *10*, 1419. [CrossRef]
80. Schroeder, J.C.; DiNatale, B.C.; Murray, I.A.; Flaveny, C.A.; Liu, Q.; Laurenzana, E.M.; Lin, J.M.; Strom, S.C.; Omiecinski, C.J.; Amin, S.; et al. The uremic toxin 3-indoxyl sulfate is a potent endogenous agonist for the human aryl hydrocarbon receptor. *Biochemistry* **2010**, *49*, 393–400. [CrossRef]
81. Tellez-Plaza, M.; Navas-Acien, A.; Crainiceanu, C.M.; Guallar, E. Cadmium exposure and hypertension in the 1999–2004 National Health and Nutrition Examination Survey (NHANES). *Environ. Health Perspect.* **2008**, *116*, 51–56. [CrossRef]
82. Mange, K.C.; Cizman, B.; Joffe, M.; Feldman, H.I. Arterial hypertension and renal allograft survival. *JAMA* **2000**, *283*, 633–638. [CrossRef]
83. Mange, K.C.; Feldman, H.I.; Joffe, M.M.; Fa, K.; Bloom, R.D. Blood Pressure and the Survival of Renal Allografts from Living Donors. *J. Am. Soc. Nephrol.* **2004**, *15*, 187–193. [CrossRef]
84. Weir, M.R.; Burgess, E.D.; Cooper, J.E.; Fenves, A.Z.; Goldsmith, D.; McKay, D.; Mehrotra, A.; Mitsnefes, M.M.; Sica, D.A.; Taler, S.J. Assessment and management of hypertension in transplant patients. *J. Am. Soc. Nephrol.* **2015**, *26*, 1248–1260. [CrossRef] [PubMed]
85. Akesson, A.; Lundh, T.; Vahter, M.; Bjellerup, P.; Lidfeldt, J.; Nerbrand, C.; Samsioe, G.; Strömberg, U.; Skerfving, S. Tubular and glomerular kidney effects in Swedish women with low environmental cadmium exposure. *Environ. Health Perspect.* **2005**, *113*, 1627–1631. [CrossRef] [PubMed]
86. Buser, M.C.; Ingber, S.Z.; Raines, N.; Fowler, D.A.; Scinicariello, F. Urinary and blood cadmium and lead and kidney function: NHANES 2007–2012. *Int. J. Hyg. Environ. Health* **2016**, *219*, 261–267. [CrossRef] [PubMed]
87. Huang, M.; Choi, S.J.; Kim, D.W.; Kim, N.Y.; Park, C.H.; Do Yu, S.; Kim, D.S.; Park, K.S.; Song, J.S.; Kim, H.; et al. Risk assessment of low-level cadmium and arsenic on the kidney. *J. Toxicol. Environ. Health A* **2009**, *72*, 1493–1498. [CrossRef] [PubMed]
88. Geeth Gunawardana, C.; Martinez, R.E.; Xiao, W.; Templeton, D.M.; Geeth, C. Cadmium inhibits both intrinsic and extrinsic apoptotic pathways in renal mesangial cells. *Am. J. Physiol. Ren. Physiol.* **2006**, *290*, 1074–1082. [CrossRef] [PubMed]
89. Prozialeck, W.C.; Edwards, J.R. Mechanisms of cadmium-induced proximal tubule injury: New insights with implications for biomonitoring and therapeutic interventions. *J. Pharm. Exp.* **2012**, *343*, 2–12. [CrossRef]
90. Shaikh, Z.A.; Vu, T.T.; Zaman, K. Oxidative stress as a mechanism of chronic cadmium-induced hepatotoxicity and renal toxicity and protection by antioxidants. *Toxicol. Appl. Pharm.* **1999**, *154*, 256–263. [CrossRef]
91. Johri, N.; Jacquillet, G.; Unwin, R. Heavy metal poisoning: The effects of cadmium on the kidney. *BioMetals* **2010**, *23*, 783–792. [CrossRef]
92. Liu, J.; Qu, W.; Kadiiska, M.B. Role of oxidative stress in cadmium toxicity and carcinogenesis. *Toxicol. Appl. Pharm.* **2009**, *238*, 209–214. [CrossRef]
93. Andersen, O. Chelation of cadmium. *Environ. Health Perspect.* **1984**, *54*, 249–266. [CrossRef]
94. Kasiske, B.L.; Guijarro, C.; Massy, Z.A.; Wiederkehr, M.R.; Ma, J.Z. Cardiovascular disease after renal transplantation. *J. Am. Coll. Cardiol.* **1996**, *7*, 158–165.
95. Kasiske, B.L.; Vazquez, M.A.; Harmon, W.E.; Brown, R.S.; Danovitch, G.M.; Gaston, R.S.; Roth, D.; Scandling, J.D.; Singer, G.G.; The American Society of Transplantation. Recommendations for the outpatient surveillance of renal transplant recipients. American Society of Transplantation. *J. Am. Soc. Nephrol.* **2000**, *11*, S1–S86. [PubMed]

96. Ducloux, D.; Kazory, A.; Chalopin, J.M. Predicting coronary heart disease in renal transplant recipients: A prospective study. *Kidney Int.* **2004**, *66*, 441–447. [CrossRef] [PubMed]
97. Kiberd, B.; Panek, R. Cardiovascular outcomes in the outpatient kidney transplant clinic: The Framingham risk score revisited. *Clin. J. Am. Soc. Nephrol.* **2008**, *3*, 822–828. [CrossRef]
98. Winkelmayer, W.C.; Lorenz, M.; Kramar, R.; Födinger, M.; Hörl, W.H.; Sunder-Plassmann, G. C-reactive protein and body mass index independently predict mortality in kidney transplant recipients. *Am. J. Transpl.* **2004**, *4*, 1148–1154. [CrossRef]
99. Hartog, J.W.L. Risk factors for chronic transplant dysfunction and cardiovascular disease are related to accumulation of advanced glycation end-products in renal transplant recipients. *Nephrol. Dial. Transpl.* **2006**, *21*, 2263–2269. [CrossRef]
100. Abedini, S.; Holme, I.; März, W.; Weihrauch, G.; Fellström, B.; Jardine, A.; Cole, E.; Maes, B.; Neumayer, H.H.; Grønhagen-Riska, C.; et al. Inflammation in renal transplantation. *Clin. J. Am. Soc. Nephrol.* **2009**, *4*, 1246–1254. [CrossRef]
101. Turkmen, K.; Tonbul, H.Z.; Toker, A.; Gaipov, A.; Erdur, F.M.; Cicekler, H.; Anil, M.; Ozbek, O.; Selcuk, N.Y.; Yeksan, M.; et al. The relationship between oxidative stress, inflammation, and atherosclerosis in renal transplant and end-stage renal disease patients. *Ren. Fail.* **2012**, *34*, 1229–1237. [CrossRef]
102. Ocak, N.; Dirican, M.; Ersoy, A.; Sarandol, E. Adiponectin, leptin, nitric oxide, and C-reactive protein levels in kidney transplant recipients: Comparison with the hemodialysis and chronic renal failure. *Ren. Fail.* **2016**, *38*, 1639–1646. [CrossRef]
103. van Gennip, A.C.E.; Broers, N.J.H.; ter Meulen, K.J.; Canaud, B.; Christiaans, M.H.L.; Cornelis, T.; Gelens, M.A.C.J.; Hermans, M.M.H.; Konings, C.J.A.M.; van der Net, J.B.; et al. Endothelial dysfunction and low-grade inflammation in the transition to renal replacement therapy. *PLoS ONE* **2019**, *14*, e0222547. [CrossRef]
104. Mazzaferro, S.; Pasquali, M.; Taggi, F.; Baldinelli, M.; Conte, C.; Muci, M.L.; Pirozzi, N.; Carbone, I.; Francone, M.; Pugliese, F. Progression of coronary artery calcification in renal transplantation and the role of secondary hyperparathyroidism and inflammation. *Clin. J. Am. Soc. Nephrol.* **2009**, *4*, 685–690. [CrossRef] [PubMed]
105. Himmelfarb, J.; Stenvinkel, P.; Ikizler, T.A.; Hakim, R.M. The elephant in uremia: Oxidant stress as a unifying concept of cardiovascular disease in uremia. *Kidney Int.* **2002**, *62*, 1524–1538. [CrossRef] [PubMed]
106. Cachofeiro, V.; Goicochea, M.; de Vinuesa, S.G.; Oubiña, P.; Lahera, V.; Luño, J. Oxidative stress and inflammation, a link between chronic kidney disease and cardiovascular disease. *Kidney Int.* **2008**, *74*, S4–S9. [CrossRef] [PubMed]
107. Liu, J.; Tian, J.; Chaudhry, M.; Maxwell, K.; Yan, Y.; Wang, X.; Shah, P.T.; Khawaja, A.A.; Martin, R.; Robinette, T.J.; et al. Attenuation of Na/K-ATPase Mediated Oxidant Amplification with pNaKtide Ameliorates Experimental Uremic Cardiomyopathy. *Sci. Rep.* **2016**, *6*, 34592. [CrossRef]
108. Jerotic, D.; Matic, M.; Suvakov, S.; Vucicevic, K.; Damjanovic, T.; Savic-Radojevic, A.; Pljesa-Ercegovac, M.; Coric, V.; Stefanovic, A.; Ivanisevic, J.; et al. Association of Nrf2, SOD2 and GPX1 Polymorphisms with Biomarkers of Oxidative Distress and Survival in End-Stage Renal Disease Patients. *Toxins* **2019**, *11*, 431. [CrossRef]
109. La Russa, D.; Pellegrino, D.; Montesanto, A.; Gigliotti, P.; Perri, A.; La Russa, A.; Bonofiglio, R. Oxidative Balance and Inflammation in Hemodialysis Patients: Biomarkers of Cardiovascular Risk? *Oxid. Med. Cell Longev.* **2019**, *2019*, 1–7. [CrossRef]
110. Sies, H. (Ed.) *Oxidative Stress II: Oxidants and Antioxidants*; Academic Press: New York, NY, USA, 1991.
111. Langlois, M.; Duprez, D.; Delanghe, J.; De Buyzere, M.; Clement, D.L. Serum vitamin C concentration is low in peripheral arterial disease and is associated with inflammation and severity of atherosclerosis. *Circulation* **2001**, *103*, 1863–1868. [CrossRef]
112. Korantzopoulos, P.; Kolettis, T.M.; Kountouris, E.; Dimitroula, V.; Karanikis, P.; Pappa, E.; Siogas, K.; Goudevenos, J.A. Oral vitamin C administration reduces early recurrence rates after electrical cardioversion of persistent atrial fibrillation and attenuates associated inflammation. *Int. J. Cardiol.* **2005**, *102*, 321–326. [CrossRef]
113. Mikirova, N.; Casciari, J.; Rogers, A.; Taylor, P. Effect of high-dose intravenous vitamin C on inflammation in cancer patients. *J. Transl. Med.* **2012**, *10*. [CrossRef]

114. Mikirova, N.; Casciari, J.; Riordan, N.; Hunninghake, R. Clinical experience with intravenous administration of ascorbic acid: Achievable levels in blood for different states of inflammation and disease in cancer patients. *J. Transl. Med.* **2013**, *11*, 191. [CrossRef]
115. Frei, B.; England, L.; Ames, B.N. Ascorbate is an outstanding antioxidant in human blood plasma. *Proc. Natl. Acad. Sci. USA* **1989**, *86*, 6377–6381. [CrossRef] [PubMed]
116. Wang, S.; Eide, T.C.; Sogn, E.M.; Berg, K.J.; Sund, R.B. Plasma ascorbic acid in patients undergoing chronic haemodialysis. *Eur. J. Clin. Pharm.* **1999**, *55*, 527–532. [CrossRef]
117. Morena, M.; Cristol, J.P.; Bosc, J.Y.; Tetta, C.; Forret, G.; Leger, C.L.; Delcourt, C.; Papoz, L.; Descomps, B.; Canaud, B. Convective and diffusive losses of vitamin C during haemodiafiltration session: A contributive factor to oxidative stress in haemodialysis patients. *Nephrol. Dial. Transpl.* **2002**, *17*, 422–427. [CrossRef] [PubMed]
118. Sullivan, J.F.; Eisenstein, A.B. Ascorbic acid depletion during hemodialysis. *JAMA* **1972**, *220*, 1697–1699. [CrossRef] [PubMed]
119. Jacob, R.A. Assessment of Human Vitamin C Status. *J. Nutr.* **1990**, *120*, 1480–1485. [CrossRef]
120. Johnston, C.S.; Solomon, R.E.; Corte, C. Vitamin C depletion is associated with alterations in blood histamine and plasma free carnitine in adults. *J. Am. Coll. Nutr.* **1996**, *15*, 586–591. [CrossRef]
121. Zhang, K.; Li, Y.; Cheng, X.; Liu, L.; Bai, W.; Guo, W.; Wu, L.; Zuo, L. Cross-over study of influence of oral vitamin C supplementation on inflammatory status in maintenance hemodialysis patients. *BMC Nephrol.* **2013**, *14*, 252. [CrossRef]
122. Attallah, N.; Osman-Malik, Y.; Frinak, S.; Besarab, A. Effect of intravenous ascorbic acid in hemodialysis patients with EPO-hyporesponsive anemia and hyperferritinemia. *Am. J. Kidney Dis.* **2006**, *47*, 644–654. [CrossRef]
123. May, J.M.; Harrison, F.E. Role of vitamin C in the function of the vascular endothelium. *Antioxid. Redox Signal.* **2013**, *19*, 2068–2083. [CrossRef]
124. Sotomayor, C.G.; Eisenga, M.F.; Gomes Neto, A.W.; Ozyilmaz, A.; Gans, R.O.B.; de Jong, W.H.A.; Zelle, D.M.; Berger, S.P.; Gaillard, C.A.J.M.; Navis, G.J.; et al. Vitamin C Depletion and All-Cause Mortality in Renal Transplant Recipients. *Nutrients* **2017**, *9*, 568. [CrossRef]
125. Gacitúa, T.A.; Sotomayor, C.G.; Groothof, D.; Eisenga, M.F.; Pol, R.A.; de Borst, M.H.; Gans, R.O.B.; Berger, S.P.; Rodrigo, R.; Navis, G.J.; et al. Plasma Vitamin C and Cancer Mortality in Kidney Transplant Recipients. *J. Clin. Med.* **2019**, *8*, 2064. [CrossRef] [PubMed]
126. Schreck, R.; Rieber, P.; Baeuerle, P.A. Reactive oxygen intermediates as apparently widely used messengers in the activation of the NF-kappa B transcription factor and HIV-1. *EMBO J.* **1991**, *10*, 2247–2258. [CrossRef]
127. Yan, S.D.; Schmidt, A.M.; Anderson, G.M.; Zhang, J.; Brett, J.; Zou, Y.S.; Pinsky, D.; Stern, D. Enhanced cellular oxidant stress by the interaction of advanced glycation end products with their receptors/binding proteins. *J. Biol. Chem.* **1994**, *269*, 9889–9897. [PubMed]
128. Linden, E.; Cai, W.; He, J.C.; Xue, C.; Li, Z.; Winston, J.; Vlassara, H.; Uribarri, J. Endothelial dysfunction in patients with chronic kidney disease results from advanced glycation end products (AGE)-mediated inhibition of endothelial nitric oxide synthase through RAGE activation. *Clin. J. Am. Soc. Nephrol.* **2008**, *3*, 691–698. [CrossRef]
129. Stinghen, A.E.M.; Massy, Z.A.; Vlassara, H.; Striker, G.E.; Boullier, A. Uremic Toxicity of Advanced Glycation End Products in CKD. *J. Am. Soc. Nephrol.* **2016**, *27*, 354–370. [CrossRef] [PubMed]
130. Stam, F.; van Guldener, C.; Becker, A.; Dekker, J.M.; Heine, R.J.; Bouter, L.M.; Stehouwer, C. DA Endothelial Dysfunction Contributes to Renal Function-Associated Cardiovascular Mortality in a Population with Mild Renal Insufficiency: The Hoorn Study. *J. Am. Soc. Nephrol.* **2006**, *17*, 537–545. [CrossRef]
131. Calviño, J.; Cigarran, S.; Gonzalez-Tabares, L.; Menendez, N.; Latorre, J.; Cillero, S.; Millan, B.; Cobelo, C.; Sanjurjo-Amado, A.; Quispe, J.; et al. Advanced glycation end products (AGEs) estimated by skin autofluorescence are related with cardiovascular risk in renal transplant. *PLoS ONE* **2018**, *13*, e0201118. [CrossRef]
132. Choi, B.S.; Shin, M.J.; Shin, S.J.; Kim, Y.S.; Choi, Y.J.; Kim, Y.-S.; Moon, I.S.; Kim, S.Y.; Koh, Y.B.; Bang, B.K.; et al. Clinical significance of an early protocol biopsy in living-donor renal transplantation: Ten-year experience at a single center. *Am. J. Transpl.* **2005**, *5*, 1354–1360. [CrossRef]

133. Heilman, R.L.; Devarapalli, Y.; Chakkera, H.A.; Mekeel, K.L.; Moss, A.A.; Mulligan, D.C.; Mazur, M.J.; Hamawi, K.; Williams, J.W.; Reddy, K.S. Impact of Subclinical Inflammation on the Development of Interstitial Fibrosis and Tubular Atrophy in Kidney Transplant Recipients. *Am. J. Transpl.* **2010**, *10*, 563–570. [CrossRef]
134. Henderson, N.C.; Mackinnon, A.C.; Farnworth, S.L.; Kipari, T.; Haslett, C.; Iredale, J.P.; Liu, F.T.; Hughes, J.; Sethi, T. Galectin-3 expression and secretion links macrophages to the promotion of renal fibrosis. *Am. J. Pathol.* **2008**, *172*, 288–298. [CrossRef]
135. Kolatsi-Joannou, M.; Price, K.L.; Winyard, P.J.; Long, D.A. Modified citrus pectin reduces galectin-3 expression and disease severity in experimental acute kidney injury. *PLoS ONE* **2011**, *6*, 18683. [CrossRef]
136. Frenay, A.-R.S.; Yu, L.; van der Velde, A.R.; Vreeswijk-Baudoin, I.; López-Andrés, N.; van Goor, H.; Silljé, H.H.; Ruifrok, W.P.; de Boer, R.A. Pharmacological inhibition of galectin-3 protects against hypertensive nephropathy. *Am. J. Physiol. Ren. Physiol.* **2015**, *308*, F500–F509. [CrossRef]
137. Martinez-Martinez, E.; Ibarrola, J.; Calvier, L.; Fernandez-Celis, A.; Leroy, C.; Cachofeiro, V.; Rossignol, P.; Lopez-Andres, N. Galectin-3 blockade reduces renal fibrosis in two normotensive experimental models of renal damage. *PLoS ONE* **2016**, *11*, e0166272. [CrossRef]
138. Dang, Z.; Mackinnon, A.; Marson, L.P.; Sethi, T. Tubular Atrophy and Interstitial Fibrosis After Renal Transplantation Is Dependent on Galectin-3. *Transplantation* **2012**, *93*, 477–484. [CrossRef]
139. O'Seaghdha, C.; Hwang, S.; Ho, J.; Vasan, R.; Levy, D.; Fox, C. Elevated Galectin-3 Precedes the Development of CKD. *J. Am. Soc. Nephrol.* **2013**, *24*, 1470–1477. [CrossRef]
140. Rebholz, C.M.; Selvin, E.; Liang, M.; Ballantyne, C.M.; Hoogeveen, R.C.; Aguilar, D.; McEvoy, J.W.; Grams, M.E.; Coresh, J. Plasma galectin-3 levels are associated with the risk of incident chronic kidney disease. *Kidney Int.* **2018**, *93*, 252–259. [CrossRef]
141. Alam, M.L.; Katz, R.; Bellovich, K.A.; Bhat, Z.Y.; Brosius, F.C.; de Boer, I.H.; Gadegbeku, C.A.; Gipson, D.S.; Hawkins, J.J.; Himmelfarb, J.; et al. Soluble ST2 and Galectin-3 and Progression of CKD. *Kidney Int. Rep.* **2018**, *4*, 103–111. [CrossRef]
142. Moe, S.M.; Drüeke, T.; Lameire, N.; Eknoyan, G. Chronic Kidney Disease-Mineral-Bone Disorder: A New Paradigm. *Adv. Chronic. Kidney Dis.* **2007**, *14*, 3–12. [CrossRef]
143. Simmons, E.M.; Langone, A.; Sezer, M.T.; Vella, J.P.; Recupero, P.; Morrow, J.D.; Ikizler, T.A.; Himmelfarb, J. Effect of renal transplantation on biomarkers of inflammation and oxidative stress in end-stage renal disease patients. *Transplantation* **2005**, *79*, 914–919. [CrossRef]
144. Yilmaz, M.I.; Sonmez, A.; Saglam, M.; Cayci, T.; Kilic, S.; Unal, H.U.; Karaman, M.; Cetinkaya, H.; Eyileten, T.; Gok, M.; et al. A longitudinal study of inflammation, CKD-mineral bone disorder, and carotid atherosclerosis after renal transplantation. *Clin. J. Am. Soc. Nephrol.* **2015**, *10*, 471–479. [CrossRef]
145. Cozzolino, M.; Mangano, M.; Stucchi, A.; Ciceri, P.; Conte, F.; Galassi, A. Cardiovascular disease in dialysis patients. *Nephrol. Dial. Transpl.* **2018**, *33*, iii28–iii34. [CrossRef] [PubMed]
146. DeLoach, S.S.; Joffe, M.M.; Mai, X.; Goral, S.; Rosas, S.E. Aortic calcification predicts cardiovascular events and all-cause mortality in renal transplantation. *Nephrol. Dial. Transpl.* **2009**, *24*, 1314–1319. [CrossRef] [PubMed]
147. Nguyen, P.T.; Henrard, S.; Coche, E.; Goffin, E.; Devuyst, O.; Jadoul, M. Coronary artery calcification: A strong predictor of cardiovascular events in renal transplant recipients. *Nephrol. Dial. Transpl.* **2010**, *25*, 3773–3778. [CrossRef] [PubMed]
148. Roe, P.; Wolfe, M.; Joffe, M.; Rosas, S.E. Inflammation, coronary artery calcification and cardiovascular events in incident renal transplant recipients. *Atherosclerosis* **2010**, *212*, 589–594. [CrossRef]
149. Claes, K.J.; Heye, S.; Bammens, B.; Kuypers, D.R.; Meijers, B.; Naesens, M.; Vanrenterghem, Y.; Evenepoel, P. Aortic calcifications and arterial stiffness as predictors of cardiovascular events in incident renal transplant recipients. *Transpl. Int.* **2013**, *26*, 973–981. [CrossRef]
150. Davis, B.; Marin, D.; Hurwitz, L.M.; Ronald, J.; Ellis, M.J.; Ravindra, K.V.; Collins, B.H.; Kim, C.Y. Application of a Novel CT-Based Iliac Artery Calcification Scoring System for Predicting Renal Transplant Outcomes. *Am. J. Roent* **2016**, *206*, 436–441. [CrossRef]
151. Benjamens, S.; Pol, R.A.; Glaudemans, A.W.J.M.; Wieringa, I.; Berger, S.P.; Bakker, S.J.L.; Slart, R.H.J.A. A high abdominal aortic calcification score by dual X-ray absorptiometry is associated with cardiovascular events after kidney transplantation. *Nephrol. Dial. Transpl.* **2018**, *33*, 2253–2259. [CrossRef]

152. Braun, J.; Oldendorf, M.; Moshage, W.; Heidler, R.; Zeitler, E.; Luft, F.C. Electron beam computed tomography in the evaluation of cardiac calcifications in chronic dialysis patients. *Am. J. Kidney Dis.* **1996**, *27*, 394–401. [CrossRef]
153. London, G.; Marty, C.; Marchais, S.J.; Guerin, A.P.; Metivier, F.; de Vernejoul, M. Arterial Calcifications and Bone Histomorphometry in End-Stage Renal Disease. *J. Am. Soc. Nephrol.* **2004**, *15*, 1943–1951. [CrossRef]
154. Seifert, M.E.; Hruska, K.A. The Kidney-Vascular-Bone Axis in the Chronic Kidney Disease-Mineral Bone Disorder. *Transplantation* **2016**, *100*, 497–505. [CrossRef]
155. Adragao, T.; Herberth, J.; Monier-Faugere, M.-C.; Branscum, A.J.; Ferreira, A.; Frazao, J.M.; Dias Curto, J.; Malluche, H.H. Low Bone Volume-A Risk Factor for Coronary Calcifications in Hemodialysis Patients. *Clin. J. Am. Soc. Nephrol.* **2009**, *4*, 450–455. [CrossRef] [PubMed]
156. Asci, G.; Ok, E.; Savas, R.; Ozkahya, M.; Duman, S.; Toz, H.; Kayikcioglu, M.; Branscum, A.J.; Monier-Faugere, M.C.; Herberth, J.; et al. The link between bone and coronary calcifications in CKD-5 patients on haemodialysis. *Nephrol. Dial. Transpl.* **2011**, *26*, 1010–1015. [CrossRef]
157. Bouquegneau, A.; Salam, S.; Delanaye, P.; Eastell, R.; Khwaja, A. Mini-Review Bone Disease after Kidney Transplantation. *Clin. J. Am. Soc. Nephrol.* **2016**, *11*, 1282–1296. [CrossRef] [PubMed]
158. Malluche, H.H.; Monier-Faugere, M.-C.; Herberth, J. Bone disease after renal transplantation. *Nat. Rev. Neprhol.* **2010**, *6*, 32–40. [CrossRef] [PubMed]
159. Drüeke, T.B.; Evenepoel, P. The Bone after Kidney Transplantation. *Clin. J. Am. Soc. Nephrol.* **2019**, *14*, 795–797. [CrossRef] [PubMed]
160. Neves, C.L.; Dos Reis, L.M.; Batista, D.G.; Custodio, M.R.; Graciolli, F.G.; Martin, R.D.C.T.; Neves, K.R.; Dominguez, W.V.; Moyses, R.M.; Jorgetti, V. Persistence of bone and mineral disorders 2 years after successful kidney transplantation. *Transplantation* **2013**, *96*, 290–296. [CrossRef]
161. Iyer, S.P.; Nikkel, L.E.; Nishiyama, K.K.; Dworakowski, E.; Cremers, S.; Zhang, C.; Mcmahon, D.J.; Boutroy, S.; Liu, X.S.; Ratner, L.E.; et al. Kidney Transplantation with Early Corticosteroid Withdrawal: Paradoxical Effects at the Central and Peripheral Skeleton. *J. Am. Soc. Nephrol.* **2014**, *25*, 1331–1341. [CrossRef]
162. Keronen, S.; Martola, L.; Finne, P.; Burton, I.S.; Kröger, H.; Honkanen, E. Changes in Bone Histomorphometry after Kidney Transplantation. *Clin. J. Am. Soc. Nephrol.* **2019**, *14*, 894–903. [CrossRef]
163. Moe, S.M. Vascular calcification and renal osteodystrophy relationship in chronic kidney disease. *Eur. J. Clin. Investig.* **2006**, *36*, 51–62. [CrossRef]
164. Sotomayor, C.G.; Benjamens, S.; Gomes-Neto, A.W.; Pol, R.A.; Groothof, D.; te Velde-Keyzer, C.A.; Chong, G.; Glaudemans, A.W.J.M.; Berger, S.P.; Bakker, S.J.L.; et al. Bone Mineral Density and Aortic Calcification. *Transplantation* **2020**. [CrossRef]
165. Czaya, B.; Faul, C. FGF23 and inflammation—a vicious coalition in CKD. *Kidney Int.* **2019**, *96*, 813–815. [CrossRef] [PubMed]
166. Singh, S.; Grabner, A.; Yanucil, C.; Schramm, K.; Czaya, B.; Krick, S.; Czaja, M.J.; Bartz, R.; Abraham, R.; Di Marco, G.S.; et al. Fibroblast growth factor 23 directly targets hepatocytes to promote inflammation in chronic kidney disease. *Kidney Int.* **2016**, *90*, 985–996. [CrossRef] [PubMed]
167. Egli-Spichtig, D.; Imenez Silva, P.H.; Glaudemans, B.; Gehring, N.; Bettoni, C.; Zhang, M.Y.H.; Pastor-Arroyo, E.M.; Schönenberger, D.; Rajski, M.; Hoogewijs, D.; et al. Tumor necrosis factor stimulates fibroblast growth factor 23 levels in chronic kidney disease and non-renal inflammation. *Kidney Int.* **2019**, *96*, 890–905. [CrossRef] [PubMed]
168. Hamano, T.; Matsui, I.; Mikami, S.; Tomida, K.; Fujii, N.; Imai, E.; Rakugi, H.; Isaka, Y. Fetuin-mineral complex reflects extraosseous calcification stress in CKD. *J. Am. Soc. Nephrol.* **2010**, *21*, 1998–2007. [CrossRef] [PubMed]
169. Kuro-O, M. Klotho and endocrine fibroblast growth factors: markers of chronic kidney disease progression and cardiovascular complications? *Nephrol. Dial. Transpl.* **2019**, *34*, 15–21. [CrossRef]
170. Cianciolo, G.; Capelli, I.; Angelini, M.L.; Valentini, C.; Baraldi, O.; Scolari, M.P.; Stefoni, S. Importance of vascular calcification in kidney transplant recipients. *Am. J. Nephrol.* **2014**, *39*, 418–426. [CrossRef]
171. Van Ballegooijen, A.J.; Cepelis, A.; Visser, M.; Brouwer, I.A.; Van Schoor, N.M.; Beulens, J.W. Joint Association of Low Vitamin D and Vitamin K Status with Blood Pressure and Hypertension. *Hypertension* **2017**, *69*, 1165–1172. [CrossRef] [PubMed]

172. Hou, Y.-C.; Lu, C.-L.; Zheng, C.-M.; Chen, R.-M.; Lin, Y.-F.; Liu, W.-C.; Yen, T.-H.; Chen, R.; Lu, K.-C. Correction: Hou et al. Emerging Role of Vitamins D and K in Modulating Uremic Vascular Calcification: The Aspect of Passive Calcification. *Nutrients* **2019**, *11*, 152. [CrossRef] [PubMed]
173. van Ballegooijen, A.J.; Beulens, J.W.J.; Keyzer, C.A.; Navis, G.J.; Berger, S.P.; de Borst, M.H.; Vervloet, M.G.; Bakker, S.J.L. Joint association of vitamins D and K status with long-term outcomes in stable kidney transplant recipients. *Nephrol. Dial. Transpl.* **2020**, *35*, 706–714. [CrossRef] [PubMed]
174. Nguyen, P.T.H.; Coche, E.; Goffin, E.; Beguin, C.; Vlassenbroek, A.; Devuyst, O.; Robert, A.; Jadoul, M. Prevalence and determinants of coronary and aortic calcifications assessed by chest CT in renal transplant recipients. *Am. J. Nephrol.* **2007**, *27*, 329–335. [CrossRef] [PubMed]
175. Shimizu, H.; Takahashi, M.; Takeda, S.I.; Inoue, S.; Fujishiro, J.; Hakamata, Y.; Kaneko, T.; Murakami, T.; Takeuchi, K.; Takeyoshi, I.; et al. Mycophenolate mofetil prevents transplant arteriosclerosis by direct inhibition of vascular smooth muscle cell proliferation. *Transplantation* **2004**, *77*, 1661–1667. [CrossRef] [PubMed]
176. Eisenga, M.F.; Gomes-Neto, A.W.; Van Londen, M.; Ziengs, A.L.; Douwes, R.M.; Stam, S.P.; Osté, M.C.J.; Knobbe, T.J.; Hessels, N.R.; Buunk, A.M.; et al. Rationale and design of TransplantLines: A prospective cohort study and biobank of solid organ transplant recipients. *BMJ Open* **2018**, *8*, 24502. [CrossRef] [PubMed]

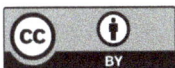

© 2020 by the authors. Licensee MDPI, Basel, Switzerland. This article is an open access article distributed under the terms and conditions of the Creative Commons Attribution (CC BY) license (http://creativecommons.org/licenses/by/4.0/).

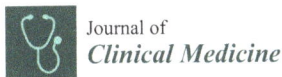

Article

Characteristics and Dysbiosis of the Gut Microbiome in Renal Transplant Recipients

J. Casper Swarte [1,2,*], Rianne M. Douwes [1], Shixian Hu [2,3], Arnau Vich Vila [2,3], Michele F. Eisenga [1], Marco van Londen [1], António W. Gomes-Neto [1], Rinse K. Weersma [2], Hermie J.M. Harmsen [4] and Stephan J.L. Bakker [1]

1. Department of Internal Medicine, Division of Nephrology, University Medical Center Groningen, University of Groningen, 9700RB Groningen, The Netherlands; r.m.douwes@umcg.nl (R.M.D.); m.f.eisenga@umcg.nl (M.F.E.); m.van.londen@umcg.nl (M.v.L.); a.w.gomes.neto@umcg.nl (A.W.G.-N.); s.j.l.bakker@umcg.nl (S.J.L.B.)
2. Department of Gastroenterology and Hepatology, University Medical Center Groningen, University of Groningen, 9700RB Groningen, The Netherlands; s.hu01@umcg.nl (S.H.); a.vich.vila@umcg.nl (A.V.V.); r.k.weersma@umcg.nl (R.K.W.)
3. Department of Genetics, University Medical Center Groningen, University of Groningen, 9700RB Groningen, The Netherlands
4. Department of Medical Microbiology, University Medical Center Groningen, University of Groningen, 9700RB Groningen, The Netherlands; h.j.m.harmsen@umcg.nl
* Correspondence: j.c.swarte@umcg.nl; Tel.: +31-50-3668893

Received: 30 December 2019; Accepted: 28 January 2020; Published: 1 February 2020

Abstract: Renal transplantation is life-changing in many aspects. This includes changes to the gut microbiome likely due to exposure to immunosuppressive drugs and antibiotics. As a consequence, renal transplant recipients (RTRs) might suffer from intestinal dysbiosis. We aimed to investigate the gut microbiome of RTRs and compare it with healthy controls and to identify determinants of the gut microbiome of RTRs. Therefore, RTRs and healthy controls participating in the TransplantLines Biobank and Cohort Study (NCT03272841) were included. We analyzed the gut microbiome using 16S rRNA sequencing and compared the composition of the gut microbiome of RTRs to healthy controls using multivariate association with linear models (MaAsLin). Fecal samples of 139 RTRs (50% male, mean age: 58.3 ± 12.8 years) and 105 healthy controls (57% male, mean age: 59.2 ± 10.6 years) were collected. Median time after transplantation of RTRs was 6.0 (1.5–12.5)years. The microbiome composition of RTRs was significantly different from that of healthy controls, and RTRs had a lower diversity of the gut microbiome ($p < 0.01$). Proton-pump inhibitors, mycophenolate mofetil, and estimated glomerular filtration rate (eGFR) are significant determinants of the gut microbiome of RTRs ($p < 0.05$). Use of mycophenolate mofetil correlated to a lower diversity ($p < 0.01$). Moreover, significant alterations were found in multiple bacterial taxa between RTRs and healthy controls. The gut microbiome of RTRs contained more Proteobacteria and less Actinobacteria, and there was a loss of butyrate-producing bacteria in the gut microbiome of RTRs. By comparing the gut microbiome of RTRs to healthy controls we have shown that RTRs suffer from dysbiosis, a disruption in the balance of the gut microbiome.

Keywords: gut microbiome; renal transplant recipient; diarrhea; immunosuppressive medication; gut microbiota; kidney transplantation; 16S rRNA sequencing; butyrate-producing bacteria; Proteobacteria

1. Introduction

It is becoming increasingly evident that the gut microbiome plays a role in various diseases such as inflammatory bowel disease, diabetes, autoimmune diseases, and cancer [1]. However, less is known about the role of the gut microbiome in the field of renal transplantation. Renal transplantation is the best available treatment for patients with end-stage renal disease (ESRD). Despite improved prognosis and quality of life (QoL) compared to dialysis treatment, renal transplant recipients (RTRs) suffer from many problems in the years after transplantation. After transplantation one out of five RTRs suffers from chronic diarrhea which is associated with a lower QoL, increased abdominal complaints, higher mortality, and gut dysbiosis [2–4]. Furthermore, all RTRs use immunosuppressive drugs and frequently require antibiotics which potentially influence the gut microbiome [5]. Chronic diarrhea and the use of immunosuppressive drugs may change the gut microbiota composition. As a consequence, this can disrupt gut homeostasis leading to a disruption in the balance of the gut microbiome called dysbiosis. This has previously been reported in mice studies. The introduction of prednisolone and tacrolimus to mice resulted in dysbiosis, an overgrowth of *Escherichia coli*, and an increased colonization with opportunistic pathogens [6]. However, the gut microbiome of RTRs has not been studied extensively.

In previous studies among allogenic stem cell transplant recipients and RTRs, a lower diversity of the gut microbiome was observed [7,8]. Furthermore, this lower diversity of the gut microbiome in allogenic stem cell recipients was associated with a higher risk of mortality [9]. In addition, Annavajhala et al. demonstrated that liver transplant recipients with a lower gut microbiome diversity have a higher risk of colonization by multidrug-resistant bacteria [10]. These studies show that the gut microbiome is clinically relevant in the field of transplantation. However, the role of the gut microbiome in renal transplantation has not been adequately studied. Characterization of the gut microbiome in the first three months after renal transplantation showed significant changes in the composition of the gut microbiome and showed that diarrhea was associated with dysbiosis and a loss of diversity [8]. It is currently unknown whether dysbiosis of the gut microbiome remains prevalent more than one year after transplantation and which factors are determinants of the gut microbiota composition in RTRs. The aim of this study was to characterize the gut microbiome of RTRs for at least more than one year post-transplantation. We compared the composition of the gut microbiome between RTRs and healthy controls and identified determinants of the gut microbiome of RTRs.

2. Experimental Section

2.1. Study Population

We included 139 RTRs who were at least one year post-transplantation and 105 healthy donors from the TransplantLines Biobank and Cohort Study (ClinicalTrials.gov Identifier NCT03272841). TransplantLines is a prospective observational cohort study in solid transplant recipients [11]. Donors underwent medical screening in the University Medical Center Groningen (UMCG) and can be considered healthy controls. All participants were included during a study visit at the outpatient clinic of the UMCG between September 2015 and April 2018. RTRs were treated with standard antihypertensive and immunosuppressive therapy. The research protocol of the TransplantLines study was approved by the independent medical ethics committee of UMCG (METC 2014/077) and was performed in adherence to the Declaration of Helsinki and the Declaration of Istanbul. All subjects provided a written informed consent.

2.2. Patient Characteristics

All measurements were performed during a study visit at the outpatient clinic. Weight, length, and waist and hip circumference were measured in duplicate. Body fat percentage was measured using the multifrequency bioelectrical impedance device (BIA, Quadscan 4000, Bodystat, Douglas, British Isles). Blood pressure was measured by qualified nurses according to a standard clinical protocol as described previously [11]. Hypertension was classified as a mean systolic pressure >140 mm Hg, and/or a mean diastolic pressure >90 mm Hg and/or use of antihypertensive medication. Diabetes mellitus was defined according to the guidelines of the American Diabetes Association [12]. Estimated glomerular filtration rate (eGFR) was calculated using the serum creatinine-based chronic kidney disease epidemiology collaboration (CKD-EPI) formula. Proteinuria was defined as urinary protein excretion >0.5 g per 24 h. Glucose and hemoglobin A1c (HbA1c) were determined using standard laboratory methods. Smoking status was recorded using a questionnaire. Medication use was retrieved from medical records and verified with patients during study visits. The study design is described in detail in the TransplantLines design paper [11].

2.3. Sample Collection

Blood samples were collected after an overnight fasting period of 8–12 h and stored at −80 °C. Participants were instructed to collect a fecal sample the day prior to the study visit at home and store the sample on ice. Upon arrival at the UMCG the fecal samples were immediately stored at −80 °C. Participants also collected 24-hour urine samples the day prior to the study visit.

2.4. DNA Extraction and 16S rRNA Sequencing

Deoxyribonucleic acid (DNA) was extracted from 0.25 g feces [13]. The genes for the 16S rRNA V4 and V5 region were amplified by polymerase chain reaction (PCR) using the TaKaRa Taq Hot start version kit (TaKaRa Bio Inc., Kusatsu, Japan). We used the 341F and 806R primers containing a 6-nucleotide Illumina-MiSeq adapter sequence. The PCR product was purified with AMPure XP beads (Beckman Coulter, USA). DNA concentrations were measured with Qubit 2.0 Fluorometer to ensure equal library presentation for each sample, dilutions were made accordingly [14]. The normalized DNA library was sequenced using the MiSeq Benchtop Sequencer.

2.5. Microbiome Profiling

Bacterial taxonomy was assigned using PAired-eND Assembler for DNA sequences (PANDAseq), Quantitative Insights Into Microbial Ecology (QIIME), and ARB [15–17]. QIIME was used to assign taxonomy to the phylum, class, order, family, and genus level. ARB was used to assign taxonomy to the species level. As previously described, PANDAseq was used to increase the quality of sequence reads. Readouts with at quality score lower than 0.9 were discarded according to the protocol followed by Heida et al. [14].

2.6. Statistical Analyses

Data are presented as mean ± standard deviation (SD) for normally distributed data and median with interquartile range (IQR) for non-normally distributed data. Differences between baseline characteristics of RTRs and healthy controls were tested using a t-test or a Mann–Whitney u-test.

Sample richness/evenness was estimated using the Shannon index using QIIME. The microbial dissimilarities matrix (Bray–Curtis) was obtained using *vegdist* from the *vegan* R-package [18]. Principal coordinates were constructed and plotted with the *cmdscale* function. We used permutational multivariate analysis of variance using distance matrices (ADONIS) to analyze the variance in the Bray–Curtis matrix that could be explained by metadata such as age, sex, body mass index (BMI), fat percentage, smoking, eGFR, and medication. Pearson correlation was used to correlate metadata to the Shannon diversity index. *p*-values <0.01 were considered statistically significant.

Multivariate analysis by linear models (MaAsLin) is a tool to find associations between clinical metadata and bacterial abundance. We used MaAsLin to find associations between microbiome data and clinical phenotype. MaAsLin performs a boosted, additive general linear model between metadata and microbial abundance [19]. Covariates including sex, body mass index (BMI), smoking, use of antihypertensive medication, use of antibiotics, use of statins, use of proton-pump inhibitor (PPI), and read depth were forced into the model. These covariates are known to influence the gut microbiome [20]. All *p*-values were corrected for multiple testing using false discovery rate (FDR). $p_{FDR} < 0.10$ was considered statistically significant for taxonomic analysis.

3. Results

3.1. Baseline Characteristics

We included 139 RTRs (age 58.3 ± 12.8 years; 50% males) at a median post-transplantation time of 6.0 (1.5–12.5) years and 105 healthy controls (age 59.2 ± 10.6 years; 57% males). Mean BMI was 27.7 ± 5.4 kg/m² for RTRs and 27.2 ± 6.0 kg/m² for controls. In total 3 (3%) healthy controls and 38 (27%) RTRs had diabetes mellitus ($p < 0.001$). RTRs had a significantly higher HbA1c, 40.0 (37.0–46.0) compared to healthy controls, 37.5 (36.0–40.0) ($p < 0.001$). RTRs had a significantly lower eGFR of 48.3 ± 16.7 mL/min/1.73 m² compared with 69.0 ± 19.2 mL/min/1.73 m² for controls ($p < 0.001$). In total 7 (5%) RTRs used antibiotics, 115 (83%) RTRs used antihypertensive medication, 96 (69%) RTRs used PPIs, and 66 (47%) RTRs used statins. Cyclosporine was used by 25 (18%) RTRs, tacrolimus by 79 (57%) RTRs, azathioprine was used by 13 (9%) RTRs, mycophenolate mofetil by 100 (72%) RTRs, and prednisolone by 133 (96%) RTRs (Table 1).

Table 1. Baseline characteristics of renal transplant recipients (RTRs) and controls.

Demographics	Control	RTRs	p-Value
Number of Subjects, n (%)	105	139	-
Age (years)	59.2 ± 10.6	58.3 ± 12.8	0.96
Male, n (%)	60 (57)	69 (50)	0.24
BMI (kg/m²)	27.2 ± 6.0	27.7 ± 5.4	0.60
Diabetes Mellitus, n (%)	3 (3)	38 (27)	<0.001
Hypertension, n (%)	10 (10)	115 (83)	<0.001
Smoking, n (%)	-	12 (9)	-
Years since Transplantation, Median (IQR)	-	6.0 (1.5–12.5)	-
Cardiovascular Parameters			
Glucose, mmol/L, Median (IQR)	5.4 (4.0–5.9)	5.4 (4.9–6.2)	0.06
HbA1c, mmol/L, Median (IQR)	37.5 (36.0–40.0)	40.0 (37.0–46.0)	<0.001
Systolic Blood Pressure (mmHg)	130.4 ± 14.2	136.5 ± 17.7	0.02
Diastolic Blood Pressure (mmHg)	75.8 ± 9.4	78.5 ± 9.6	0.03
Heart Frequency (bpm)	69.7 ± 25.8	72.1 ± 13.1	0.02
Renal Function Parameters			
Serum Creatinine (μmol/L)	97.3 ± 22.1	133.1 ± 42.6	<0.001
eGFR (mL/min/1.73 m²)	69.0 ± 19.2	48.3 ± 16.7	<0.001
Proteinuria (0.5 g/24 h), n (%)	0 (0)	11 (7.9)	-
Medication, n (%)			
Antibiotics (n = 1)	0 (0)	7 (5)	-
Antihypertensive Agents (n = 8)	10 (10)	115 (83)	<0.001
Proton-pump Inhibitors	8 (8)	96 (69)	<0.001
Statins	8 (8)	66 (47)	<0.001
Cyclosporine	-	25 (18)	-
Tacrolimus	-	79 (57)	-
Azathioprine	-	13 (9)	-
Mycophenolate mofetil	-	100 (72)	-
Prednisolone	-	133 (96)	-

All characteristics are presented as means ± standard deviation unless otherwise stated. IQR—interquartile range.

3.2. Diversity of the Gut Microbiome

The median Shannon diversity index, a measure for the diversity of the gut microbiome, was significantly lower in RTR samples with 3.4 (3.1–3.8) vs. 3.7 (3.5–4.0) for healthy controls ($p < 0.001$). The median operational taxonomic units (OTUs) per sample was 256 (214–304) for RTRs and 314 (260–351) for healthy controls ($p < 0.001$) (Figure 1). The diversity between samples was further assessed using beta diversity analysis. The gut microbiome was significantly different between RTRs and healthy controls ($p < 0.01$). A separation in gut microbiota composition can be observed between RTRs and healthy controls in the principal coordinate plot (Figure 2). A permutational multivariate analysis of variance using distance matrices (ADONIS) was performed to estimate the variation explained in the gut microbiome by different variables. In total, 5.8% of the variation of the gut microbiome of RTRs and healthy controls was significantly explained by sample type (RTR or healthy control, $p < 0.001$). Furthermore, using ADONIS, baseline characteristics including medication use were tested in the gut microbiome of RTRs. Within the gut microbiome of RTRs age (1.2%), BMI (1.1%), and eGFR (1.0%) significantly explained variation within the gut microbiome. Furthermore, the use of PPIs (1.2%) and the use of mycophenolate mofetil (1.0%) significantly explained variation within the gut microbiome of RTRs. Age was positively correlated to the Shannon diversity index ($p < 0.01$). Use of mycophenolate mofetil and use of antibiotics was negatively correlated to the Shannon diversity index ($p < 0.01$) (Figure 3).

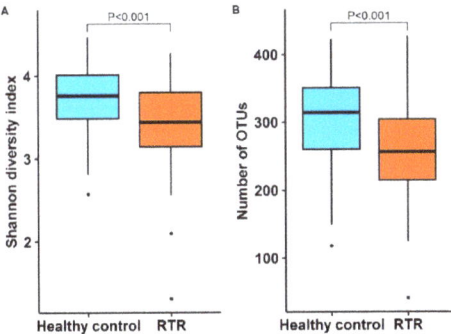

Figure 1. This is a figure showing the diversity of the gut microbiome of renal transplant recipients (RTRs) compared to healthy controls: (**A**) a boxplot depicting the Shannon diversity index, which is a measure for the diversity of the gut microbiome, was significantly lower in RTRs compared to healthy controls ($p < 0.001$); (**B**) a boxplot showing the number of observed operation taxonomic units (OTUs) between RTRs and healthy controls ($p < 0.001$).

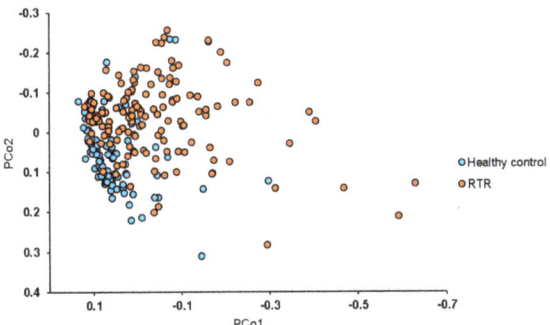

Figure 2. Principal coordinate analysis of 139 RTRs and 105 healthy controls. The principal coordinates plot shows principal coordinates for the Bray–Curtis distance, a measure for the composition of the gut microbiome, for RTRs and healthy controls. Separation in the composition of the gut microbiome between RTRs and healthy controls can be observed. PCo1 is principal coordinate 1 and PCo2 is principal coordinate 2. The gut microbiome of RTRs is significantly different from that of healthy controls in the first coordinate (PCo1 vs. PCo2: $p < 0.01$). RTR or healthy control status significantly explained 5.8% of variation in the gut microbiome ($p < 0.001$).

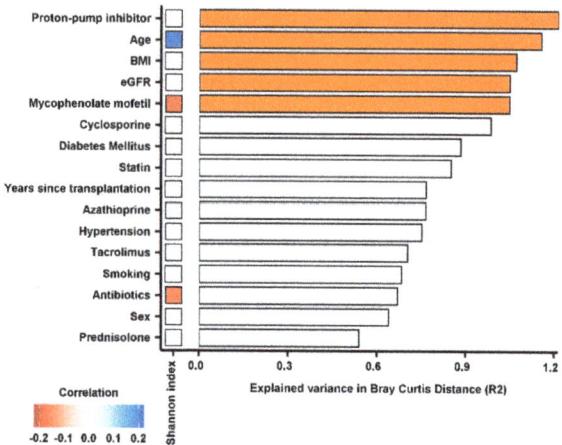

Figure 3. Depiction of variables that are associated with variation in the gut microbiome within RTRs. In the bar plots, the x-axis represents the percentage of explained variance in the gut microbiome of RTRs expressed as the Bray–Curtis distance. The heatmap depicts significant negative correlations (red) and positive correlations (blue) with the Shannon diversity index ($p < 0.01$). These variables were tested only in the gut microbiome of RTRs. Bars in orange represent variables which significantly explain variance in gut microbiota composition ($p < 0.05$).

3.3. Composition of the Gut Microbiome

We analyzed the gut microbiome at different taxonomic levels: phylum, class, order, family, genus, and species. Using MaAsLin, we were able to identify significant differences in taxa abundances between RTRs and healthy controls while correcting for age, sex, BMI, smoking, use of antihypertensive medication, use of antibiotics, use of statins, use of PPIs, and read depth. In total, we found significant alterations in 127 of the 447 bacterial taxa abundances in the gut microbiome of RTRs ($p_{FDR} < 0.10$) (Table 2). On the phylum level we found that RTRs have significantly higher levels of Proteobacteria and lower levels of Actinobacteria ($p_{FDR} < 0.10$) (Figure 4). Within the phylum Proteobacteria, the species *E. coli* was significantly more abundant in the gut microbiome of RTRs ($p_{FDR} < 0.10$). Within the phylum Actinobacteria multiple species had a lower abundance within the gut microbiome of RTRs, especially multiple *Bifidobacterium* species ($p_{FDR} < 0.10$). The predominant phylum Firmicutes was not significantly different in RTRs compared to healthy controls. However, within the phylum Firmicutes there were many significantly different species in the gut microbiome of RTRs compared to healthy controls (Figure 4 and Table S1). An extensive overview of MaAsLin results for complete taxonomy is provided in Table S1.

Table 2. Overview of significantly altered taxa between renal transplant recipients and healthy controls.

Taxonomic Level	Total Number of Taxa [1]	Number of Significant Taxa [2]
Phylum	6	2
Class	17	5
Order	31	8
Family	60	18
Genus	123	27
Species	205	63
Total	442	123

[1] Total number of taxa with an abundance >0.1%; [2] $p_{FDR} < 0.10$.

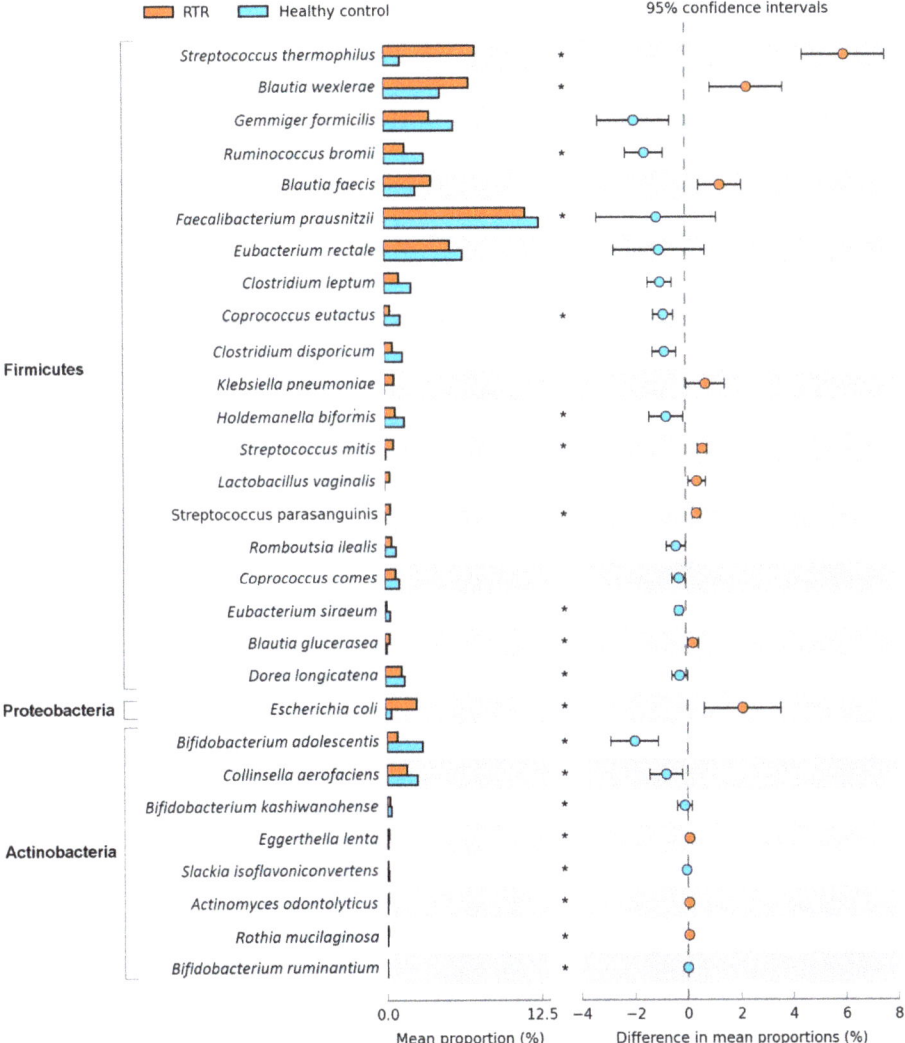

Figure 4. This figure depicts the abundance of phyla and species for RTRs and healthy controls. Bar plots represent the mean proportion and differences in mean proportions with 95% confidence intervals are depicted on the right. Taxa that are depicted were filtered for a difference in mean proportion >0.2%. $p_{FDR} < 0.10$ was considered as statistically significant and indicated in the plot with a star (*).

4. Discussion

We have shown that the gut microbiome of RTRs is different compared to the gut microbiome of healthy controls. Interestingly, we demonstrated that RTRs have dysbiosis characterized by general loss of microbial diversity. We found that RTRs have an increased abundance of Proteobacteria, a decrease in Actinobacteria, and a loss of butyrate-producing bacteria. Finally, we found that age, BMI, eGFR, the use of PPIs, and the use of mycophenolate mofetil are determinants of the gut microbiome of RTRs and that age, BMI, and the use of mycophenolate mofetil correlate to the diversity of the gut microbiome.

In a pilot study of Lee et al., significant changes were seen in the gut microbiome of RTRs when pre-transplantation samples were compared to post-transplantation samples. The diversity, although not significant, was lower after transplantation. Proteobacteria and Enterobacteriales were increased in the gut microbiome post-transplantation [8]. We observed a significant loss of diversity in the composition of the gut microbiome in RTRs with a similar increase in Proteobacteria. It is known that a lower diversity is associated with various diseases such as inflammatory bowel disease (IBD), metabolic disease and cardiovascular disease, as stated by the Human Microbiome Consortium [21]. Previous research in a cohort of allogeneic hematopoietic stem cell transplantation (allo-HSCT) recipients demonstrated that a lower diversity of the gut microbiome was associated with a higher mortality risk [9]. Additionally, allo-HSCT recipients who were deceased had a higher level of Gammaproteobacteria, Enterobacteriales, and Enterobacteriaceae [7]. These findings are strikingly similar to the results of our study. We also observed a lower diversity and higher levels of Proteobacteria, Gammaproteobacteria, Enterobacteriaceae, *Escherichia*, *Streptococcus*, and *Lactobacillus* in the gut microbiome of RTRs. However, it is unknown whether these changes in the composition of the gut microbiome are associated with mortality in RTRs.

The lower diversity observed in the gut microbiome of RTRs suggest that RTRs suffer from dysbiosis. We found increased levels of Proteobacteria which has previously been proposed as a marker for dysbiosis in the gut microbiome [22]. Furthermore, we observed a loss of butyrate-producing bacteria in RTRs. Butyrate is a short-chain fatty acid (SCFA) that plays a key role in maintaining gut health. Butyrate is associated with trans-epithelial fluid transport, reduction of inflammation and oxidative stress, reinforcement of the epithelial barrier, and has potential protective properties against colorectal cancer [23]. In this study, lower levels of *Faecalibacterium prausnitzii*, *Gemmiger formicilis*, *Eubacterium rectale*, *Coprococcus catus*, *Coprococcus comes* and *Roseburia* were observed in the gut microbiome of RTRs. These are all well-known butyrate-producing bacteria [24]. The decrease of butyrate production in RTRs could be detrimental to their gut health. Furthermore, animal studies show that butyrate has immunomodulatory properties through the effect on regulatory T-cells (Treg), which in turn plays a key role in suppressing inflammatory responses. Increasing butyrate in the gut improved renal dysfunction and reduced local and systemic inflammation in mice [25,26]. These results have also been observed in allogeneic bone marrow transplant recipients. Reduced butyrate altered gene regulation and resulted in fewer Treg cells. Restoring butyrate levels led to improved junction integrity, decreased apoptosis, and improved graft versus host disease [27]. Dysbiosis and a loss of butyrate-producing bacteria in the gut microbiome of RTRs could therefore have detrimental effects on gut health. Further research is needed to study the clinical consequences of the loss of butyrate-producing bacteria in RTRs.

In another study of Lee et al., a loss of diversity and a loss of butyrate-producing bacteria was also observed in RTRs with post-transplantation diarrhea. In this study, post-transplantation diarrhea was not associated with common infectious diarrheal pathogens but rather with dysbiosis [4]. RTRs had lower levels of *Ruminococcus*, *Coprococcus*, and *Dorea* in this study. These findings are in accordance with results from our study, which also demonstrated lower levels of *Ruminococcus* in the microbiome of RTRs. However, we did not observe higher levels of *Coprococcus* and *Dorea* in RTRs. One reason for this might be that we included patients more than one year after transplantation while Lee et al. included patients within the first year after transplantation. In addition, we corrected for various factors that influence the composition of the gut microbiome, which was not done in the study by Lee et al. [8].

We found many significant differences in taxa abundance in RTRs compared to healthy controls. Some of these differences in the composition of the gut microbiome might indicate that RTRs suffer from increased inflammation in the gut. For example, the abundance of Proteobacteria was much higher in RTRs compared to healthy controls. This was also observed in patients with severe intestinal inflammation and inflammatory bowel disease (IBD), colorectal cancer, necrotizing enterocolitis, and irritable bowel syndrome (IBS) [28]. Increased oxygen availability in the gut colonocytes could explain these findings, since it is associated with inflammation in the gut and drives the expansion of aerobic Proteobacteria, Enterobacteriaceae, and *E. coli* while lowering the levels of anaerobic bacteria such as *Bifidobacterium* and butyrate-producing bacteria [22,28]. In this study, RTRs indeed had an increased abundance of Proteobacteria, Enterobacteriaceae, and *E. coli*, and lower levels of Clostridia and Bifidobacteria. These similarities in the gut microbiome composition of RTRs and IBD patients suggest that RTRs may be suffering from inflammation in the gut, which could lead to a loss of epithelial barrier function and diarrhea [29].

In this study, we showed that use of PPIs and mycophenolate mofetil was associated with variation within the gut microbiome of RTR. Imhann et al. demonstrated that the use of PPIs changes the gut microbiome, especially an increase of *Streptococcus* species was found in PPI users [30]. We found multiple *Streptococcus* species that had a higher abundance in the gut microbiome of RTRs. This could be due to the use of PPIs. The influence of immunosuppressive medication on the gut microbiome is not yet well studied in RTRs. In a previous murine study, prednisolone, tacrolimus, and mycophenolate mofetil changed the gut microbiome [6]. Mycophenolate mofetil has multiple side effects including diarrhea [31]. In our study, the use of mycophenolate mofetil was significantly correlated to a lower diversity of the gut microbiome. A lower diversity of the gut microbiome is more prevalent in less healthy individuals. More research is needed to investigate the interplay between the use of mycophenolate mofetil, the gut microbiome, and clinical outcomes.

Improving the observed dysbiotic state of RTRs might have clinical implications concerning long-term outcome after renal transplantation. Important issues are that many RTRs suffer from cognitive decline and development of skin cancer [32,33]. Dysbiosis might contribute to cognitive decline due to an effect of the gut microbiome on the gut–brain axis [34]. The same mechanism might apply to the occurrence of skin cancer, due to an effect of the gut microbiome on the gut–skin axis [33,35]. Improving the dysbiotic state of the gut microbiome in RTRs may therefore be a modifiable factor that allows for inhibition of cognitive decline and skin cancer after renal transplantation. Changing the diet of RTRs might be an intervention that allows for improvement of the gut dysbiosis of RTRs. Diet has been identified as an important potentially modifiable factor influencing the gut microbiome [20]. After transplantation, many RTRs adhere to the diet that was prescribed prior to transplantation [36]. This diet includes a protein restriction, which is meant to limit and prevent uremic symptoms and progression of decline of renal function [37]. It also includes a phosphorus restriction to prevent hypophosphatemia, and a potassium restriction to prevent occurrence of hyperkaliemia, cardiac arrhythmias, and acute cardiac death [37]. Improving diet and eating habits may have a positive effect on the composition of the gut microbiome, which could ultimately translate into a beneficial effect on cognitive function [38]. Future, larger cohort studies could focus on the influence of diet on the gut microbiome in RTRs, and on potential sex differences therein. Potential sex differences in the gut microbiome might be of interest, but cohorts to allow for determining those likely need to be large, because previously reported sex differences in the gut microbiome are small [20,39].

We showed that there are many differences in the gut microbiome of RTRs compared to healthy controls. However, the current study should be interpreted within its limitations. The main indication for renal transplantation is chronic kidney disease (CKD). Alterations in the gut microbiome of patients with CKD are already present before transplantation. Patients with CKD also suffer from a lower diversity of the gut microbiome and dysbiosis. A lower colonization by Bifidobacteria and an increase in Enterobacteriaceae was observed in patients with CKD [26]. These findings are similar to our findings which suggest that the dysbiosis observed in RTRs may already be present pre-transplantation and does not recover post-transplantation [8]. Moreover, we measured the composition of the gut microbiome using 16S rRNA sequencing instead of metagenomic sequencing. Therefore, we were unable to analyze metabolic pathways of bacteria. Furthermore, SCFA were not measured in the current study. Therefore, it remains unknown whether the observed loss of butyrate-producing bacteria also leads to a decreased production of butyrate. Future studies should include pre-transplantation patients and study how the gut microbiome develops after transplantation. Focus should be on the metagenome of RTRs to study the effects of dysbiosis, the metabolism genes, and metabolites. Furthermore, current studies of the gut microbiome mainly focus on bacteria. However, at the kingdom level of the gut microbiome, there are many more micro-organisms such as archaea, fungi, eukaryotes, as well as viruses which could also play an important role in the gut microbiome of immunosuppressed patients [40].

In conclusion, the gut microbiome of RTRs more than one year post-transplantation is significantly different from that of healthy controls. The gut microbiome of RTRs contains more Proteobacteria and less Actinobacteria and there is a loss of butyrate-producing bacteria which could be detrimental to gut health. The use of mycophenolate mofetil and antibiotics is associated with variation in the gut microbiome of RTRs and correlated to a lower diversity. The results of this study are preliminary and require replication in a larger cohort. Nevertheless, we demonstrate that RTRs suffer from dysbiosis more than one year post-transplantation and that the use of mycophenolate mofetil correlates to a lower diversity.

Supplementary Materials: The following are available online at http://www.mdpi.com/2077-0383/9/2/386/s1, Table S1: MaAsLin results for RTRs compared to healthy controls.

Author Contributions: Conceptualization, J.C.S., H.J.M.H., and S.J.L.B.; data curation, J.C.S., M.F.E., M.v.L., and A.W.G.-N.; formal analysis, J.C.S., S.H., and S.J.L.B.; investigation, J.C.S.; methodology, J.C.S., S.H., A.V.V., H.J.M.H., and S.J.L.B.; resources, H.J.M.H. and S.J.L.B.; software, J.C.S. and S.H.; supervision, R.K.W., H.J.M.H., and S.J.L.B.; writing—original draft, J.C.S.; writing—review and editing, J.C.S., R.M.D., S.H., M.F.E., A.V.V., M.v.L., A.W.G.-N., R.K.W., H.J.M.H., and S.J.L.B. All authors have read and agreed to the published version of the manuscript.

Funding: R.M. Douwes is supported by NWO/TTW in a partnership program with DSM, Animal Nutrition and Health, The Netherlands; grant number: 14939.

Acknowledgments: The authors thank Rebekka van den Bosch, Rudi Tonk, Carien Bus-Spoor, and Ranko Gacesa for technical assistance.

Conflicts of Interest: The authors declare no conflict of interest.

References

1. Thursby, E.; Juge, N. Introduction to the human gut microbiota. *Biochem. J.* **2017**, *474*, 1823–1836. [CrossRef]
2. Ekberg, H.; Kyllönen, L.; Madsen, S.; Grave, G.; Solbu, D.; Holdaas, H. Clinicians underestimate gastrointestinal symptoms and overestimate quality of life in renal transplant recipients: A multinational survey of nephrologists. *Transplantation* **2007**, *84*, 1052–1054. [CrossRef] [PubMed]
3. Bunnapradist, S.; Neri, L.; Wong, W.; Lentine, K.L.; Burroughs, T.E.; Pinsky, B.W.; Takemoto, S.K.; Schnitzler, M.A. Incidence and Risk Factors for Diarrhea Following Kidney Transplantation and Association with Graft Loss and Mortality. *Am. J. Kidney Dis.* **2008**, *51*, 478–486. [CrossRef] [PubMed]
4. Lee, J.R.; Magruder, M.; Zhang, L.; Westblade, L.F.; Satlin, M.J.; Robertson, A.; Edusei, E.; Crawford, C.; Ling, L.; Taur, Y.; et al. Gut microbiota dysbiosis and diarrhea in kidney transplant recipients. *Am. J. Transplant.* **2019**, *19*, 488–500. [CrossRef] [PubMed]
5. Zimmermann, M.; Zimmermann-Kogadeeva, M.; Wegmann, R.; Goodman, A.L. Mapping human microbiome drug metabolism by gut bacteria and their genes. *Nature* **2019**, *570*, 462–467. [CrossRef] [PubMed]
6. Tourret, J.; Willing, B.P.; Dion, S.; MacPherson, J.; Denamur, E.; Finlay, B.B. Immunosuppressive treatment alters secretion of ileal antimicrobial peptides and gut microbiota, and favors subsequent colonization by uropathogenic Escherichia coli. *Transplantation* **2017**, *101*, 74–82. [CrossRef] [PubMed]
7. Taur, Y.; Jenq, R.R.; Perales, M.A.; Littmann, E.R.; Morjaria, S.; Ling, L.; No, D.; Gobourne, A.; Viale, A.; Dahi, P.B.; et al. The effects of intestinal tract bacterial diversity on mortality following allogeneic hematopoietic stem cell transplantation. *Blood* **2014**, *124*, 1174–1182. [CrossRef] [PubMed]
8. Lee, J.R.; Muthukumar, T.; Dadhania, D.; Toussaint, N.C.; Ling, L.; Pamer, E.; Suthanthiran, M. Gut microbial community structure and complications after kidney transplantation: A pilot study. *Transplantation* **2014**, *98*, 697–705. [CrossRef]
9. Taur, Y.; Jenq, R.R.; Ubeda, C.; Van Den Brink, M.; Pamer, E.G. Role of intestinal microbiota in transplantation outcomes. *Best Pract. Res. Clin. Haematol.* **2015**, *28*, 155–161. [CrossRef]

10. Annavajhala, M.K.; Gomez-Simmonds, A.; Macesic, N.; Sullivan, S.B.; Kress, A.; Khan, S.D.; Giddins, M.J.; Stump, S.; Kim, G.I.; Narain, R.; et al. Colonizing multidrug-resistant bacteria and the longitudinal evolution of the intestinal microbiome after liver transplantation. *Nat. Commun.* **2019**, *10*, 1–12. [CrossRef]
11. Eisenga, M.F.; Gomes-Neto, A.W.; Van Londen, M.; Ziengs, A.L.; Douwes, R.M.; Stam, S.P.; Osté, M.C.J.; Knobbe, T.J.; Hessels, N.R.; Buunk, A.M.; et al. Rationale and design of TransplantLines: A prospective cohort study and biobank of solid organ transplant recipients. *BMJ Open* **2018**, *8*, 1–13. [CrossRef] [PubMed]
12. Gavin, J.R.; Alberti, K.G.M.M.; Davidson, M.B.; DeFronzo, R.A.; Drash, A.; Gabbe, S.G.; Genuth, S.; Harris, M.I.; Kahn, R.; Keen, H.; et al. Report of the expert committee on the diagnosis and classification of diabetes mellitus. *Diabetes Care* **2002**, *25*, 5–20.
13. De Goffau, M.C.; Luopajärvi, K.; Knip, M.; Ilonen, J.; Ruohtula, T.; Härkönen, T.; Orivuori, L.; Hakala, S.; Welling, G.W.; Harmsen, H.J.; et al. Fecal microbiota composition differs between children with β-cell autoimmunity and those without. *Diabetes* **2013**, *62*, 1238–1244. [CrossRef]
14. Heida, F.H.; Van Zoonen, A.G.J.F.; Hulscher, J.B.F.; Te Kiefte, B.J.C.; Wessels, R.; Kooi, E.M.W.; Bos, A.F.; Harmsen, H.J.M.; De Goffau, M.C. A necrotizing enterocolitis-associated gut microbiota is present in the meconium: Results of a prospective study. *Clin. Infect. Dis.* **2016**, *62*, 863–870. [CrossRef]
15. Caporaso, J.G.; Kuczynski, J.; Stombaugh, J.; Bittinger, K.; Bushman, F.D.; Costello, E.K.; Fierer, N.; Pena, A.G.; Goodrich, J.K.; Gordon, J.I.; et al. QIIME allows analysis of high-throughput community sequencing data. *Nat. Methods* **2011**, *7*, 1–12. [CrossRef] [PubMed]
16. Masella, A.P.; Bartram, A.K.; Truszkowski, J.M.; Brown, D.G.; Neufeld, J.D. PANDAseq: Paired-end assembler for illumina sequences. *BMC Bioinformatics* **2012**, *13*, 31. [CrossRef] [PubMed]
17. Ludwig, W.; Strunk, O.; Westram, R.; Richter, L.; Meier, H.; Yadhukumar, A.; Buchner, A.; Lai, T.; Steppi, S.; Jacob, G.; et al. ARB: A software environment for sequence data. *Nucleic Acids Res.* **2004**, *32*, 1363–1371. [CrossRef] [PubMed]
18. Oksanen, J.; Blanchet, F.G.; Kindt, R.; Legendre, P.; Minchin, P.R.; O'hara, R.B.; Simpson, G.L.; Solymos, P.; Stevens, M.H.H.; Wagner, H. Package 'vegan'. Community Ecology Package. **2018**. Available online: https://cran.ism.ac.jp/web/packages/vegan/vegan.pdf (accessed on 1 February 2020).
19. Morgan, X.C.; Tickle, T.L.; Sokol, H.; Gevers, D.; Devaney, K.L.; Ward, D.V.; Reyes, J.A.; Shah, S.A.; LeLeiko, N.; Snapper, S.B.; et al. Dysfunction of the intestinal microbiome in inflammatory bowel disease and treatment. *Genome Biol.* **2012**, *13*, R79. [CrossRef]
20. Zhernakova, A.; Kurilshikov, A.; Bonder, M.J.; Tigchelaar, E.F.; Schirmer, M.; Vatanen, T.; Mujagic, Z.; Vila, A.V.; Falony, G.; Vieira-Silva, S.; et al. Population-based metagenomics analysis reveals markers for gut microbiome composition and diversity. *Science* **2016**, *352*, 565–569. [CrossRef]
21. Consortium, T.H.M.P. Structure, Function and Diversity of the Healthy Human Microbiome. *Nature* **2013**, *486*, 1049–1058.
22. Shin, N.R.; Whon, T.W.; Bae, J.W. Proteobacteria: Microbial signature of dysbiosis in gut microbiota. *Trends Biotechnol.* **2015**, *33*, 496–503. [CrossRef] [PubMed]
23. Canani, R.B.; Costanzo, M.; Di Leone, L.; Pedata, M.; Meli, R.; Calignano, A. Potential beneficial effects of butyrate in intestinal and extraintestinal diseases. *World J. Gastroenterol.* **2011**, *17*, 1519–1528. [CrossRef]
24. Flint, H.J.; Duncan, S.H.; Scott, K.P.; Louis, P. Links between diet, gut microbiota composition and gut metabolism. *Proc. Nutr. Soc.* **2014**, *760*, 13–22. [CrossRef] [PubMed]
25. Furusawa, Y.; Obata, Y.; Fukuda, S.; Endo, T.A.; Nakato, G.; Takahashi, D.; Nakanishi, Y.; Uetake, C.; Kato, K.; Kato, T.; et al. Commensal microbe-derived butyrate induces the differentiation of colonic regulatory T cells. *Nature* **2013**, *504*, 446–450. [CrossRef]
26. Sampaio-Maia, B.; Simões-Silva, L.; Pestana, M.; Araujo, R.; Soares-Silva, I.J. The Role of the Gut Microbiome on Chronic Kidney Disease. *Adv. Appl. Microbiol.* **2016**, *96*, 65–94. [PubMed]
27. Mathewson, N.D.; Jenq, R.; Mathew, A.V.; Koenigsknecht, M.; Hanash, A.; Toubai, T.; Oravecz-Wilson, K.; Wu, S.R.; Sun, Y.; Rossi, C.; et al. Gut microbiome-derived metabolites modulate intestinal epithelial cell damage and mitigate graft-versus-host disease. *Nat. Immunol.* **2016**, *17*, 505–513. [CrossRef]
28. Litvak, Y.; Byndloss, M.X.; Tsolis, R.M.; Bäumler, A.J. Dysbiotic Proteobacteria expansion: A microbial signature of epithelial dysfunction. *Curr. Opin. Microbiol.* **2017**, *39*, 1–6. [CrossRef]
29. Tang, Y.; Forsyth, C.B.; Keshavarzian, A. New molecular insights into inflammatory bowel disease-induced diarrhea. *Expert Rev. Gastroenterol. Hepatol.* **2011**, *5*, 615–625. [CrossRef]

30. Imhann, F.; Bonder, M.J.; Vila, A.V.; Fu, J.; Mujagic, Z.; Vork, L.; Tigchelaar, E.F.; Jankipersadsing, S.A.; Cenit, M.C.; Harmsen, H.J.M.; et al. Proton pump inhibitors affect the gut microbiome. *Gut* **2016**, *65*, 740–748. [CrossRef]
31. Spasić, A.; Catić-Đorđević, A.; Veličković-Radovanović, R.; Stefanović, N.; Džodić, P.; Cvetković, T. Adverse effects of mycophenolic acid in renal transplant recipients: Gender differences. *Int. J. Clin. Pharm.* **2019**, *41*, 776–784. [CrossRef] [PubMed]
32. Chu, N.M.; Gross, A.L.; Shaffer, A.A.; Haugen, C.E.; Norman, S.P.; Xue, Q.L.; Sharrett, A.R.; Carlson, M.C.; Bandeen-Roche, K.; Segev, D.L.; et al. Frailty and changes in cognitive function after kidney transplantation. *J. Am. Soc. Nephrol.* **2019**, *30*, 336–345. [CrossRef] [PubMed]
33. Pruett, T. Spectrum of Cancer Risk Among US Solid Organ Transplant Recipients. *Yearb. Surg.* **2012**, *2012*, 105–106. [CrossRef]
34. Appleton, J. The gut-brain axis: Influence of microbiota on mood and mental health. *Integr. Med.* **2018**, *17*, 28–32.
35. Salem, I.; Ramser, A.; Isham, N.; Ghannoum, M.A. The gut microbiome as a major regulator of the gut-skin axis. *Front. Microbiol.* **2018**, *9*, 1–14. [CrossRef]
36. Eisenga, M.F.; Kieneker, L.M.; Soedamah-Muthu, S.S.; Van Den Berg, E.; Deetman, P.E.; Navis, G.J.; Gans, R.O.B.; Gaillard, C.A.J.M.; Bakker, S.J.L.; Joosten, M.M. Urinary potassium excretion, renal ammoniagenesis, and risk of graft failure and mortality in renal transplant recipients1-3. *Am. J. Clin. Nutr.* **2016**, *104*, 1703–1711. [CrossRef]
37. Kalantar-Zadeh, K.; Fouque, D. Nutritional management of chronic kidney disease. *N. Engl. J. Med.* **2017**, *377*, 1765–1776. [CrossRef]
38. Novotný, M.; Klimova, B.; Valis, M. Microbiome and cognitive impairment: Can any diets influence learning processes in a positive way? *Front. Aging Neurosci.* **2019**, *11*, 1–7. [CrossRef]
39. de la Cuesta-Zuluaga, J.; Kelley, S.T.; Chen, Y.; Escobar, J.S.; Mueller, N.T.; Ley, R.E.; McDonald, D.; Huang, S.; Swafford, A.D.; Knight, R.; et al. Age- and Sex-Dependent Patterns of Gut Microbial Diversity in Human Adults. *mSystems* **2019**, *4*, 1–12. [CrossRef]
40. Lozupone, C.A.; Stombaugh, J.I.; Gordon, J.I.; Jansson, J.K.; Knight, R. Diversity, stability and resilience of the human gut microbiota. *Nature* **2012**, *489*, 220–230. [CrossRef]

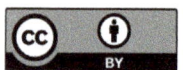

© 2020 by the authors. Licensee MDPI, Basel, Switzerland. This article is an open access article distributed under the terms and conditions of the Creative Commons Attribution (CC BY) license (http://creativecommons.org/licenses/by/4.0/).

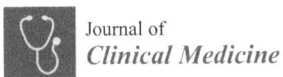

Article

Conversion to Everolimus was Beneficial and Safe for Fast and Slow Tacrolimus Metabolizers after Renal Transplantation

Gerold Thölking [1,2,*], Nils Hendrik Gillhaus [2], Katharina Schütte-Nütgen [2], Hermann Pavenstädt [2], Raphael Koch [3], Barbara Suwelack [2] and Stefan Reuter [2]

1. Department of Internal Medicine and Nephrology, University Hospital of Münster Marienhospital Steinfurt, 48565 Steinfurt, Germany
2. Department of Medicine D, Division of General Internal Medicine, Nephrology and Rheumatology, University Hospital of Münster, 48149 Münster, Germany; nilshendrik.gillhaus@ukmuenster.de (N.H.G.); katharina.schuette-nuetgen@ukmuenster.de (K.S.-N.); hermann.pavenstaedt@ukmuenster.de (H.P.); barbara.suwelack@ukmuenster.de (B.S.); stefan.reuter@ukmuenster.de (S.R.)
3. Institute of Biostatistics and Clinical Research, University of Münster, 48149 Münster, Germany; raphael.koch@ukmuenster.de
* Correspondence: gerold.thoelking@ukmuenster.de; Tel.: +49-2552-791226; Fax: +49-2552-791181

Received: 29 December 2019; Accepted: 20 January 2020; Published: 23 January 2020

Abstract: Fast tacrolimus (TAC) metabolism (concentration/dose (C/D) ratio <1.05 ng/mL/mg) is a risk factor for inferior outcomes after renal transplantation (RTx) as it fosters, e.g., TAC-related nephrotoxicity. TAC minimization or conversion to calcineurin-inhibitor free immunosuppression are strategies to improve graft function. Hence, we hypothesized that especially patients with a low C/D ratio profit from a switch to everolimus (EVR). We analyzed data of 34 RTx recipients (17 patients with a C/D ratio <1.05 ng/mL/mg vs. 17 patients with a C/D ratio ≥1.05 ng/mL/mg) who were converted to EVR within 24 months after RTx. The initial immunosuppression consisted of TAC, mycophenolate, prednisolone, and basiliximab induction. During an observation time of 36 months after changing immunosuppression from TAC to EVR, renal function, laboratory values, and adverse effects were compared between the groups. Fast TAC metabolizers were switched to EVR 4.6 (1.5–21.9) months and slow metabolizers 3.3 (1.8–23.0) months after RTx ($p = 0.838$). Estimated glomerular filtration rate (eGFR) did not differ between the groups at the time of conversion (baseline). Thereafter, the eGFR in all patients increased noticeably (fast metabolizers eGFR 36 months: + 11.0 ± 11.7 ($p = 0.005$); and slow metabolizers eGFR 36 months: + 9.4 ± 15.9 mL/min/1.73 m^2 ($p = 0.049$)) vs. baseline. Adverse events were not different between the groups. After the switch, eGFR values of all patients increased statistically noticeably with a tendency towards a higher increase in fast TAC metabolizers. Since conversion to EVR was safe in a three-year follow-up for slow and fast TAC metabolizers, this could be an option to protect fast metabolizers from TAC-related issues.

Keywords: tacrolimus; C/D ratio; tacrolimus metabolism; everolimus; conversion; kidney transplantation

1. Introduction

Tarolimus (TAC)-based therapy is the recommended immunosuppressive standard therapy after renal transplantation (RTx), although its numerous adverse effects include the development of acute and chronic nephrotoxicity [1]. Unfortunately, TAC has a narrow therapeutic window and a high inter- and intraindividual variable pharmacokinetics, which requires therapeutic drug monitoring (TDM). TAC metabolism is subject to several non-modifiable factors such as age, sex, and CYP3A4/5 genotype of the RTx recipient as well as parameters that may vary, e.g., hematocrit, serum albumin, and steroid doses [2]. In view of the variety of impacting factors, transplant physicians are waiting for a stratification method to identify individuals with a high risk to develop TAC-related adverse effects.

Recently, we and others described a simple and cost-effective tool, the TAC concentration/dose ratio (C/D ratio), to address this problem [3,4]. The C/D ratio is calculated by dividing the TAC trough level by the daily TAC dose. To keep the tool as simple and practical as possible for clinical application, we decided to use only two different C/D ratio categories, although our first approach involved three [4]. A TAC C/D ratio < 1.05 ng/mL/mg assessed three months after RTx indicates fast TAC metabolism, whereas a C/D ratio ≥ 1.05 ng/mL/mg is suggestive of individuals with slow Tac clearance [5]. Using this C/D ratio cut off, we and others showed that the renal function of fast metabolizers is inferior to that of slow metabolizers after RTx and liver transplantation (cut off 1.09 ng/mL/mg), which is due to, e.g., higher incidences of TAC-related nephrotoxicity and rejections [4–10]. This resulted in decreased graft and patient survival [5,7]. In view of the data, modifications of the immunosuppressive regime of patients with a C/D ratio < 1.05 ng/mL/mg should be considered.

The ZEUS study showed that conversion of RTx recipients from calcineurin inhibitor (CNI) to everolimus (EVR) 4.5 months posttransplant is associated with a significant improvement in renal function, which is maintained for at least five years after RTx [11]. Despite increased rates of early mild acute rejections, long-term graft function was not affected in patients who switched to EVR. A positive effect of conversion from CNI to EVR on renal function was even shown for late conversion after RTx (after a mean of 82.6 months) [12]. However, in none of these studies was a C/D ratio-based stratification investigated in this regard.

Due to the negative impact of TAC on the outcomes of fast metabolizers, we hypothesized that these patients, after conversion to EVR, might have greater benefits than slow metabolizers.

2. Patients and Methods

2.1. Patients

This retrospective study included 17 fast metabolizers and 17 slow metabolizers undergoing RTx at the University Hospital of Münster, Germany, between December 2007 and November 2013. The inclusion criteria comprised: age ≥ 18 years of age, intake of immediate release TAC since RTx, and switch from TAC to EVR within 24 months after RTx. All patients received an initial immunosuppression with TAC (Prograf®), mycophenolate mofetil (CellCept®), prednisolone (Decortin H®/Soludecortin H®), and an induction therapy with basiliximab (Simulect®) at Days 0 and 4. TAC target trough levels were 7–12 ng/mL until the end of Month 1, 6–10 ng/mL for Months 2–3, and 3–8 ng/mL subsequently. The starting dose of mycophenolate mofetil 1 g twice a day (b.i.d.) was adjusted in case of adverse effects. Prednisolone was started with 250 mg before and directly after RTx and tapered to a maintenance dosage of 5 mg once daily (q.d.) after six months. The recipient's data were taken from the electronic health records of the hospital information system. Patients were switched from TAC to EVR with a target trough level of 3–8 ng/mL.

Renal function and complications were observed in a 36-month follow-up after conversion to EVR. Renal function was expressed as the estimated glomerular filtration rate (eGFR) calculated by the CKD-EPI formula [13]. Creatinine was analyzed in a whole blood sample (enzymatic assay; Creatinine-Pap, Roche Diagnostics, Mannheim, Germany). Proteinuria was assessed using spot urine. TAC levels were determined using the automated tacrolimus (TACR) assay (Dimension Clinical Chemistry System, Siemens Healthcare Diagnostic GmbH, Eschborn, Germany). EVR levels were measured by LC-MS/MS. Only 12-h TAC and EVR trough levels were used for analysis. Donor-specific antibodies (DSA) were assessed by single beat antigen assay (Luminex).

The C/D ratio was calculated using the following formula:

$$C/D \text{ ratio (ng/mL * 1/mg)} = \frac{\text{blood TAC trough level (ng/mL)}}{\text{daily TAC dose (mg)}} \quad (1)$$

The TAC C/D ratio was calculated one month after RTx and used for grouping [14]. RTx recipients with a C/D ratio <1.05 ng/mL/mg were defined as fast and with a C/D ratio ≥1.05 ng/mL/mg as slow metabolizers.

Histologic results on rejections were obtained only from indication biopsies. All biopsy specimens had been reviewed by two pathologists in the local Institute of Pathology according to the revised Banff criteria [15].

The data of all RTx recipients were anonymized prior to analysis. The study was approved by the local ethics committee (Ethik Kommission der Ärztekammer Westfalen-Lippe und der Medizinischen Fakultät der Westfälischen Wilhelms-Universität, No. 2014-381-f-N). All participants in this study had given written informed consent to record their clinical data and to use it in anonymized analyses at the time of transplantation.

2.2. Statistical Analyses

IBM SPSS Statistics 26 for Windows (IBM Corporation, Somers, NY, USA) were used for statistical analyses of all data. All p-values were two-sided and were intended to be exploratory, not confirmatory. Exploratory p-values ≤0.05 were denoted as statistically noticeable. Absolute and relative frequencies are given for categorical variables. Normally-distributed continuous variables are shown as mean ± standard deviation and not normally-distributed continuous variables as median (minimum–maximum). The corresponding pairwise comparisons between fast and slow metabolizers were performed using Welch's t-tests for normally distributed data, exact Mann–Whitney U tests for skewed distributed continuous variables, and Fisher's exact tests for categorical variables without adjusting for multiple testing. Intra-group changes between two points in time were analyzed using Wilcoxon signed-rank tests for related samples. Boxplots were used for graphical representation.

3. Results

3.1. Descriptive Statistics

Patient characteristics, transplantation data, and immunosuppression after the first month are given in Table 1. Slow metabolizers tended to be older and had a lighter body weight, but all characteristics did not differ noticeably between groups. Fast metabolizers were converted from TAC to EVR after a median of 4.6 (1.5–21.9) months, slow metabolizers 3.3 (1.8–23.0) months after RTx (p = 0.832). Despite similar TAC trough levels after the first month (M1), TAC doses were noticeably higher and C/D ratio values were lower for fast metabolizers than for slow metabolizers (both p < 0.001), due to group classification.

Table 1. Patient characteristics and immunosuppression.

	Fast Metabolizers (n = 17)	Slow Metabolizers (n = 17)	p-Values
Recipient Characteristics			
Sex (m/f)	11 (65%)/6 (35%)	10 (59%)/7 (41%)	1 [a]
Age (year)	48.0 ± 15.7	54.6 ± 12.8	0.187 [b]
Height (cm)	175.0 ± 10.7	171.4 ± 10.2	0.317 [b]
Weight (kg)	79.0 ± 20.6	69.0 ± 11.9	0.095 [b]
BMI (kg/m^2)	24.7 (18.7–35.8)	22.3 (18.9–32.6)	0.114 [c]
Transplant characteristics			
Number of RTx			
1	15 (88%)	13 (77%)	
2	2 (12%)	3 (18%)	0.511 [a]
3	0	1 (6%)	

Table 1. Cont.

	Fast Metabolizers (n = 17)	Slow Metabolizers (n = 17)	p-Values
Transplant characteristics			
Living donor transplantation	6 (35%)	7 (41%)	1 [a]
ABOi	0	2 (12%)	0.485 [a]
ESP	1 (6%)	2 (12%)	1 [a]
CIT (h)	6.8 (1.6–17.4)	5.5 (1.6–19.3)	0.838 [c]
WIT (min)	35 (20–45)	30 (25–50)	0.858 [c]
CMV risk			
Low	6 (35%)	2 (12%)	
Intermediate	7 (41%)	13 (77%)	0.139 [a]
High	4 (24%)	2 (12%)	
Donor characteristics			
Donor sex (m/f)	10 (59%)/7 (41%)	6 (35%)/11 (66%)	0.303 [a]
Donor age (year)	56.8 ± 8.8	57.4 ± 10.9	0.877 [b]
Immunosuppression at M1			
TAC dose (mg)	12 (7–23)	7 (4–12)	<0.001 [c]
TAC trough level (ng/mL)	8.5 (4.6–17.6)	10.0 (5.6–14.1)	0.208 [c]
TAC C/D ratio (ng/mL*1/mg)	0.77 (0.40–1.00)	1.35 (1.05–2.56)	<0.001 [b]
Prednisolone dose (mg)	20 (15–40)	20 (15–50)	0.422 [c]
Mycophenolate mofetil dose (mg)	1000 (750–2000)	1000 (1000–2000)	0.501 [c]

BMI, body mass index; RTx, renal transplantation; ABOi, ABO incompatible transplantation; ESP, European senior program; CIT, cold ischemia time; WIT, warm ischemia time; CMV, cytomegalovirus; TAC, tacrolimus; C/D, concentration/dose. Statistics: Variables are reported as absolute and relative frequencies, mean ± standard deviation or median (minimum–maximum). [a] Fisher's exact test; [b] Welch's t-test; [c] Mann–Whitney U-test.

The main reason for a conversion from TAC to EVR was CNI-nephrotoxicity in both metabolism groups (Table 2).

Table 2. Reasons for the conversion to everolimus.

	Fast Metabolizers (n = 17)	Slow Metabolizers (n = 17)	p-Value
CNI-nephrotoxicity	13 (77%)	10 (59%)	
chronic rejection	0	2 (12%)	
DGF	1 (6%)	2 (12%)	
NODAT	2 (12%)	0	0.277
BKV-infection	0	1 (6%)	
neutropenia	0	1 (6%)	
neurotoxicity	0	1 (6%)	
study	1 (6%)	0	

CNI, calcineurin inhibitor; DGF, delayed graft function; NODAT, new onset diabetes mellitus after transplantation; BKV, BK virus. Statistics: Fisher's exact test.

3.2. Renal Function

The renal function of fast and slow metabolizers was similar ten days after RTx (39.2 ± 19.7 vs. 33.7 ± 22.5 mL/min/1.73 m^2, $p = 0.456$), one month after RTx (39.4 ± 18.8 vs. 34.2 ± 13.5 mL/min/1.73 m^2, $p = 0.367$), and at the time of conversion of TAC to EVR (35.1 ± 15.2 vs. 34.2 ± 13.2 mL/min/1.73 m^2, $p = 0.850$, Figure 1A). Figure 1B provides the renal function at different time points minus the baseline eGFR (eGFR at the time of conversion, Month 0 (M0)). At the end of the follow-up, the eGFR of the fast TAC metabolizers increased considerably by 11.0 ± 11.7 mL/min/1.73 m^2 ($p = 0.005$, Figure 1B) compared to 9.4 ± 15.9 mL/min/1.73 m^2 in slow metabolizers ($p = 0.049$). These changes were not statistically noticeably different between both groups ($p = 0.691$), but more homogenous in fast metabolizers.

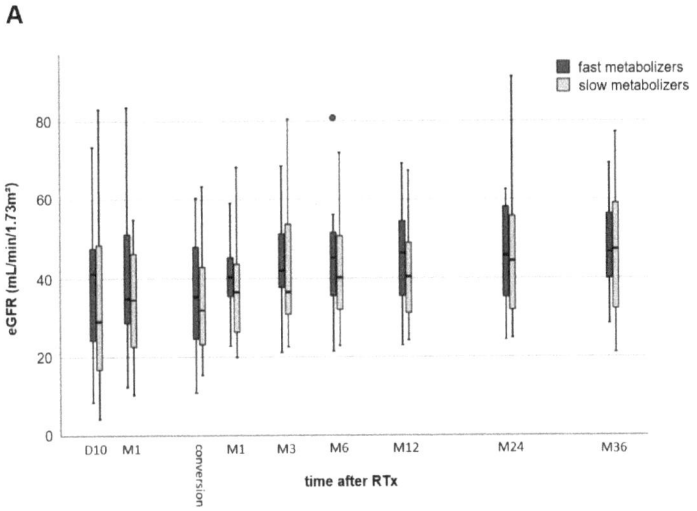

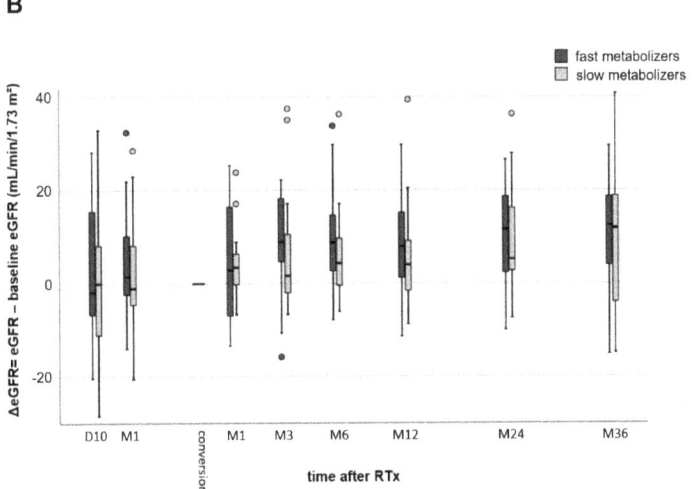

Figure 1. Comparison of renal function (eGFR values) of fast and slow TAC metabolizers. Both groups showed a considerable increase in renal function from Day 10 after kidney transplantation to 36 months after conversion from TAC to EVR (no differences between the groups) (**A**). Comparison of eGFR values to baseline eGFR (time of conversion from TAC to EVR) (**B**). Thirty-six months after transplantation, renal function of slow metabolizers showed a noticeable increase ($p = 0.049$), while fast metabolizers a highly noticeable increase ($p = 0.005$).

3.3. Adverse Events

The median proteinuria value of fast metabolizers was 193 (19–665) mg/g creatinine at M1 after RTx and 361 (97–831) mg/g creatinine at M6 (maximum values) after conversion (Figure 2). The proteinuria in slow metabolizers was 218 (137–664) mg/g creatinine at M1 after RTx and 344 (167–665) mg/g creatinine at M6 (maximum values). At M36, proteinuria had declined to the baseline values without difference between the groups at all time points.

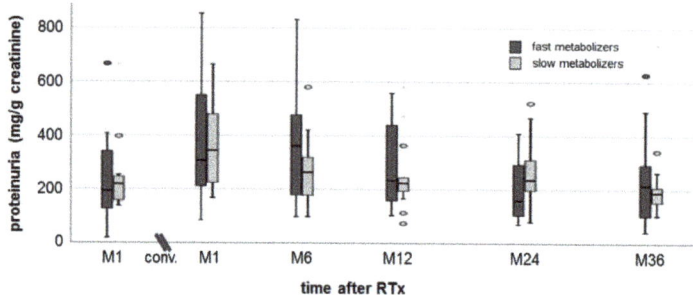

Figure 2. Proteinuria. There was a slight increase in proteinuria in both groups from M1 after RTx to M1 after conversion. At a follow-up of 36 months post-conversion, proteinuria recovered to values measured at M1 after RTx.

Table 3 shows the adverse events before and after conversion to EVR. There was no graft loss and no differences in outcomes such as delayed graft function (DGF) or overall survival between the groups. The DSA number in all patient groups before and after conversion was low and did not change noticeably. Although it was 9 vs. 6 biopsy-proven acute rejection (BPAR) cases in fast vs. slow metabolizers before conversion to EVR, BPAR rates were considerably lower during follow-up (two episodes (12%) in fast metabolizers and one episode (6%) in slow metabolizer) than before conversion. Cytomegalovirus (CMV) and BK virus (BKV) infections did not occur at different frequencies in fast or slow TAC metabolizers and were uncommon after conversion to EVR.

Table 3. Adverse events.

	Fast Metabolizers ($n = 17$)	Slow Metabolizers ($n = 17$)	p-Value
DGF	4 (24%)	5 (29%)	1 [a]
Antibodies and rejection			
Preformed Class II DSA	1 (6%)	1 (6%)	1 [a]
Class II DSA before conversion	1 (6%)	1 (6%)	1 [a]
Class I DSA after conversion	1 (6%)	0	1 [a]
BPAR before conversion to EVR			
AMR	1 (6%)	1 (6%)	
TCMR	1 (6%)	2 (12%)	0.490 [b]
Combined AMR + TCMR	7 (41%)	3 (18%)	
BPAR after conversion to EVR			
AMR	0	0	
TCMR	2 (12%)	0	0.485 [a]
Combined AMR + TCMR	0	1 (6%)	
Infections			
CMV infection before conversion	2 (12%)	4 (24%)	0.656 [a]
CMV infection after conversion	1 (6%)	0	1 [a]
BKV infection before conversion	2 (12%)	1 (6%)	1 [a]
BKV infection after conversion	0	0	-
Death	0	1 (6%)	1 [a]

DGF, delayed graft function; DSA, donor-specific antibody; BPAR, biopsy-proven acute rejection; AMR, antibody-mediated rejection; TCMR, T-cell mediated rejection; EVR, everolimus. Statistics: Adverse events are reported as absolute and relative frequencies. [a] Fisher's exact test.

Cholesterol and triglycerides tended to be higher in fast than slow metabolizers (no noticeable differences, Figure 3A,B) and increased to a similar extent (approximately 20 mg/dL) in both groups after conversion to EVR. Platelets slightly increased after RTx but without differences between fast and slow metabolizers (Figure 3C). Hemoglobin levels decreased by 1 g/dL on average in both groups one month after RTx, but increased from 10.8 ± 1.7 g/dL (M1) to 12.5 ± 1.4 g/dL (M36 after conversion) in fast metabolizers and from 10.6 ± 1.6 g/dL (M1) to 13.9 ± 1.1 g/dL (M36 after conversion) in slow metabolizers (Figure 3D). Three years after conversion, hemoglobin levels were noticeably higher in slow metabolizers ($p = 0.019$). None of the RTx recipients needed erythropoiesis-stimulating agents. HbA1c levels increased slightly from 5.3% (4.5–6.4%) at RTx to 6.3% (5.3–9.1%) at M6 after conversion in fast metabolizers and from 5.3% (4.6–6.0%) at RTx to 5.5% (5.0–7.1%) at M6 in slow metabolizers (Figure 3E). HbA1c values decreased only slightly in both groups to a comparable extent until M36.

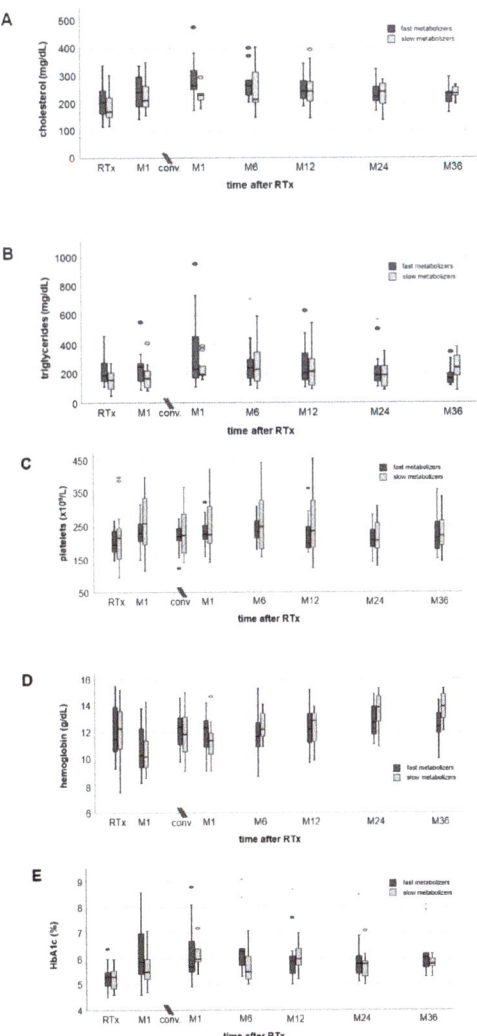

Figure 3. Courses of laboratory values. Cholesterol (**A**) and triglyceride (**B**) levels showed an increase after transplantation, but in a 36-month follow-up values decreased close to values measured at RTx (no noticeable differences between fast and slow metabolizers at any time). Mean platelets (**C**) and hemoglobin (**D**) remained in the normal range at all times without noticeable differences between the groups. Hemoglobin values dropped more than 1 g/dL at M1 after RTx, but had recovered already at the time of conversion from TAC to EVR (no noticeable differences between fast and slow metabolizers at all times). HbA1c levels (**E**) showed an increase one month after RTx without a relevant recovery during a 36-month follow-up after conversion. There were no noticeable differences in HbA1c values between the groups.

4. Discussion

The outcome of fast TAC metabolizers was shown to be inferior compared to the outcomes of slow TAC metabolizers when standard immunosuppression (immediate-release TAC, mycophenolate mofetil (MMF), and prednisolone) is used after RTx [4,5]. This finding was confirmed by others, even when higher C/D ratios were used for group definitions or when including patients receiving extended-release TAC [7,16]. In addition to increased rejection rates in patients with a low C/D ratio, increased rates of BK virus infection, CNI-related nephrotoxicity, and IF/TA were responsible for the lower eGFR of fast metabolizers [4,5,7–10]. In accordance with these data, Stegall et al. recently demonstrated in a large prospective cohort study using TAC-based immunosuppression that almost all kidney allografts have developed severe histological damage within ten years of RTx. However, the most frequently observed histological pathologies were arterial hyalinosis and glomerulosclerosis [17]. Both injuries can be linked to, e.g., CNI exposure [18]. Thus, CNI-induced nephrotoxicity remains a serious problem during CNI treatment [19]. Since only small case studies with patients who had CNI nephrotoxicity have investigated this conversion approach before and did not provide information regarding the TAC metabolism type of their patients, we herein investigated whether a conversion from TAC to EVR could be beneficial and safe for these patients [20,21].

In previous studies, we observed that as early as one month after RTx the kidney function of fast metabolizers is noticeably inferior to the kidney function of slow metabolizers [4]. Since TAC trough level and doses are usually higher within the first year after RTx and both can contribute to CNI nephrotoxicity, it is not surprising that CNI nephrotoxicity was the main reason for the conversion of TAC to EVR in our study cohort [10]. This disadvantage of fast metabolizers with respect to a lower eGFR persists over time and can still be observed to a large extent many years after Tx leading to inferior outcomes [5]. A comparable observation was made in liver transplanted patients [6]. However, in our present study, we were not able to show considerable advantages in fast metabolizers compared to slow metabolizers in relation to the eGFR after conversion of TAC to EVR. The change in eGFR from switching to M36 was similar in both, although a trend toward a higher increase in fast TAC metabolizers was observed. Two reasons might be responsible for this observation. First, the small number of cases could have masked the effect, especially when considering that a conversion of CNI to EVR usually leads to a small increase in eGRF. (This is independent of the type of TAC metabolism, although that has not been specifically studied before. For the first time, we present data relating to the C/D ratio before conversion.) [22] Notably, this effect may be more pronounced in cyclosporine-treated patients because cyclosporine A is a more potent vasoconstrictor than TAC [23,24]. Second, the time of the conversion could be relevant. Since renal function usually improves within the first year after transplantation due to the recovery from the transplant procedure and due to adaption of the kidney, these effects could also have an impact on the outcomes after conversion, since one may speculate that these processes might develop differently when using antiproliferative acting mechanistic target of rapamycin (mTOR)-inhibitors instead of CNIs [25–27]. In contrast to sirolimus-containing regimens [28,29], EVR-based immunosuppression was not found to lead to increased rates of delayed graft function or to poor results in terms of eGFR recovery after transplantation [30–33]. It was even postulated that progression of allograft fibrosis can be reduced by using mTOR-inhibition to down-regulate TGF-β signaling that is relevant for development of fibrosis [34]. However, even the large ELEVATE trial, which compared early conversion from TAC to EVR after RTx vs. CNI therapy, was not able to show differences between TAC- and EVR-treated patients in regards to the eGFR 12 months after RTx [35].

Nevertheless, we were able to show that conversion from TAC to EVR can improve eGFR even in RTx patients who had developed already CNI-induced side effects such as CNI nephrotoxcity—the main reason for conversion to EVR in our study. These data are in line with data from a small case series and a study showing reduced loss or even improvement of renal function after conversion to EVR in patients with CNI nephrotoxicity or chronic allograft nephropathy [20,21,36].

The overall rejection rate was low after conversion and not different between groups. No antibody-mediated rejection was observed until M36 and only one T-cell-mediated rejection occurred. Most importantly, we could not find any differences in (de novo) DSA. Based on our analyses at M36, class I DSA had occurred in only one patient (6%) of fast metabolizers. Due to previous transplantations, preformed Class II DSA were detectable in equal frequencies in both groups. The occurrence of de novo DSA apparently did not result in antibody-mediated rejection episodes within the three-year study period, as far as we know. However, rejections can occur later, as it is known from retrospective data that EVR-based regimens increase the risk of developing de novo DSA after RTx [37,38]. Interestingly, the prospective ELEVATE trial evaluated RTx patients with low immunological risk who were switched approximately three months after transplantation from CNI-based to EVR-based immunosuppression. One conclusion from the trial was that rejection rates in patients on the EVR-based regimen compared to patients receiving TAC had been higher; de novo DSA were not different between groups [35].

Consistent to previous data [27,35,39], after switching to EVR, we found no safety issues in either slow or fast TAC metabolizers (Table 3). However, others report high rates of adverse events and treatment discontinuation after conversion [30,40]. For example, the change in the lipid profile was as expected to occur for EVR, and showed no new safety concerns [35]. Notably, blood count and proteinuria even improved after conversion. It is known that mTOR-inhibition can be associated with a higher incidence of proteinuria compared to CNI treatment, an effect that is potentially dose-dependent [41–43]. However, it was suggested that especially late conversion promotes proteinuria. Our result is at least in line with the published results of others [44].

Of note, in this study, only one case of CMV infection occurred in fast metabolizers and no BKV infection after conversion. These data are consistent with randomized controlled trial data showing lower viral infection rates after switching to EVR [35].

The limitations of our study are the retrospective design and the limited sample size of our single-center study. However, we believe that our results are encouraging to design a prospective trial that can further evaluate our hypotheses.

In summary, we conclude from our data that selected RTx patients may benefit from a conversion from an immediate-release TAC-based immunosuppressive regimen to an EVR-based protocol to avoid further impair of kidney function associated with TAC treatment in these patients. This option could be especially interesting for patients who have already developed TAC-related adverse effects such as nephrotoxicity. Conversion to EVR is safe in selected slow and fast TAC metabolizers as the outcomes and the rate of adverse event did not noticeably differ between both TAC metabolizer types. However, these results must be confirmed in a prospective study.

Author Contributions: Conceptualization, G.T. and S.R.; Data curation, N.H.G.; Formal analysis, N.H.G. and R.K.; Methodology, G.T., S.R., and R.K.; Resources, H.P. and B.S.; Supervision, G.T.; Writing—original draft, G.T. and S.R.; and Writing—review and editing, K.S.-N., H.P., R.K., and B.S. All authors have read and agreed to the published version of the manuscript.

Funding: The APC was funded by the Open Access Fund of the University of Münster.

Conflicts of Interest: The authors declare no conflict of interest. The funders had no role in the design of the study; in the collection, analyses, or interpretation of data; in the writing of the manuscript, or in the decision to publish the results.

References

1. Kidney Disease: Improving Global Outcomes Transplant Work, G. KDIGO clinical practice guideline for the care of kidney transplant recipients. *Am. J. Transplant.* **2009**, *9* (Suppl. S3), S1–S155.
2. Schutte-Nutgen, K.; Tholking, G.; Suwelack, B.; Reuter, S. Tacrolimus—Pharmacokinetic Considerations for Clinicians. *Curr. Drug Metab.* **2018**, *19*, 342–350. [CrossRef] [PubMed]

3. Ji, E.; Choi, L.; Suh, K.S.; Cho, J.Y.; Han, N.; Oh, J.M. Combinational effect of intestinal and hepatic CYP3A5 genotypes on tacrolimus pharmacokinetics in recipients of living donor liver transplantation. *Transplantation* **2012**, *94*, 866–872. [CrossRef] [PubMed]
4. Tholking, G.; Fortmann, C.; Koch, R.; Gerth, H.U.; Pabst, D.; Pavenstadt, H.; Kabar, I.; Husing, A.; Wolters, H.; Reuter, S.; et al. The tacrolimus metabolism rate influences renal function after kidney transplantation. *PLoS ONE* **2014**, *9*, e111128. [CrossRef] [PubMed]
5. Schutte-Nutgen, K.; Tholking, G.; Steinke, J.; Pavenstadt, H.; Schmidt, R.; Suwelack, B.; Reuter, S. Fast Tac Metabolizers at Risk (-) It is Time for a C/D Ratio Calculation. *J. Clin. Med.* **2019**, *8*, 587. [CrossRef] [PubMed]
6. Tholking, G.; Siats, L.; Fortmann, C.; Koch, R.; Husing, A.; Cicinnati, V.R.; Gerth, H.U.; Wolters, H.H.; Anthoni, C.; Pavenstadt, H.; et al. Tacrolimus Concentration/Dose Ratio is Associated with Renal Function After Liver Transplantation. *Ann. Transplant.* **2016**, *21*, 167–179. [CrossRef]
7. Jouve, T.; Fonrose, X.; Noble, J.; Janbon, B.; Fiard, G.; Malvezzi, P.; Stanke-Labesque, F.; Rostaing, L. The TOMATO study (TacrOlimus MetabolizAtion in kidney TransplantatiOn): Impact of the concentration-dose ratio on death-censored graft survival. *Transplantation* **2019**. [CrossRef]
8. Egeland, E.J.; Reisaeter, A.V.; Robertsen, I.; Midtvedt, K.; Strom, E.H.; Holdaas, H.; Hartmann, A.; Asberg, A. High tacrolimus clearance—A risk factor for development of interstitial fibrosis and tubular atrophy in the transplanted kidney: A retrospective single-center cohort study. *Trans. Int.* **2019**, *32*, 257–269. [CrossRef] [PubMed]
9. Egeland, E.J.; Robertsen, I.; Hermann, M.; Midtvedt, K.; Storset, E.; Gustavsen, M.T.; Reisaeter, A.V.; Klaasen, R.; Bergan, S.; Holdaas, H.; et al. High Tacrolimus Clearance Is a Risk Factor for Acute Rejection in the Early Phase After Renal Transplantation. *Transplantation* **2017**, *101*, e273–e279. [CrossRef] [PubMed]
10. Tholking, G.; Schutte-Nutgen, K.; Schmitz, J.; Rovas, A.; Dahmen, M.; Bautz, J.; Jehn, U.; Pavenstadt, H.; Heitplatz, B.; Van Marck, V.; et al. A Low Tacrolimus Concentration/Dose Ratio Increases the Risk for the Development of Acute Calcineurin Inhibitor-Induced Nephrotoxicity. *J. Clin. Med.* **2019**, *8*, 1586. [CrossRef]
11. Budde, K.; Lehner, F.; Sommerer, C.; Reinke, P.; Arns, W.; Eisenberger, U.; Wuthrich, R.P.; Muhlfeld, A.; Heller, K.; Porstner, M.; et al. Five-year outcomes in kidney transplant patients converted from cyclosporine to everolimus: The randomized ZEUS study. *Am. J. Transplant.* **2015**, *15*, 119–128. [CrossRef] [PubMed]
12. Budde, K.; Sommerer, C.; Rath, T.; Reinke, P.; Haller, H.; Witzke, O.; Suwelack, B.; Baeumer, D.; Sieder, C.; Porstner, M.; et al. Renal function to 5 years after late conversion of kidney transplant patients to everolimus: A randomized trial. *J. Nephrol.* **2015**, *28*, 115–123. [CrossRef] [PubMed]
13. Levey, A.S.; Stevens, L.A.; Schmid, C.H.; Zhang, Y.L.; Castro, A.F.; Feldman, H.I.; Kusek, J.W.; Eggers, P.; Van Lente, F.; Greene, T.; et al. A new equation to estimate glomerular filtration rate. *Ann. Intern. Med.* **2009**, *150*, 604–612. [CrossRef] [PubMed]
14. Tholking, G.; Schmidt, C.; Koch, R.; Schuette-Nuetgen, K.; Pabst, D.; Wolters, H.; Kabar, I.; Husing, A.; Pavenstadt, H.; Reuter, S.; et al. Influence of tacrolimus metabolism rate on BKV infection after kidney transplantation. *Sci. Rep.* **2016**, *6*, 32273. [CrossRef] [PubMed]
15. Haas, M.; Loupy, A.; Lefaucheur, C.; Roufosse, C.; Glotz, D.; Seron, D.; Nankivell, B.J.; Halloran, P.F.; Colvin, R.B.; Akalin, E.; et al. The Banff 2017 Kidney Meeting Report: Revised diagnostic criteria for chronic active T cell-mediated rejection, antibody-mediated rejection, and prospects for integrative endpoints for next-generation clinical trials. *Am. J. Transplant.* **2018**, *18*, 293–307. [CrossRef]
16. Nowicka, M.; Gorska, M.; Nowicka, Z.; Edyko, K.; Edyko, P.; Wislicki, S.; Zawiasa-Bryszewska, A.; Strzelczyk, J.; Matych, J.; Kurnatowska, I. Tacrolimus: Influence of the Posttransplant Concentration/Dose Ratio on Kidney Graft Function in a Two-Year Follow-Up. *Kidney Blood Press. Res.* **2019**, *44*, 1075–1088. [CrossRef]
17. Stegall, M.D.; Cornell, L.D.; Park, W.D.; Smith, B.H.; Cosio, F.G. Renal Allograft Histology at 10 Years After Transplantation in the Tacrolimus Era: Evidence of Pervasive Chronic Injury. *Am. J. Transplant.* **2018**, *18*, 180–188. [CrossRef]
18. Einecke, G.; Reeve, J.; Halloran, P.F. Hyalinosis Lesions in Renal Transplant Biopsies: Time-Dependent Complexity of Interpretation. *Am. J. Transplant.* **2017**, *17*, 1346–1357. [CrossRef]
19. Naesens, M.; Kuypers, D.R.; Sarwal, M. Calcineurin inhibitor nephrotoxicity. *Clin. J. Am. Soc. Nephrol.* **2009**, *4*, 481–508. [CrossRef]

20. Nanmoku, K.; Shinzato, T.; Kubo, T.; Shimizu, T.; Yagisawa, T. Conversion to Everolimus in Kidney Transplant Recipients with Calcineurin Inhibitor-Induced Nephropathy: 3 Case Reports. *Trans. Proc.* **2019**, *51*, 1424–1427. [CrossRef]
21. Morales, J.; Fierro, A.; Benavente, D.; Zehnder, C.; Ferrario, M.; Contreras, L.; Herzog, C.; Buckel, E. Conversion from a calcineurin inhibitor-based immunosuppressive regimen to everolimus in renal transplant recipients: Effect on renal function and proteinuria. *Trans. Proc.* **2007**, *39*, 591–593. [CrossRef]
22. Hoskova, L.; Malek, I.; Kopkan, L.; Kautzner, J. Pathophysiological mechanisms of calcineurin inhibitor-induced nephrotoxicity and arterial hypertension. *Physiol. Res.* **2017**, *66*, 167–180. [CrossRef]
23. Gardiner, S.M.; March, J.E.; Kemp, P.A.; Fallgren, B.; Bennett, T. Regional haemodynamic effects of cyclosporine A, tacrolimus and sirolimus in conscious rats. *Br. J. Pharmacol.* **2004**, *141*, 634–643. [CrossRef]
24. Zaltzman, J.S. A comparison of short-term exposure of once-daily extended release tacrolimus and twice-daily cyclosporine on renal function in healthy volunteers. *Transplantation* **2010**, *90*, 1185–1191. [CrossRef]
25. Alperovich, G.; Maldonado, R.; Moreso, F.; Fulladosa, X.; Grinyo, J.M.; Seron, D. Glomerular enlargement assessed by paired donor and early protocol renal allograft biopsies. *Am. J. Transplant.* **2004**, *4*, 650–654. [CrossRef]
26. Ma, M.K.M.; Yung, S.; Chan, T.M. mTOR Inhibition and Kidney Diseases. *Transplantation* **2018**, *102*, S32–S40. [CrossRef]
27. Husing, A.; Schmidt, M.; Beckebaum, S.; Cicinnati, V.R.; Koch, R.; Tholking, G.; Stella, J.; Heinzow, H.; Schmidt, H.H.; Kabar, I. Long-Term Renal Function in Liver Transplant Recipients After Conversion from Calcineurin Inhibitors to mTOR Inhibitors. *Ann. Transplant.* **2015**, *20*, 707–713. [CrossRef]
28. Lui, S.L.; Chan, K.W.; Tsang, R.; Yung, S.; Lai, K.N.; Chan, T.M. Effect of rapamycin on renal ischemia-reperfusion injury in mice. *Trans. Int.* **2006**, *19*, 834–839. [CrossRef]
29. Smith, K.D.; Wrenshall, L.E.; Nicosia, R.F.; Pichler, R.; Marsh, C.L.; Alpers, C.E.; Polissar, N.; Davis, C.L. Delayed graft function and cast nephropathy associated with tacrolimus plus rapamycin use. *J. Am. Soc. Nephrol.* **2003**, *14*, 1037–1045. [CrossRef]
30. Sanchez-Escuredo, A.; Diekmann, F.; Revuelta, I.; Esforzado, N.; Ricart, M.J.; Cofan, F.; Torregrosa, J.V.; Peri, L.; Ruiz, A.; Campistol, J.M.; et al. An mTOR-inhibitor-based protocol and calcineurin inhibitor (CNI)-free treatment in kidney transplant recipients from donors after cardiac death: Good renal function, but high incidence of conversion to CNI. *Trans. Int.* **2016**, *29*, 362–368. [CrossRef]
31. Sommerer, C.; Suwelack, B.; Dragun, D.; Schenker, P.; Hauser, I.A.; Witzke, O.; Hugo, C.; Kamar, N.; Merville, P.; Junge, M.; et al. An open-label, randomized trial indicates that everolimus with tacrolimus or cyclosporine is comparable to standard immunosuppression in de novo kidney transplant patients. *Kidney Int.* **2019**, *96*, 231–244. [CrossRef]
32. Tedesco-Silva, H.; Pascual, J.; Viklicky, O.; Basic-Jukic, N.; Cassuto, E.; Kim, D.Y.; Cruzado, J.M.; Sommerer, C.; Adel Bakr, M.; Garcia, V.D.; et al. Safety of Everolimus with Reduced Calcineurin Inhibitor Exposure in De Novo Kidney Transplants: An Analysis from the Randomized TRANSFORM Study. *Transplantation* **2019**, *103*, 1953–1963. [CrossRef]
33. Manzia, T.M.; Carmellini, M.; Todeschini, P.; Secchi, A.; Sandrini, S.; Minetti, E.; Furian, L.; Spagnoletti, G.; Pisani, F.P.; Piredda, G.B.P.; et al. A 3-month, multicenter, randomized, open-label study to evaluate the impact on wound healing of the early [vs. delayed] introduction of everolimus in de novo kidney transplant recipients, with a follow-up evaluation at 12 month after transplant (NEVERWOUND study). *Transplantation* **2019**. [CrossRef]
34. Rivelli, R.F.; Goncalves, R.T.; Leite, M., Jr.; Santos, M.A.; Delgado, A.G.; Cardoso, L.R.; Takiya, C.M. Early withdrawal of calcineurin inhibitor from a sirolimus-based immunosuppression stabilizes fibrosis and the transforming growth factor-beta signalling pathway in kidney transplant. *Nephrology* **2015**, *20*, 168–176. [CrossRef] [PubMed]
35. de Fijter, J.W.; Holdaas, H.; Oyen, O.; Sanders, J.S.; Sundar, S.; Bemelman, F.J.; Sommerer, C.; Pascual, J.; Avihingsanon, Y.; Pongskul, C.; et al. Early Conversion from Calcineurin Inhibitor—To Everolimus-Based Therapy Following Kidney Transplantation: Results of the Randomized ELEVATE Trial. *Am. J. Transplant.* **2017**, *17*, 1853–1867. [CrossRef]
36. Cataneo-Davila, A.; Zuniga-Varga, J.; Correa-Rotter, R.; Alberu, J. Renal function outcomes in kidney transplant recipients after conversion to everolimus-based immunosuppression regimen with CNI reduction or elimination. *Trans. Proc.* **2009**, *41*, 4138–4146. [CrossRef]

37. Kamar, N.; Del Bello, A.; Congy-Jolivet, N.; Guilbeau-Frugier, C.; Cardeau-Desangles, I.; Fort, M.; Esposito, L.; Guitard, J.; Game, X.; Rostaing, L. Incidence of donor-specific antibodies in kidney transplant patients following conversion to an everolimus-based calcineurin inhibitor-free regimen. *Clin. Transplant.* **2013**, *27*, 455–462. [CrossRef] [PubMed]
38. Croze, L.E.; Tetaz, R.; Roustit, M.; Malvezzi, P.; Janbon, B.; Jouve, T.; Pinel, N.; Masson, D.; Quesada, J.L.; Bayle, F.; et al. Conversion to mammalian target of rapamycin inhibitors increases risk of de novo donor-specific antibodies. *Trans. Int.* **2014**, *27*, 775–783. [CrossRef]
39. Fischer, L.; Klempnauer, J.; Beckebaum, S.; Metselaar, H.J.; Neuhaus, P.; Schemmer, P.; Settmacher, U.; Heyne, N.; Clavien, P.A.; Muehlbacher, F.; et al. A randomized, controlled study to assess the conversion from calcineurin-inhibitors to everolimus after liver transplantation–PROTECT. *Am. J. Transplant.* **2012**, *12*, 1855–1865. [CrossRef]
40. Budde, K.; Lehner, F.; Sommerer, C.; Arns, W.; Reinke, P.; Eisenberger, U.; Wuthrich, R.P.; Scheidl, S.; May, C.; Paulus, E.M.; et al. Conversion from cyclosporine to everolimus at 4.5 months posttransplant: 3-year results from the randomized ZEUS study. *Am. J. Transplant.* **2012**, *12*, 1528–1540. [CrossRef]
41. Diekmann, F.; Andres, A.; Oppenheimer, F. mTOR inhibitor-associated proteinuria in kidney transplant recipients. *Transplant. Rev.* **2012**, *26*, 27–29. [CrossRef] [PubMed]
42. Wiseman, A.C.; McCague, K.; Kim, Y.; Geissler, F.; Cooper, M. The effect of everolimus versus mycophenolate upon proteinuria following kidney transplant and relationship to graft outcomes. *Am. J. Transplant.* **2013**, *13*, 442–449. [CrossRef]
43. Ponticelli, C.; Graziani, G. Proteinuria after kidney transplantation. *Trans. Int.* **2012**, *25*, 909–917. [CrossRef] [PubMed]
44. Giron, F.; Baez, Y.; Nino-Murcia, A.; Rodriguez, J.; Salcedo, S. Conversion therapy to everolimus in renal transplant recipients: Results after one year. *Transplant. Proc.* **2008**, *40*, 711–713. [CrossRef]

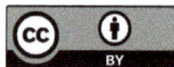

© 2020 by the authors. Licensee MDPI, Basel, Switzerland. This article is an open access article distributed under the terms and conditions of the Creative Commons Attribution (CC BY) license (http://creativecommons.org/licenses/by/4.0/).

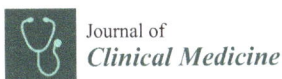

Article

Serum Klotho in Living Kidney Donors and Kidney Transplant Recipients: A Meta-Analysis

Charat Thongprayoon [1,*], Javier A. Neyra [2,3,4], Panupong Hansrivijit [5], Juan Medaura [6], Napat Leeaphorn [7], Paul W. Davis [6], Wisit Kaewput [8], Tarun Bathini [9], Sohail Abdul Salim [6], Api Chewcharat [1], Narothama Reddy Aeddula [10], Saraschandra Vallabhajosyula [11], Michael A. Mao [12] and Wisit Cheungpasitporn [6,*]

1. Division of Nephrology and Hypertension, Mayo Clinic, Rochester, MN 55905, USA; chewcharat.api@mayo.edu
2. Division of Nephrology, Bone and Mineral Metabolism, Department of Internal Medicine, University of Kentucky, Lexington, KY 40506, USA; javier.neyra@uky.edu
3. Charles and Jane Pak Center for Mineral Metabolism and Clinical Research, Dallas, TX 75390, USA
4. Division of Nephrology, Department of Internal Medicine, University of Texas Southwestern Medical Center, Dallas, TX 75390, USA
5. Department of Internal Medicine, University of Pittsburgh Medical Center Pinnacle, Harrisburg, PA 17105, USA; hansrivijitp@upmc.edu
6. Division of Nephrology, Department of Medicine, University of Mississippi Medical Center, Jackson, MS 39216, USA; jmedaura@umc.edu (J.M.); pwdavis@umc.edu (P.W.D.); sohail3553@gmail.com (S.A.S.)
7. Renal Transplant Program, University of Missouri-Kansas City School of Medicine/Saint Luke's Health System, Kansas City, MO 64110, USA; napat.leeaphorn@gmail.com
8. Department of Military and Community Medicine, Phramongkutklao College of Medicine, Bangkok 10400, Thailand; wisitnephro@gmail.com
9. Department of Internal Medicine, University of Arizona, Tucson, AZ 85721, USA; tarunjacobb@gmail.com
10. Division of Nephrology, Department of Medicine, Deaconess Health System, Evansville, IN 47710, USA; dr.anreddy@gmail.com
11. Department of Cardiovascular Medicine, Mayo Clinic, Rochester, MN 55905, USA; Vallabhajosyula.Saraschandra@mayo.edu
12. Division of Nephrology and Hypertension, Mayo Clinic, Jacksonville, FL 32224, USA; mao.michael@mayo.edu
* Correspondence: charat.thongprayoon@gmail.com (C.T.); wcheungpasitporn@gmail.com (W.C.)

Received: 21 May 2020; Accepted: 9 June 2020; Published: 12 June 2020

Abstract: α-Klotho is a known anti-aging protein that exerts diverse physiological effects, including phosphate homeostasis. Klotho expression occurs predominantly in the kidney and is significantly decreased in patients with chronic kidney disease. However, changes in serum klotho levels and impacts of klotho on outcomes among kidney transplant (KTx) recipients and kidney donors remain unclear. A literature search was conducted using MEDLINE, EMBASE, and Cochrane Database from inception through October 2019 to identify studies evaluating serum klotho levels and impacts of klotho on outcomes among KTx recipients and kidney donors. Study results were pooled and analyzed utilizing a random-effects model. Ten cohort studies with a total of 431 KTx recipients and 5 cohort studies with a total of 108 living kidney donors and were identified. After KTx, recipients had a significant increase in serum klotho levels (at 4 to 13 months post-KTx) with a mean difference (MD) of 243.11 pg/mL (three studies; 95% CI 67.41 to 418.81 pg/mL). Although KTx recipients had a lower serum klotho level with a MD of = −234.50 pg/mL (five studies; 95% CI −444.84 to −24.16 pg/mL) compared to healthy unmatched volunteers, one study demonstrated comparable klotho levels between KTx recipients and eGFR-matched controls. Among kidney donors, there was a significant decrease in serum klotho levels post-nephrectomy (day 3 to day 5) with a mean difference (MD) of −232.24 pg/mL (three studies; 95% CI −299.41 to −165.07 pg/mL). At one year following kidney donation, serum klotho levels remained lower than baseline before nephrectomy with a MD of = −110.80 pg/mL (two studies; 95% CI 166.35 to 55.24 pg/mL). Compared to healthy volunteers, living kidney donors had lower serum klotho levels with a MD of = −92.41 pg/mL (two studies; 95% CI −180.53 to −4.29 pg/mL). There is a significant reduction in serum klotho levels after living kidney donation and an increase in serum klotho levels after KTx. Future prospective studies are needed to assess the impact of changes in klotho on clinical outcomes in KTx recipients and living kidney donors.

Keywords: klotho; α-Klotho; FGF-23; kidney transplantation; kidney donor; renal transplantation; transplantation; Nephrology; CKD-MBD; CKD-Mineral and Bone Disorder

1. Introduction

α-Klotho (klotho) is a membrane protein that is highly expressed in the kidney, especially in the distal tubular epithelial cells [1–10]. Membrane-bound klotho regulates phosphate homeostasis by acting as a co-factor of fibroblast growth factor 23 (FGF23) [11–14]. FGF23-Klotho signaling promotes urinary phosphate excretion and suppresses the expression of renal 1α-hydroxylase, resulting in reduced vitamin D-dependent intestinal absorption of calcium and phosphate [11,15]. Altogether, FGF23-Klotho signaling regulates phosphate metabolism and prevents phosphate retention [16–20]. Soluble klotho can be detected in the circulation in two forms: (1) cleaved klotho, which is derived from cleavage of the extracellular domain of membrane klotho, and potentially (2) secreted klotho, which is derived from an alternatively spliced klotho mRNA transcript [21,22].

Soluble klotho displays diverse physiological effects and hormonal functions, including the reduction of oxidative stress and the inhibition of intracellular insulin and insulin-like growth factor 1 (IGF-1) signaling [15,23–28]. Klotho protects the kidney by suppression of apoptosis [29,30] and cell senescence [31,32], suppression of fibrosis [33–37], and upregulation of autophagy [3,38] in renal tubular cells. Klotho-deficient mice develop premature aging, hyperphosphatemia, vascular calcification and endothelial dysfunction, and have shorter lifespans, while klotho overexpressing mice have 20–30% longer lifespans than wild type mice [2,24,39]. Since klotho expression is the most abundant in the kidney [40], patients with kidney diseases, including acute kidney injury (AKI) and chronic kidney disease (CKD), are found to have a significant reduction in klotho expression and soluble levels [41–51]. Studies have demonstrated that serum klotho declines in progressive human CKD with the lowest serum klotho levels among patients with end-stage kidney disease (ESKD) on dialysis [41,48]. Low serum klotho is associated with increased mortality and cardiovascular events among patients with ESKD [52].

When compared to treatment with chronic dialysis, kidney transplantation (KTx) is the best therapeutic option for patients with ESKD and is associated with increased survival and better quality of life [53–56]. In addition, living donor KTx provides greater allograft longevity than those transplanted from a deceased donor [57]. However, changes in serum klotho levels and the impact of klotho on outcomes among KTx recipients and kidney donors remain unclear [58–75]. Thus, we conducted this systematic review and meta-analysis to assess serum klotho levels and the impact of klotho on outcomes among KTx recipients and kidney donors.

2. Methods

2.1. Search Strategy and Literature Review

A systematic literature search of MEDLINE (1946 to October 2019), EMBASE (1988 to October 2019), and the Cochrane Database of Systematic Reviews (database inception to October 2019) was conducted (1) to assess studies evaluating serum klotho levels and effects of klotho on outcomes among KTx recipients and kidney donors. The systematic literature review was undertaken independently by two investigators (C.T. and W.C.) using a search strategy that combined the terms of ("klotho" OR "klotho protein" OR "klotho gene") AND ("kidney transplantation" OR "renal transplantation" OR "kidney donor") which is provided in online Supplementary Materials (Table S1). No language limitation was applied. A manual search for conceivably relevant studies using references of the included articles was also performed. This study was conducted by the PRISMA (Preferred Reporting Items for Systematic Reviews and Meta-Analysis) statement [76]. The data for this meta-analysis are publicly available through the Open Science Framework (URL: https://osf.io/kx9we/).

2.2. Selection Criteria

Eligible studies must have been (1) clinical trials or observational studies (cohort, case-control, or cross-sectional studies) that evaluated serum klotho levels and effects of klotho on outcomes among KTx recipients or kidney donors, and (2) studies that presented data to calculate mean differences (MDs) with 95% confidence intervals (CIs) that evaluated changes in serum klotho before and after KTx/kidney donation or compared serum klotho between KTx patients/donors and a control group composed of non-KTx or non-donor controls. Retrieved articles were individually reviewed for eligibility by the two investigators (C.T. and W.C.). Discrepancies were addressed and solved by joint consensus. Inclusion was not limited by the size of the study.

2.3. Data Abstraction

A structured data collecting form was used to obtain the following information from each study including the title, name of the first author, publication year, year of the study, country where the study was conducted, demographic data of kidney transplant recipients and donors, methods used to measure serum klotho, serum klotho levels, estimated glomerular filtration rate (eGFR), control group, and adjusted effect estimates with 95% CI and covariates that were adjusted for in the multivariable analysis. This data extraction process was independently performed by two investigators (C.T. and W.C.).

2.4. Statistical Analysis

Analyses were performed utilizing the Comprehensive Meta-Analysis 3.3 software (version 3; Biostat Inc., Englewood, NJ, USA). Adjusted point estimates from each study were consolidated by the generic inverse variance approach of DerSimonian and Laird, which designated the weight of each study based on its variance [77]. The summary statistics for each outcome were the mean change from baseline and standard deviation (SD) of the mean change. The mean change in each group was obtained by subtracting the final mean from the baseline mean. The MDs were preferred since all studies use the same continuous outcome and unit of measure (pg/mL) of serum klotho and FGF-23 levels. The SD of mean change was computed, assuming a conservative correlation coefficient of 0.5 [78]. Effects sizes of 0.2 were interpreted as small, those of 0.5 as moderate, and of 0.8 as large [79]. Given the possibility of between-study variance, we used a random-effect model rather than a fixed-effect model. Cochran's Q test and I^2 statistics were applied to determine between-study heterogeneity. A value of I^2 of 0% to 25% represents insignificant heterogeneity, 26% to 50% low heterogeneity, 51% to 75% moderate heterogeneity and 76–100% high heterogeneity [80]. The presence of publication bias was assessed by the Egger test [81].

3. Results

A total of 132 potentially eligible articles were identified using our search strategy. After the exclusion of 93 articles based on title and abstract for clearly not fulfilling inclusion criteria on the basis of the type of article, study design, population or outcome of interest, or due to being duplicates, 39 articles were left for full-length review. Eighteen of these were excluded from the full-length review as they did not report the outcome of interest, while six articles were excluded because they were not observational studies. Thus, 15 studies (10 cohort studies [58–67] with a total of 431 KTx recipients and 5 cohort studies [68–72] with a total of 108 living kidney donors) were included. The literature retrieval, review, and selection process are demonstrated in Figure 1.

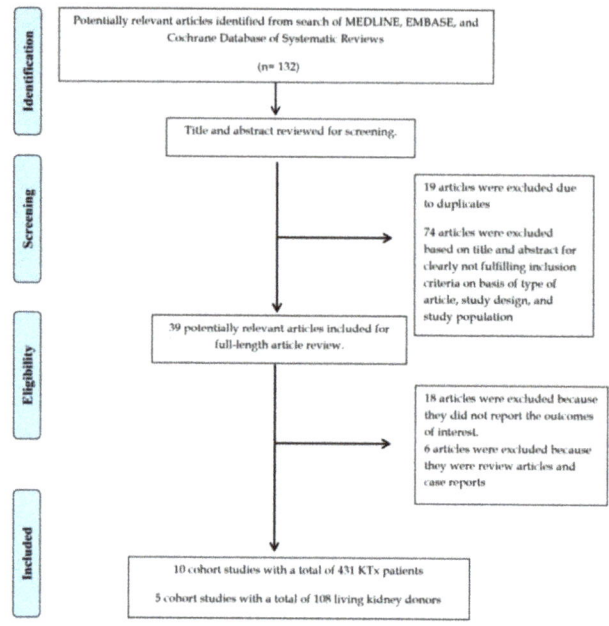

Figure 1. Outline of our search methodology. Abbreviation: KTx, kidney transplant.

3.1. Serum Klotho after Kidney Transplantation

The characteristics of the included studies assessing serum klotho after kidney transplantation are presented in Tables 1 and 2. After KTx, there was a significant increase in serum klotho levels in recipients (at 4 to 13 months post-KTx) in reference to baseline levels before KTx with a mean difference (MD) of 243.11 pg/mL (three studies; 95% CI 67.41 to 418.81 pg/mL, I^2 = 93%), Figure 2A. There were significant reductions in serum PTH and phosphate levels with MDs of −134.65 pg/mL (95% CI −176.09 to −93.21 pg/mL, I^2 = 0%) and −2.81 mg/dL (95% CI −3.46 to −2.16 mg/dL, I^2 = 97%), respectively. There was no significant change in serum calcium levels with a MD of 0.37 mg/dL (95% CI, −0.05 to 0.79 mg/dL, I^2 = 83%). Although KTx recipients had lower serum klotho levels with a MD of = −234.50 pg/mL (five studies; 95% CI −444.84 to −24.16 pg/mL, I^2 = 93%, Figure 2B) compared to healthy unmatched volunteers, one study demonstrated comparable klotho level between KTx recipients and eGFR-matched controls [66]. Two studies demonstrated high serum klotho levels in deceased donors as a prognostic marker for good allograft function within one year after KTx ($p < 0.05$) [59,60].

Table 1. Characteristics of the included studies assessing serum klotho after kidney transplantation.

Study	Year	Country	N-KTx	Characteristics-KTx	Klotho before KTx (pg/mL)	Other Markers before KTx	Klotho after KTx (pg/mL)	Other Markers after KTx
Kubota et al.		Japan	20	Age 6.9 ± 4.5 years Male 12 (60%)	988 ± 122	FGF23 5343 ± 1350 pg/mL	At 4 months 1405 ± 125	N/A
Tan et al.	2017	Australia	29	Age 49 (35–55) years Male 17 (59%)	307 (279–460)	iFGF23 2060 (825–5075) pg/mL eGFR 7.4 (6.5–8.7) mL/min/1.73 m^2	At 52 weeks 460 (311–525)	At 52 weeks iFGF23 64 (34–88) pg/mL eGFR 60.4 (50.5–71.6) mL/min/1.73 m^2
Mizusaki et al.	2019	Japan	36	Age 38.1 ± 14 years Male 15 (42%)	211.8	eGFR 3.8 ± 0.8 mL/min/1.73 m^2	At 1 year 369.3	At 1 year eGFR 49 ± 17 mL/min/1.73 m^2

Abbreviations: eGFR, estimated glomerular filtration rate; iFGF23, intact fibroblast growth factor-23; KTx, kidney transplant; N/A, not available.

Table 2. Characteristics of the included studies comparing serum klotho between KTx recipients and healthy volunteers.

Study	Year	Country	N-KTx	Characteristics-KTx	Klotho-KTx (pg/mL)	Other Markers-KTx	N-Control	Klotho-Control (pg/mL)	Other Markers-Control
Balogu et al.		Turkey	40	N/A	153 ± 170	FGF23 47.4 ± 61 pg/mL eGFR 56.3 ± 1.6 mL/min/1.73 m^2	20 healthy subjects	641 ± 1797	FGF23 1.6 ± 1.3 pg/mL eGFR 97.3 ± 13.5 mL/min/1.73 m^2
Malyszko et al.	2014	Poland	84	Median time from KTx 37 (13–72) months Age 47.9 ± 12.0 years Male 64 (76%)	228 (161–384)	FGF23 16.7 (13.8–21.2) pg/mL	22 healthy subjects	757 (632–839)	FGF23 11.7 (10.8–17.2) pg/mL GFR-matched control eGFR 62 (57–73) mL/min/1.73 m^2
Bleskestad et al.	2015	Norway	40	Median time from KTx	605 (506–784)	eGFR	39 GFR-matched controls	GFR-matched controls	iFGF23 63 (52–87) pg/mL Healthy volunteer eGFR 99.5 (89.5–110.8) mL/min/1.73 m^2
Tartaglione et al.	2017	Italy	80	18.3 (IQR 12.2–26.2) years Age 61.3 ± 11.8 years Male 29 (73%) Time for KTx 77.6 (37.6–119.5) months Age 54.7 ± 10.3 years Male 49 (61%) Time from KTx	449 (388–534)	62 (52–72) mL/min/1.73 m^2 iFGF23 75 (53–108) pg/mL eGFR 46.3 (36.2–58.3) mL/min/1.73 m^2 FGF23 41 (25–59) pg/mL	20 healthy subjects 30 healthy subjects	660 (536–847) Healthy volunteers 692 (618–866) 795 (619–901)	iFGF23 51 (36–68) pg/mL eGFR 109.1 ± 14.1 mL/min/1.73 m^2 FGF23 34 (28–441) pg/mL
Nahandi et al.	2017	Iran	30	6.42 ± 2.44 years Age 30.9 ± 5.3 years	276 ± 241	eGFR 64.53 ± 17.83 mL/min/1.73 m^2	27 healthy subjects	N/A	N/A

Abbreviations: eGFR, estimated glomerular filtration rate; FGF23, fibroblast growth factor-23; KTx, kidney transplant; N/A, not available.

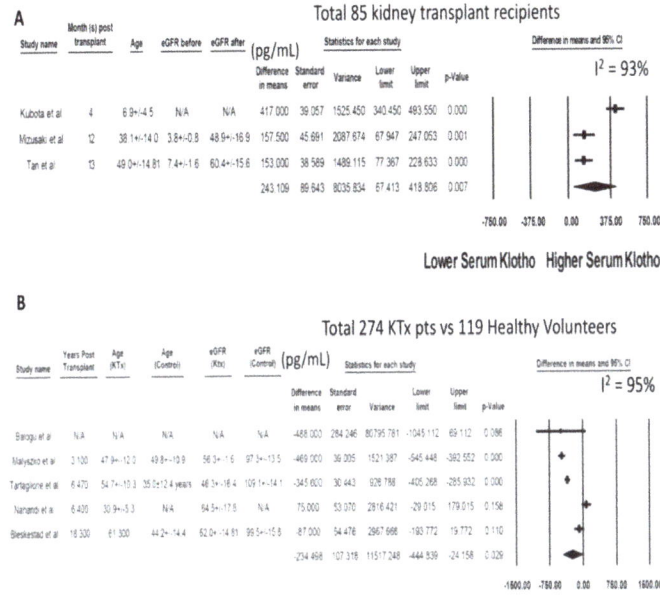

Figure 2. (**A**) Change in Serum Klotho in KTx Recipients after Kidney Transplant. (**B**) Serum Klotho in KTx Recipients Compared to Unmatched Healthy Volunteers.

3.2. Serum Klotho after Living Kidney Donation

The characteristics of the included studies assessing serum klotho after kidney transplantation are presented in Tables 3 and 4. A total of 108 living kidney donors were identified from five cohort studies. After kidney donation, there was a significant decrease in serum klotho levels post-nephrectomy (day 3 to day 5) with a mean difference (MD) of −232.24 pg/mL (three studies; 95% CI −299.41 to −165.07 pg/mL, $I^2 = 0$), Figure 3A. At one year following the kidney donation, serum klotho levels remained lower than baseline before nephrectomy with a MD of = −110.80 pg/mL (two studies; 95% CI −166.35 to −55.24 pg/mL, $I^2 = 5$), Figure 3B.

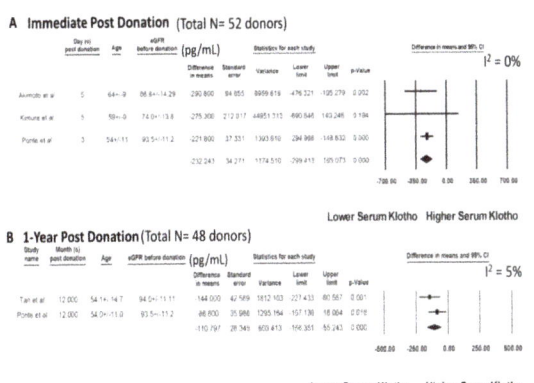

Figure 3. Changes in serum klotho after living kidney donation: (**A**) immediate post-donation and (**B**) one year post-donation.

Table 3. Characteristics of the included studies evaluating serum klotho after living kidney donation.

Study	Year	Country	N-Donor	Characteristics-Donor	Klotho before Donor Nephrectomy (pg/mL)	Other Markers before Donor Nephrectomy	Klotho after Donor Nephrectomy (pg/mL)	Other Markers after Donor Nephrectomy
Akimoto et al.	2013	Japan	10	Age 64 ± 9 years Male 4 (40%) Living donor	910 (755–1132)	eGFR 87 (72–92) mL/min/1.73 m^2	At day 5 619 (544.6–688.5)	N/A
Ponte et al.	2014	Switzerland	27	Age 54 ± 11 years	526 (482–615)	eGFR	At day 3	At day 3 FGF23 26.9 (22.1–38.0) pg/mL At day 360 eGFR
				Male 15 (57%) Living donor		95 ± 11 mL/min/1.73 m^2 FGF23 48.1 (37.4–60.0) pg/mL eGFR	304 (266–491) At day 360 440 (398–613) At day 5	63 ± 13 mL/min/1.73 m^2 FGF23 45.2 (37.7–56.4) pg/mL
Kimura et al.	2015	Japan	15	Age 59 ± 9 years Male 8 (53%) Living donor	1084 (795–1638)	74 ± 14 mL/min/1.73 m^2	809 (638–1357)	N/A
Tan et al.	2017	Australia	21	Age 54.1 ± 14.7 Male 13 (62%) Living donor	564 (468–663)	eGFR 94 (82–97) mL/min/1.73 m^2 iFGF23 52 ± 15 pg/mL	At 12 months 420 (378–555)	At 12 months eGFR 61 (49–69) mL/min/1.73 m^2 iFGF23 72 ± 22 pg/mL

Abbreviations: eGFR, estimated glomerular filtration rate; FGF23, fibroblast growth factor-23; N/A, not available.

Table 4. Characteristics of the included studies comparing serum klotho between living kidney donors and healthy volunteers.

Study	Year	Country	N-Donor	Characteristics-Donor	Klotho-Donor (pg/mL)	Other Markers-Donor	N-Control	Klotho-Control (pg/mL)	Other Markers-Control
Thorsen et al.	2016	Norway	35	Age 56.5 ± 9.4 years	669 (409–1161)	FGF23	35 healthy subjects	725 (458–1222)	FGF23
				Male 21 (60%)		62.6 (6.6–112) pg/mL			51.8 (25.9–90) pg/mL
				Living donor		eGFR			eGFR
				Time from donor nephrectomy					
				Median 15 years		75.8 ± 12.3 mL/min/1.73 m^2			99.0 ± 13.1 mL/min/1.73 m^2
Tan et al.	2017	Australia	21	Age 54.1 ± 14.7 years	420 (378–555)	eGFR	20 healthy subjects	517 (434–667)	eGFR
				Male 13 (62%)		61 (49–69) mL/min/1.73 m^2			97 (89–102) mL/min/1.73 m^2
				Living donor		iFGF23			iFGF
				Time from donor nephrectomy 1 year		72 ± 22 pg/mL			52 ± 15 pg/mL

Abbreviations: eGFR, estimated glomerular filtration rate; FGF23, fibroblast growth factor-23.

There was no significant change in serum FGF-23 at one year post-donation with a MD of = 8.19 pg/mL (two studies; 95% CI −14.24 to 30.62 pg/mL, I^2 = 85%), Figure 4A. Compared to unmatched healthy volunteers, living kidney donors had lower serum klotho levels with a MD of = −92.41 pg/mL (two studies; 95% CI −180.53 to −4.29 pg/mL, I^2 = 44%), Figure 4B.

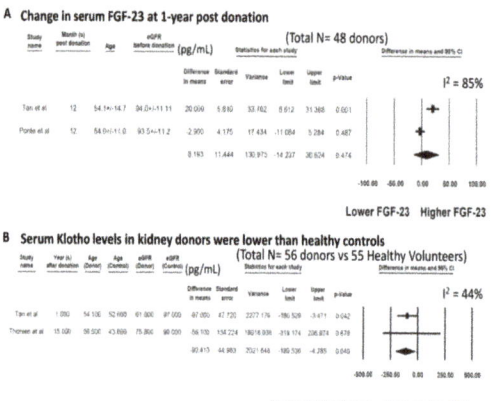

Figure 4. (**A**) Changes in Serum FGF-23 at one year post-donation and (**B**) Serum klotho levels in kidney donors compared to unmatched healthy controls.

3.3. Evaluation for Publication Bias

A funnel plot was not drawn because of the limited number of studies in each analysis. Generally, tests for funnel plot asymmetry should be used only when there are at least ten study groups, because the power of the test is too low to distinguish chance from real asymmetry [82]. Egger's regression test demonstrated no significant publication bias in all analyses ($p > 0.05$).

4. Discussion

In this meta-analysis, we demonstrated that serum klotho levels were significantly increased after successful KTx. While KTx recipients had lower serum klotho levels compared to unmatched healthy volunteers, serum klotho levels in kidney transplant recipients were comparable to those in eGFR-matched controls. Among kidney donors, we found a significant decrease in serum klotho levels post-nephrectomy at day 3 to day 5, which remained lower than baseline before nephrectomy at one year following kidney donation. Compared to healthy volunteers, living kidney donors had lower serum klotho levels.

The findings from our meta-analysis support that klotho is primarily synthesized in the kidneys [40], and transplanting a new kidney into ESKD patients would result in an increase in renal klotho and serum klotho levels post-KTx. In addition to the oligo-anuric state, patients with advanced CKD/ESKD have a significant reduction in klotho and progressively lose the ability to prevent phosphate retention, resulting in hyperphosphatemia, vascular calcification, and cardiovascular disease [83,84]. After successful KTx, in addition to improvement in eGFR, there is also a significant increase in klotho, altogether leading to an improvement in phosphate homeostasis. Recent studies have demonstrated that post-transplant hypophosphatemia after KTx is associated with good kidney allograft function [85,86]. Although the actual underlying mechanisms remain unclear, this is likely because excellent quality transplanted kidneys have higher eGFR and klotho expression, resulting in a reduction in phosphate levels post-KTx.

We identified two cohorts of KTx patients who received their kidneys from deceased donors; higher serum klotho levels in these donors were prognostic for good allograft function at one year after KTx [59,60]. In the ischemia-reperfusion injury (IRI), which is unavoidable to a certain degree in all KTx surgeries, soluble klotho protects renal tubular cells from oxidative damage by inhibiting the insulin/IGF-1 signaling pathway and by inhibition of TGF-β1 for decreasing renal fibrosis [87,88], and upregulation of autophagy in renal tubular cells [3,89]. In addition, klotho is also involved in the inhibition of Wnt pathway-associated β-catenin activation, thus improving renal fibrosis [87]. Compared to patients with early graft function, a lower level of klotho is observed in implantation biopsies among patients with delayed graft function (DGF) [90]. Although data on the effects of klotho on long-term allograft outcomes are limited, it is well known that poor allograft function at one year after KTx and DGF is associated with renal allograft loss [91,92]. Following successful KTx, patients regain functions of klotho via FGF23-Klotho signaling, and with the previously accumulated FGF23, residual hyperparathyroidism, and the use of calcineurin inhibitors (especially cyclosporine) [93–95], post-KTx hypophosphatemia can commonly occur up to 86% [85,96,97]. Post-KTx hypophosphatemia is known to be associated with lower risks of death-censored graft failure and cardiovascular mortality [85]. The association between post-KTx hypophosphatemia and reduced cardiovascular mortality among KTx recipients could be related to the reduction of calcium phosphate product, an important factor associated with vascular calcification and cardiovascular events [98,99]. Our study demonstrated that successful KTx can result in a significant increase in serum klotho levels among KTx recipients [85]. In addition, previous literature has demonstrated trending towards normal FGF-23 levels after successful KTx [42,100]. Thus, regaining function in FGF23-Klotho signaling after KTx helps promote urinary phosphate excretion and reduced vitamin D-dependent intestinal absorption of calcium and phosphate [11,15], which might explain the association between post-KTx hypophosphatemia and reduced cardiovascular mortality. Future studies are needed to assess the impact of klotho levels on long-term cardiovascular health in KTx recipients, allograft, and patient survival.

Living donors supply approximately 40% of kidney allografts in the United States [101]. Overall, living kidney donation is considered safe and does not appear to increase long-term mortality compared with controls [102–107]. A recent systematic review of 52 studies comprising 118,426 living kidney donors reassured the safety of living kidney donations with the finding of no difference in all-cause mortality among donors and controls [108]. In addition, a large retrospective population-based matched cohort study of 2028 kidney donors in comparison with 20,280 matched non-donor controls (followed for a median of 6.5 years) demonstrated no difference in the rate of cardiovascular events between the two groups [109]. Although the findings of our study showed a significant reduction in serum klotho at post-operative day 3 to 5 and at one year following kidney donation, the degree of klotho reduction seemed to be attenuated at one year post-donation compared to the early post-operative period. In addition, we found no significant change in serum FGF-23 at one year post-donation. It is possible that after living kidney donation serum klotho is not severely reduced enough to stimulate the rise in serum FGF-23, which occurred in patients with advanced CKD [41,110]. Elevated FGF-23 levels have been shown to be associated with increased mortality and cardiovascular events [111–113]. Thus, no significant increase in FGF-23 levels after living kidney donation is consistent with the findings of no difference in all-cause mortality among donors and controls in previous literature [108,109].

Despite these published reassuring findings of donor safety [108,109], a recent small multicenter study of living kidney donors and healthy controls ($n = 124$) demonstrated an association between living kidney donation and a significant increase in left ventricular mass and reduced aortic distensibility [114]. In addition to functions of klotho via FGF23-Klotho signaling, soluble klotho also has FGF23-independent effects, including endothelial protection from senescence, anti-fibrotic properties, cardioprotection, and prevention of vascular calcifications [84,115,116]. Klotho-deficient CKD mice have significant left ventricular hypertrophy (LVH) and cardiac fibrosis compared with wild-type mice [117]. Soluble klotho also provides cardioprotection against stress-induced exaggerated cardiac remodeling through downregulation of transient receptor potential cation channel 6 (TRPC6) [118]. Although an increased LVH and reduced aortic distensibility in living kidney donors could be related to an increased risk of hypertension post living kidney donation [102,103], future studies are required to assess whether a reduction in serum klotho levels after living kidney donation may play a role in the higher risk of LVH, and reduced aortic distensibility observed among living kidney donors.

Our meta-analysis is subject to certain limitations. First, although there were comparative groups, all studies are observational, making them susceptible to selection bias. Second, many variables may influence klotho levels in the post-transplant period that may contribute to the heterogeneity between the included studies evaluating changes in serum klotho levels among KTx recipients. Data on medications that may affect endogenous klotho expression in the kidney and soluble levels such as angiotensin II inhibitors and hydroxymethylglutaryl-CoA (HMG-CoA) reductase inhibitors [17,21,119,120] as well as data on immunosuppression were limited in included studies. Lifestyle, diet, psychological stress, and activities such as exercises may also affect serum klotho levels [121–124]. Thus, future prospective studies are needed to assess the impact of changes in klotho on clinical outcomes in KTx recipients and living kidney donors. Third, the follow-up duration of included studies was limited to only one year, and future studies are required to evaluate the impacts of serum klotho levels on long-term clinical outcomes. Fourth, serum klotho is also affected by the aging process and declines with older age [125]. However, we demonstrated an increase in serum klotho levels after KTx at one year and a decrease in klotho levels at immediate postoperative (which is less likely to be affected by the aging process). Lastly, all included studies measured serum klotho levels by ELISA. Recently, immunoprecipitation-immunoblot (IP-IB) assay is shown to be superior to the ELISA and highly correlated with eGFR [126]. However, this technique requires the labor-intensive nature of the IP-IB assay, and further research is needed to evaluate the use of the IP-IB assay in KTx patients.

In conclusion, compared to patients' baseline, serum klotho levels increase early after successful KTx and decrease after living kidney donation, respectively. Future studies are required to assess the impact of serum klotho levels on risk-stratification and patient-centered outcomes in both living donors and KTx recipients.

Supplementary Materials: The following are available online at http://www.mdpi.com/2077-0383/9/6/1834/s1, Table S1: Search strategy.

Author Contributions: Conceptualization, C.T., J.A.N., J.M., N.L., P.W.D., W.K., T.B., S.A.S., A.C., N.R.A., S.V., M.A.M. and W.C.; Data curation, C.T., N.L. and W.C.; Formal analysis, C.T. and W.C.; Funding acquisition, J.M.; Investigation, C.T., P.H., N.L., W.K. and W.C.; Methodology, C.T., J.A.N., P.H., W.K. and W.C.; Project administration, C.T. and T.B.; Resources, T.B.; Software, T.B.; Supervision, J.A.N., J.M., P.W.D., S.A.S., A.C., S.V., M.A.M. and W.C.; Validation, C.T., P.W.D., W.K., N.R.A. and W.C.; Visualization, J.A.N., P.H., J.M. and N.L.; Writing—original draft, C.T. and W.C.; Writing—review and editing, J.A.N., P.H., J.M., N.L., P.W.D., W.K., T.B., S.A.S., A.C., N.R.A., S.V., M.A.M. and W.C. All authors have read and agreed to the published version of the manuscript.

Funding: This research received no external funding.

Acknowledgments: None. All authors had access to the data and played essential roles in writing of the manuscript. Neyra is currently supported by an Early Career Pilot Grant from the National Center for Advancing Translational Sciences (NCATS), National Institutes of Health (NIH), through Grant UL1 TR001998.

Conflicts of Interest: The authors deny any conflict of interest.

References

1. Hu, M.C.; Shi, M.; Zhang, J.; Pastor, J.; Nakatani, T.; Lanske, B.; Razzaque, M.S.; Rosenblatt, K.P.; Baum, M.G.; Kuro-o, M.; et al. Klotho: A novel phosphaturic substance acting as an autocrine enzyme in the renal proximal tubule. *FASEB J.* **2010**, *24*, 3438–3450. [CrossRef]
2. Kuro-o, M. Klotho and aging. *Biochim. Biophys. Acta* **2009**, *1790*, 1049–1058. [CrossRef]
3. Bian, A.; Neyra, J.A.; Zhan, M.; Hu, M.C. Klotho, stem cells, and aging. *Clin. Interv. Aging* **2015**, *10*, 1233–1243. [PubMed]
4. Hu, M.C.; Shi, M.; Cho, H.J.; Adams-Huet, B.; Paek, J.; Hill, K.; Shelton, J.; Amaral, A.P.; Faul, C.; Taniguchi, M.; et al. Klotho and phosphate are modulators of pathologic uremic cardiac remodeling. *J. Am. Soc. Nephrol.* **2015**, *26*, 1290–1302. [CrossRef] [PubMed]

5. Henao Agudelo, J.S.; Baia, L.C.; Ormanji, M.S.; Santos, A.R.P.; Machado, J.R.; Saraiva Câmara, N.O.; Navis, G.J.; de Borst, M.H.; Heilberg, I.P. Fish Oil Supplementation Reduces Inflammation but Does Not Restore Renal Function and Klotho Expression in an Adenine-Induced CKD Model. *Nutrients* **2018**, *10*, 1283. [CrossRef]
6. Huang, X.; Liu, T.; Zhao, M.; Fu, H.; Wang, J.; Xu, Q. Protective Effects of Moderate Ca Supplementation against Cd-Induced Bone Damage under Different Population-Relevant Doses in Young Female Rats. *Nutrients* **2019**, *11*, 849. [CrossRef] [PubMed]
7. Muñoz-Castañeda, J.R.; Rodelo-Haad, C.; Pendon-Ruiz de Mier, M.V.; Martin-Malo, A.; Santamaria, R.; Rodriguez, M. Klotho/FGF23 and Wnt Signaling as Important Players in the Comorbidities Associated with Chronic Kidney Disease. *Toxins (Basel)* **2020**, *12*, 185.
8. Buendía, P.; Carracedo, J.; Soriano, S.; Madueño, J.A.; Ortiz, A.; Martín-Malo, A.; Aljama, P.; Ramírez, R. Klotho Prevents NFκB Translocation and Protects Endothelial Cell From Senescence Induced by Uremia. *J. Gerontol. A Biol. Sci. Med. Sci.* **2015**, *70*, 1198–1209. [CrossRef] [PubMed]
9. Carracedo, J.; Buendía, P.; Merino, A.; Madueño, J.A.; Peralbo, E.; Ortiz, A.; Martín-Malo, A.; Aljama, P.; Rodríguez, M.; Ramírez, R. Klotho modulates the stress response in human senescent endothelial cells. *Mech. Ageing Dev.* **2012**, *133*, 647–654. [CrossRef] [PubMed]
10. Donate-Correa, J.; Martín-Núñez, E.; Ferri, C.; Hernández-Carballo, C.; Tagua, V.G.; Delgado-Molinos, A.; López-Castillo, Á.; Rodríguez-Ramos, S.; Cerro-López, P.; López-Tarruella, V.C.; et al. FGF23 and Klotho Levels are Independently Associated with Diabetic Foot Syndrome in Type 2 Diabetes Mellitus. *J. Clin. Med.* **2019**, *8*. [CrossRef] [PubMed]
11. Shimada, T.; Hasegawa, H.; Yamazaki, Y.; Muto, T.; Hino, R.; Takeuchi, Y.; Fujita, T.; Nakahara, K.; Fukumoto, S.; Yamashita, T. FGF-23 is a potent regulator of vitamin D metabolism and phosphate homeostasis. *J. Bone Miner. Res.* **2004**, *19*, 429–435. [CrossRef] [PubMed]
12. Komaba, H.; Fukagawa, M. FGF23-parathyroid interaction: Implications in chronic kidney disease. *Kidney Int.* **2010**, *77*, 292–298. [CrossRef] [PubMed]
13. Rodelo-Haad, C.; Santamaria, R.; Muñoz-Castañeda, J.R.; Pendón-Ruiz de Mier, M.V.; Martin-Malo, A.; Rodriguez, M. FGF23, Biomarker or Target? *Toxins (Basel)* **2019**, *11*, 175. [CrossRef] [PubMed]
14. Liu, Y.C.; Tsai, J.P.; Wang, L.H.; Lee, M.C.; Hsu, B.G. Positive correlation of serum fibroblast growth factor 23 with peripheral arterial stiffness in kidney transplantation patients. *Clin. Chim. Acta* **2020**, *505*, 9–14. [CrossRef]
15. Razzaque, M.S. The FGF23-Klotho axis: Endocrine regulation of phosphate homeostasis. *Nat. Rev. Endocrinol.* **2009**, *5*, 611–619. [CrossRef]
16. Shimada, T.; Kakitani, M.; Yamazaki, Y.; Hasegawa, H.; Takeuchi, Y.; Fujita, T.; Fukumoto, S.; Tomizuka, K.; Yamashita, T. Targeted ablation of Fgf23 demonstrates an essential physiological role of FGF23 in phosphate and vitamin D metabolism. *J. Clin. Investig.* **2004**, *113*, 561–568. [CrossRef]
17. Zou, D.; Wu, W.; He, Y.; Ma, S.; Gao, J. The role of klotho in chronic kidney disease. *BMC Nephrol.* **2018**, *19*, 285. [CrossRef] [PubMed]
18. Erben, R.G.; Andrukhova, O. FGF23-Klotho signaling axis in the kidney. *Bone* **2017**, *100*, 62–68. [CrossRef] [PubMed]
19. Olauson, H.; Lindberg, K.; Amin, R.; Jia, T.; Wernerson, A.; Andersson, G.; Larsson, T.E. Targeted deletion of Klotho in kidney distal tubule disrupts mineral metabolism. *J. Am. Soc. Nephrol.* **2012**, *23*, 1641–1651. [CrossRef] [PubMed]
20. Martin, A.; David, V.; Quarles, L.D. Regulation and function of the FGF23/klotho endocrine pathways. *Physiol. Rev.* **2012**, *92*, 131–155. [CrossRef] [PubMed]
21. Hu, M.C.; Kuro-o, M.; Moe, O.W. Secreted klotho and chronic kidney disease. *Adv. Exp. Med. Biol.* **2012**, *728*, 126–157. [PubMed]
22. Takeshita, A.; Kawakami, K.; Furushima, K.; Miyajima, M.; Sakaguchi, K. Central role of the proximal tubular αKlotho/FGF receptor complex in FGF23-regulated phosphate and vitamin D metabolism. *Sci. Rep.* **2018**, *8*, 6917. [CrossRef] [PubMed]
23. Mencke, R.; Olauson, H.; Hillebrands, J.L. Effects of Klotho on fibrosis and cancer: A renal focus on mechanisms and therapeutic strategies. *Adv. Drug Deliv. Rev.* **2017**, *121*, 85–100. [PubMed]
24. Kuro-o, M.; Matsumura, Y.; Aizawa, H.; Kawaguchi, H.; Suga, T.; Utsugi, T.; Ohyama, Y.; Kurabayashi, M.; Kaname, T.; Kume, E.; et al. Mutation of the mouse klotho gene leads to a syndrome resembling ageing. *Nature* **1997**, *390*, 45–51. [PubMed]

25. Maekawa, Y.; Ishikawa, K.; Yasuda, O.; Oguro, R.; Hanasaki, H.; Kida, I.; Takemura, Y.; Ohishi, M.; Katsuya, T.; Rakugi, H. Klotho suppresses TNF-alpha-induced expression of adhesion molecules in the endothelium and attenuates NF-kappaB activation. *Endocrine* **2009**, *35*, 341–346.
26. Nabeshima, Y. Toward a better understanding of Klotho. *Sci. Aging Knowl. Environ.* **2006**, *2006*, pe11.
27. Jin, M.; Lv, P.; Chen, G.; Wang, P.; Zuo, Z.; Ren, L.; Bi, J.; Yang, C.W.; Mei, X.; Han, D. Klotho ameliorates cyclosporine A-induced nephropathy via PDLIM2/NF-kB p65 signaling pathway. *Biochem. Biophys. Res. Commun.* **2017**, *486*, 451–457. [PubMed]
28. Wang, Y.; Kuro-o, M.; Sun, Z. Klotho gene delivery suppresses Nox2 expression and attenuates oxidative stress in rat aortic smooth muscle cells via the cAMP-PKA pathway. *Aging Cell* **2012**, *11*, 410–417. [CrossRef] [PubMed]
29. Panesso, M.C.; Shi, M.; Cho, H.J.; Paek, J.; Ye, J.; Moe, O.W.; Hu, M.C. Klotho has dual protective effects on cisplatin-induced acute kidney injury. *Kidney Int.* **2014**, *85*, 855–870.
30. Hu, M.C.; Shi, M.; Zhang, J.; Quinones, H.; Griffith, C.; Kuro-o, M.; Moe, O.W. Klotho deficiency causes vascular calcification in chronic kidney disease. *J. Am. Soc. Nephrol.* **2011**, *22*, 124–136.
31. Kuro-o, M. Klotho as a regulator of oxidative stress and senescence. *Biol. Chem.* **2008**, *389*, 233–241. [CrossRef]
32. Liu, F.; Wu, S.; Ren, H.; Gu, J. Klotho suppresses RIG-I-mediated senescence-associated inflammation. *Nat. Cell Biol.* **2011**, *13*, 254–262. [CrossRef] [PubMed]
33. Doi, S.; Zou, Y.; Togao, O.; Pastor, J.V.; John, G.B.; Wang, L.; Shiizaki, K.; Gotschall, R.; Schiavi, S.; Yorioka, N.; et al. Klotho inhibits transforming growth factor-beta1 (TGF-beta1) signaling and suppresses renal fibrosis and cancer metastasis in mice. *J. Biol. Chem.* **2011**, *286*, 8655–8665. [PubMed]
34. Zhou, L.; Li, Y.; Zhou, D.; Tan, R.J.; Liu, Y. Loss of Klotho contributes to kidney injury by derepression of Wnt/beta-catenin signaling. *J. Am. Soc. Nephrol.* **2013**, *24*, 771–785. [CrossRef]
35. Sugiura, H.; Yoshida, T.; Shiohira, S.; Kohei, J.; Mitobe, M.; Kurosu, H.; Kuro-o, M.; Nitta, K.; Tsuchiya, K. Reduced Klotho expression level in kidney aggravates renal interstitial fibrosis. *Am. J. Physiol. Renal Physiol.* **2012**, *302*, F1252–F1264. [CrossRef]
36. Guan, X.; Nie, L.; He, T.; Yang, K.; Xiao, T.; Wang, S.; Huang, Y.; Zhang, J.; Wang, J.; Sharma, K.; et al. Klotho suppresses renal tubulo-interstitial fibrosis by controlling basic fibroblast growth factor-2 signalling. *J. Pathol.* **2014**, *234*, 560–572. [PubMed]
37. Huang, J.S.; Chuang, C.T.; Liu, M.H.; Lin, S.H.; Guh, J.Y.; Chuang, L.Y. Klotho attenuates high glucose-induced fibronectin and cell hypertrophy via the ERK1/2-p38 kinase signaling pathway in renal interstitial fibroblasts. *Mol. Cell Endocrinol.* **2014**, *390*, 45–53.
38. Shi, M.; Flores, B.; Gillings, N.; Bian, A.; Cho, H.J.; Yan, S.; Liu, Y.; Levine, B.; Moe, O.W.; Hu, M.C. AlphaKlotho Mitigates Progression of AKI to CKD through Activation of Autophagy. *J. Am. Soc. Nephrol.* **2016**, *27*, 2331–2345. [CrossRef]
39. Wang, Y.; Sun, Z. Current understanding of klotho. *Ageing Res. Rev.* **2009**, *8*, 43–51. [CrossRef]
40. Olauson, H.; Mencke, R.; Hillebrands, J.L.; Larsson, T.E. Tissue expression and source of circulating αKlotho. *Bone* **2017**, *100*, 19–35. [CrossRef]
41. Hu, M.C.; Kuro-o, M.; Moe, O.W. The emerging role of Klotho in clinical nephrology. *Nephrol. Dial. Transplant.* **2012**, *27*, 2650–2657. [CrossRef] [PubMed]
42. Amiri, F.S.; Khatami, M.R. Fibroblast Growth Factor 23 in Postrenal Transplant: An Often Forgotten Hormone. *Exp. Clin. Transplant.* **2016**, *14*, 606–616. [PubMed]
43. Neyra, J.A.; Li, X.; Mescia, F.; Ortiz-Soriano, V.; Adams-Huet, B.; Pastor, J.; Hu, M.C.; Toto, R.D.; Moe, O.W. Urine Klotho Is Lower in Critically Ill Patients With Versus Without Acute Kidney Injury and Associates With Major Adverse Kidney Events. *Crit. Care Explor.* **2019**, *1*, e0016. [CrossRef]
44. Sanchez-Niño, M.D.; Fernandez-Fernandez, B.; Ortiz, A. Klotho, the elusive kidney-derived anti-ageing factor. *Clin. Kidney J.* **2019**, *13*, 125–127.
45. Christov, M.; Neyra, J.A.; Gupta, S.; Leaf, D.E. Fibroblast Growth Factor 23 and Klotho in AKI. *Semin. Nephrol.* **2019**, *39*, 57–75. [CrossRef] [PubMed]
46. Neyra, J.A.; Hu, M.C. αKlotho and Chronic Kidney Disease. *Vitam. Horm.* **2016**, *101*, 257–310. [PubMed]
47. Hu, M.C.; Kuro-o, M.; Moe, O.W. Klotho and chronic kidney disease. *Contrib. Nephrol.* **2013**, *180*, 47–63. [PubMed]
48. Barker, S.L.; Pastor, J.; Carranza, D.; Quiñones, H.; Griffith, C.; Goetz, R.; Mohammadi, M.; Ye, J.; Zhang, J.; Hu, M.C.; et al. The demonstration of αKlotho deficiency in human chronic kidney disease with a novel synthetic antibody. *Nephrol. Dial. Transplant.* **2015**, *30*, 223–233. [CrossRef]

49. Seiler, S.; Rogacev, K.S.; Roth, H.J.; Shafein, P.; Emrich, I.; Neuhaus, S.; Floege, J.; Fliser, D.; Heine, G.H. Associations of FGF-23 and sKlotho with cardiovascular outcomes among patients with CKD stages 2–4. *Clin. J. Am. Soc. Nephrol.* **2014**, *9*, 1049–1058. [CrossRef]
50. Wang, Q.; Su, W.; Shen, Z.; Wang, R. Correlation between Soluble α-Klotho and Renal Function in Patients with Chronic Kidney Disease: A Review and Meta-Analysis. *Biomed. Res. Int.* **2018**, *2018*, 9481475. [CrossRef]
51. Sari, F.; Inci, A.; Dolu, S.; Ellidag, H.Y.; Cetinkaya, R.; Ersoy, F.F. High serum soluble α-Klotho levels in patients with autosomal dominant polycystic kidney disease. *J. Investig. Med.* **2017**, *65*, 358–362. [CrossRef]
52. Memmos, E.; Sarafidis, P.; Pateinakis, P.; Tsiantoulas, A.; Faitatzidou, D.; Giamalis, P.; Vasilikos, V.; Papagianni, A. Soluble Klotho is associated with mortality and cardiovascular events in hemodialysis. *BMC Nephrol.* **2019**, *20*, 217. [CrossRef] [PubMed]
53. Thongprayoon, C.; Hansrivijit, P.; Leeaphorn, N.; Acharya, P.; Torres-Ortiz, A.; Kaewput, W.; Kovvuru, K.; Kanduri, S.R.; Bathini, T.; Cheungpasitporn, W. Recent Advances and Clinical Outcomes of Kidney Transplantation. *J. Clin. Med.* **2020**, *9*, 1193. [CrossRef]
54. Thongprayoon, C.; Kaewput, W.; Kovvuru, K.; Hansrivijit, P.; Kanduri, S.R.; Bathini, T.; Chewcharat, A.; Leeaphorn, N.; Gonzalez-Suarez, M.L.; Cheungpasitporn, W. Promises of Big Data and Artificial Intelligence in Nephrology and Transplantation. *J. Clin. Med.* **2020**, *9*, 1107. [CrossRef]
55. Cheungpasitporn, W.; Thongprayoon, C.; Vaitla, P.K.; Chewcharat, A.; Hansrivijit, P.; Koller, F.L.; Mao, M.A.; Bathini, T.; Salim, S.A.; Katari, S.; et al. Degree of Glomerulosclerosis in Procurement Kidney Biopsies from Marginal Donor Kidneys and Their Implications in Predicting Graft Outcomes. *J. Clin. Med.* **2020**, *9*, 1469. [CrossRef]
56. Leeaphorn, N.; Thongprayoon, C.; Chon, W.J.; Cummings, L.S.; Mao, M.A.; Cheungpasitporn, W. Outcomes of kidney retransplantation after graft loss as a result of BK virus nephropathy in the era of newer immunosuppressant agents. *Am. J. Transplant.* **2020**, *20*, 1334–1340. [CrossRef] [PubMed]
57. Davis, C.L.; Delmonico, F.L. Living-donor kidney transplantation: a review of the current practices for the live donor. *J. Am. Soc. Nephrol.* **2005**, *16*, 2098–2110. [CrossRef] [PubMed]
58. Mizusaki, K.; Hasuike, Y.; Kimura, T.; Nagasawa, Y.; Kuragano, T.; Yamada, Y.; Nojima, M.; Yamamoto, S.; Nakanishi, T.; Ishihara, M. Inhibition of the Mammalian Target of Rapamycin May Augment the Increase in Soluble Klotho Levels in Renal Transplantation Recipients. *Blood Purif.* **2019**, *47* (Suppl. 2), 12–18. [CrossRef] [PubMed]
59. Deng, G.; Yang, A.; Wu, J.; Zhou, J.; Meng, S.; Zhu, C.; Wang, J.; Shen, S.; Ma, J.; Liu, D. The Value of Older Donors' Klotho Level in Predicting Recipients' Short-Term Renal Function. *Med. Sci. Monit.* **2018**, *24*, 7936–7943. [CrossRef] [PubMed]
60. Kim, S.M.; Kim, S.J.; Ahn, S.; Min, S.-I.; Min, S.-K.; Ha, J. The Potential Role of Klotho as a Prognostic Biomarker in Deceased Donor Kidney Transplantation. *Transplantation* **2018**, *102*, S539. [CrossRef]
61. Kubota, M.; Hamasaki, Y.; Masuda, T.; Hashimoto, J.; Takahashi, Y.; Saito, A.; Yuasa, R.; Muramatsu, M.; Sakai, K.; Shishido, S. Fgf 23-Aklotho axis and phosphate metabolism in the early post-kidney transplantation period. In *Pediatric Transplantation*; Wiley: Hoboken, NJ, USA, 2019.
62. Tan, S.J.; Crosthwaite, A.; Langsford, D.; Obeysekere, V.; Ierino, F.L.; Roberts, M.A.; Hughes, P.D.; Hewitson, T.D.; Dwyer, K.M.; Toussaint, N.D. Mineral adaptations following kidney transplantation. *Transpl. Int.* **2017**, *30*, 463–473. [CrossRef] [PubMed]
63. Baloglu, İ.; Turkmen, K.; Selçuk, N.Y.; Tonbul, H.Z.; Erdur, F.M. Fgf-23 and Klotho Levels in Renal Transplant Patients and Comparison with Hemodialysis Patients. In *Nephrology Dialysis Transplantation*; Oxford University Press: Oxford, UK, 2017.
64. Tartaglione, L.; Pasquali, M.; Rotondi, S.; Muci, M.L.; Leonangeli, C.; Farcomeni, A.; Fassino, V.; Mazzaferro, S. Interactions of sclerostin with FGF23, soluble klotho and vitamin D in renal transplantation. *PLoS ONE* **2017**, *12*, e0178637. [CrossRef] [PubMed]
65. Zaare Nahandi, M.; Ardalan, M.R.; Banagozar Mohamadi, A.; Ghorbani Haghjo, A.; Jabbarpor Bonyadi, M.; Mohamadian, T. Relationship of Serum Klotho Level With ACE Gene Polymorphism in Stable Kidney Allograft Recipients. *Iran. J. Kidney Dis.* **2017**, *11*, 151–156. [PubMed]
66. Bleskestad, I.H.; Thorsen, I.S.; Jonsson, G.; Skadberg, Ø.; Bergrem, H.; Gøransson, L.G. Soluble Klotho and intact fibroblast growth factor 23 in long-term kidney transplant patients. *Eur. J. Endocrinol.* **2015**, *172*, 343–350. [CrossRef]

67. Malyszko, J.; Koc-Zorawska, E.; Matuszkiewicz-Rowinska, J. FGF23 and Klotho in relation to markers of endothelial dysfunction in kidney transplant recipients. *Transplant. Proc.* **2014**, *46*, 2647–2650. [CrossRef]
68. Akimoto, T.; Kimura, T.; Watanabe, Y.; Ishikawa, N.; Iwazu, Y.; Saito, O.; Muto, S.; Yagisawa, T.; Kusano, E. The impact of nephrectomy and renal transplantation on serum levels of soluble Klotho protein. *Transplant. Proc.* **2013**, *45*, 134–136. [CrossRef]
69. Kimura, T.; Akimoto, T.; Watanabe, Y.; Kurosawa, A.; Nanmoku, K.; Muto, S.; Kusano, E.; Yagisawa, T.; Nagata, D. Impact of Renal Transplantation and Nephrectomy on Urinary Soluble Klotho Protein. *Transplant. Proc.* **2015**, *47*, 1697–1699. [CrossRef]
70. Ponte, B.; Trombetti, A.; Hadaya, K.; Ernandez, T.; Fumeaux, D.; Iselin, C.; Martin, P.Y.; de Seigneux, S. Acute and long term mineral metabolism adaptation in living kidney donors: A prospective study. *Bone* **2014**, *62*, 36–42. [CrossRef]
71. Tan, S.J.; Hewitson, T.D.; Hughes, P.D.; Holt, S.G.; Toussaint, N.D. Changes in Markers of Mineral Metabolism After Living Kidney Donation. *Transplant. Direct* **2017**, *3*, e150. [CrossRef]
72. Thorsen, I.S.; Bleskestad, I.H.; Jonsson, G.; Skadberg, Ø.; Gøransson, L.G. Neutrophil Gelatinase-Associated Lipocalin, Fibroblast Growth Factor 23, and Soluble Klotho in Long-Term Kidney Donors. *Nephron Extra* **2016**, *6*, 31–39. [CrossRef]
73. Hong, Y.A.; Choi, D.E.; Lim, S.W.; Yang, C.W.; Chang, Y.K. Decreased parathyroid Klotho expression is associated with persistent hyperparathyroidism after kidney transplantation. *Transplant. Proc.* **2013**, *45*, 2957–2962. [CrossRef]
74. Ozdem, S.; Yılmaz, V.T.; Ozdem, S.S.; Donmez, L.; Cetinkaya, R.; Suleymanlar, G.; Ersoy, F.F. Is Klotho F352V Polymorphism the Missing Piece of the Bone Loss Puzzle in Renal Transplant Recipients? *Pharmacology* **2015**, *95*, 271–278. [CrossRef]
75. Krajisnik, T.; Olauson, H.; Mirza, M.A.; Hellman, P.; Akerström, G.; Westin, G.; Larsson, T.E.; Björklund, P. Parathyroid Klotho and FGF-receptor 1 expression decline with renal function in hyperparathyroid patients with chronic kidney disease and kidney transplant recipients. *Kidney Int.* **2010**, *78*, 1024–1032. [CrossRef] [PubMed]
76. Moher, D.; Liberati, A.; Tetzlaff, J.; Altman, D.G. Preferred reporting items for systematic reviews and meta-analyses: The PRISMA statement. *PLoS Med.* **2009**, *6*, e1000097. [CrossRef]
77. DerSimonian, R.; Laird, N. Meta-analysis in clinical trials. *Control. Clin. Trials* **1986**, *7*, 177–188. [CrossRef]
78. Follmann, D.; Elliott, P.; Suh, I.; Cutler, J. Variance imputation for overviews of clinical trials with continuous response. *J. Clin. Epidemiol.* **1992**, *45*, 769–773. [CrossRef]
79. Cohen, J. Statistical power analysis. *Curr. Dir. Psychol. Sci.* **1992**, *1*, 98–101. [CrossRef]
80. Higgins, J.P.; Thompson, S.G.; Deeks, J.J.; Altman, D.G. Measuring inconsistency in meta-analyses. *BMJ* **2003**, *327*, 557–560. [CrossRef] [PubMed]
81. Easterbrook, P.J.; Berlin, J.A.; Gopalan, R.; Matthews, D.R. Publication bias in clinical research. *Lancet* **1991**, *337*, 867–872. [CrossRef]
82. Egger, M.; Davey Smith, G.; Schneider, M.; Minder, C. Bias in meta-analysis detected by a simple, graphical test. *BMJ* **1997**, *315*, 629–634. [CrossRef]
83. John, G.B.; Cheng, C.Y.; Kuro-o, M. Role of Klotho in aging, phosphate metabolism, and CKD. *Am. J. Kidney Dis.* **2011**, *58*, 127–134. [CrossRef] [PubMed]
84. Kalaitzidis, R.G.; Duni, A.; Siamopoulos, K.C. Klotho, the Holy Grail of the kidney: from salt sensitivity to chronic kidney disease. *Int. Urol. Nephrol.* **2016**, *48*, 1657–1666. [CrossRef] [PubMed]
85. Van Londen, M.; Aarts, B.M.; Deetman, P.E.; van der Weijden, J.; Eisenga, M.F.; Navis, G.; Bakker, S.J.L.; de Borst, M.H. Post-Transplant Hypophosphatemia and the Risk of Death-Censored Graft Failure and Mortality after Kidney Transplantation. *Clin. J. Am. Soc. Nephrol.* **2017**, *12*, 1301–1310. [CrossRef] [PubMed]
86. Nakai, K.; Mitsuiki, K.; Kuroki, Y.; Nishiki, T.; Motoyama, K.; Nakano, T.; Kitazono, T. Relative hypophosphatemia early after transplantation is a predictor of good kidney graft function. *Clin. Exp. Nephrol.* **2019**, *23*, 1161–1168. [CrossRef]
87. Hu, M.C.; Moe, O.W. Klotho as a potential biomarker and therapy for acute kidney injury. *Nat. Rev. Nephrol.* **2012**, *8*, 423–429. [CrossRef] [PubMed]
88. Aiello, S.; Noris, M. Klotho in acute kidney injury: Biomarker, therapy, or a bit of both? *Kidney Int.* **2010**, *78*, 1208–1210. [CrossRef] [PubMed]

89. Li, P.; Shi, M.; Maique, J.; Shaffer, J.; Yan, S.; Moe, O.W.; Hu, M.C. Beclin 1/Bcl-2 complex-dependent autophagy activity modulates renal susceptibility to ischemia-reperfusion injury and mediates renoprotection by Klotho. American journal of physiology. *Am. J. Physiol. Renal Physiol.* **2020**, *318*, F772–F792. [CrossRef] [PubMed]
90. Castellano, G.; Intini, A.; Stasi, A.; Divella, C.; Gigante, M.; Pontrelli, P.; Franzin, R.; Accetturo, M.; Zito, A.; Fiorentino, M.; et al. Complement Modulation of Anti-Aging Factor Klotho in Ischemia/Reperfusion Injury and Delayed Graft Function. *Am. J. Transplant.* **2016**, *16*, 325–333. [CrossRef]
91. De Sandes-Freitas, T.V.; Felipe, C.R.; Aguiar, W.F.; Cristelli, M.P.; Tedesco-Silva, H.; Medina-Pestana, J.O. Prolonged Delayed Graft Function Is Associated with Inferior Patient and Kidney Allograft Survivals. *PLoS ONE* **2015**, *10*, e0144188. [CrossRef] [PubMed]
92. Weber, S.; Dienemann, T.; Jacobi, J.; Eckardt, K.U.; Weidemann, A. Delayed graft function is associated with an increased rate of renal allograft rejection: A retrospective single center analysis. *PLoS ONE* **2018**, *13*, e0199445. [CrossRef] [PubMed]
93. Lee, C.H.; Kim, G.H. Electrolyte and Acid-base disturbances induced by clacineurin inhibitors. *Electrolyte Blood Press* **2007**, *5*, 126–130. [PubMed]
94. Demeule, M.; Béliveau, R. Cyclosporin inhibits phosphate transport and stimulates alkaline phosphatase activity in renal BBMV. *Am. J. Physiol.* **1991**, *260*, F518–F524. [PubMed]
95. Falkiewicz, K.; Nahaczewska, W.; Boratynska, M.; Owczarek, H.; Klinger, M.; Kaminska, D.; Wozniak, M.; Szepietowski, T.; Patrzalek, D. Tacrolimus decreases tubular phosphate wasting in renal allograft recipients. *Transplant. Proc.* **2003**, *35*, 2213–2215.
96. Messa, P.; Cafforio, C.; Alfieri, C. Calcium and phosphate changes after renal transplantation. *J. Nephrol.* **2010**, *23* (Suppl. 16), S175–S181. [PubMed]
97. Sakhaee, K. Post-renal transplantation hypophosphatemia. *Pediatr. Nephrol.* **2010**, *25*, 213–220.
98. Cheungpasitporn, W.; Thongprayoon, C.; Hansrivijit, P.; Medaura, J.; Chewcharat, A.; Bathini, T.; Mao, M.; Erickson, S. Impact of admission calcium-phosphate product on 1-year mortality among hospitalized patients. *Adv. Biomed. Res.* **2020**, *9*, 14.
99. Thongprayoon, C.; Cheungpasitporn, W.; Mao, M.A.; Erickson, S.B. Calcium-phosphate product and its impact on mortality in hospitalized patients. *Nephrology (Carlton)* **2020**, *25*, 22–28. [PubMed]
100. Pichler, G.; Haller, M.C.; Kainz, A.; Wolf, M.; Redon, J.; Oberbauer, R. Prognostic value of bone- and vascular-derived molecular biomarkers in hemodialysis and renal transplant patients: A systematic review and meta-analysis. *Nephrol. Dial. Transplant.* **2017**, *32*, 1566–1578.
101. Lentine, K.L.; Patel, A. Risks and outcomes of living donation. *Adv. Chronic Kidney Dis.* **2012**, *19*, 220–228.
102. Ommen, E.S.; Winston, J.A.; Murphy, B. Medical risks in living kidney donors: absence of proof is not proof of absence. *Clin. J. Am. Soc. Nephrol.* **2006**, *1*, 885–895.
103. Asgari, E.; Hilton, R.M. One size does not fit all: Understanding individual living kidney donor risk. *Pediatr. Nephrol.* **2020**. [CrossRef] [PubMed]
104. Fehrman-Ekholm, I.; Elinder, C.G.; Stenbeck, M.; Tydén, G.; Groth, C.G. Kidney donors live longer. *Transplantation* **1997**, *64*, 976–978. [CrossRef]
105. Okamoto, M.; Akioka, K.; Nobori, S.; Ushigome, H.; Kozaki, K.; Kaihara, S.; Yoshimura, N. Short- and long-term donor outcomes after kidney donation: analysis of 601 cases over a 35-year period at Japanese single center. *Transplantation* **2009**, *87*, 419–423. [CrossRef] [PubMed]
106. Ibrahim, H.N.; Foley, R.; Tan, L.; Rogers, T.; Bailey, R.F.; Guo, H.; Gross, C.R.; Matas, A.J. Long-term consequences of kidney donation. *N. Engl. J. Med.* **2009**, *360*, 459–469. [CrossRef] [PubMed]
107. Segev, D.L.; Muzaale, A.D.; Caffo, B.S.; Mehta, S.H.; Singer, A.L.; Taranto, S.E.; McBride, M.A.; Montgomery, R.A. Perioperative mortality and long-term survival following live kidney donation. *JAMA* **2010**, *303*, 959–966. [CrossRef] [PubMed]
108. O'Keeffe, L.M.; Ramond, A.; Oliver-Williams, C.; Willeit, P.; Paige, E.; Trotter, P.; Evans, J.; Wadström, J.; Nicholson, M.; Collett, D.; et al. Mid- and Long-Term Health Risks in Living Kidney Donors: A Systematic Review and Meta-analysis. *Ann. Intern. Med.* **2018**, *168*, 276–284. [CrossRef] [PubMed]
109. Garg, A.X.; Meirambayeva, A.; Huang, A.; Kim, J.; Prasad, G.V.; Knoll, G.; Boudville, N.; Lok, C.; McFarlane, P.; Karpinski, M.; et al. Cardiovascular disease in kidney donors: Matched cohort study. *BMJ* **2012**, *344*, e1203. [CrossRef]
110. Musgrove, J.; Wolf, M. Regulation and Effects of FGF23 in Chronic Kidney Disease. *Annu. Rev. Physiol.* **2020**, *82*, 365–390. [CrossRef]

111. Wolf, M. Forging forward with 10 burning questions on FGF23 in kidney disease. *J. Am. Soc. Nephrol.* **2010**, *21*, 1427–1435. [CrossRef]
112. Marthi, A.; Donovan, K.; Haynes, R.; Wheeler, D.C.; Baigent, C.; Rooney, C.M.; Landray, M.J.; Moe, S.M.; Yang, J.; Holland, L.; et al. Fibroblast Growth Factor-23 and Risks of Cardiovascular and Noncardiovascular Diseases: A Meta-Analysis. *J. Am. Soc. Nephrol.* **2018**, *29*, 2015–2027. [CrossRef]
113. Grabner, A.; Amaral, A.P.; Schramm, K.; Singh, S.; Sloan, A.; Yanucil, C.; Li, J.; Shehadeh, L.A.; Hare, J.M.; David, V.; et al. Activation of Cardiac Fibroblast Growth Factor Receptor 4 Causes Left Ventricular Hypertrophy. *Cell Metab.* **2015**, *22*, 1020–1032. [CrossRef] [PubMed]
114. Moody, W.E.; Ferro, C.J.; Edwards, N.C.; Chue, C.D.; Lin, E.L.; Taylor, R.J.; Cockwell, P.; Steeds, R.P.; Townend, J.N. Cardiovascular Effects of Unilateral Nephrectomy in Living Kidney Donors. *Hypertension* **2016**, *67*, 368–377. [CrossRef] [PubMed]
115. Vervloet, M.G.; Massy, Z.A.; Brandenburg, V.M.; Mazzaferro, S.; Cozzolino, M.; Ureña-Torres, P.; Bover, J.; Goldsmith, D. Bone: A new endocrine organ at the heart of chronic kidney disease and mineral and bone disorders. *Lancet Diabetes Endocrinol.* **2014**, *2*, 427–436. [CrossRef]
116. Hum, J.M.; O'Bryan, L.M.; Tatiparthi, A.K.; Cass, T.A.; Clinkenbeard, E.L.; Cramer, M.S.; Bhaskaran, M.; Johnson, R.L.; Wilson, J.M.; Smith, R.C.; et al. Chronic Hyperphosphatemia and Vascular Calcification Are Reduced by Stable Delivery of Soluble Klotho. *J. Am. Soc. Nephrol.* **2017**, *28*, 1162–1174. [CrossRef] [PubMed]
117. Xie, J.; Yoon, J.; An, S.W.; Kuro-o, M.; Huang, C.L. Soluble Klotho Protects against Uremic Cardiomyopathy Independently of Fibroblast Growth Factor 23 and Phosphate. *J. Am. Soc. Nephrol.* **2015**, *26*, 1150–1160. [CrossRef] [PubMed]
118. Xie, J.; Cha, S.K.; An, S.W.; Kuro, O.M.; Birnbaumer, L.; Huang, C.L. Cardioprotection by Klotho through downregulation of TRPC6 channels in the mouse heart. *Nat. Commun.* **2012**, *3*, 1238. [CrossRef] [PubMed]
119. Leone, F.; Lofaro, D.; Gigliotti, P.; Perri, A.; Vizza, D.; Toteda, G.; Lupinacci, S.; Armentano, F.; Papalia, T.; Bonofiglio, R. Soluble Klotho levels in adult renal transplant recipients are modulated by recombinant human erythropoietin. *J. Nephrol.* **2014**, *27*, 577–585. [CrossRef]
120. Donate-Correa, J.; Henríquez-Palop, F.; Martín-Núñez, E.; Pérez-Delgado, N.; Muros-de-Fuentes, M.; Mora-Fernández, C.; Navarro-González, J.F. Effect of Paricalcitol on FGF-23 and Klotho in Kidney Transplant Recipients. *Transplantation* **2016**, *100*, 2432–2438. [CrossRef]
121. Prather, A.A.; Epel, E.S.; Arenander, J.; Broestl, L.; Garay, B.I.; Wang, D.; Dubal, D.B. Longevity factor klotho and chronic psychological stress. *Transl. Psychiatry* **2015**, *5*, e585. [CrossRef]
122. Jurado-Fasoli, L.; Amaro-Gahete, F.J.; De-la, O.A.; Gutiérrez, Á.; Castillo, M.J. Alcohol consumption and S-Klotho plasma levels in sedentary healthy middle-aged adults: A cross sectional study. *Drug Alcohol Depend.* **2019**, *194*, 107–111. [CrossRef]
123. Amaro-Gahete, F.J.; De-la, O.A.; Jurado-Fasoli, L.; Ruiz, J.R.; Castillo, M.J.; Gutiérrez, Á. Role of Exercise on S-Klotho Protein Regulation: A Systematic Review. *Curr. Aging Sci.* **2018**, *11*, 100–107. [CrossRef] [PubMed]
124. Jurado-Fasoli, L.; Amaro-Gahete, F.J.; De-la, O.A.; Martinez-Tellez, B.; Ruiz, J.R.; Gutiérrez, Á.; Castillo, M.J. Adherence to the Mediterranean diet, dietary factors, and S-Klotho plasma levels in sedentary middle-aged adults. *Exp. Gerontol.* **2019**, *119*, 25–32. [CrossRef] [PubMed]
125. Deng, G.; Liu, D. Klotho: A Promising Biomarker Closely Related to Kidney Transplant. *Exp. Clin. Transplant.* **2018**, *16*, 253–258. [PubMed]
126. Neyra, J.A.; Moe, O.W.; Pastor, J.; Gianella, F.; Sidhu, S.S.; Sarnak, M.J.; Ix, J.H.; Drew, D.A. Performance of soluble Klotho assays in clinical samples of kidney disease. *Clin. Kidney J.* **2020**, *13*, 235–244. [CrossRef] [PubMed]

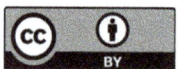

© 2020 by the authors. Licensee MDPI, Basel, Switzerland. This article is an open access article distributed under the terms and conditions of the Creative Commons Attribution (CC BY) license (http://creativecommons.org/licenses/by/4.0/).

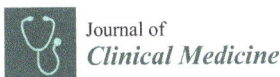

Article

Conversion from Standard-Release Tacrolimus to MeltDose® Tacrolimus (LCPT) Improves Renal Function after Liver Transplantation

Johannes von Einsiedel [1,†], Gerold Thölking [2,*,†], Christian Wilms [1], Elena Vorona [1], Arne Bokemeyer [1], Hartmut H. Schmidt [1], Iyad Kabar [1,‡] and Anna Hüsing-Kabar [1,‡]

1. Department of Medicine B, Gastroenterology and Hepatology, University Hospital Münster, 48149 Münster, Germany; johannes.voneinsiedel@ukmuenster.de (J.v.E.); Christian.Wilms@ukmuenster.de (C.W.); Elena.Vorona@ukmuenster.de (E.V.); Arne.Bokemeyer@ukmuenster.de (A.B.); hepar@ukmuenster.de (H.H.S.); iyad.kabar@ukmuenster.de (I.K.); Anna.Huesing-Kabar@ukmuenster.de (A.H.-K.)
2. Department of Internal Medicine and Nephrology, University Hospital of Münster Marienhospital Steinfurt, 48565 Steinfurt, Germany
* Correspondence: Gerold.Thoelking@ukmuenster.de; Tel.: +49-2552-791226; Fax: +49-2552-791181
† These authors contributed equally and are both considered first authors.
‡ These authors contributed equally and are both considered last authors.

Received: 17 April 2020; Accepted: 28 May 2020; Published: 1 June 2020

Abstract: Renal impairment is a typical side effect of tacrolimus (Tac) treatment in liver transplant (LT) recipients. One strategy to avoid renal dysfunction is to increase the concentration/dose (C/D) ratio by improving drug bioavailability. LT recipients converted from standard-release Tac to MeltDose® Tac (LCPT), a novel technological formulation, were able to reduce the required Tac dose due to higher bioavailability. Hence, we hypothesize that such a conversion increases the C/D ratio, resulting in a preservation of renal function. In the intervention group, patients were switched from standard-release Tac to LCPT. Clinical data were collected for 12 months after conversion. Patients maintained on standard-release Tac were enrolled as a control group. Twelve months after conversion to LCPT, median C/D ratio had increased significantly by 50% ($p < 0.001$), with the first significant increase seen 3 months after conversion ($p = 0.008$). In contrast, C/D ratio in the control group was unchanged after 12 months (1.75 vs. 1.76; $p = 0.847$). Estimated glomerular filtration rate (eGFR) had already significantly deteriorated in the control group at 9 months (65.6 vs. 70.6 mL/min/1.73 m^2 at study onset; $p = 0.006$). Notably, patients converted to LCPT already had significant recovery of mean eGFR 6 months after conversion (67.5 vs. 65.3 mL/min/1.73 m^2 at study onset; $p = 0.029$). In summary, conversion of LT recipients to LCPT increased C/D ratio associated with renal function improvement.

Keywords: MeltDose®; LCPT; tacrolimus; renal function; liver transplantation; C/D ratio; metabolism

---

1. Introduction

The calcineurin inhibitor tacrolimus (Tac) is considered a first-line immunosuppressant in liver transplant (LT) recipients [1–4]. Because of its small therapeutic window, therapy with Tac requires close drug monitoring [5]. In addition, deterioration of renal function induced by acute or chronic calcineurin inhibitor nephrotoxicity (CNIT) is a common side effect [6]. Recent studies have reported characteristics of chronic CNIT in up to 70% of LT recipients [7,8]. Furthermore, up to 8.5% of patients develop end-stage renal disease in long-term follow-up [9].

Several studies have revealed that the risk of CNIT is associated with both high Tac trough concentration and high daily Tac dose [10,11], although CNIT may occur even with low-dose regimens [12]. One potential explanation for this association is the correlation between CNIT and a fast metabolism rate of twice-daily immediate-release Tac (IR-Tac). The Tac blood concentration to daily dose ratio (C/D ratio) has been identified as a simple tool to describe patients' metabolism rate in a steady state, in which a low C/D ratio reflects a high rate of metabolism [13–15]. A low IR-Tac C/D ratio is linked with higher C2 Tac blood concentrations despite comparable trough levels in patients with high C/D ratios [16]. In this regard, a low C/D ratio is strongly associated with an increased risk of CNIT and a faster decline of renal function in both kidney transplant (KT) and LT recipients [13,16–19]. Thus, increasing the C/D ratio by improving Tac bioavailability may result in better nephroprotection. One way of potentially influencing the pharmacokinetics of Tac is to change the formulation of the drug [20].

LCPT is a novel Tac formulation using MeltDose® technology, in which the particle size of the drug is reduced from 10 µm to the smallest possible units (<0.1 µm), resulting in increased dissolution and thus better absorption [21]. This feature, combined with drug release over the entire intestinal tract, results in LCPT having significantly better bioavailability than other Tac formulations. Tremblay et al. showed that the intraday peak-to-trough fluctuation was approximately 30% lower for LCPT than for standard-release Tac (IR-Tac and once- daily extended-release Tac (ER-Tac)) [20]. A dose reduction of up to 30% has been observed in KT and LT recipients on LCPT [22].

Hence, we hypothesize that conversion from standard-release Tac to LCPT increases C/D ratio and thereby preserves renal function.

2. Materials and Methods

2.1. Patients and Study Design

Figure 1 illustrates the enrolment of the subjects in the study. This observational study was performed on patients who had undergone cadaveric liver transplantation at the University Hospital of Münster. LT recipients were included at the time of presentation at our Outpatient Transplant Clinic between March 2017 and August 2018. The study start was defined as the first appointment in this period.

At this time point, the treating physicians made a decision to either leave the patients on their usual immunosuppressive treatment (control group) or to switch them from standard-release Tac (IR- or ER-Tac) to LCPT (intervention group). Data were analysed over a 12-month follow-up. Inclusion criteria were aged over 18 years, intake of standard-release Tac before enrolment, stable graft function and an interval between transplantation and inclusion in the study of at least 1 month. LT recipients were not allowed to receive any medications or agents that could interfere with Tac. The decision about drug conversion was made by treating physicians at their own discretion.

The initial immunosuppressive regimen consisted of Tac (Prograf or Advagraf), mycophenolate mofetil (CellCept, MMF) and prednisolone (Decortin H/Soludecortin H). Tac was given at a dose of 0.1 mg/kg twice daily with a target trough concentration of 8–10 ng/mL during the first month, 6–8 ng/mL from months 2 to 3, and 3–5 ng/mL thereafter. MMF was started at a dose of 1 g twice daily and was adjusted in case of adverse effects. Initial prednisolone was given at a dose of 250 mg once daily intravenously before and immediately after LTx and was tapered stepwise. In most cases, prednisolone had been discontinued within 6–12 months after LTx.

Laboratory data were collected at study onset (at the time of conversion to LCPT or the first presentation during the above-mentioned period in the control group (t_0)) and after 3 (t_3), 6 (t_6), 9 (t_9) and 12 (t_{12}) months. Serum bilirubin, alanine transaminase (ALT) and international normalized ratio (INR) were measured to assess graft function. General demographic data and information on transplantation and diagnoses were obtained from the patient records.

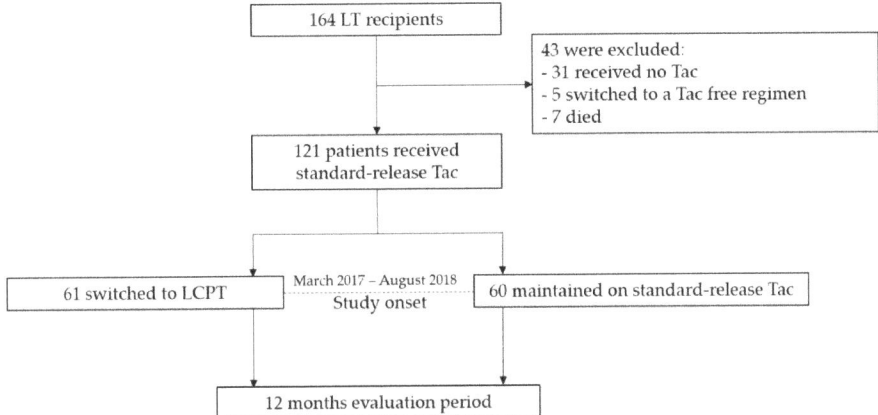

Figure 1. Study design and patient enrolment. A total of 164 liver transplant (LT) recipients were screened for eligibility. Only LT recipients who were started on IR- or ER-Tac (standard-release tacrolimus) and continued taking this drug until the beginning of the study were included. During the enrolment period (March 2017–August 2018), 121 patients met the inclusion criteria and were either switched to LCPT (once-daily MeltDose® tacrolimus (Tac); intervention group) or maintained on standard-release tacrolimus (control group). Clinical data were analysed in a 12-month follow-up. We hypothesized that conversion from standard-release Tac to LCPT increases concentration/dose (C/D) ratio and thereby preserves renal function

The C/D ratio, calculated as the ratio of Tac trough level to the corresponding daily dose, was determined 3 months before study start, at the study start and at subsequent evaluation time points. The t_0 C/D ratio in the intervention group was determined the day before first LCPT intake. Renal function was calculated using the estimated glomerular filtration rate (eGFR) in accordance with the Chronic Kidney Disease Epidemiology Collaboration equation at the corresponding time points. The difference from baseline eGFR (t_0) was determined at the time points of t_3, t_6, t_9 and t_{12}. A negative value indicates deterioration of eGFR, while a positive value indicates improvement.

The study was conducted in accordance with current medical guidelines and the Declarations of Istanbul and Helsinki. The study was also approved by the local ethics committee (Ethik Kommission der Ärztekammer Westfalen-Lippe und der Medizinischen Fakultät der Westfälischen Wilhelms-Universität Münster, No. 2016-046-f-S). Collected patient data were anonymized and written consent for collection and use of the clinical data was obtained.

2.2. Statistical Analysis

Statistical analysis was performed with IBM SPSS® Statistics 25 for Windows (IBM Corporation, Somers, NY, USA). Normally distributed data are shown as mean ± standard deviation; non-normally distributed data are shown as median (minimum–maximum). For unrelated groups, normally distributed data were compared with a *t*-test, non-normally distributed data with the Mann–Whitney U-test and categorical variables with Fisher's exact test. Comparison of continuous variables within a connected group was performed with the Wilcoxon signed-rank test. Pearson's test was used to describe normally distributed data, whereas Spearman's test was applied to non-normally distributed data. In all statistical evaluations, two-sided tests were used; a *p*-value of ≤ 0.05 was considered significant for all tests performed.

The study onset was defined as the baseline (t_0). In the first approach, eGFR changes (t_3-t_{12}) from baseline were compared between the intervention group and the control group. In the next step, eGFR changes from every time point to baseline were compared within each group (eGFR slope).

A negative value indicates deterioration in eGFR, whereas a positive value indicates an improvement in renal function.

Multivariable analysis was performed to identify independent predictors of alterations in renal function (ΔeGFR) after 12 months compared with that at baseline. For this purpose, univariable analysis with factors known to potentially influence renal function was initially performed. Variables that showed a p-value < 0.15 in univariable analysis were included in the multivariable analysis. Variables with a significance of <0.05 in multivariable analysis were considered significant.

3. Results

3.1. Study Population

A total of 121 patients were included in this study: 61 in the intervention group and 60 in the control group. An overview of patient characteristics, underlying diagnoses for LTx, comorbidities and immunosuppression is shown in Tables 1 and 2. There were only small differences in the demographic data between the study groups. The control group had a more extended warm ischemic time ($p = 0.005$). As coimmunosuppression, patients received mycophenolate mofetil (MMF) at a daily dose of 1000 (500–2000) mg (LCPT) and 1500 (500–2000) mg (control), everolimus at 2.0 (0.5–5.0) mg (LCPT) and 2.0 (2.0–4.0) mg (control), prednisolone at 5.0 (5.0–7.5) mg (LCPT and control) and sirolimus at 1.0 mg (control). In the intervention group, 45 patients suffered from chronic kidney disease (CKD, categories 2–4). The control group showed a similar distribution in 39 LT recipients. No patients were in CKD category 5 or on dialysis. In the absence of kidney biopsies, the underlying renal disease remained unclear. The median interval between transplantation and study onset was 2.8 (0.1–20.8) years in the intervention group and 6.6 (0.2–16.5) years in the control group ($p < 0.001$). The reasons for a conversion from standard-release Tac to LCPT were CNIT (n = 7), neurotoxicity (n = 5) and prevention of side effects via better bioavailability of LCPT (n = 49).

Table 1. Patient characteristics.

	LCPT (n = 61)	Standard-Release Tac (n = 60)	p-Value
Age at LTx (years)	46.3 ± 16.7	48.8 ± 12.4	0.348 [a]
Age at study onset (years)	51.0 ± 15.9	56.1 ± 12.7	0.054 [a]
Height (m)	1.72 ± 0.087	1.73 ± 0.094	0.714 [a]
Weight (kg)	79.4 ± 20.8	76.7 ± 16.5	0.420 [a]
BMI (kg/m^2)	26.7 ± 6.1	25.6 ± 5.0	0.310 [a]
Sex (male/female)	29 (47.5%)/32 (52.5%)	38 (63.3%)/22 (36.7%)	0.101 [b]
CIT (h)	11.3 ± 2.6	10.5 ± 2.4	0.065 [a]
WIT (min)	38.9 ± 9.2	43.8 ± 8.7	0.005 [a]
Number of grafts			0.255 [b]
One	56 (91.8%)	49 (81.7%)	
Two	4 (6.6%)	8 (13.3%)	
Three	1 (1.6%)	3 (5.0%)	
Blood type			0.545 [b]
A	28 (47.5%)	30 (50.0%)	
B	6 (10.2%)	6 (10.0%)	
AB	6 (10.2%)	2 (3.3%)	
O	19 (32.2%)	22 (36.7%)	
Hepatitis B antigen (positive)	5 (8.2%)	7 (11.9%)	0.556 [b]
Hepatitis C antibody (positive)	9 (14.8%)	8 (13.6%)	1.000 [b]
Recipient CMV IgG (positive)	34 (57.6%)	27 (45.0%)	0.201 [b]
Donor CMV IgG (positive)	32 (56.1%)	37 (63.8%)	0.450 [b]

Statistics: Values shown as mean ± standard deviation or number (percentage). [a] t-test, [b] Fisher's exact test. LCPT, once-daily MeltDose® tacrolimus; Tac, tacrolimus; LTx, liver transplantation; BMI, body mass index; CIT, cold ischemic time; WIT, warm ischemic time; CMV, cytomegalovirus.

Table 2. Underlying diagnoses for LTx, comorbidities and immunosuppression at study start.

	LCPT (n = 61)	Standard-Release Tac (n = 60)	p-Value
Principal diagnosis			0.455
Alcoholism	9 (14.8%)	16 (26.7%)	
Viral hepatitis	15 (24.6%)	15 (25.0%)	
Genetically related metabolic disease	7 (11.5%)	5 (8.3%)	
Toxic: nutritional or NASH	3 (4.9%)	1 (1.7%)	
Autoimmune liver disease	11 (18.0%)	13 (21.7%)	
Other	16 (26.2%)	10 (16.7%)	
Arterial hypertension	36 (59.0%)	37 (61.7%)	0.853
Diabetes mellitus	18 (29.5%)	17 (28.3%)	1.000
Hyperlipidaemia	19 (31.1%)	14 (23.3%)	0.415
CKD at study start			0.598
CKD 2	18 (29.5%)	21 (35.0%)	
CKD 3a	16 (26.2%)	10 (16.7%)	
CKD 3b	9 (14.8%)	7 (11.7%)	
CKD 4	2 (3.3%)	1 (1.7%)	
Tac formulation at study onset			<0.001
Immediate-release Tac	43 (70.5%)	22 (36.7%)	
Extended-release Tac	18 (29.5%)	38 (63.3%)	
Co-immunosuppression			0.060
MMF	34 (55.7%)	35 (58.3%)	
Everolimus	13 (21.3%)	5 (8.3%)	
Prednisolone	3 (4.9%)	10 (16.7%)	
Sirolimus	0	1 (1.7%)	
None	11 (18.0%)	9 (15.0%)	
Reasons for a switch to LCPT			
CNIT	7		
Neurotoxicity	5		
Preventions of side effects	49		

Statistics: Values shown as number (percentage). All p-values from Fisher's exact tests. LCPT, once-daily MeltDose® tacrolimus; Tac, tacrolimus; LTx, liver transplantation; NASH, nonalcoholic steatohepatitis; CKD, chronic kidney disease (categories set with reference to [23]). MMF, mycophenolate mofetil; CNIT, calcineurin inhibitor nephrotoxicity.

3.2. C/D Ratio

At study start (baseline), the C/D ratio in the intervention group was comparable to that in the control group (1.68 (0.30–13.45) vs. 1.76 (0.38–7.40) ng/mL×1/mg, respectively; $p = 0.362$, Table 3). During the 12-month evaluation period, no significant changes in the C/D ratio were observed in the control group. After 12 months, the median C/D ratio was approximately at the baseline level (1.75 (0.49–6.40) ng/mL × 1/mg; $p = 0.847$). In the control group, there was a slight decrease in both the daily Tac dose at study end compared with that at baseline (2.5 (0.5–10.0) vs. 2.8 (0.5–10.0) mg, respectively; $p = 0.084$), as well as in the median Tac trough level (4.7 (1.5–14.3) ng/mL at study onset to 4.1 (1.6–15.6) ng/mL after 12 months; $p = 0.082$). However, the differences in both cases were not significant.

In contrast, the C/D ratio in patients switched to LCPT was 50% higher 12 months after conversion than that at baseline (2.52 (0.58–6.40) vs. 1.68 (0.30–13.45) ng/mL × 1/mg, respectively; $p < 0.001$). A significant increase in the C/D ratio was already observed in this group 3 months after study onset (2.03 (0.33–13.60) ng/mL × 1/mg; $p = 0.008$). Regarding the daily Tac dose, a significant reduction of 33.3% was observed after 12 months compared with that at baseline (2.0 (0.4–7.8) vs. 3.0 (1.0–22.0) mg, respectively; $p < 0.001$)). Moreover, the Tac trough level was significantly reduced at study end (4.4 (2.2–11.8) vs. 6.0 (1.5–26.9) ng/mL at study onset; $p < 0.001$).

To confirm that conditions were stable before study onset, C/D ratios, Tac doses and trough level 3 months before enrolment were also obtained. There were no significant differences between the groups at t_{-3} (Table 3) nor between study start and 3 months earlier within a group. Patients in the intervention group showed similar median C/D ratio compared with that at baseline (1.44 (0.24–6.20) vs. 1.68 (0.30–13.45) ng/mL × 1/mg, respectively; $p = 0.204$). Daily Tac dose differed significantly due to single outlier values shortly after transplant (3.0 (0.5–12.0) (t_{-3}) vs. 3.0 (1.0–22.0) (t_0) mg; $p = 0.049$), while Tac trough level showed no considerable differences (5.0 (2.4–15.3) (t_{-3}) vs. 6.0 (1.5–26.9) (t_0) ng/mL; $p = 0.722$).

No significant differences were detectable in the control group between baseline and 3 months before: C/D ratio (1.69 (0.40–9.20) vs. 1.76 (0.38–7.40) ng/mL × 1/mg, respectively; $p = 0.626$), Tac daily dose (2.5 (0.5–9.0) vs. 2.8 (0.5–10.0) mg, respectively; $p = 0.362$) and Tac trough level (4.4 (1.5–14.7) vs. 4.7 (1.5–14.3) ng/mL, respectively; $p = 0.742$).

Table 3. Tacrolimus concentration/dose (C/D) ratio, daily dose and blood trough concentration.

	LCPT	Standard-Release Tac	p-Value
Tac C/D ratio (ng/mL × 1/mg)			
3 months before (n = 54 vs. 58)	1.44 (0.24–6.20) on s-r-Tac	1.69 (0.40–9.20)	0.344
At study onset (n = 61 vs. 60)	1.68 (0.30–13.45) on s-r-Tac	1.76 (0.38–7.40)	0.362
After 3 months (n = 61 vs. 60)	2.03 (0.33–13.60)	1.83 (0.41–7.00)	0.735
After 6 months (n = 61 vs. 60)	2.33 (0.77–8.47)	1.63 (0.68–7.40)	0.011
After 9 months (n = 61 vs. 60)	2.13 (0.60–9.33)	1.70 (0.54–7.20)	0.136
After 12 months (n = 61 vs. 60)	2.52 (0.58–6.40)	1.75 (0.49–6.40)	0.009
Tac daily dose (mg)			
3 months before (n = 54 vs. 58)	3.0 (0.5–12.0) on s-r-Tac	2.5 (0.5–9.0)	0.056
At study onset (n = 61 vs. 60)	3.0 (1.0–22.0) on s-r-Tac	2.8 (0.5–10.0)	0.044
After 3 months (n = 61 vs. 60)	2.0 (0.8–8.0)	2.5 (0.5–9.0)	0.330
After 6 months (n = 61 vs. 60)	2.0 (0.8–5.0)	2.5 (0.5–7.0)	0.248
After 9 months (n = 61 vs. 60)	2.0 (0.4–6.0)	2.5 (0.5–9.0)	0.060
After 12 months (n = 61 vs. 60)	2.0 (0.4–7.8)	2.5 (0.5–10.0)	0.047
Tac trough level (ng/mL)			
3 months before (n = 54 vs. 58)	5.0 (2.4–15.3) on s-r-Tac	4.4 (1.5–14.7)	0.087
At study onset (n = 61 vs. 60)	6.0 (1.5–26.9) on s-r-Tac	4.7 (1.5–14.3)	0.005
After 3 months (n = 61 vs. 60)	4.6 (0.5–13.1)	4.4 (2.2–10.4)	0.863
After 6 months (n = 61 vs. 60)	4.7 (1.5–12.7)	4.1 (2.0–10.9)	0.022
After 9 months (n = 61 vs. 60)	4.3 (1.5–15.1)	4.0 (1.9–10.1)	0.867
After 12 months (n = 61 vs. 60)	4.4 (2.2–11.8)	4.1 (1.6–15.6)	0.283

To confirm that conditions were stable before enrolment, values 3 months prior to study onset are given for all patients who had already undergone liver transplantation (n = 54 vs. 58). In the intervention group (LCPT), values 3 months before and the day before the first LCPT intake (study onset) were determined when s-r-Tac was administered. LCPT, once-daily MeltDose® tacrolimus; Tac, tacrolimus; s-r-Tac, standard-release tacrolimus. p-values from Mann–Whitney U-test.

As shown in Figure 2, the C/D ratio at study end was significantly higher in patients on LCPT than in the control group (2.52 (0.58–6.40) vs. 1.75 (0.49–6.40) ng/mL × 1/mg, respectively; $p = 0.009$). The median Tac trough level and the daily dose were significantly higher in the intervention group at study onset (Table 3). After 12-month follow-up, the Tac dose in the LCPT group was significantly reduced compared with that in the control group (2.0 (0.4–7.8) vs. 2.5 (0.5–10.0) mg, respectively; $p = 0.047$). However, the Tac trough level was comparable in the two groups at study end (4.4 (2.2–11.8) vs. 4.1 (1.6–15.6) ng/mL, respectively; $p = 0.283$).

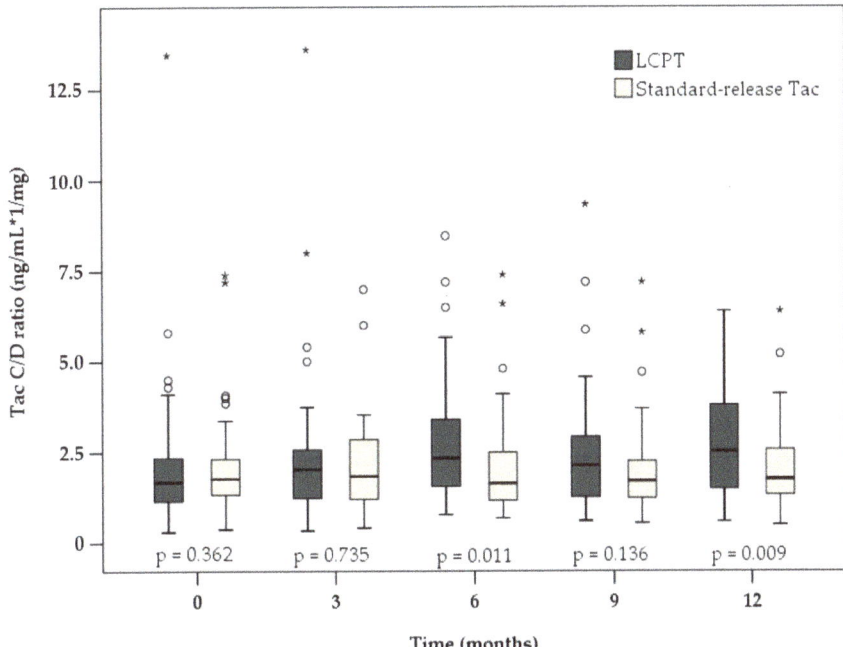

Figure 2. Boxplots of C/D ratio among patients receiving LCPT (dark grey) or standard-release Tac (light brown) at baseline and 3, 6, 9 and 12 months later. There were significant differences between the two study groups at 6 and 12 months after conversion. *p*-values reflect differences between the groups at each time point.

3.3. Renal Function

At baseline (study onset, t_0), patients in the control group had a higher mean eGFR than patients switched to LCPT (Figure 3), although the difference (ΔeGFR) was not significant ($p = 0.157$). However, mean ΔeGFR in patients on LCPT had significantly improved at 6 months after conversion ($p = 0.029$). In contrast, patients on standard-release Tac showed a significant decline of mean ΔeGFR 9 months after study initiation ($p = 0.006$). Over the 12-month evaluation period, mean ΔeGFR continued to improve significantly in patients receiving LCPT ($p = 0.001$), whereas mean ΔeGFR continued to deteriorate in the control group ($p < 0.001$). In a pairwise comparison between the groups, eGFR values did not differ significantly (Supplementary Table S1).

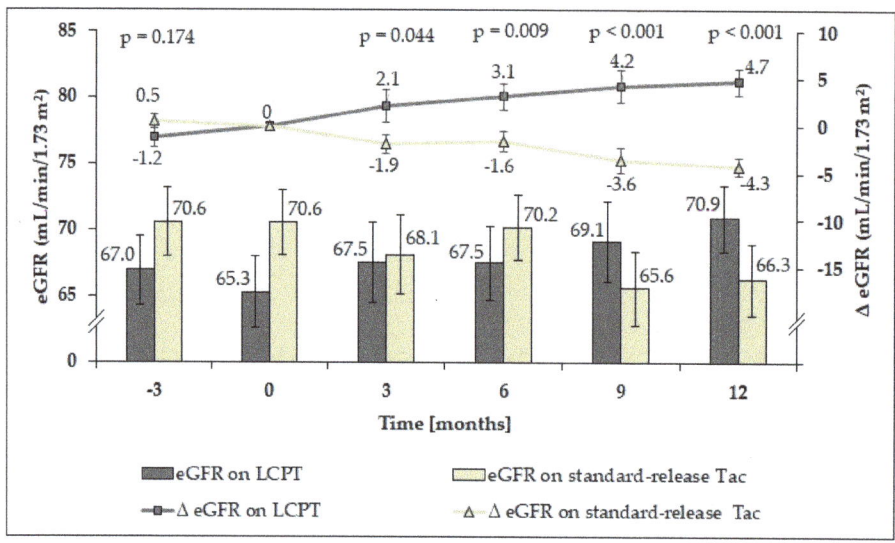

Figure 3. Glomerular filtration rate (eGFR; mL/min/1.73 m^2) over time and the difference from baseline at each time point (ΔeGFR ± SEM) in each study group. Improved renal function with a significantly increased mean ΔeGFR was already observed 3 months after conversion to LCPT (dark grey). *p*-values reflect comparison of ΔeGFR between the study groups.

While absolute eGFR values are meaningful to only a limited extent, eGFR slope (ΔeGFR) relative to the baseline can be used as additional empirical support (Table 4). Three months before study onset, there were no significant differences within the study groups relative to baseline. In the intervention group, renal function increased 6 months after conversion ($p = 0.029$). In contrast, LT recipients in the control group showed a significant decline of eGFR 9 months after study initiation ($p = 0.006$). Over the 12-month evaluation period, renal function continued to significantly improve in patients receiving LCPT ($p = 0.001$), whereas eGFR continued to deteriorate in the control group ($p < 0.001$).

Table 4. Slope analysis (ΔeGFR) of glomerular filtration rate (eGFR; mL/min/1.73 m^2).

Time Point	Estimate	95% Confidence Limit		*p*-Value
		Lower	Upper	
LCPT				
−3 months vs. baseline	−1.2	−3.2	0.8	0.223
3 months vs. baseline	2.1	−1.3	5.5	0.219
6 months vs. baseline	3.1	0.3	6.0	0.029
9 months vs. baseline	4.2	0.8	7.6	0.015
12 months vs. baseline	4.7	1.9	7.5	0.001
Standard-release Tac				
−3 months vs. baseline	0.5	−1.0	1.9	0.547
3 months vs. baseline	−1.9	−3.9	0.0	0.053
6 months vs. baseline	−1.6	−3.8	0.6	0.154
9 months vs. baseline	−3.6	−6.1	−1.1	0.006
12 months vs. baseline	−4.3	−6.2	−2.3	<0.001

The "estimate" value describes the difference between the respective time point and the baseline (ΔeGFR). A negative value shows a decline and a positive value an improvement of eGFR. LCPT, once-daily MeltDose® tacrolimus; Tac, tacrolimus; *p*-values within a group are relative to the baseline.

In further analysis, the eGFR values of the patients suffering from diabetes mellitus and arterial hypertension were compared between the groups.

At every time point, patients with diabetes mellitus had significantly lower eGFR than patients without it, regardless of the study group (Table 5). However, eGFR among diabetic patients recovered in a manner similar to that of nondiabetics upon switching to LCPT. In contrast, renal function deteriorated in patients maintained on standard-release Tac in a similar fashion, regardless of diabetes.

Table 5. Glomerular filtration rate (eGFR; mL/min/1.73 m^2) in diabetic and nondiabetic patients.

Time Point	LCPT			Standard-Release Tac		
	Diabetics (n = 18)	Non-Diabetics (n = 43)	p-Value	Diabetics (n = 17)	Non-Diabetics (n = 43)	p-Value
t_0	52.6 ± 21.3	70.3 ± 19.0	0.003	56.0 ± 20.3	76.3 ± 15.6	<0.001
t_3	56.2 ± 21.2	72.3 ± 20.0	0.013	51.2 ± 17.6	74.9 ± 18.1	<0.001
t_6	56.3 ± 19.2	73.0 ± 18.4	0.004	56.5 ± 20.3	75.5 ± 15.1	<0.001
t_9	57.1 ± 22.1	74.4 ± 17.7	0.007	53.2 ± 22.2	71.5 ± 16.5	0.002
t_{12}	56.3 ± 19.5	77.2 ± 13.4	<0.001	49.9 ± 22.5	72.7 ± 16.6	<0.001

LCPT, once-daily MeltDose® tacrolimus; Tac, tacrolimus; t_0 to t_{12}, time points (months). eGFR values shown as mean ± standard deviation. p-values from t-test.

Patients with arterial hypertension in both study groups had a lower mean eGFR than patients with normal blood pressure at each time point (Table 6). However, renal function recovered in patients treated with LCPT and deteriorated in those maintained on standard-release Tac over the course of the study, regardless of the presence of arterial hypertension.

Table 6. Glomerular filtration rate (eGFR; mL/min/1.73 m^2) in patients with and without arterial hypertension.

Time Point	LCPT			Standard-Release Tac		
	Arterial Hypertension (n = 36)	Normal Blood Pressure (n = 25)	p-Value	Arterial Hypertension (n = 37)	Normal Blood Pressure (n = 23)	p-Value
t_0	59.3 ± 20.7	74.3 ± 18.7	0.006	66.8 ± 21.0	76.6 ± 14.5	0.056
t_3	63.4 ± 22.4	73.1 ± 19.2	0.111	64.6 ± 22.4	74.2 ± 16.7	0.121
t_6	62.6 ± 20.1	74.2 ± 18.5	0.038	65.5 ± 20.4	77.6 ± 12.7	0.015
t_9	65.1 ± 19.9	74.7 ± 20.7	0.120	63.2 ± 21.8	70.4 ± 16.3	0.222
t_{12}	66.7 ± 17.0	76.9 ± 18.3	0.042	61.2 ± 22.4	74.5 ± 15.6	0.015

LCPT, once-daily MeltDose® tacrolimus; Tac, tacrolimus; t_0 to t_{12}, time points (months). eGFR values shown as mean ± standard deviation. p-values from t-test.

Multivariable analysis was performed to identify independent predictors of alterations in renal function expressed as ΔeGFR (Supplementary Table S2). Conversion to LCPT was the only identified independent predictor of significant changes in eGFR.

3.4. Liver Function

During the entire follow-up, we monitored the graft function (Table 7). LT recipients in the LCPT group showed significantly lower serum bilirubin concentrations than the control group at all time points. However, the median values in both study groups remained within the lower part of the normal range throughout the course of the study. Regarding the parameters ALT and INR, no differences were observed between the groups.

Table 7. Assessment of liver function over time in each study group.

	LCPT (n = 61)	Standard-Release Tac (n = 60)	p-Value
Bilirubin (mg/dL)			
At study onset	0.4 (0.2–1.3)	0.6 (0.2–2.0)	0.001
After 3 months	0.4 (0.2–2.2)	0.5 (0.2–4.0)	0.006
After 6 months	0.4 (0.2–1.2)	0.6 (0.2–2.1)	0.010
After 9 months	0.4 (0.2–1.2)	0.5 (0.2–1.9)	0.001
After 12 months	0.5 (0.2–1.2)	0.6 (0.2–2.7)	0.011
ALT (U/L)			
At study onset	20 (8–102)	21 (9–117)	0.431
After 3 months	24 (8–78)	22 (10–140)	0.348
After 6 months	20 (6–92)	18 (8–448)	0.406
After 9 months	20 (7–202)	20 (7–138)	0.997
After 12 months	20 (9–104)	20 (7–380)	0.696
INR			
At study onset	1.0 (0.9–2.2)	1.0 (0.9–1.6)	0.765
After 3 months	1.0 (0.9–2.3)	1.0 (0.9–1.3)	0.871
After 6 months	1.0 (0.9–1.3)	1.0 (0.9–1.6)	0.969
After 9 months	1.0 (0.9–1.3)	1.0 (0.9–1.5)	0.634
After 12 months	1.0 (0.9–1.3)	1.0 (0.9–1.5)	0.217

LCPT, once-daily MeltDose® tacrolimus; Tac, tacrolimus; ALT, alanine transaminase; INR, international normalized ratio; p-values from Mann–Whitney U-test.

4. Discussion

The present study shows that the conversion of LT recipients from standard-release Tac to LCPT was beneficial in regard to renal function. This may be due to the improved bioavailability of LCPT which led to a significant increase in C/D ratio.

Notably, the median daily Tac dose declined by 33.3% among LT recipients after conversion. A dose reduction of approximately 30% with a comparable area under the curve (AUC) was reported in recent studies of KT and LT recipients [20,24,25]. In those studies, this finding was also attributed to the greater bioavailability of LCPT.

In our cohort, the median C/D ratio among LT recipients who switched to LCPT had increased by 50% at 12 months after conversion. The C/D ratio among patients maintained on standard-release Tac remained unchanged over the 12-month period. In accordance with these data, Franco et al. described a 35% increase in the C/D ratio among KT recipients after conversion from IR-Tac and a 83.3% increase among those who were switched from ER-Tac to LCPT [26]. In the study by Rostaing et al., KT recipients had a 20% higher C/D ratio 12 months after conversion to LCPT and a 24.4% higher C/D ratio 24 months after conversion [27]. In contrast, Kamińska et al. showed that the C/D ratio of KT recipients converted from IR-Tac to ER-Tac did not change significantly [28]. To our knowledge, the present study is the first to describe a significant increase in the C/D ratio after a switch to LCPT among LT recipients.

In a previous study, we explored the impact of the C/D ratio on renal function after kidney transplantation (KTx) [14]. Fast metabolizers, defined as patients with a C/D ratio < 1.05 ng/mL × 1/mg, showed a strong association with decreased renal function compared with slow metabolizers in a 24-month follow-up. Similar results were confirmed among LT recipients in a 36-month follow-up study [13]. In that cohort, the cut-off value for fast metabolizers was defined as a C/D ratio < 1.09 ng/mL × 1/mg. In a 5-year follow-up, KT recipients with a lower Tac C/D ratio showed a higher risk of renal impairment as well as higher mortality rates [17]. Recently, several studies confirmed these findings [19,29,30] and a further negative impact of fast Tac metabolism on increased kidney allograft rejection rates and BK virus infections was demonstrated [17,18,31].

Given these results, we postulated that a higher C/D ratio after conversion to LCPT is associated with nephroprotection. Surprisingly, we already observed significant improvement of renal function 6 months after conversion. Twelve months after conversion, the mean ΔeGFR was 4.7 mL/min/1.73 m^2 higher than at baseline. In contrast, eGFR had deteriorated significantly in patients maintained on standard-release Tac 9 months after study onset and ΔeGFR had decreased by 4.3 mL/min/1.73 m^2 at 12 months.

After conversion to LCPT, the median trough level declined from 6.0 ng/mL at study onset to 4.6 ng/mL (month 3) without a subsequent decrease until month 12. A lower Tac trough level in the LCPT group has already been reported in a prospective study, although the same target trough level was given [27]. Alongside better bioavailability of LCPT, trough level reduction might be another reason for the increase in renal function. However, median trough levels did not vary considerably between subsequent time points (t_3–t_{12}) while renal function showed further recovery. Notably, median Tac trough levels were also slightly reduced in the control group (t_0–t_{12}), although eGFR showed further decline over the 12-month follow-up. Therefore, we postulate that improvement of bioavailability and a reduced peak Tac level after conversion to LCPT are factors more relevant to the increase in eGFR than the reduction in Tac trough levels alone.

As an explanation for the nephroprotective potential of LCPT, Schütte-Nütgen et al. hypothesized that a lower daily Tac dose results in a lower peak serum concentration (C_{max}), which in turn reduces the side effects of Tac overdosing within the first hours after drug intake [17]. In a review article on LT recipients, Baraldo reported that LCPT had a similar AUC after 24 h and a similar minimal blood concentration (C_{min}), but had a significantly lower C_{max} and a smaller C_{max}/C_{min} fluctuation ratio when compared with IR-Tac [32]. In addition, Bunnadaprist et al. postulated that there is a reduced cumulative Tac dose in KT recipients receiving LCPT [33]. In a recent study, we also showed that fast metabolizers with a C/D ratio < 1.05 ng/mL × 1/mg had significantly higher Tac blood concentrations than slow metabolizers 2 h after Tac intake [16]. In the same study, we showed that a low C/D ratio was significantly associated with acute CNIT. Although renal biopsy is not routinely performed in LT recipients, we can assume that patients converted to LCPT suffered less frequently from CNIT. In contrast, Kamar et al. reported similar renal function in de novo KTx recipients who were randomized to LCPT or ER-Tac in a 4-week follow-up [34]. Notably, C_{min} and AUC_{0-24} were slightly higher in the LCPT group (at days 3, 7 and 14), a fact that might have influenced the results.

In the current study, the control group had an increased warm ischemic time (WIT) compared with the intervention group (~5 min). Prolonged cold and warm ischemic times can be associated with long-term allograft dysfunction [32]. Nevertheless, at the beginning of our study, the liver function parameters ALT and INR did not differ between the groups and median bilirubin was within the normal range. In a study by Laskey et al., increasing WIT during LTx was associated with a lack of renal recovery in the presence of pretransplant subacute kidney injury [35]. It was concluded that minimization of WIT could potentially avoid renal replacement therapy or the need for subsequent kidney transplantation. At the study start in our cohort, the control group showed even higher eGFR values despite increased WIT compared with the intervention group. Notably, the control group had a more extended interval between LTx and study onset than patients switched to LCPT (6.6 (0.2–16.5) vs.2.8 (0.1–20.8) years, respectively).

In regard to the Tac formulations used before study onset, IR-Tac was administered more frequently than ER-Tac in the intervention group and vice versa in the control group. A recent study on pharmacokinetics in a large transplant cohort showed similar Tac trough levels and bioavailability between these two formulations [36]. Notably, C/D ratio as well as C/D intrapatient variability was reported not to change considerably during conversion from IR-Tac to ER-Tac in KT recipients [28]. These findings justify our and others' approach of including patients taking either one of these formulations [19,29].

In the current study, patients suffering from diabetes mellitus or arterial hypertension had reduced renal function. Interestingly, patients who were switched to LCPT (median C/D ratio increased from 1.68 to 2.52 ng/mL × 1/mg) showed considerable recovery of eGFR independent of the presence of both conditions. In accordance with these findings, Bardou et al. showed that slow Tac metabolizers (C/D ratio > 1.8 ng/mL × 1/mg) were less likely to suffer from diabetes and hypertension after LTx [37].

Finally, we recognize that our study has limitations due to its retrospective design and the limited sample size from a single-centre. In addition, in this study, we cannot provide Tac C_{max}, C_2 (2 h after Tac intake) nor AUC, although higher C_{max} or C_2 could potentially induce higher CNIT. Therefore, we can only hypothesize that, after conversion to LCPT, lower C_2 was a more relevant factor to the improvement of renal function than trough level reduction. Further investigations should also include data on the concentrations of different Tac metabolites, which could be responsible for adverse effects, such as CNIT, infections and myelotoxicity [38,39]. Furthermore, given the retrospective design of this study, the study beginning in the control group had a wide range from March 2017 until August 2018 and the time period from LTx to the beginning of the study was significantly increased compared with that in the intervention group. The longer Tac exposure in the control group might have had a negative influence on renal function in this cohort. However, at t_0, the control group showed even higher eGFR values than patients converted to LCPT (70.6 ± 19.3 vs. 65.3 ± 21.1, respectively).

Another limitation of the study is that the reasons for conversion to LCPT in our study were taken only from the clinical reports from our Outpatient Transplant Clinic. In addition, in contrast to the case for KTx recipients, renal biopsy is not routinely performed in LT recipients which limits our ability to analyse CNIT before study onset.

5. Conclusions

To the best of our knowledge, this is the first study to show that conversion from standard-release Tac to LCPT increases the C/D ratio in LT recipients associated with renal recovery. This finding was independent of known risk factors for renal impairment. Prospective studies are needed to confirm our findings.

Supplementary Materials: The following are available online at http://www.mdpi.com/2077-0383/9/6/1654/s1, Table S1: Glomerular filtration rate (eGFR; mL/min/1.73 m^2) over time. Table S2: Univariate and multivariate analysis of variance on eGFR at 12 months relative to baseline (study onset; t_0).

Author Contributions: Conceptualization, J.v.E., G.T., I.K. and A.H.-K.; Methodology, J.v.E., G.T., I.K. and A.H.-K.; Formal analysis, J.v.E., G.T., A.B., I.K. and A.H.-K.; Investigation, J.v.E., G.T., I.K. and A.H.-K.; Resources, H.H.S., I.K. and A.H.-K.; Data curation, J.v.E., G.T., I.K., C.W. and A.H.-K.; Writing—original draft preparation, J.v.E., G.T., I.K. and A.H.-K.; writing—review and editing, C.W., E.V., A.B. and H.H.S.; Visualization, J.v.E. and I.K.; Supervision, J.v.E., G.T., I.K. and A.H.-K.; Project administration, H.H.S., I.K. and A.H.-K.; funding acquisition, J.v.E., E.V. and I.K. All authors have read and agreed to the published version of the manuscript.

Funding: This study was supported by Chiesi GmbH, Hamburg, Germany, as local representative of the marketing authorisation holder Chiesi Farmaceutici S.p.A. of LCPT. Chiesi supported creation of a database and infrastructure costs (including the wage for a study nurse who helped in database creation and data collection, as well as costs for statistical consultation and publication fees).

Conflicts of Interest: The underlying study represents an investigator-initiated trial. The study was designed by the authors alone without any external input regarding design, analysis or approval for the manuscript either by Chiesi GmbH or by any other unmentioned party. The authors themselves did not receive any financial support with regard to this study.

References

1. Wiesner, R.H.; Fung, J.J. Present state of immunosuppressive therapy in liver transplant recipients. *Liver Transpl.* **2011**, *17* (Suppl. S3), S1–S9. [CrossRef]
2. McAlister, V.C.; Haddad, E.; Renouf, E.; Malthaner, R.A.; Kjaer, M.S.; Gluud, L.L. Cyclosporin versus tacrolimus as primary immunosuppressant after liver transplantation: A meta-analysis. *Am. J. Transplant.* **2006**, *6*, 1578–1585. [CrossRef] [PubMed]

3. European Association for the Study of the Liver. EASL Clinical Practice Guidelines: Liver transplantation. *J. Hepatol.* **2016**, *64*, 433–485. [CrossRef] [PubMed]
4. O'Grady, J.G.; Hardy, P.; Burroughs, A.K.; Elbourne, D.; UK and Ireland Liver Transplant Study Group. Randomized controlled trial of tacrolimus versus microemulsified cyclosporin (TMC) in liver transplantation: Poststudy surveillance to 3 years. *Am. J. Transplant.* **2007**, *7*, 137–141. [CrossRef] [PubMed]
5. Naesens, M.; Kuypers, D.R.; Sarwal, M. Calcineurin inhibitor nephrotoxicity. *Clin. J. Am. Soc. Nephrol.* **2009**, *4*, 481–508. [CrossRef] [PubMed]
6. Beckebaum, S.; Cicinnati, V.R.; Radtke, A.; Kabar, I. Calcineurin inhibitors in liver transplantation - still champions or threatened by serious competitors? *Liver Int.* **2013**, *33*, 656–665. [CrossRef] [PubMed]
7. Ziolkowski, J.; Paczek, L.; Senatorski, G.; Niewczas, M.; Oldakowska-Jedynak, U.; Wyzgal, J.; Sanko-Resmer, J.; Pilecki, T.; Zieniewicz, K.; Nyckowski, P.; et al. Renal function after liver transplantation: Calcineurin inhibitor nephrotoxicity. *Transplant. Proc.* **2003**, *35*, 2307–2309. [CrossRef]
8. Afonso, R.C.; Hidalgo, R.; Zurstrassen, M.P.; Fonseca, L.E.; Pandullo, F.L.; Rezende, M.B.; Meira-Filho, S.P.; Ferraz-Neto, B.H. Impact of renal failure on liver transplantation survival. *Transplant. Proc.* **2008**, *40*, 808–810. [CrossRef]
9. Gonwa, T.A.; Mai, M.L.; Melton, L.B.; Hays, S.R.; Goldstein, R.M.; Levy, M.F.; Klintmalm, G.B. End-stage renal disease (ESRD) after orthotopic liver transplantation (OLTX) using calcineurin-based immunotherapy: Risk of development and treatment. *Transplantation* **2001**, *72*, 1934–1939. [CrossRef]
10. Kuypers, D.R.; de Jonge, H.; Naesens, M.; Lerut, E.; Verbeke, K.; Vanrenterghem, Y. CYP3A5 and CYP3A4 but not MDR1 single-nucleotide polymorphisms determine long-term tacrolimus disposition and drug-related nephrotoxicity in renal recipients. *Clin. Pharmacol. Ther.* **2007**, *82*, 711–725. [CrossRef]
11. Kershner, R.P.; Fitzsimmons, W.E. Relationship of FK506 whole blood concentrations and efficacy and toxicity after liver and kidney transplantation. *Transplantation* **1996**, *62*, 920–926. [CrossRef] [PubMed]
12. Tsuchiya, T.; Ishida, H.; Tanabe, T.; Shimizu, T.; Honda, K.; Omoto, K.; Tanabe, K. Comparison of pharmacokinetics and pathology for low-dose tacrolimus once-daily and twice-daily in living kidney transplantation: Prospective trial in once-daily versus twice-daily tacrolimus. *Transplantation* **2013**, *96*, 198–204. [CrossRef] [PubMed]
13. Tholking, G.; Siats, L.; Fortmann, C.; Koch, R.; Husing, A.; Cicinnati, V.R.; Gerth, H.U.; Wolters, H.H.; Anthoni, C.; Pavenstadt, H.; et al. Tacrolimus Concentration/Dose Ratio is Associated with Renal Function After Liver Transplantation. *Ann. Transplant.* **2016**, *21*, 167–179. [CrossRef] [PubMed]
14. Tholking, G.; Fortmann, C.; Koch, R.; Gerth, H.U.; Pabst, D.; Pavenstadt, H.; Kabar, I.; Husing, A.; Wolters, H.; Reuter, S.; et al. The tacrolimus metabolism rate influences renal function after kidney transplantation. *PLoS ONE* **2014**, *9*, e111128. [CrossRef] [PubMed]
15. Rancic, N.; Dragojevic-Simic, V.; Vavic, N.; Kovacevic, A.; Segrt, Z.; Draskovic-Pavlovic, B.; Mikov, M. Tacrolimus concentration/dose ratio as a therapeutic drug monitoring strategy: The influence of gender and comedication. *Vojnosanit. Pregl.* **2015**, *72*, 813–822. [CrossRef] [PubMed]
16. Tholking, G.; Schutte-Nutgen, K.; Schmitz, J.; Rovas, A.; Dahmen, M.; Bautz, J.; Jehn, U.; Pavenstadt, H.; Heitplatz, B.; Van Marck, V.; et al. A Low Tacrolimus Concentration/Dose Ratio Increases the Risk for the Development of Acute Calcineurin Inhibitor-Induced Nephrotoxicity. *J. Clin. Med.* **2019**, *8*, 1586. [CrossRef]
17. Schutte-Nutgen, K.; Tholking, G.; Steinke, J.; Pavenstadt, H.; Schmidt, R.; Suwelack, B.; Reuter, S. Fast Tac Metabolizers at Risk (-) It is Time for a C/D Ratio Calculation. *J. Clin. Med.* **2019**, *8*, 587. [CrossRef]
18. Egeland, E.J.; Robertsen, I.; Hermann, M.; Midtvedt, K.; Storset, E.; Gustavsen, M.T.; Reisaeter, A.V.; Klaasen, R.; Bergan, S.; Holdaas, H.; et al. High Tacrolimus Clearance Is a Risk Factor for Acute Rejection in the Early Phase After Renal Transplantation. *Transplantation* **2017**, *101*, e273–e279. [CrossRef]
19. Nowicka, M.; Gorska, M.; Nowicka, Z.; Edyko, K.; Edyko, P.; Wislicki, S.; Zawiasa-Bryszewska, A.; Strzelczyk, J.; Matych, J.; Kurnatowska, I. Tacrolimus: Influence of the Posttransplant Concentration/Dose Ratio on Kidney Graft Function in a Two-Year Follow-Up. *Kidney Blood Press. Res.* **2019**, *44*, 1075–1088. [CrossRef]

20. Tremblay, S.; Nigro, V.; Weinberg, J.; Woodle, E.S.; Alloway, R.R. A Steady-State Head-to-Head Pharmacokinetic Comparison of All FK-506 (Tacrolimus) Formulations (ASTCOFF): An Open-Label, Prospective, Randomized, Two-Arm, Three-Period Crossover Study. *Am. J. Transplant.* **2017**, *17*, 432–442. [CrossRef]
21. Grinyo, J.M.; Petruzzelli, S. Once-daily LCP-Tacro MeltDose tacrolimus for the prophylaxis of organ rejection in kidney and liver transplantations. *Expert Rev. Clin. Immunol.* **2014**, *10*, 1567–1579. [CrossRef] [PubMed]
22. Garnock-Jones, K.P. Tacrolimus prolonged release (Envarsus(R)): A review of its use in kidney and liver transplant recipients. *Drugs* **2015**, *75*, 309–320. [CrossRef] [PubMed]
23. Levin, A.; Stevens, P.E. Summary of KDIGO 2012 CKD Guideline: Behind the scenes, need for guidance, and a framework for moving forward. *Kidney Int.* **2014**, *85*, 49–61. [CrossRef] [PubMed]
24. DuBay, D.A.; Teperman, L.; Ueda, K.; Silverman, A.; Chapman, W.; Alsina, A.E.; Tyler, C.; Stevens, D.R. Pharmacokinetics of Once-Daily Extended-Release Tacrolimus Tablets Versus Twice-Daily Capsules in De Novo Liver Transplant. *Clin. Pharmacol. Drug Dev.* **2019**, *8*, 995–1008. [CrossRef] [PubMed]
25. Alloway, R.R.; Eckhoff, D.E.; Washburn, W.K.; Teperman, L.W. Conversion from twice daily tacrolimus capsules to once daily extended-release tacrolimus (LCP-Tacro): Phase 2 trial of stable liver transplant recipients. *Liver Transpl.* **2014**, *20*, 564–575. [CrossRef] [PubMed]
26. Franco, A.; Mas-Serrano, P.; Balibrea, N.; Rodriguez, D.; Javaloyes, A.; Diaz, M.; Gascon, I.; Ramon-Lopez, A.; Perez-Contreras, J.; Selva, J.; et al. Envarsus, a novelty for transplant nephrologists: Observational retrospective study. *Nefrologia* **2019**, *39*, 506–512. [CrossRef]
27. Rostaing, L.; Bunnapradist, S.; Grinyo, J.M.; Ciechanowski, K.; Denny, J.E.; Silva, H.T., Jr.; Budde, K.; Envarsus Study, G. Novel Once-Daily Extended-Release Tacrolimus Versus Twice-Daily Tacrolimus in De Novo Kidney Transplant Recipients: Two-Year Results of Phase 3, Double-Blind, Randomized Trial. *Am. J. Kidney Dis.* **2016**, *67*, 648–659. [CrossRef]
28. Kaminska, D.; Poznanski, P.; Kuriata-Kordek, M.; Zielinska, D.; Mazanowska, O.; Koscielska-Kasprzak, K.; Krajewska, M. Conversion From a Twice-Daily to a Once-Daily Tacrolimus Formulation in Kidney Transplant Recipients. *Transplant. Proc.* **2020**. [CrossRef]
29. Jouve, T.; Fonrose, X.; Noble, J.; Janbon, B.; Fiard, G.; Malvezzi, P.; Stanke-Labesque, F.; Rostaing, L. The TOMATO study (TacrOlimus MetabolizAtion in kidney TransplantatiOn): Impact of the concentration-dose ratio on death-censored graft survival. *Transplantation* **2019**. [CrossRef]
30. Kwiatkowska, E.; Kwiatkowski, S.; Wahler, F.; Gryczman, M.; Domanki, L.; Marchelk-Mysliwiec, M.; Ciechanowski, K.; Drozd-Dabrowska, M. C/D Ratio in Long-Term Renal Function. *Transplant. Proc.* **2019**, *51*, 3265–3270. [CrossRef]
31. Tholking, G.; Schmidt, C.; Koch, R.; Schuette-Nuetgen, K.; Pabst, D.; Wolters, H.; Kabar, I.; Husing, A.; Pavenstadt, H.; Reuter, S.; et al. Influence of tacrolimus metabolism rate on BKV infection after kidney transplantation. *Sci. Rep.* **2016**, *6*, 32273. [CrossRef] [PubMed]
32. Baraldo, M. Meltdose Tacrolimus Pharmacokinetics. *Transplant. Proc.* **2016**, *48*, 420–423. [CrossRef]
33. Bunnapradist, S.; Rostaing, L.; Alloway, R.R.; West-Thielke, P.; Denny, J.; Mulgaonkar, S.; Budde, K. LCPT once-daily extended-release tacrolimus tablets versus twice-daily capsules: A pooled analysis of two phase 3 trials in important de novo and stable kidney transplant recipient subgroups. *Transpl. Int.* **2016**, *29*, 603–611. [CrossRef] [PubMed]
34. Kamar, N.; Cassuto, E.; Piotti, G.; Govoni, M.; Ciurlia, G.; Geraci, S.; Poli, G.; Nicolini, G.; Mariat, C.; Essig, M.; et al. Pharmacokinetics of Prolonged-Release Once-Daily Formulations of Tacrolimus in De Novo Kidney Transplant Recipients: A Randomized, Parallel-Group, Open-Label, Multicenter Study. *Adv. Ther.* **2019**, *36*, 462–477. [CrossRef]
35. Laskey, H.L.; Schomaker, N.; Hung, K.W.; Asrani, S.K.; Jennings, L.; Nydam, T.L.; Gralla, J.; Wiseman, A.; Rosen, H.R.; Biggins, S.W. Predicting renal recovery after liver transplant with severe pretransplant subacute kidney injury: The impact of warm ischemia time. *Liver Transpl.* **2016**, *22*, 1085–1091. [CrossRef] [PubMed]
36. Lu, Z.; Bonate, P.; Keirns, J. Population pharmacokinetics of immediate- and prolonged-release tacrolimus formulations in liver, kidney and heart transplant recipients. *Br. J. Clin. Pharmacol.* **2019**, *85*, 1692–1703. [CrossRef]
37. Bardou, F.N.; Guillaud, O.; Erard-Poinsot, D.; Chambon-Augoyard, C.; Thimonier, E.; Vallin, M.; Boillot, O.; Dumortier, J. Tacrolimus exposure after liver transplantation for alcohol-related liver disease: Impact on complications. *Transpl. Immunol.* **2019**, *56*, 101227. [CrossRef]

38. Zegarska, J.; Hryniewiecka, E.; Zochowska, D.; Samborowska, E.; Jazwiec, R.; Borowiec, A.; Tszyrsznic, W.; Chmura, A.; Nazarewski, S.; Dadlez, M.; et al. Tacrolimus Metabolite M-III May Have Nephrotoxic and Myelotoxic Effects and Increase the Incidence of Infections in Kidney Transplant Recipients. *Transplant. Proc.* **2016**, *48*, 1539–1542. [CrossRef]
39. Vanhove, T.; de Jonge, H.; de Loor, H.; Oorts, M.; de Hoon, J.; Pohanka, A.; Annaert, P.; Kuypers, D.R.J. Relationship between In Vivo CYP3A4 Activity, CYP3A5 Genotype, and Systemic Tacrolimus Metabolite/Parent Drug Ratio in Renal Transplant Recipients and Healthy Volunteers. *Drug Metab. Dispos.* **2018**, *46*, 1507–1513. [CrossRef]

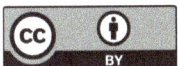

© 2020 by the authors. Licensee MDPI, Basel, Switzerland. This article is an open access article distributed under the terms and conditions of the Creative Commons Attribution (CC BY) license (http://creativecommons.org/licenses/by/4.0/).

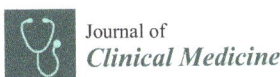

Article

Optimized Identification of Advanced Chronic Kidney Disease and Absence of Kidney Disease by Combining Different Electronic Health Data Resources and by Applying Machine Learning Strategies

Christoph Weber [1,†], Lena Röschke [1,†], Luise Modersohn [2], Christina Lohr [2], Tobias Kolditz [2], Udo Hahn [2], Danny Ammon [3], Boris Betz [1,*,‡] and Michael Kiehntopf [1,*,‡]

1. Department of Clinical Chemistry and Laboratory Diagnostics and Integrated Biobank Jena (IBBJ), Jena University Hospital, 07747 Jena, Germany; christoph.weber@med.uni-jena.de (C.W.); lena.marie.roeschke@uni-jena.de (L.R.)
2. Jena University Language & Information Engineering (JULIE) Lab, Friedrich Schiller University Jena, 07743 Jena, Germany; luise.modersohn@uni-jena.de (L.M.); christina.lohr@uni-jena.de (C.L.); tbs.kldtz@gmail.com (T.K.); udo.hahn@uni-jena.de (U.H.)
3. Data Integration Center, Jena University Hospital, 07743 Jena, Germany; danny.ammon@med.uni-jena.de
* Correspondence: Boris.Betz@med.uni-jena.de (B.B.); Michael.Kiehntopf@med.uni-jena.de (M.K.); Tel.: +49-3641-9-325074 (B.B.); +49-3641-9-325001 (M.K.)
† Christoph Weber and Lena Röschke contributed equally.
‡ Boris Betz and Michael Kiehntopf contributed equally.

Received: 25 June 2020; Accepted: 28 August 2020; Published: 12 September 2020

Abstract: Automated identification of advanced chronic kidney disease (CKD ≥ III) and of no known kidney disease (NKD) can support both clinicians and researchers. We hypothesized that identification of CKD and NKD can be improved, by combining information from different electronic health record (EHR) resources, comprising laboratory values, discharge summaries and ICD-10 billing codes, compared to using each component alone. We included EHRs from 785 elderly multimorbid patients, hospitalized between 2010 and 2015, that were divided into a training and a test (n = 156) dataset. We used both the area under the receiver operating characteristic (AUROC) and under the precision-recall curve (AUCPR) with a 95% confidence interval for evaluation of different classification models. In the test dataset, the combination of EHR components as a simple classifier identified CKD ≥ III (AUROC 0.96[0.93–0.98]) and NKD (AUROC 0.94[0.91–0.97]) better than laboratory values (AUROC CKD 0.85[0.79–0.90], NKD 0.91[0.87–0.94]), discharge summaries (AUROC CKD 0.87[0.82–0.92], NKD 0.84[0.79–0.89]) or ICD-10 billing codes (AUROC CKD 0.85[0.80–0.91], NKD 0.77[0.72–0.83]) alone. Logistic regression and machine learning models improved recognition of CKD ≥ III compared to the simple classifier if only laboratory values were used (AUROC 0.96[0.92–0.99] vs. 0.86[0.81–0.91], $p < 0.05$) and improved recognition of NKD if information from previous hospital stays was used (AUROC 0.99[0.98–1.00] vs. 0.95[0.92–0.97]], $p < 0.05$). Depending on the availability of data, correct automated identification of CKD ≥ III and NKD from EHRs can be improved by generating classification models based on the combination of different EHR components.

Keywords: chronic kidney disease (CKD); no known kidney disease (NKD); ICD-10 billing codes; phenotyping; electronic health record (EHR); estimated glomerular filtration rate (eGFR); machine learning (ML); generalized linear model network (GLMnet); random forest (RF); artificial neural network (ANN); clinical natural language processing (clinical NLP); discharge summaries; laboratory values; area under the receiver operating characteristic (AUROC); area under the precision-recall curve (AUCPR)

1. Introduction

Chronic kidney disease (CKD) is a major public health concern characterized by an increasing prevalence and associated with a high level of morbidity and mortality [1,2]. Correct identification of CKD is crucial, e.g., for appropriate dosing of drugs and for early intervention, including the prevention of progression [3]. For clinical research, accurate identification of CKD or absence of kidney disease (NKD = no known kidney disease) is essential for clinical trials and epidemiological studies. In this context, a particular challenge is to store samples from hospitalized patients with known kidney status in clinical biorepositories, as part of Healthcare-Integrated Biobanking (HIB). At the time point of sample selection and storage, only a limited range of information regarding the respective patient phenotype is available.

Administrative data such as ICD-10 billing codes are often used in research trails to identify patients with CKD [4]. However, administrative databases are not maintained with the primary purpose of supporting research; thus, it might be that, e.g., mild impairment of kidney function will be underrepresented because they cannot be billed [5]. Indeed, many studies have demonstrated that ICD-10 billing codes considerably underestimate the prevalence of CKD [6]. Moreover, there is no ICD-10 billing code for NKD, as the purpose of ICD-10 billing codes is to indicate the presence of a disease.

Electronic health records (EHRs) are a promising source for the diagnosis or exclusion of CKD. EHRs contain structured data (laboratory values, epidemiological data) and unstructured data (narrative discharge summaries).

The laboratory assessment of kidney function is based on an equation to estimate the glomerular filtration rate (GFR) [3]. This equation, Chronic Kidney Disease Epidemiology Collaboration (CKD-EPI), includes the blood creatinine level, age, sex and ethnicity [7]. According to the Kidney Disease: Improving Global Outcomes (KDIGO) definition, CKD Stage III and higher can be diagnosed by an eGFR below 60 mL/min/1.73m^2 for a time period of at least 90 days [3]. However, previous laboratory data on hospitalized patients are often not fully available, e.g., they were recorded in other hospitals or in outpatient clinics.

Unstructured data such as discharge summaries can fill the gap of missing medical information. Letters are available in a digital form for every hospitalized patient and often contain complementary information, not only about the current hospital stay, but also about the clinical history of the patient including chronic diseases. Information can be extracted from narrative discharge summaries for example by reusing SNOMED CT codes from EHRs [8], screening the letters for disease-specific keywords [9,10], or using mL based natural language processing (NLP) technology for ICD-10 billing codes [11] or SNOMED CT [12] coding, named entity recognition [13], or relation extraction [14].

Data analysis from EHRs can be performed in a rule-based format for example by strictly adhering to the KDIGO definition of CKD ≥ III. In recent years, various machine learning (ML) methods have been applied to improve the automated recognition of chronic kidney disease, using mainly laboratory values and demographic information [15–20]. However, to the best of our knowledge, no study specifically targeted advanced CKD ≥ III or NKD.

In this study, we hypothesize that combining structured (laboratory values, ICD-10 billing codes) and unstructured (discharge summaries) information from EHRs and applying mL for data analysis can reliably distinguish between patients with advanced CKD (stage ≥ III) and patients with no known kidney disease (NKD) in different scenarios of data availability.

2. Materials and Methods

2.1. Study Population

The dataset of this retrospective study has been derived from the Jena Part of the 3000 PA text corpus of the Smart Medical Information Technology for Healthcare (SMITH) consortium (part of the Medical Informatics Initiative founded by the German Federal Ministry of Education and

Research) [21–23]. The dataset consisted of EHRs from 785 individuals who were from European descent and had an index hospital stay for at least five days on a ward for internal medicine or in an intensive care unit between 2010 and 2015. No individual deceased during the index hospital stay. At the time point of retrospective data collection, all individuals were deceased. The EHRs included discharge summaries, laboratory values and ICD-10 billing codes. The study was approved by the local ethics committee (4639-12/15); data were collected retrospectively and anonymized, individual-level informed consent of participants was waived by the ethics review board. The study was also approved by the data protection officer of Jena University Hospital.

2.2. Classification of CKD and NKD by ICD-10 Billing Codes

For classification of CKD and NKD, ICD-10 billing codes of the index hospital stay, extracted from the hospital accounting system and from hospital discharge summaries, were used. For extraction of kidney diseases from discharge summaries the HEALTH DISCOVERY text mining tool v5.7.0 from AVERBIS (https://health-discovery.io/) was applied using the discharge pipeline with default settings to extract basic medical information (detailed information can be found in the AVERBIS HEALTH DISCOVERY User Manual Version 5.7, 4 December 2018). Subsequently, a Python script was applied to extract the ICD-10 billing codes from these output files. ICD-10 billing codes for CKD classification were used according to ICD-10 billing codes for moderate to severe kidney disease from the Charlson comorbidity index [24] (Supplementary Materials). For the definition of no kidney disease (NKD), none of these codes as well as further ICD-10 billing codes for kidney disease published by the Centers for Disease Control and Prevention (CDC, http://www.cdc.gov/ckd) (Supplementary Materials) should be present.

2.3. Laboratory and Demographic Data

Laboratory values and demographics of the patients were extracted from the laboratory information system (LIS) of the University Hospital of Jena. The following values were considered in the analysis and classification of the study cohort:

- Numerical variables: age, eGFR at admission, eGFR at discharge, eGFR over index hospital stay. Measurements of albumin in urine were available in less than 5% of the cohort and therefore excluded from further analysis.
- Categorical variable: sex.

Descriptive statistics were reported as the mean [SD] or median [I quartile–III quartile] for continuous variables and absolute numbers (percentages) for categorical variables.

2.4. Classification of CKD and NKD by Blood Creatinine and eGFR

In order to define CKD and NKD by laboratory values from the current hospital index stay, we created the following rules. If all eGFR values during the index stay were below 60 mL/min/1.73 m^2, the case was assigned to CKD. If all eGFR values during the index hospital stay were above 60 mL/min/1.73m^2 and there was no presence of AKI (definition see below), the case was assigned to NKD.

2.5. Classification of CKD and NKD by Manual Review

CKD stage III or higher was defined according to the KDIGO guidelines. This included an eGFR, based on the formula CKD-EPI [7], which had to be less than 60 mL/min/1.73 m^2 for at least 3 months (90 days) or by an additional proof of kidney damage [3].

We defined NKD, adapted from James et al. [25], as the complete absence of GFR less than 60 mL/min/1.73m^2, stable serum creatinine measurements, e.g., no fulfillment of acute kidney disease criteria, median absence of proteinuria when multiple measurements were made before and the absence of AKI in patient laboratory history. AKI was present, if serum creatinine had increased by more than 26.5 mmol/L within 48 h or increased more than 1.5-fold over 7 days [26]. In addition, adapted from the publication by Duff et al. [27], we included AKI recovery defined as a decline in creatinine for more than 33% over 7 days.

All cases were reviewed by an advanced medical student and a physician to assess the underlying kidney status based on individual EHRs, including discharge summaries, ICD-10 billing codes and laboratory test results performed before, subsequent to, and during the index hospital stay. Of note, for clarification of difficult cases, the reviewers used information not available to the rule-based or statistical algorithms (e.g., laboratory values after index hospital stay). The review was used as a reference standard for comparison with automated classification.

2.6. Dataset for the Machine Learning Methods

The dataset used for logistic regression and the different mL models is composed of 11 to 19 different categorical and numerical variables. Three of them are derived variables to improve classification.

1. Numerical variables: age; first eGFR of the index hospital stay; last eGFR of the index hospital stay; time difference between the first and last blood measurement of the index hospital stay as an indicator for the length of hospital stay; mean eGFR over index hospital stay; mean eGFR over all available laboratory values.
2. Due to the varying distribution of eGFR measurements, additionally derived numerical variables were defined for usage in mL algorithms: the ratio between the number of hospital visits with eGFR measurements and the number of total visits; the ratio between the number of total eGFR measurements and hospital visits with eGFR measurements; the ratio between the number of eGFR measurements lower than 60 mL/min/1.73 m^2 and hospital visits with eGFR measurements.
3. Categorical variables: sex; occurrence of AKI and AKI recovery over laboratory history; occurrence of AKI and AKI recovery over index stay.

All of these variables were used in all mL models. Further categorical variables, listed below, were added in different combinations, as described in the results.

CKD: eGFR at admission below 60 mL/min/1.73 m^2 (eGFR_admission), eGFR at discharge below 60 mL/min/1.73 m^2 (eGFR_discharge), and all eGFR measurements during index stay below 60 mL/min/1.73 m^2 (eGFR).

NKD: eGFR at admission above 60 mL/min/1.73 m^2 (eGFR_admission), eGFR at discharge above 60 mL/min/1.73 m^2 (eGFR_discharge), eGFR always above 60 mL/min/1.73 m^2 (eGFR_history), all eGFR during index stay above 60 mL/min/1.73 m^2 (eGFR); classification by ICD-10 billing codes (ICD); classification by ICD-10 codes from discharge summaries.

2.7. Classification of CKD and NKD Using Machine Learning Methods

We applied three different mL methods—generalized linear model via penalized maximum likelihood (GLMnet) [28], random forests (RF) [29] and artificial neural network (ANN) [30]. These are all well-established approaches that represent different types of mL methods.

GLMnet is a statistical method in which different models generalize to the concept of a penalty parameter and in which different models have different loss functions. A penalty parameter constrains the size of the model coefficients such that the only way the coefficients can increase is if a comparable decrease in the models loss function is experienced. A loss function essentially calculates how poorly a model is performing by comparing what the model is predicting with the actual value it is supposed to output. If both values are very similar, the loss value will be very low. There are three common penalty parameters (ridge regression, lasso penalty, elastic-net penalty). We used the elastic-net penalty which is controlled by the *alpha* parameter. It bridges the gap between the ridge regression (alpha = 0), which is good for retaining all features while reducing the noise that less influential variables may create and the lasso (alpha = 1) penalty, which actually excludes features from the model.

Like a simple rule-based decision tree, random forests are tree-based models and part of a class of non-parametric algorithms that work by partitioning the feature space into a number of smaller regions. The predictions are obtained by fitting a simpler model in each region. Random forests use the same principles as bagging trees, which grow many trees (*ntree*) on bootstrapped copies of the training data, and extend it with an additional random component through split-variable randomization, where each time a split is to be performed the search for the split variable is limited to a random subset (*mtry*) of the original features.

Artificial neural networks are designed to simulate the biological neural networks of animal brains. They process input examples of a given task and map them against the desired output by forming probability-weighted associations between the two, storing these in the net data structure itself. In its basic form a neural network has three layers. An input layer which consists of all of the original input features, a hidden layer where the majority of the learning process takes place and an output layer [31].

The dataset was randomly split into 80% training and 20% test data. The prevalence for CKD or NKD respectively was similar in the two datasets (Supplementary Materials).

To properly adapt the mL algorithms, we optimized the hyperparameters that are used to control the learning process of a model and cannot be directly estimated from the data. We used a grid search method, which is simply an exhaustive search through a manually specified subset of the hyperparameter space of the learning algorithm. We specified these hyperparameters for every type of model, trailed all combinations and selected the model with the best results (see Supplementary Materials for details). For the GLMnet, the regularization parameter *lambda*, which controls the overall strength of the penalty term and helps to control the model from overfitting to the training data, was calculated during a pre-training of the model. Subsequently the best alpha parameter was determined. It ranges between [0,1] and was divided into steps of 0.1.

Random forest was tuned on the *mtry* parameter in a range between [1,18] depending on the number of features of the model, divided into steps of 1. The *ntree* parameter was set to its default value $ntree = 100$.

The artificial neural network is a fully connected feed-forward network with a single hidden layer. We use a fixed number of units between 11 and 19 in the input layer depending on the number of features of the model and a single unit with a sigmoid activation function for binary classification as the output layer. We optimized the number of units in the hidden layer as a hyperparameter (*size*) for every model in a range between [1,10] divided into steps of 1 (see Supplementary Materials for details).

In addition, all models were evaluated using three separate 10-fold cross-validations as the resampling scheme and were trained to optimize the F1 score. The final F1 score for each model is averaged over the resamples.

Classifications were assessed using sensitivity, specificity, positive predictive value (PPV), negative predictive value (NPV), F1 score, accuracy, area under the receiver operating characteristics (AUROC) and precision-recall curve (AUCPR). For AUROC and AUCPR, the 95% confidence interval was calculated (see Supplementary Materials for formulas and for detailed classification performances regarding the different models).

Area under the precision–recall curve is known to be more informative for class-imbalanced predictive tasks [32], as it is more sensitive to changes in the number of false-positive predictions. Comparison between AUROC was calculated according to DeLong et al. [33].

Analyses were implemented using R STUDIO (version 1.2.5001), the R SOFTWARE (version 3.6.1) [34] and the following packages: *limma* [35] for plots, *rio* [36], *plyr* [37], *nlme* [38], *tidyverse* bundle [39], *pROC* [40], *ROCR* [41] for data management, data analysis and functional programming and *caret* [42] for all mL models. Graphs were generated by GraphPad Prism (version 8.4.2).

3. Results

The study cohort comprises 785 cases, with an average age of 75 years, the majority of individuals were male (61%), and 95% and 49% of the patients had at least one or three severe disease(s) of the Charlson comorbidity index, respectively. Most patients were hospitalized due to cardiovascular disease (40%), gastrointestinal/liver diseases (15%) or oncology disorders (15%). The prevalence of

CKD in this elderly morbid cohort was comparable to other studies that included probably less morbid non-hospitalized patients ([43,44]). The prevalence for patients with no known kidney disease (NKD) was lower than for CKD. NKD was associated with younger age, better kidney function and fewer co-morbidities compared to CKD ≥ III. (Table 1).

Table 1. Epidemiological Characteristics from all Individuals and from Individuals with CKD ≥ III or NKD Identified by the Reference Standard, Respectively.

Characteristics	Cohort (n = 785)	CKD ≥ III (n = 373)	NKD (n = 129)
Age, years, mean [SD]	74.6 [12.2]	77.9 [10]	68.4 [13.7]
Sex, male	476 (60.6%)	215 (57.6%)	79 (61.2%)
eGFR at admission, median, [quartiles], mL/min/1.73 m^2	(n = 780) [1] 49.6 [28.6–77.3] (n = 748)	(n = 372) [1] 28.9 [18.1–41.8]	88.6 [78.5–99.6]
Charlson morbidity category ≥1	711 (95.3%)	366 (98.1%)	113 (87.6%)
≥3	387 (49.3%)	224 (60.1%)	36 (27.9%)
Median	2	3	2
Myocardial infarction	128 (16.3%)	75 (20.1%)	11 (8.5%)
Chronic heart failure	419 (54.4)	247 (66.2%)	33 (25.6%)
Peripheral vascular disease	131 (16.7%)	75 (20.1%)	17 (13.2%)
Cerebrovascular disease	51 (6.5%)	28 (7.5%)	7 (5.4%)
Dementia	31 (3.9%)	18 (4.8%)	4 (3.1%)
Chronic pulmonary disease	183 (23.3%)	73 (16.9%)	23 (17.8%)
Rheumatic diseases	13 (1.7%)	4 (1.1%)	3 (2.3%)
Peptic ulcer disease	21 (2.7%)	11 (2.9%)	1 (0.8%)
Hemiplegia or paraplegia	29 (3.7%)	8 (2.1%)	6 (4.7%)
Liver disease	137 (17.5%)	44 (11.8%)	35 (25.1%)
Diabetes mellitus	332 (42.3%)	152 (40.7%)	51 (39.5%)
Any malignancy	137 (17.5%)	32 (8.6%)	38 (29.5%)
Hypertension	567 (72.3%)	270 (72.4%)	93 (72.1%)
Major cause for admission			
Infectious diseases	58 (7.4%)	28 (7.5%)	6 (4.7%)
Oncology disorders	119 (15.2%)	30 (8.0%)	34 (26.4%)
Cardiovascular Diseases	315 (40.1%)	192 (51.5%)	40 (31.0%)
Pulmonary diseases	82 (10.4%)	25 (6.7%)	12 (9.3%)
Gastrointestinal and liver diseases	118 (15.0%)	35 (9.4%)	27 (20.9%)
Kidney diseases	47 (6.0%)	36 (9.7%)	2 (1.6%)
other	46 (5.9%)	27 (7.2%)	8 (6.2%)

[1] eGFR at admission could not be calculated for all individuals because creatinine was massively interfered with by bilirubin or hemoglobin at admission.

In 128 (34%) of patients, the cause of CKD ≥ III was further specified by ICD-10 billing codes. In the remaining cohort of 245 patients with CKD ≥ III, 90% suffered from diabetes mellitus II and/or hypertension. More than 33% of etiologies for CKD ≥ III had been documented only in discharge summaries (Supplementary Materials).

There was a high incidence for AKI (33.6%) and AKI recovery (27.4%) in the CKD ≥ III cohort (Supplementary Materials).

Most patients were assigned to CKD status by discharge summaries, followed by eGFR and ICD-10 billing codes (Figure 1a). After manual review, less than 1% of the CKD cases identified by discharge summaries and eGFR and ICD-10 billing codes did not suffer from CKD III–V (Figure 1b). Patients identified by discharge summaries seemed to have a better kidney function at admission, while patients assigned to CKD by eGFR or ICD-10 billing codes had a worse kidney function compared to the reference standard. Similarly, patients identified by eGFR and discharge summaries were less morbid than patients characterized as CKD by ICD-10 billing codes, as indicated by Charlson morbidity categories (Table 2). Of note, 19 patients were identified by manual review only, while each of the three formal criteria failed.

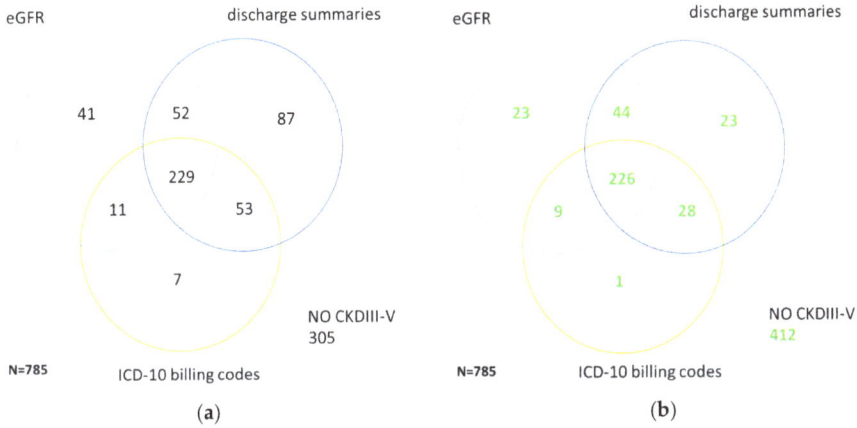

Figure 1. Venn diagrams comparing identification of CKD ≥ III by laboratory results (eGFR values), discharge summaries or ICD-10 billing codes within all patients (**a**) and within patients with CKD ≥ III according to reference standard (**b**). (**a**) Numbers of patients from the study cohort with CKD recognized by laboratory results (eGFR values), discharge summaries or ICD-10 billing codes. (**b**) Numbers of patients from the study cohort with CKD *correctly* recognized by laboratory results (eGFR values), discharge summaries or ICD-10 billing codes. A total of 19 patients were recognized by neither of the three formal criteria, but by manual review only.

Table 2. Epidemiological characteristics from patients with CKD identified by reference standard or recognized by laboratory results (eGFR values), discharge summaries or ICD-10 billing codes.

Characteristics	Reference Standard (n = 373)	eGFR (n = 333)	Discharge Summaries (n = 421)	ICD-10 Billing Codes (n = 300)
Age, years, mean [SD]	77.9 [10]	78.0 [9.7]	76.4 [10.9]	77.2 [10.3]
Sex, male	215 (57.6%)	189 (56.8%)	258 (61.3%)	182 (60.7%)
eGFR at admission, median, [quartiles], mL/min/1.73 m²	(n = 372)[1] 28.9 [18.1–41.8]	26.8 [17.5–39.4]	(n = 420)[1] 32.9 [19.6–50]	25.7 [15.2–39.6]
Charlson morbidity category ≥1	366 (98.1%)	326 (97.9%)	413 (98.1%)	297 (99%)
≥3	224 (60.1%)	198 (59.5%)	257 (61.1%)	220 (73.3%)
Median	3	3	3	3

[1] eGFR could not be calculated for all individuals because creatinine was massively interfered with by bilirubin or hemoglobin at admission.

Similar to CKD, the patient cohort was investigated for patients with no known kidney disease (NKD). Numbers of patients assigned to NKD by laboratory values, ICD-10 billing codes or discharge summaries are depicted in Figure 2a. Comparison with the reference standard (Figure 2b) confirms 65% of the patients assigned to NKD by all three categories. Patients identified by the laboratory NKD criteria were younger, had a higher eGFR at admission and did therefore better correspond with the reference standard compared to patients assigned to NKD by discharge summaries or ICD-10 billing codes (Table 3).

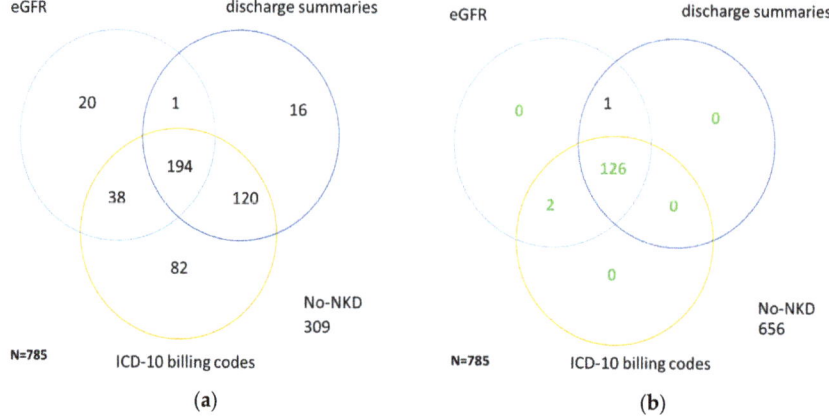

Figure 2. Venn diagrams comparing identification of no known kidney disease (NKD) by laboratory results (eGFR values), discharge summaries or ICD -10 billing codes within all patients (**a**) and within patients with CKD ≥ III according to reference standard (**b**). (**a**) Numbers of patients from the study cohort with NKD recognized via the eHealth sources laboratory results (eGFR values), discharge summaries or ICD-10 billing codes. (**b**) Numbers of patients from the study cohort with NKD *correctly* recognized via laboratory results (eGFR values), discharge summaries or ICD-10 billing codes.

Table 3. Epidemiological characteristics from patients with NKD identified by reference standard or recognized by sources laboratory results (eGFR values), discharge summaries or ICD-10 billing codes.

Chracteristics	Reference Standard (n = 129)	eGFR (n = 253)	Discharge Summaries (n = 334)	ICD-10 Billing Codes (n = 437)
Age, years, mean [SD]	68.4 [13.7]	69.3 [13.3]	72.9 [13.3]	73.3 [13.0]
Sex, male	79 (61.2%)	161 (63.6%)	196 (58.7%)	265 (60.6%)
eGFR at admission, median, [quartiles], mL/min/1.73 m²	88.6 [78.6–99.3]	84.5 [75.7–96.2]	76.0 *,1 [53.8–89.5]	69.9 *,2 [50.0–87.7]
Charlson morbidity score ≥1	113 (87.6%)	232 (91.7%)	308 (92.2%)	403 (92.2%)
≥3	36 (27.9%)	91 (36.0%)	116 (34.7%)	145 (33.2%)
Median	2	2	2	2

* eGFR could not be calculated for all individuals because creatinine was massively interfered with by bilirubin or hemoglobin at admission. ¹ n = 331; ² n = 434.

Tables 4 and 5 depict the specificities and sensitivities of the different rules applied for identification of CKD or NKD, respectively. While ICD-10 billing codes show excellent specificity for identification of CKD, the sensitivity was lower compared to discharge summaries and eGFR. Discharge summaries had a better sensitivity, but a reduced specificity compared to ICD-10 billing codes (Table 4). Using eGFR < 60 mL/min/1.73 m² during the whole hospital stay results in good sensitivity and specificity. If only the first eGFR at admission or the last eGFR measurement at discharge were used, overall performance (AUROC) did only minimally change compared to the original rule.

Table 4. Performance of different rules for identification of patients with CKD compared to the reference standard.

Category	Sensitivity	Specificity	PPV	NPV	AUROC (CI)	AUCPR (CI)
ICD-10 billing codes	0.71	0.91	0.88	0.78	0.81 (0.78–0.84)	0.86 (0.83–0.90)
Discharge summary	0.86	0.76	0.76	0.86	0.81 (0.78–0.84)	0.84 (0.81–0.88)
eGFR <60 mL/min/1.73 m² during Index hospital stay	0.81	0.92	0.91	0.84	0.87 (0.84–0.90)	0.90 (0.87–0.93)
eGFR_at_admission <60 mL/min/1.73 m²	0.96	0.75	0.77	0.95	0.85 (0.83–0.87)	0.88 (0.84–0.91)
eGFR_at_discharge <60 mL/min/1.73 m²	0.91	0.82	0.82	0.91	0.86 (0.84–0.89)	0.89 (0.85–0.92)

Table 5. Performance of different rules for identification of patients with NKD compared to the reference standard.

Category	Sensitivity	Specificity	PPV	NPV	AUROC (CI)	AUPR (CI)
ICD-10 billing codes	0.99	0.53	0.29	1	0.76 (0.74–0.78)	0.64 (0.56–0.73)
Discharge summary	0.98	0.68	0.38	1	0.83 (0.81–0.86)	0.68 (0.60–0.76)
eGFR ≥ 60 mL/min/1.73m² during Index hospital stay	1.00	0.82	0.52	1	0.91 (0.89–0.92)	0.75 (0.68–0.83)
eGFR_at_admission ≥ 60 mL/min/1.73 m²	1.00	0.71	0.41	1.00	0.86 (0.84–0.87)	0.70 (0.62–0.78)
eGFR_at_discharge ≥ 60 mL/min/1.73 m²	1.00	0.64	0.35	1.00	0.82 (0.80–0.84)	0.68 (0.59–0.76)

Regarding NKD, ICD-10 billing codes, discharge summaries and creatinine blood values, at admission, at discharge and during hospital stay, have all excellent sensitivity. However, acceptable specificity (>80%) was achieved only by using eGFR < 60 mL/min/1.73m² during the whole hospital stay. However, the PPV was still low at 0.52 (Table 5).

Combining laboratory measurements with discharge summaries and ICD-10 billing codes using logistic regression developed in a training dataset resulted in a better overall performance for identification of CKD (AUROC: 0.96[0.93–0.98]) or NKD (AUROC: 0.94[0.91–0.97]) in the test dataset compared to estimated glomerular filtration rate (eGFR) values (CKD: AUROC 0.85[0.79–0.90]; NKD: AUROC 0.91[0.87–0.94]), discharge summaries (CKD: AUROC 0.87[0.82–0.92], NKD: AUROC 0.84[0.79–0.89]) or ICD-10 billing codes (CKD: AUROC 0.85[0.80–0.91], NKD: AUROC 0.77[0.72–0.83]) alone (Figure 3 and Supplementary Materials). Interestingly, the combination of all three categories, however, did not (NKD) or only minimally (CKD ≥ III) increase the performance in comparison with the combination of laboratory results and discharge summaries (CKD: AUROC 0.94[0.9–0.97]; NKD: AUROC 0.95[0.92–0.97]).

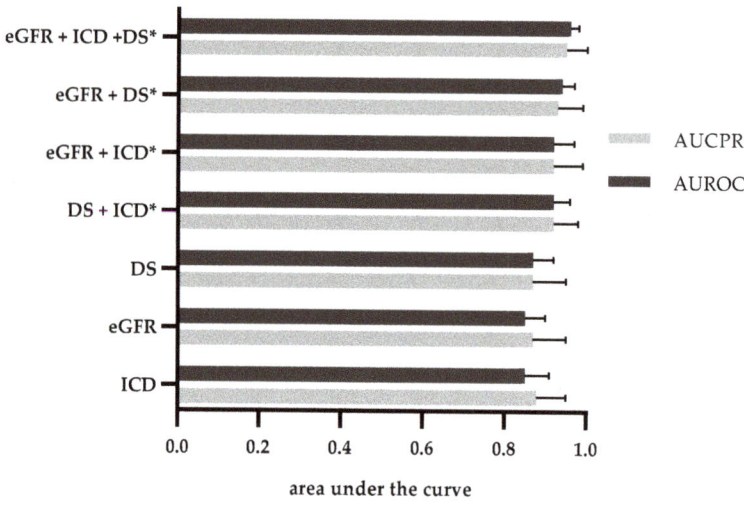

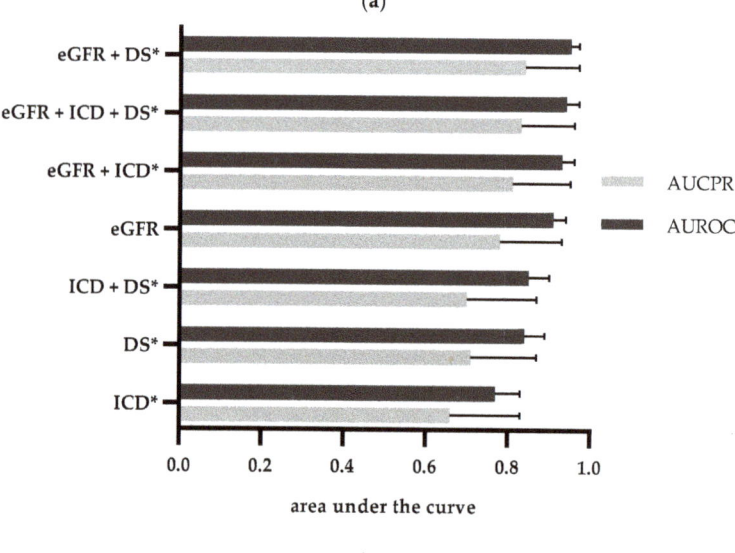

Figure 3. Area under the receiver operating characteristic (AUROC) and under the precision-recall curve (AUCPR) for simple categorical classifiers based on combinations of EHR components for CKD ≥ III (**a**) and NKD (**b**) on the test dataset. eGFR values = "eGFR", discharge summaries = "DS" and ICD-10 billing codes = "ICD". For the complete list of all combinations, see Supplementary Materials. Logistic regression was calculated on the training dataset. Performance is calculated on the test dataset (n = 156). * Indicates $p < 0.05$ for difference in AUROC compared to eGFR.

In NKD, AUROC values were quite high. However, AUCPR values that include sensitivity and PPV were lower. It is therefore helpful to include several parameters, e.g., AUROC and AUCPR for assessing test performance, particularly in imbalanced data [32].

To further improve performance for correct assignment of patients to CKD ≥ III or NKD, we developed a logistic regression and three mL models using (1) all data from the index hospital stay including laboratory values with incidence of AKI and AKI recovery including staging, demographics, ICD-billing codes and ICDs from discharge summaries; (2) laboratory values and demographics from the index hospital stay; (3) and (4) in addition to (1) or (2) includes laboratory values from previous hospital stays, respectively (for a detailed listing of variables, see Supplementary Materials).

Figure 4 shows the AUROCs and AUCPRs of the respective best logistic regression (LR) and best different mL models for identification of CKD ≥ III and NKD compared to the best simple categorical classifier for each scenario. In general, AUROCs of LR and of the different mL models were only slightly different between each other (see Supplementary Materials for more details).

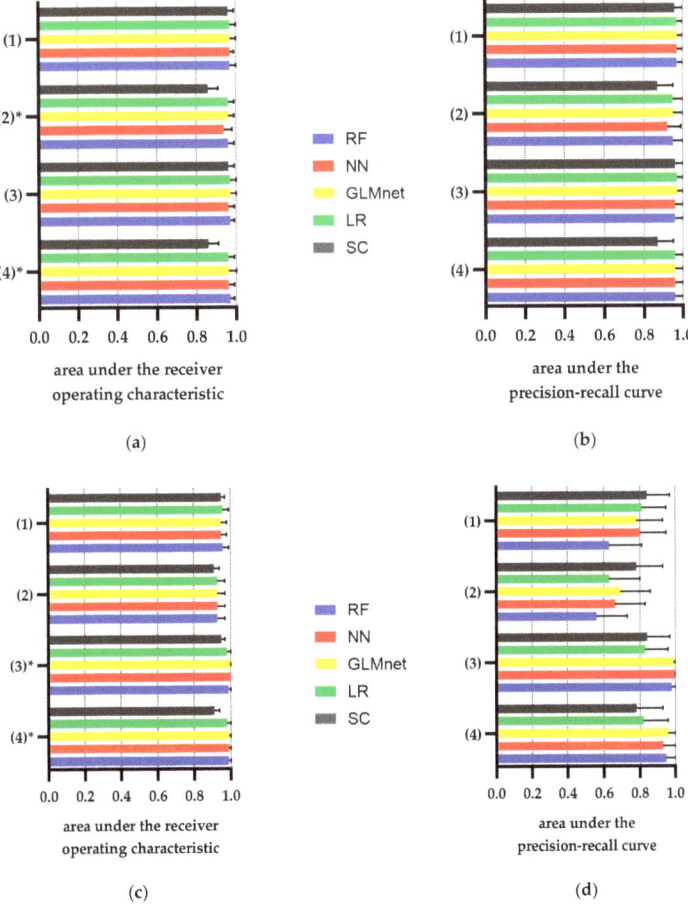

Figure 4. AUROC (**a**,**c**) and AUCPR (**b**,**d**) of the simple categorical classifier and of models calculated from logistic regression and the three mL methods for identification of CKD (**a**,**b**) and NKD (**c**,**d**) in different scenarios of data availability. (**a**) AUROC and (**b**) AUCPR for identification of CKD ≥ III; (**c**) AUROC and (**d**) AUCPR for identification of NKD. SC = simple categorical classifier, LR = logistic regression, GLMnet = generalized linear machine network, RF = random forest, NN = Artificial Neuronal Network. N = 156 patients (test dataset). Scenarios: (1) All data from the index hospital stay including laboratory values, demographics, ICD-billing codes and ICDs from discharge summaries; (2) laboratory values and demographics from the index hospital stay; (3) and (4) includes, in addition to (1) or (2), laboratory values from previous hospital stays, respectively. * Indicates $p < 0.05$ for difference in AUROC between SC and all other models.

For identification of CKD ≥ III, the AUROCs of the LR and machine learning models were not significantly better in scenario 1 (LR/ML: 0.97[0.95–1.00]) and scenario 3 (LR/ML: 0.97[0.94–1.00]) compared to the simple classifier in scenario 1 and 3 (0.96[0.94–0.99]), respectively. AUROCs of the LR and mL models significantly ($p < 0.05$) improved in scenario 2 (LR/ML: 0.96[0.92–0.99]) and scenario 4 (LR: 0.96[0.93–0.99]/ML 0.97[0.94–0.99]) compared to the simple classifier in scenario 2 and 4 (0.86[0.81–0.91]), respectively. In scenarios 2 and 4, data were restricted to laboratory values alone.

For identification of NKD, AUROCs of the LR and mL models significantly ($p < 0.05$) improved in scenario 3 (LR: 0.98[0.96–1.00]/ML: 1.00[1.00–1.00]) and scenario 4 (LR: 0.98[0.96–1.00]/ML: 0.99[0.98–1.00]) compared to the simple classifier in scenario 3 (0.95[0.92–0.97]) and scenario 4 (0.91[0.87–0.94]), respectively (Figure 4c). In scenarios 3 and 4, data from previous hospital stays were included. AUCPRs of the logistic regression and mL models for identification of NKD also improved in scenarios 3 and 4 compared to the simple classifier (Figure 4d, see Supplementary Materials for more details). AUROCs of LR and mL models slightly improved in scenario 1 (LR/ML: 0.96[0.93–0.99]) and scenario 2 (LR/ML: 0.93[0.89–0.97]) compared to the simple classifier in scenario 1 (0.95[0.92–0.97]) and scenario 2 (0.91[0.87–0.94]), respectively (Figure 4c). However, AUCPR of LR and mL models decreased in scenario 1 and 2 compared to the simple classifier.

In conclusion, the best LR and mL models slightly improved AUROCs for identification of CKD ≥ III and NKD compared to the best simple categorical classifier in each scenario. However, we observed a significant improvement by models compared to the simple classifier for CKD ≥ III only in scenarios 2 and 4 and for NKD only in scenarios 3 and 4.

4. Discussion

The results of our study demonstrate that laboratory values have the best performance for identifying CKD ≥ III and NKD from EHRs compared to discharge summaries and ICD-10 billing codes in an elderly multimorbid cohort of hospitalized patients. Combining classifiers based on laboratory values (creatinine/eGFR), ICD-10 billing codes or ICD-10 codes extracted from discharge summaries outperformed each component alone for identification of CKD ≥ III and NKD. Classification could be further improved by calculation of logistic regression and mL models if data were restricted to laboratory values (CKD ≥ III) or if additional values from previous hospital stays were added (NKD).

Although each of the mentioned EHR components have been investigated before, we could demonstrate the extent to which the classification is improved by combining laboratory values with ICD-10 billing codes and discharge summaries. Furthermore, we are the first, to our knowledge, to describe classification performance for NKD.

The good sensitivity and specificity of laboratory values for the identification of CKD ≥ III and NKD can be explained by the fact that both entities are mainly defined by blood creatinine and eGFR values [3,26]. However, many epidemiological studies and clinical trials have utilized ICD-10 billing codes for defining CKD status [4]—more than 50% of cardiovascular trials do not report eGFR measurement in respective study populations [45].

Previous studies have demonstrated a high specificity of billing codes. However, many CKD patients will be overlooked by using billing codes alone and the identified cohort is biased towards more advanced CKD stages with higher creatinine values [5,46,47]. These results have been replicated and confirmed in the current study. A sensitivity of 75% indicates that approximately one-quarter of patients with advanced CKD ≥ III had been missed by ICD-10 billing codes. Patients recognized by ICD-10 billing codes had a lower eGFR and showed a higher morbidity in comparison to the reference standard.

However, the sensitivity of ICD-10 billing codes was much better in our study than in a recent study by Diamantidis et al. who reported a very low sensitivity of ICD-10 billing codes for recognizing CKD > III [43]. The discrepancy might be explained by differences in the patient cohorts as the latter study included non-hospitalized patients.

Gomez-Salgado et al., in contrast, recently showed good correlation between ICD-10 billing codes and researchers' judgment based on clinical documentation [48]. A possible explanation for the conflicting results between our study and Gomez-Salgado et al. could be the extent to which laboratory values were considered for identification of CKD.

Our study also confirms previous findings of slight under-documentation of CKD using discharge summaries [49]. Indeed approximately 20% of patients with advanced CKD ≥ III were not identified by discharge summaries. However, in line with the study of Singh et al., we could also show that the sensitivity of discharge summaries is higher than the sensitivity of billing codes for CKD [9]. The reduced specificity of discharge summaries could be explained by the fact that many patients with CKD stage I and II were counted as CKD ≥ III. Differing definitions for chronic kidney disease might also be the reason why a recent study by Hernandez-Boussard et al. observed a better accuracy for unstructured discharge summaries for recognizing CKD compared to our study [50]. Other possible explanations are different information sources and a different study cohort.

In a study by Nadkarni et al., an algorithm was developed and evaluated to identify patients with CKD Stage III caused by hypertension or diabetes, using structured and unstructured information from EHRs [51]. The algorithm based on keywords from medical notes and laboratory values outperformed phenotyping by ICD-10 billing codes by a margin. These results resonate with the outcome of our study that included advanced CKD from any cause in hospitalized patients.

Missing previous health records is a common problem in clinical studies and might affect correct identification of diseases [52]. However, in contrast to the identification of patients with diabetes mellitus [53], we can demonstrate good F1 score (>0.8), although using datasets restricted to the current hospital stay for simple classifiers. For CKD ≥ III, mL models based on laboratory values alone had a similar AUROC as the simple categorical classifiers including discharge summaries and ICD-10 billing codes. This indicates that mL models might be able to—at least partly—compensate for missing information.

The results of our study are encouraging, not only for stratification of patients for clinical and epidemiological studies, but also in the context of, e.g., Healthcare-Integrated Biobanking, where automated classifiers based on minimal clinical information are of great importance for early selection of samples of specific disease entities.

Structured information such as laboratory values and billing codes are often readily available. Results from our study show that a PPV of 0.77, 0.82 or 0.91 can be achieved for the identification of CKD by using eGFR values at admission, at discharge or from the complete hospital stay, respectively. This is in line with other studies demonstrating that a single measurement of eGFR might overestimate the number of CKD cases [54]. The slightly higher PPV when using eGFR values at discharge compared to admission can be explained by the fact that interfering acute kidney injury is more likely to be present at admission than after a successful treatment at discharge.

Suboptimal PPV values associated with false classification can significantly impact the phenotyping process and thus might cause severe bias in the outcomes of subsequent studies. Consequently, there is a need for further optimization of CKD and NKD classification.

Wei et al. combined different sources of information (primary notes, medication and billing codes) to improve phenotyping based on EHR for several chronic diseases (not CKD though) and demonstrated that PPV and F1 score can be increased by combining different information sources [55]. Results from Wei et al. can be confirmed in our study in relation to CKD and NKD with the caveat that eGFR should be included in any combination.

The addition of discharge summaries and/or ICD-10 billing codes to laboratory values not only increases the performance of correct identification of CKD ≥ III but also helped to further specify the cause of the disease in at least one-third of the cohort. There were more etiologies for CKD in the discharge summaries compared to the ICD-10 billing codes.

Another novelty of this study is that, to the best of the authors' knowledge, for the first time the entity of NKD (no known kidney disease) was investigated using EHRs. Identifying NKD is a challenging task because ICD-10 billing codes and discharge summaries are designed to describe the presence of illness rather than its absence. However, the question of NKD might be of particular interest for scientific reasons. The validity of association studies and clinical trials depends on the correct assignment of co-morbidities. If large cohorts of CKD patients are counted as NKD, studies might be biased and results might thus be flawed. Our study demonstrates that single EHR sources had low PPV and AUCPR for NKD assignment. Combining laboratory values with discharge summaries improved PPV and AUCPR. Interestingly, the further addition of ICD-10 billing codes to this combination did not result in a further improvement of PPV and AUCPR. Future epidemiological studies should take these results in consideration for classification of NKD.

Finally, we demonstrated that logistic regression and mL algorithms have the potential to improve recognition of CKD ≥ III and NKD, particularly in certain scenarios of data availability. This might be helpful for the development of clinical decision support systems (CDSS) in the near future that ultimately will allow clinicians and researches almost instantly to evaluate the chronic kidney status of patients.

Direct comparison with other studies applying mL strategies for the detection of CKD is hampered due to different definitions of CKD, different patient cohorts and data variables used. Almansour et al. described an Artificial Neural Network with an accuracy of more than 99% [20]. Salekin et al. used the same cohort and reduced the number of variables down to 12 and achieved an F1 score of 99% by using a wrapper approach to identify the best subset of attributes and a random forest classifier [56]. However, both studies rely on the same data source comprising 24 variables of 400 patients to build a predictive model. In contrast to our study, the dataset does not include series of creatinine measurements or information from discharge summaries or ICD-10 billing codes about CKD. Rashidian et al. used laboratory values, demographics and ICD-10 billing codes to identify patients with CKD achieving a F1 score of approximately 0.8 [57]. In our study, AUROC and AUCPR for identification of CKD from mL algorithms surpassed 0.95 in all scenarios of unrestricted or restricted data availability. One reason for these differences could be that the study by Rashidian et al. did not use discharge letters as source of information. As mentioned before, in our study discharge summaries can add valuable information to the classification process. This is also reflected by the result that mL algorithms did not significantly improve performance of CKD ≥ III identification (AUROC 0.97) compared to a simple classifier based on laboratory values, discharge summaries and ICD-10 billing codes (AUROC 0.96).

The mL algorithms used in our study failed to outperform rule-based classifiers for identification of NKD if data were restricted to the index hospital stay: although AUROC is (non-significantly) increasing, PPV is declining and thus superiority of the models has to be rejected. An explanation for this result could be that the correct assignment of NKD mainly depends on the availability of the complete dataset. Additionally, we cannot exclude that the low prevalence of NKD in our morbid patient cohort affected the efficacy of mL strategies.

To the best of our knowledge, this is the first study trying to detect specifically CKD Stage ≥ III and NKD by mL methods. Therefore, it is mandatory that the proof-of-concept presented here needs further elaboration in larger independent patient cohorts.

The strength of the study is the comprehensive dataset including discharge summaries of the index hospital stay and laboratory values with a reviewed reference standard.

Several limitations need to be acknowledged. The patient cohort included in the study was quite morbid and not representative of a general hospital population or, even more so, an outpatient population. Therefore, the extent of improvement by combining different information sources needs to be prospectively validated in other independent cohorts.

The AVERBIS HEALTH DISCOVERY software tool was used for the extraction of information attributes from discharge summaries that have been predefined by the authors. The use of natural language processing (NLP) methods for information extraction and automated feature selection could have resulted in an increased performance of the data extraction method.

Similarly, the total number of patients was rather small for training mL classifiers. We may guess that, in a larger patient cohort, the performance of the different models might further increase. However, the scope of the present study was to demonstrate the feasibility and potential of using eHealth sources and mL models to improve phenotyping of CKD and NKD.

The models presented in this manuscript focus on the detection of advanced CKD (Stage III or higher) or on the absence of kidney disease. Patients with mild CKD (Stage I and II) are not taken into consideration although the correct identification of this group might be important for clinical treatment and research purpose. Future studies with larger patient cohorts might be able to develop more granular models differentiating between mild and advanced CKD.

Another limitation is that neither a single rule nor a combination of them achieved a sensitivity for identification of CKD ≥ III of 100%. This could be explained by the fact that most patients were treated primarily for non-nephrological reasons during the index hospital stay and thus CKD was not mentioned at all in the current discharge summaries or by the ICD-10 billing codes, although they had a documented eGFR < 60 mL/min/1.73m^2 for a period longer than 90 days.

Furthermore, data included in the analysis were incomplete, since laboratory results from primary care or other institutions (for example, from general practitioners or other hospitals) were not available. Most importantly albuminuria was available in less than 5% of the whole cohort and could therefore not included in the analysis.

Missing data, however, reflects "real-world" conditions. Missing data can be, at least partly, compensated for—as shown in our study—by the extraction of unstructured information from the discharge summaries that usually contain a multitude of pre-existing health data from other healthcare providers.

5. Conclusions

In summary, combining laboratory results (creatinine and eGFR) with discharge summaries and ICD-10 billing codes had the best performance in a simple categorical classifier for phenotyping of CKD ≥ III and NKD. Logistic regression or mL models had the potential to further improve the correct identification of CKD ≥ III if only laboratory values were used and of NKD if data from previous hospital stays were included into models.

Supplementary Materials: Supplementary Materials are available online. http://www.mdpi.com/2077-0383/9/9/2955/s1, Table S1: Characteristics of the study cohort; Additional characteristics of the study cohort; Table S2: ICD-10 billing codes for definition of CKD; Table S3: ICD-10 billing codes for exclusion of NKD; Table S4: detailed performance characteristics for combinations of simple classifiers for identification of CKD and NKD; Table S5: Detailed AUC-ROC and -PR for combinations of different classifiers for identification of CKD and NKD; Table S6: Cause for CKD in the CKD>III cohort; detailed cause for CKD ≥ III and source of information; Table S7: Incidence of AKI and AKI Recovery in the complete study cohort with creati-nine values (n=780) and in CKD>III cohort with creatinine values (n=372); Table S8: Source of information for etiologies of CKD>III; Table S9: Distribution of true positives and true negatives for CKD and NKD, in the training and test datasets; Table S10: Detailed performance characteristics for combinations of different classifiers for identification of CKD and NKD; Table S11: Detailed AUC-ROC and -PR for combinations of different classifiers for identification of CKD and NKD; Table S12: Detailed performance characteristics for different generalized linear model networks for identification of CKD and NKD; Table S13: Detailed AUC-ROC and -PR for different generalized linear model networks for identification of CKD and NKD; Table S14: Detailed performance characteristics for different gen-eralized linear model networks for identification of CKD and NKD; Table S15: Detailed AUC-ROC and -PR for different generalized linear model networks for identification of CKD and NKD; Table S16: Detailed performance characteristics for different random forest models for identification of CKD and NKD; Table S17: Detailed AUC-ROC and -PR for different random forest models for identification of CKD and NKD; Table S18: Detailed performance characteristics for different random forest models for identification of CKD and NKD; Table S19: Detailed AUC-ROC and -PR for different random forest models for identification of CKD and NKD; Table S20: Detailed performance characteristics for different neural networks models for identification of CKD and NKD; Table S21: Detailed AUC-ROC and -PR for for different neural networks models for identification of CKD and NKD; Table S22: Detailed performance characteristics for different neural networks models for identification of CKD and NKD; Table S23: Detailed AUC-ROC and -PR for for different neural networks models for identification of CKD and NKD; Table S24: Detailed performance characteristics for different generalized linear mod-els for identification of CKD and NKD; Table S25: Detailed AUC-ROC and -PR for for different generalized linear models for identification of CKD and NKD; Table S26: Detailed performance characteristics for different generalized linear models for identification of

CKD and NKD; Table S27: Detailed AUC-ROC and -PR for for different generalized linear models for identification of CKD and NKD; Table S28: Detailed hyperparameters of different machine learning models; Table S29: Detailed hyperparameters of different machine learning models.

Author Contributions: Conceptualization, U.H., B.B. and M.K.; data curation, C.W. and L.R.; formal analysis, C.W., L.R. and L.M.; funding acquisition, U.H. and M.K.; investigation, C.W., L.R., C.L., T.K., B.B. and M.K.; methodology, C.W., B.B. and M.K.; project administration, M.K.; resources, L.M., C.L., T.K., U.H., D.A. and M.K.; software, C.W.; supervision, U.H. and M.K.; validation, C.W., L.R. and B.B.; visualization, C.W., B.B. and M.K.; writing—original draft, C.W. and B.B.; writing—review & editing, U.H., B.B. and M.K. All authors have read and agreed to the published version of the manuscript.

Funding: This work was supported by the Deutsche Forschungsgemeinschaft (DFG) under grant KI 564/2-1 and HA 2079/8-1 within the STAKI^{2}B^2 project (Semantic Text Analysis for Quality-controlled Extraction of Clinical Phenotype Information within the Framework of Healthcare-Integrated Biobanking).

Conflicts of Interest: The authors declare no conflict of interest.

References

1. Wang, J.; Wang, F.; Saran, R.; He, Z.; Zhao, M.H.; Li, Y.; Zhang, L.; Bragg-Gresham, J. Mortality risk of chronic kidney disease: A comparison between the adult populations in urban China and the United States. *PLoS ONE* **2018**, *13*, e0193734. [CrossRef]
2. Xie, Y.; Bowe, B.; Mokdad, A.H.; Xian, H.; Yan, Y.; Li, T.; Maddukuri, G.; Tsai, C.Y.; Floyd, T.; Al-Aly, Z. Analysis of the Global Burden of Disease study highlights the global, regional, and national trends of chronic kidney disease epidemiology from 1990 to 2016. *Kidney Int.* **2018**, *94*, 567–581. [CrossRef] [PubMed]
3. Kidney Disease: Improving Global Outcomes (KDIGO) CKD Work Group. KDIGO 2012 Clinical Practice Guideline for the Evaluation and Management of Chronic Kidney Disease. *Kidney Int. Suppl.* **2013**, *3*, 1–150.
4. Anderson, J.; Glynn, L.G. Definition of chronic kidney disease and measurement of kidney function in original research papers: A review of the literature. *Nephrol. Dial. Transplant.* **2011**, *26*, 2793–2798. [CrossRef] [PubMed]
5. Jalal, K.; Anand, E.J.; Venuto, R.; Eberle, J.; Arora, P. Can billing codes accurately identify rapidly progressing stage 3 and stage 4 chronic kidney disease patients: A diagnostic test study. *BMC Nephrol.* **2019**, *20*, 260. [CrossRef]
6. Vlasschaert, M.E.; Bejaimal, S.A.; Hackam, D.G.; Quinn, R.; Cuerden, M.S.; Oliver, M.J.; Iansavichus, A.; Sultan, N.; Mills, A.; Garg, A.X. Validity of administrative database coding for kidney disease: A systematic review. *Am. J. Kidney Dis.* **2011**, *57*, 29–43. [CrossRef]
7. Levey, A.S.; Stevens, L.A.; Schmid, C.H.; Zhang, Y.L.; Castro, A.F., 3rd; Feldman, H.I.; Kusek, J.W.; Eggers, P.; Van Lente, F.; Greene, T.; et al. A new equation to estimate glomerular filtration rate. *Ann. Intern. Med.* **2009**, *150*, 604–612. [CrossRef]
8. Bhattacharya, M.; Jurkovitz, C.; Shatkay, H. Co-occurrence of medical conditions: Exposing patterns through probabilistic topic modeling of snomed codes. *J. Biomed. Inform.* **2018**, *82*, 31–40. [CrossRef]
9. Singh, B.; Singh, A.; Ahmed, A.; Wilson, G.A.; Pickering, B.W.; Herasevich, V.; Gajic, O.; Li, G. Derivation and validation of automated electronic search strategies to extract Charlson comorbidities from electronic medical records. *Mayo Clin. Proc.* **2012**, *87*, 817–824. [CrossRef]
10. Upadhyaya, S.G.; Murphree, D.H., Jr.; Ngufor, C.G.; Knight, A.M.; Cronk, D.J.; Cima, R.R.; Curry, T.B.; Pathak, J.; Carter, R.E.; Kor, D.J. Automated Diabetes Case Identification Using Electronic Health Record Data at a Tertiary Care Facility. *Mayo Clin. Proc. Innov. Qual. Outcomes* **2017**, *1*, 100–110. [CrossRef]
11. Lin, C.; Lou, Y.S.; Tsai, D.J.; Lee, C.C.; Hsu, C.J.; Wu, D.C.; Wang, M.C.; Fang, W.H. Projection Word Embedding Model With Hybrid Sampling Training for Classifying ICD-10-CM Codes: Longitudinal Observational Study. *JMIR Med. Inform.* **2019**, *7*, e14499. [CrossRef] [PubMed]
12. Batool, R.; Khattak, A.M.; Kim, T.-S.; Lee, S. Automatic extraction and mapping of discharge summary's concepts into SNOMED CT. In Proceedings of the 35th Annual International Conference of the IEEE Engineering in Medicine and Biology Society, Osaka, Japan, 3–7 July 2013.
13. Tang, B.; Cao, H.; Wu, Y.; Jiang, M.; Xu, H. Recognizing clinical entities in hospital discharge summaries using Structural Support Vector Machines with word representation features. *BMC Med. Inform. Decis. Mak.* **2013**, *13* (Suppl. 1), S1. [CrossRef] [PubMed]

14. Sahu, S.K.; Anand, A.; Oruganty, K.; Gattu, M. Relation extraction from clinical texts using domain invariant convolutional neural network. In Proceedings of the 15th Workshop on Biomedical Natural Language Processing, BioNLP@ACL 2016, Berlin, Germany, 12 August 2016; pp. 206–215.
15. Xiao, J.; Ding, R.; Xu, X.; Guan, H.; Feng, X.; Sun, T.; Zhu, S.; Ye, Z. Comparison and development of machine learning tools in the prediction of chronic kidney disease progression. *J. Transl. Med.* **2019**, *17*, 119. [CrossRef] [PubMed]
16. Polat, H.; Danaei Mehr, H.; Cetin, A. Diagnosis of Chronic Kidney Disease Based on Support Vector Machine by Feature Selection Methods. *J. Med. Syst.* **2017**, *41*, 55. [CrossRef] [PubMed]
17. Chen, Z.; Zhang, Z.; Zhu, R.; Xiang, Y.; Harrington, P.B. Diagnosis of patients with chronic kidney disease by using two fuzzy classifiers. *Chemom. Intell. Lab. Syst.* **2016**, *153*, 140–145. [CrossRef]
18. Alexander Arman, S. Diagnosis Rule Extraction from Patient Data for Chronic Kidney Disease Using Machine Learning. *Int. J. Biomed. Clin. Eng. IJBCE* **2016**, *5*, 64–72. [CrossRef]
19. Elhoseny, M.; Shankar, K.; Uthayakumar, J. Intelligent Diagnostic Prediction and Classification System for Chronic Kidney Disease. *Sci. Rep.* **2019**, *9*, 9583. [CrossRef]
20. Almansour, N.A.; Syed, H.F.; Khayat, N.R.; Altheeb, R.K.; Juri, R.E.; Alhiyafi, J.; Alrashed, S.; Olatunji, S.O. Neural network and support vector machine for the prediction of chronic kidney disease: A comparative study. *Comput. Biol. Med.* **2019**, *109*, 101–111. [CrossRef]
21. Winter, A.; Staubert, S.; Ammon, D.; Aiche, S.; Beyan, O.; Bischoff, V.; Daumke, P.; Decker, S.; Funkat, G.; Gewehr, J.E.; et al. Smart Medical Information Technology for Healthcare (SMITH). *Methods Inf. Med.* **2018**, *57*, e92–e105. [CrossRef]
22. Hahn, U.; Matthies, F.; Lohr, C.; Loffler, M. 3000PA-Towards a National Reference Corpus of German Clinical Language. *Stud. Health Technol. Inform.* **2018**, *247*, 26–30.
23. Lohr, C.; Luther, S.; Matthies, F.; Modersohn, L.; Ammon, D.; Saleh, K.; Henkel, A.G.; Kiehntopf, M.; Hahn, U. CDA-Compliant Section Annotation of German-Language Discharge Summaries: Guideline Development, Annotation Campaign, Section Classification. *AMIA Annu. Symp. Proc.* **2018**, *2018*, 770–779. [PubMed]
24. Quan, H.; Sundararajan, V.; Halfon, P.; Fong, A.; Burnand, B.; Luthi, J.C.; Saunders, L.D.; Beck, C.A.; Feasby, T.E.; Ghali, W.A. Coding algorithms for defining comorbidities in ICD-9-CM and ICD-10 administrative data. *Med. Care* **2005**, *43*, 1130–1139. [CrossRef] [PubMed]
25. James, M.T.; Levey, A.S.; Tonelli, M.; Tan, Z.; Barry, R.; Pannu, N.; Ravani, P.; Klarenbach, S.W.; Manns, B.J.; Hemmelgarn, B.R. Incidence and Prognosis of Acute Kidney Diseases and Disorders Using an Integrated Approach to Laboratory Measurements in a Universal Health Care System. *JAMA Netw. Open* **2019**, *2*, e191795. [CrossRef] [PubMed]
26. Kidney Disease: Improving Global Outcomes AKI Work Group. KDIGO clinical practice guideline for acute kidney injury. *Kidney Int. Suppl.* **2012**, *2*, 1–138.
27. Duff, S.; Murray, P.T. Defining Early Recovery of Acute Kidney Injury. *Clin. J. Am. Soc. Nephrol.* **2020**, *15*. [CrossRef]
28. Friedman, J.; Hastie, T.; Tibshirani, R. Regularization Paths for Generalized Lin, ear Models via Coordinate Descent. *J. Stat. Softw.* **2010**, *33*, 1–22. [CrossRef]
29. Liaw, A.; Wiener, M. Classification and Regression by randomForest. *R News* **2002**, *2*, 18–22.
30. Hagan, M.T.; Demuth, H.B.; Beale, M. *Neural Network Design*, 1st ed.; PWS Pub.: Boston, MA, USA, 1996.
31. Boehmke, B.; Greenwell, B.M. *Hands-on Machine Learning with R*; CRC Press: Boca Raton, FL, USA, 2019.
32. Saito, T.; Rehmsmeier, M. The precision-recall plot is more informative than the ROC plot when evaluating binary classifiers on imbalanced datasets. *PLoS ONE* **2015**, *10*, e0118432. [CrossRef]
33. DeLong, E.R.; DeLong, D.M.; Clarke-Pearson, D.L. Comparing the areas under two or more correlated receiver operating characteristic curves: A nonparametric approach. *Biometrics* **1988**, *44*, 837–845. [CrossRef]
34. RStudio Team. *RStudio: Integrated Development for R*; RStudio, PBC: Boston, MA, USA, 2019; Available online: http://www.rstudio.com/ (accessed on 12 September 2020).
35. Ritchie, M.E.; Phipson, B.; Wu, D.; Hu, Y.; Law, C.W.; Shi, W.; Smyth, G.K. Limma powers differential expression analyses for RNA-sequencing and microarray studies. *Nucleic Acids Res.* **2015**, *43*, e47. [CrossRef]
36. Chan, C.-H.; Chan, G.C.; Leeper, T.J.; Becker, J. *Rio: A Swiss-Army Knife for Data File I/O*; R package version 0.5.16; 2018. Available online: https://cran.r-project.org/web/packages/rio/index.html (accessed on 12 September 2020).
37. Wickham, H. The Split-Apply-Combine Strategy for Data Analysis. *J. Stat. Softw.* **2011**, *40*, 1–29. [CrossRef]

38. Pinheiro, J.; Bates, D.; DebRoy, S.; Sarkar, D.; Team, R.C. *Nlme: Linear and Nonlinear Mixed Effects Models*; R package version 3.1-142; 2019. Available online: https://CRAN.R-project.org/package=nlme (accessed on 12 September 2020).
39. Wickham, H.; Averick, M.; Bryan, J.; Chang, W.; McGowan, L.; François, R.; Grolemund, G.; Hayes, A.; Henry, L.; Hester, J.; et al. Welcome to the Tidyverse. *J. Open Sour. Softw.* **2019**, *4*, 1686. [CrossRef]
40. Robin, X.; Turck, N.; Hainard, A.; Tiberti, N.; Lisacek, F.; Sanchez, J.-C.; Müller, M. pROC: An open-source package for R and S+ to analyze and compare ROC curves. *BMC Bioinform.* **2011**, *12*, 1–8. [CrossRef] [PubMed]
41. Sing, T.; Sander, O.; Beerenwinkel, N.; Lengauer, T. ROCR: Visualizing classifier performance in R. *Bioinformatics* **2005**, *21*, 3940–3941. [CrossRef] [PubMed]
42. Kuhn, M. *Caret: Classification and Regression Training*; R package version 6.0-86; 2020. Available online: https://cran.r-project.org/web/packages/caret/index.html (accessed on 12 September 2020).
43. Diamantidis, C.J.; Hale, S.L.; Wang, V.; Smith, V.A.; Scholle, S.H.; Maciejewski, M.L. Lab-based and diagnosis-based chronic kidney disease recognition and staging concordance. *BMC Nephrol.* **2019**, *20*, 357. [CrossRef]
44. Stevens, L.A.; Li, S.; Wang, C.; Huang, C.; Becker, B.N.; Bomback, A.S.; Brown, W.W.; Burrows, N.R.; Jurkovitz, C.T.; McFarlane, S.I.; et al. Prevalence of CKD and comorbid illness in elderly patients in the United States: Results from the Kidney Early Evaluation Program (KEEP). *Am. J. Kidney Dis.* **2010**, *55*, S23–S33. [CrossRef]
45. Konstantinidis, I.; Nadkarni, G.N.; Yacoub, R.; Saha, A.; Simoes, P.; Parikh, C.R.; Coca, S.G. Representation of Patients With Kidney Disease in Trials of Cardiovascular Interventions: An Updated Systematic Review. *JAMA Intern. Med.* **2016**, *176*, 121–124. [CrossRef]
46. Ronksley, P.E.; Tonelli, M.; Quan, H.; Manns, B.J.; James, M.T.; Clement, F.M.; Samuel, S.; Quinn, R.R.; Ravani, P.; Brar, S.S.; et al. Validating a case definition for chronic kidney disease using administrative data. *Nephrol. Dial. Transplant.* **2012**, *27*, 1826–1831. [CrossRef]
47. Kern, E.F.; Maney, M.; Miller, D.R.; Tseng, C.L.; Tiwari, A.; Rajan, M.; Aron, D.; Pogach, L. Failure of ICD-9-CM codes to identify patients with comorbid chronic kidney disease in diabetes. *Health Serv. Res.* **2006**, *41*, 564–580. [CrossRef]
48. Gomez-Salgado, J.; Bernabeu-Wittel, M.; Aguilera-Gonzalez, C.; Goicoechea-Salazar, J.A.; Larrocha, D.; Nieto-Martin, M.D.; Moreno-Gavino, L.; Ollero-Baturone, M. Concordance between the Clinical Definition of Polypathological Patient versus Automated Detection by Means of Combined Identification through ICD-9-CM Codes. *J. Clin. Med.* **2019**, *8*, 613. [CrossRef]
49. Chase, H.S.; Radhakrishnan, J.; Shirazian, S.; Rao, M.K.; Vawdrey, D.K. Under-documentation of chronic kidney disease in the electronic health record in outpatients. *J. Am. Med. Inform. Assoc.* **2010**, *17*, 588–594. [CrossRef] [PubMed]
50. Hernandez-Boussard, T.; Monda, K.L.; Crespo, B.C.; Riskin, D. Real world evidence in cardiovascular medicine: Ensuring data validity in electronic health record-based studies. *J. Am. Med. Inform. Assoc.* **2019**, *26*, 1189–1194. [CrossRef] [PubMed]
51. Nadkarni, G.N.; Gottesman, O.; Linneman, J.G.; Chase, H.; Berg, R.L.; Farouk, S.; Nadukuru, R.; Lotay, V.; Ellis, S.; Hripcsak, G.; et al. Development and validation of an electronic phenotyping algorithm for chronic kidney disease. *AMIA Annu. Symp. Proc.* **2014**, *2014*, 907–916. [PubMed]
52. Wei, W.Q.; Leibson, C.L.; Ransom, J.E.; Kho, A.N.; Caraballo, P.J.; Chai, H.S.; Yawn, B.P.; Pacheco, J.A.; Chute, C.G. Impact of data fragmentation across healthcare centers on the accuracy of a high-throughput clinical phenotyping algorithm for specifying subjects with type 2 diabetes mellitus. *J. Am. Med. Inform. Assoc.* **2012**, *19*, 219–224. [CrossRef]
53. Wei, W.Q.; Leibson, C.L.; Ransom, J.E.; Kho, A.N.; Chute, C.G. The absence of longitudinal data limits the accuracy of high-throughput clinical phenotyping for identifying type 2 diabetes mellitus subjects. *Int. J. Med. Inform.* **2013**, *82*, 239–247. [CrossRef]
54. Delanaye, P.; Glassock, R.J.; De Broe, M.E. Epidemiology of chronic kidney disease: Think (at least) twice! *Clin. Kidney J.* **2017**, *10*, 370–374. [CrossRef]
55. Wei, W.Q.; Teixeira, P.L.; Mo, H.; Cronin, R.M.; Warner, J.L.; Denny, J.C. Combining billing codes, clinical notes, and medications from electronic health records provides superior phenotyping performance. *J. Am. Med. Inform. Assoc.* **2016**, *23*, e20–e27. [CrossRef]

56. Salekin, A.; Stankovic, J. Detection of Chronic Kidney Disease and Selecting Important Predictive Attributes. In Proceedings of the 2016 IEEE International Conference on Healthcare Informatics (ICHI), Chicago, IL, USA, 4–7 October 2016; pp. 262–270.
57. Rashidian, S.; Hajagos, J.; Moffitt, R.A.; Wang, F.; Noel, K.M.; Gupta, R.R.; Tharakan, M.A.; Saltz, J.H.; Saltz, M.M. Deep Learning on Electronic Health Records to Improve Disease Coding Accuracy. *AMIA Summits Transl. Sci. Proc.* **2019**, *2019*, 620–629.

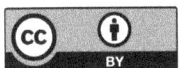

© 2020 by the authors. Licensee MDPI, Basel, Switzerland. This article is an open access article distributed under the terms and conditions of the Creative Commons Attribution (CC BY) license (http://creativecommons.org/licenses/by/4.0/).

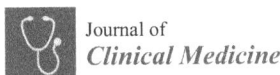

Article

Investigating Ethnic Disparity in Living-Donor Kidney Transplantation in the UK: Patient-Identified Reasons for Non-Donation among Family Members

Katie Wong [1,2,*], Amanda Owen-Smith [1], Fergus Caskey [1,2], Stephanie MacNeill [1], Charles R.V. Tomson [3], Frank J.M.F. Dor [4], Yoav Ben-Shlomo [1], Soumeya Bouacida [5], Dela Idowu [6] and Pippa Bailey [1,2]

1. Bristol Medical School: Population Health Sciences, University of Bristol, Bristol BS8 2PS, UK; a.owen-smith@bristol.ac.uk (A.O.-S.); fergus.caskey@bristol.ac.uk (F.C.); stephanie.macneill@bristol.ac.uk (S.M.); y.ben-shlomo@bristol.ac.uk (Y.B.-S.); pippa.bailey@bristol.ac.uk (P.B.)
2. Southmead Hospital, North Bristol NHS Trust, Bristol BS10 5NB, UK
3. The Newcastle upon Tyne Hospitals NHS Foundation Trust, Newcastle upon Tyne NE7 7DN, UK; ctomson@doctors.org.uk
4. Imperial College Healthcare NHS Trust, London W12 0HS, UK; frank.dor@nhs.net
5. Bristol Health Partners' Chronic Kidney Disease Health Integration Team, Bristol BS1 2NT, UK
6. Gift of Living Donation (GOLD), London NW10 0NS, UK
* Correspondence: katie.wong@bristol.ac.uk

Received: 30 September 2020; Accepted: 17 November 2020; Published: 21 November 2020

Abstract: There is ethnic inequity in access to living-donor kidney transplants in the UK. This study asked kidney patients from Black, Asian and minority ethnic groups why members of their family were not able to be living kidney donors. Responses were compared with responses from White individuals. This questionnaire-based mixed-methods study included adults transplanted between 1/4/13–31/3/17 at 14 UK hospitals. Participants were asked to indicate why relatives could not donate, selecting all options applicable from: Age; Health; Weight; Location; Financial/Cost; Job; Blood group; No-one to care for them after donation. A box entitled 'Other—please give details' was provided for free-text entries. Multivariable logistic regression was used to analyse the association between the likelihood of selecting each reason for non-donation and the participant's self-reported ethnicity. Qualitative responses were analysed using inductive thematic analysis. In total, 1240 questionnaires were returned (40% response). There was strong evidence that Black, Asian and minority ethnic group individuals were more likely than White people to indicate that family members lived too far away to donate (adjusted odds ratio (aOR) = 3.25, 95% Confidence Interval (CI) 2.30–4.58), were prevented from donating by financial concerns (aOR = 2.95, 95% CI 2.02–4.29), were unable to take time off work (aOR = 1.88, 95% CI 1.18–3.02), were "not the right blood group" (aOR = 1.65, 95% CI 1.35–2.01), or had no-one to care for them post-donation (aOR = 3.73, 95% CI 2.60–5.35). Four qualitative themes were identified from responses from Black, Asian and minority ethnic group participants: 'Burden of disease within the family'; 'Differing religious interpretations'; 'Geographical concerns'; and 'A culture of silence'. Patients perceive barriers to living kidney donation in the UK Black, Asian and minority ethnic population. If confirmed, these could be targeted by interventions to redress the observed ethnic inequity.

Keywords: living kidney donation; living-donor kidney transplantation; ethnic disparity

1. Introduction

Living-donor kidney transplantation is the optimal treatment for most people with kidney failure in terms of patient survival, graft survival and quality of life [1–6]. The healthcare costs associated with living-donor kidney transplants (LDKTs) are less than for dialysis and deceased-donor kidney transplants (DDKTs) [7,8]. The medium-term risks of donating a kidney are small [9–12], and the quality of life of donors usually returns to pre-donation levels after donation [13,14].

Only 28% of all kidney transplants performed in the UK each year are from a living donor [6], a proportion below that of the USA and the Netherlands [15]. Individuals from Black, Asian and minority ethnic populations in the UK appear to be particularly disadvantaged as they are less likely to receive a LDKT compared to White people with kidney disease [16,17]; only 18% of living donor kidney transplant recipients in the UK between April 2019–March 2020 were from Black, Asian and minority ethnic group backgrounds, despite individuals from these groups constituting 36% of the kidney transplant waiting list [6]. Improving equity in living-donor kidney transplantation has been highlighted as a UK and international research priority by patients and clinicians [18,19].

Specific religious and cultural beliefs, as well as a lack of specific knowledge about donation, have been identified as reasons for ethnic disparity in deceased organ donation [20,21]. The barriers specifically encountered by Black, Asian and minority ethnic group patients in accessing LDKTs in the UK are not well described.

We have previously investigated reasons why individuals who start assessment for kidney donation do not go on to donate in the UK. In this multicentre study, individuals from Black, Asian and minority ethnic groups were more likely to withdraw from donor evaluation [22]. However, transplant candidates and their families often make decisions regarding the suitability of potential donors before they make contact with hospital services. The perceptions of transplant candidates, regarding the suitability of family members for donation, function as an initial stage of donor screening. Transplant candidates are often uncomfortable broaching the subject of organ donation and make assumptions as to why individuals may or may not be able to donate. Transplant candidates may perceive barriers to donation that prevent potential donors from starting donor assessment. It is important to understand these perceptions in order to fully understand barriers to living-donor kidney transplantation. In this multi-centre questionnaire-based study, we investigated the reasons why family members were perceived by kidney patients as unsuitable as living kidney donors, comparing responses between individuals from White and Black, Asian and minority ethnic groups. Ultimately we aimed to identify potentially modifiable barriers to LDKTs specific to the UK Black, Asian and minority ethnic populations that could be targeted to redress the observed disparity.

2. Experimental Section

2.1. Study Design

We designed this multi-centre questionnaire-based study to investigate the patient-identified and reported reasons potential donors did not donate. We collected both quantitative (checklist item selection) and qualitative (free-text) questionnaire data to gain a greater understanding than that provided by one data type [23]. We collected data on whether participants asked potential donors to donate, whether any offered, and whether any started donor assessment. We collected data from both LDKT and DDKT recipients—LDKT recipients may have had other potential donors who volunteered but did not donate, and we wanted to ensure we captured the reasons for non-donation for all. We compared the responses of Black, Asian and minority ethnic individuals with White individuals to identify barriers that might be specific to Black, Asian and minority ethnic populations and therefore might explain the observed ethnic inequity.

2.2. Participants

The study was based at 14 hospitals in England and Northern Ireland (Supplementary Study Sites). We obtained from each hospital an anonymised list of all individuals who received kidney transplants between 1/4/13 and 31/3/17, stratified by LDKT/DDKT status. Individuals < 18 years at time of transplantation, or who lacked mental capacity according to the Mental Capacity Act 2005 were excluded. We calculated the study sample size using a variable not analysed here: the patient activation variable [24]. The study was designed to detect a 7-point difference in a continuous measure of patient activation (analysis of this variable not presented here) between LDKT cases and DDKT controls with 90% power, assuming a 5% significance level. The calculation indicated that 170 patients would be needed, and that, therefore, a total of 944 would be needed to allow analyses stratified by Index of Multiple Deprivation rank quintile and allow for 10% missing data. This sample size allows for the detection of a far smaller difference (0.16 Standard Deviation) for a dichotomous exposure or between 6–8% for a categorical outcome [24]. We performed stratified random sampling to select, on average, 110 LDKTs and 110 DDKTs from each site, weighted by the number of transplants performed at each study site. Sex and 5-year age group strata matched sampling was used to try to ensure a similar sample distribution by age and sex.

Between October 2017-November 2018, collaborators at study sites mailed paper questionnaires to participants. Questionnaires were accompanied by an invitation letter, a return postage-paid envelope, and a patient information sheet. A website-address was provided for participants who preferred to complete the questionnaire online. Non-responders were sent a second questionnaire after 4–6 weeks. We extracted anonymised data from returned paper questionnaires at the University of Bristol, and uploaded these onto a secure REDCap database [25].

2.3. Questionnaire Content

We have previously reported the development of the questionnaire alongside the findings of a single centre pilot study [24]. Participants were asked to indicate the number of living relatives ≥18 years from a list (spouse/partner, parents, sisters/brothers, children, aunts/uncles, first cousins) as a proxy for their potential living-donor pool. Friends and colleagues were not included, as they contribute very small numbers to the donor pool: between 2006–2017 only 8% of UK living donors were in this category (unpublished data provided by NHS Blood and Transplant to co-author P.B). We asked participants how many relatives had (i) offered to donate, (ii) been asked to donate by the respondent, and (iii) started donor assessment. Participants were asked for the reasons why any of the listed relatives could not donate; individuals were asked to tick all options that applied and were allowed to select multiple reasons from the following list, derived from previous qualitative research into barriers to donation [26]: Age—too old or too young to donate; Health—not healthy enough to donate; Weight—too over or underweight to donate; Location—they live too far away to be able to donate; Financial/Cost—the financial impact of donation would be too much; Job—not able to take the time off work to donate; Blood group—not the right blood group to donate; No-one to care for them after donation. A box entitled "Other—please give details" was provided for free-text entries. Individuals who the respondent considered suitable for donation but who did not donate because another person did were not considered as "not able" to donate. The responses indicated the patient-reported, and therefore the patient-identified, reasons for non-donation.

2.4. Main Exposure and Other Demographics

We collected data on self-reported ethnicity, religion, age, sex, and marital status. Participants could select "Would rather not answer" for all demographic questions. Participants indicated their ethnicity according to the UK's Office for National Statistics (ONS) 2011 census categories [27]: White; Asian/Asian British (Indian, Pakistani, Bangladeshi, Chinese); Black/African/Caribbean/Black British; Mixed/Multiple (White and Black Caribbean, White and Black African, Any other Mixed/Multiple ethnic background);

Other (Arab, Any other ethnic group). For the religion variable, participants were asked to select one option from the following: No religion; Christian; Muslim; Jewish; Hindu; Sikh; Buddhist; Other. Age was a categorical variable in 10-year age groups.

2.5. Statistical Analysis

We used descriptive statistics to summarise the characteristics of transplant recipients and their reported reasons for non-donation from family members. Black, Asian and minority ethnic group participants comprised "Asian/Asian-British", "Black/African/Caribbean/Black British", "Mixed/Multiple ethnic groups", and "Other Ethnic group". We derived a binary variable of Black, Asian and minority ethnicity (code = 1) versus White ethnicity (code = 0) as our primary exposure. The Chi2 test was used to compare the characteristics of White and Black, Asian and minority ethnic group participants, and the reasons given for non-donation. We used multivariable logistic regression to describe the association between the reporting of each reason for non-donation with respondent self-reported ethnicity. We used two models: (i) unadjusted and (ii) adjusted for potential confounders. We specified, a priori, potential confounders including sex and age. We considered socioeconomic position as a mediator on the causal pathway between ethnicity and living donation, rather than a potential confounder: we did not adjust for it in our model as this would result in potential over-adjustment and attenuation of the effect of ethnicity. We used robust standard errors to account for clustering within kidney centres. We tested for interactions between ethnicity and age and sex. We identified missing data and described patterns of missingness. We performed both a complete case analysis and a sensitivity analysis using multiple imputation using chained equations to derive 40 imputed datasets per group, for the exposure variable and potential confounders and then combined using Rubin's rules. All statistical analyses were undertaken using Stata 15 [28].

2.6. Qualitative Analysis

Individuals were able to provide free-text qualitative data responses to the question "Thinking about those people you think could not donate a kidney to you, what are the reasons for this?". All free-text responses from Black, Asian and minority ethnic group respondents were analysed, so no sampling was required. The written free-text responses were typed onto the REDCap database [25]. Free-text responses and participant demographics were then downloaded from REDCap onto an Excel spreadsheet file. NVivo qualitative software was used to facilitate analysis. Data were analysed using inductive thematic analysis [29], as described by Braun and Clarke [30]. After familiarization with the data, sections of text within the responses were coded by assigning descriptive labels. Codes were collated on the basis of shared properties to create initial potential themes, which were then refined. Themes were revisited and finalised during the preparation of the report for publication. Coding and thematic analysis were undertaken independently by both K.W. and P.B. Coding discrepancies were resolved by discussion to enhance rigour and reliability. All themes were reported using a minimum of three illustrative quotes. After completing analysis for Black, Asian and minority group respondents ($n = 56$), a matching number of White participants ($n = 56$) were purposively sampled aiming for diversity in terms of age, sex and socioeconomic status, and qualitative responses analysed for comparison.

The Strengthening The Reporting of OBservational studies in Epidemiology (STROBE) and COnsolidated criteria for REporting Qualitative studies (COREQ) guidelines were used to prepare the manuscript [31,32].

2.7. Ethical Approval and Consent

We received NHS Research Ethics Committee (REC) (REC reference 17/LO/1602) and Health Research Authority (HRA) approval. A consent form formed the first page of the questionnaire. The study was funded by a Kidney Research UK Project Grant (RP_028_20170302). The clinical and

3. Results

3.1. Quantitative Findings

A total of 1240 questionnaires were returned from 3103 patients (40% response). The characteristics of all respondents are described in Table 1. LDKT recipients were more likely to respond than DDKT recipients and women were more likely to respond than men (Table S1). Study participants appeared to be generally similar to the National population of DDKT and LDKT recipients though the study sample had fewer Black, Asian and minority ethnic group participants (largest difference 9% for DDKT) (Table S2). Overall, the proportion of missing data was small (<10% for all demographic variables) (Table S3).

Table 1. Participant demographics.

Characteristics		Participants (n = 1240) n (%)
Sex	Female	514 (41.5)
	Male	705 (56.9)
	Missing	21 (1.7)
Type of transplant	Living-donor kidney transplant	672 (54.2)
	Deceased-donor kidney transplant	565 (45.6)
	Missing	3 (0.2)
Age group (years) [a]	20–29	74 (6.0)
	30–39	137 (11.1)
	40–49	209 (16.9)
	50–59	331 (26.7)
	60–69	299 (24.1)
	70–79	150 (12.1)
	80–89	6 (0.5)
	Missing	34 (2.7)
Self-reported Ethnicity [b]	White	1027 (82.8)
	Asian/Asian-British	79 (6.4)
	Black/African/Caribbean/Black British	58 (4.7)
	Mixed/Multiple ethnic groups	10 (0.8)
	Other Ethnic groups	24 (1.9)
	Missing	42 (3.4)
Religion	Christian	717 (57.8)
	Hindu	27 (2.2)
	Sikh	13 (1.1)
	Muslim	21 (1.7)
	Jewish	6 (0.5)
	No religion	335 (27.0)
	Other	38 (3.1)
	Missing	74 (6.0)

[a] No participants aged <20 years. [b] UK's Office for National Statistics 2011 census categories.

White participants were older than Black, Asian and minority ethnic group participants, and a greater proportion of White participants were LDKT recipients compared to Black, Asian and minority ethnic group respondents. Black, Asian and minority ethnic group participants were more likely to report having a religion than White participants: of those with a religion, the majority of Black, Asian and minority ethnic group participants reported a religion other than Christianity, whereas the majority of White participants reported being Christian (Table S4). Black, Asian and minority ethnic group participants reported a larger number of potential donors compared to White respondents (median number of family members ≥ 18 years: 19 versus 16, Wilcoxon rank-sum test $p = 0.02$).

Most participants had not asked any of their relatives to donate ($n = 848/1181$, 71.8%). In total, 81.8% ($n = 973/1189$) reported that one or more relative had offered to donate, with 85.6% of these actually starting donor assessment (representing 14.4% attrition).

Participant responses to the question "Thinking about those people you think could not donate a kidney to you, what are the reasons for this?" differed by ethnicity (Table 2). Black, Asian and minority ethnic group individuals were more likely than White respondents to indicate that family members lived too far away to donate ($p < 0.001$), were prevented from donating by financial concerns ($p < 0.001$), were unable to take time off work ($p < 0.001$), were not the right blood group ($p = 0.002$), or had no-one to care for them after donation ($p < 0.001$). We found no evidence that the proportion of respondents who indicated that age ($p = 0.96$), donor health ($p = 0.88$), or donor weight ($p = 0.36$) were reasons for non-donation differed between White and Black, Asian and minority ethnic group respondents.

Table 2. Participant reported reasons relatives could not donate a kidney to them.

Reported Reason Potential Donor not Suitable for Donation	White $n = 1027$, n (%)	Black, Asian and Minority Ethnic Group $n = 171$, n (%)	White vs. Black, Asian and Minority Ethnic Group Chi^2 p-Value
Age—too old or too young to donate	562 (54.8)	94 (55.0)	0.96
Health—not healthy enough to donate	648 (63.2)	109 (63.7)	0.88
Weight—too over or underweight to donate	152 (14.8)	30 (17.5)	0.36
Location—they live too far away to be able to donate	188 (18.3)	72 (42.1)	<0.001
Financial/cost—the financial impact of donation would be too much	98 (9.6)	40 (23.4)	<0.001
Job—not able to take the time off work to donate	106 (10.3)	29 (17.0)	<0.001
Blood group—not the right blood group to donate	199 (19.4)	51 (29.8)	0.002
No-one to care for them after donation	63 (6.1)	32 (18.7)	<0.001

There was strong evidence that even after adjustment for potential confounders of sex and age, Black, Asian and minority ethnic group individuals were more likely than White respondents to indicate that family members lived too far away to donate (adjusted odds ratio (aOR) 3.25 (95% Confidence Interval (CI) 2.30–4.58)), were prevented from donating by financial concerns (aOR 2.95 (95% CI 2.02–4.29)), were unable to take time off work (aOR 1.88 (95% CI 1.18–3.02)), were not the right blood group (aOR 1.65 (95% CI 1.35–2.01)), or had no-one to care for them after donation (aOR 3.73 (95% CI 2.60–5.35)) (Table 3). The associations did not differ substantially between the complete cases analysis and the analyses with missing variables imputed (Table S5). In total, 11 individuals who had not selected the "Health – not healthy enough to donate" response indicated in the free-text that potential donors had or might develop the same kidney disease as them. In a sensitivity analysis, when these individuals were recoded as selecting "Health" as a reason for non-donation, there was no change in the direction or the size of associations observed in Table 3.

Table 3. Multivariable logistic regression analysis comparing reasons potential donor unsuitability between White and Black, Asian and minority ethnic participants [a].

Reported Reason Potential Donor Not Suitable for Donation	Black, Asian and Minority Ethnicities vs. White Unadjusted Odds Ratio (OR) [95% Confidence Interval (CI)]	Black, Asian and Minority Ethnicities vs. White Adjusted for Sex and Age OR [95% CI]
Age—too old or too young	1.00 [0.75–1.34]	0.98 [0.73–1.32]
Health—not healthy enough	1.02 [0.78–1.34]	0.96 [0.71–1.31]
Weight—too over or underweight	1.22 [0.84–1.77]	1.13 [0.78–1.65]
Location—live too far away	3.23 [2.23–4.68]	3.25 [2.30–4.58]
Financial/cost—financial impact of donation would be too much	2.89 [2.07–4.03]	2.95 [2.02–4.29]
Job—not able to take time off work	1.77 [1.15–2.71]	1.88 [1.18–3.02]
Blood group—not the right blood group	1.76 [1.43–2.17]	1.65 [1.35–2.01]
No-one to care for them after donation	3.51 [2.47–4.99]	3.73 [2.60–5.35]

[a] Complete case analysis.

There was a modest suggestion of interaction between sex and ethnicity (likelihood ratio test $p = 0.03$) in the reporting of "no-one to care for them after donation" as a reason for non-donation (Supplementary Interactions) so the increased risk seen for Black, Asian and minority ethnic group was only seen in men.

3.2. Qualitative Findings

In total, 56 Black, Asian and minority ethnicity individuals provided free-text reasons for potential donor unsuitability: respondent characteristics are presented in Table S6. Four overall themes were identified (Table 4): (i) Burden of disease within the family, (ii) Differing religious interpretations, (iii) Specific geographical concerns, and (iv) A Culture of Silence.

Table 4. UK Black, Asian and minority ethnic participant qualitative analysis themes and illustrative quotes.

Theme	Representative Quote
Burden of disease within family	"Very healthy but slight amount of protein in urine so not able to donate." (Male, 50–59 years, Asian, Hindu, Living-donor kidney transplant (LDKT)) "They all have slight renal problem" (Female, 50–59 years, Black, Deceased-donor kidney transplant (DDKT)) "Hereditary illness in the family" (Male, 50–59 years, Asian, DDKT) "Mother and 2 sibling have same condition as mine (1 sister & 1 brother)." (Male, 30–38 years, Black, Christian, DDKT)
Differing religious interpretations	"Their religion/faith forbids them to donate 1. thought they were Christians like me. 2. our culture forbids them to donate ... 3. some forbid blood transfusion and the unbelievable reasons for that." (Female, 60–69 years, Black, LDKT) "Superstition/religion (distorted beliefs). Myth." (Female, 50–59 years, Black, Christian, DDKT) "Their religion would not allow them to donate a kidney." (Female, 40–49 years, Black, Christian, LDKT) "Religious/cultural ... " (Male, 50–59 years, Asian, Hindu, LDKT)
Geographical concerns	"All of my family apart from my spouse live in Ethiopia and other countries and would not have access to healthcare or the means to come to the UK" (Male, 40–49 years, Black, Muslim, LDKT) "All my people are in Nigeria, some of them, lack of transport to help them home is the problem some of them have." (Male, 70–79 years, Black, Christian, DDKT) "I had a word with my mum, wife and my son but they couldn't come to the UK due to financial and other reasons." (Male, 40–49 years, Black, Christian, DDKT)
A culture of silence	"I did not ask for a donation so do not have a reason." (Female, 60–69 years, Asian, Sikh, DDKT) "I would not ask my cousins" (Female, 30–39 years, Asian, Muslim, LDKT) "Other 3 cousins from my mother's half sister do not have PKD but they would not offer, they didn't before, I would certainly not ask." (Female, 60–69 years, Other ethnic group, No religion, LDKT) "Are unaware of my current condition." (Male, 20–29 years, Asian, Hindu, LDKT)

3.2.1. Burden of Disease within the Family

A large number of Black, Asian and minority ethnic group respondents stated that potential donors were unable to donate due to presumed or perceived ill health. Respondents reported a heavy burden of both hereditary and non-hereditary kidney disease precluding donation:

"Family history of PKD [polycystic kidney disease]—all siblings, all children and uncles affected." (Female|50–59 years|Asian|LDKT)

"Too old and unhealthy. Heart problem, Diabetes, high blood pressure, inheritance." (Male|60–69 years|Asian|Sikh|DDKT)

Participants also reported that health problems were identified during donor assessment that prevented donation:

"There were genetic issues that were contra-indications such as a cause of cancer which was discovered during screening ... " (Male|20–29 years|Asian|Muslim|DDKT)

3.2.2. Differing Religious Interpretations

Several participants reported that a relative's religion or faith had prevented them from donating:

"Their religion would not allow them to donate a kidney." (Female|40–49 years|Black|Christian| LDKT)

However, most participants considered the beliefs as unorthodox, describing what they perceived as a distortion of a religious belief:

"Superstition/religion (distorted beliefs). Myth." (Female|60–69 years|Black|LDKT)

and a discordance between the participants' and their relatives' interpretations of their faith:

"Their religion/faith forbids them to donate ... thought they were Christians like me." (Female|60–69 years|Black|LDKT)

No participants who reported religion as a barrier to donation for their relatives reported that they shared their relatives' beliefs. All but one of the respondents who reported religion as a reason for non-donation self-identified as Christian and was Black/African/Caribbean/Black British.

3.2.3. Geographical Concerns

Several participants reported relatives being unable to donate due to geographical separation. However, it was not the distance alone that was considered a barrier to donation for some:

"While some are abroad they were willing to travel." (Male|60–69 years|Black|Christian|LDKT)

Rather, participants reported difficulties with immigration rules:

"Immigration rules can be problematic too." (Male|40–49 years|Black|Muslim|LDKT)

prohibitive financial concerns:

"My blood relatives live outside the UK. The financial cost has been a major issue." (Male|50–59 years|Other ethnic group|DDKT)

and concerns about the quality of post-donation healthcare in their potential donor's country of residence:

"I come from Papua New Guinea and health services are poor. People are afraid of death during and after donating of their kidneys. After operations the care given is not very good and people end up dying. We lost two relatives from sepsis." (Female|50–59 years| Other ethnic group|Christian|LDKT)

3.2.4. A culture of Silence

Several participants described a "culture of silence" around their illness, reporting that their family were not aware they had kidney disease:

"Are unaware of my current condition." (Male|20–29 years|Asian|Hindu|LDKT)

This was reported as a result of some participants personally not disclosing this information to relatives:

" … my reluctance to show how ill I was, to soldier on, accept my fate and manage accordingly." (Male|50–59 years|Asian|Sikh|LDKT)

As well as other family members controlling the disclosure of information to the wider family:

"The majority of my extended family do not 'officially' know that I am unwell/having dialysis or had a transplant as my parents did not want them to know." (Male|30–39 years|Other ethnic group|Other religion|DDKT)

A summary model of barriers identified is presented in Figure 1.

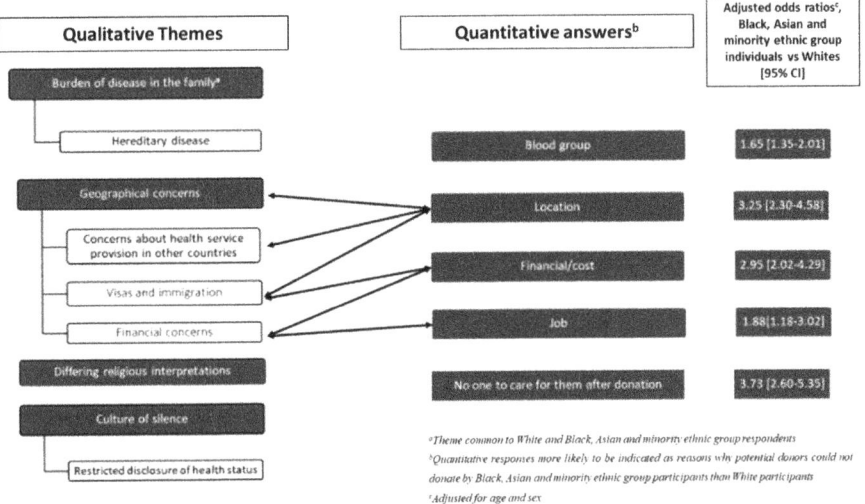

Figure 1. A summary model of barriers to living kidney donation as reported by UK Black, Asian and Minority Ethnic individuals.

3.2.5. Responses from White Participants

Comparing these free-text responses against those from the 56 purposively sampled White participants (Table S7), only one theme proved common to both White and Black, Asian and minority ethnic group respondents—"Burden of disease within the family". Two further themes were identified amongst White respondents that were not evident in the Black, Asian and minority ethnic group dataset: (i) Lack of close family relationships—through relationship breakdown or dysfunction and (ii) Protecting others. These themes and illustrative quotes are presented as Supplementary Material (Table S7).

4. Discussion

The majority of respondents indicated that they had not asked potential donors to donate, suggesting that transplant candidates may make assumptions as to why individuals may or may not be able to donate. Although 81.8% reported that one or more individuals had offered to donate, 14.4% of these participants did not have a potential donor that proceeded to donor assessment. Whilst some of these individuals may have received a DDKT before their potential donor started assessment, others may have been deemed unsuitable for donation by the transplant candidate. These findings highlight the importance of understanding patient-identified reasons as to why individuals are deemed unsuitable as living kidney donors.

Black, Asian and minority ethnic group participants were more likely than White participants to indicate that family members lived too far away to donate, and to report financial concerns in part linked to geographical distance. The qualitative data provided insight into these identified barriers, and as described they would appear to be surmountable. In the UK, NHS England allows potential donors from overseas to be reimbursed for travel, accommodation and visa costs after the event [33]. However these large "up-front" costs may be prohibitive to potential donors, and previous qualitative research has shown that many patients are unaware of the reimbursement policy [26]. Clarifying UK immigration policy and highlighting the reimbursement scheme may help potential Black, Asian and minority ethnic group recipients access their potential donor pool.

Previous research by the authors has suggested that Black, Asian and minority ethnic group ethnicity and non-Christian religious affiliation are associated with greater uncertainty in beliefs about living donation [34]. No respondents in our study reported perceiving a specific religion as forbidding living donation. This may reflect the success of work by faith leaders to clarify positions on living donation within the UK, including a new fatwa clarifying Islamic approval of organ donation and transplantation published in the UK in 2019 [35]. However, the participants' responses indicated that some of their potential donors did perceive religion as a barrier to donation. In particular there were several references to the distortion of religious beliefs being a barrier to donation. This highlights the need to better understand and consider the beliefs of potential donors who belong to non-mainstream religions, who may be outside the remit of denominational faith leaders.

A "culture of silence" about illness was an important theme identified in responses from Black, Asian and minority ethnic group participants. Although not directly comparable to the UK Black, Asian and minority ethnic group population, qualitative research in African-American LDKT recipients and donors has suggested that restricting disclosure and maintaining privacy of health status can protect against feelings of vulnerability [36], help to maintain self-perception and public identity, and is linked with rejection of the sick role which is sometimes associated with better coping skills in patients with kidney disease [37]. Potential African-American donors have also reported negative responses from family and friends regarding donation, and encouraging the recipient not to disclose their health status may be perceived as a protective act in that context [36]. We found that Black, Asian and minority ethnic group participants have larger potential donor pools than White participants, but this "culture of silence" may mean that Black, Asian and minority ethnic group individuals are less able to access their pool and therefore a LDKT. It may also mean that Black, Asian and minority ethnic group individuals are less able to access their social network during time of chronic illness: lack of social support and lack of an informed social network are associated with reduced access to transplantation [26,38–40], and worse transplant outcomes [41]. Interestingly, in White participants, lack of close relationships was identified as reason for non-donation, but this was not reported by Black, Asian and minority ethnic group participants, despite the geographical separation. Strategies to overcome this culture of silence could include interventions that engage with a patient's social network, such as the Dutch home-education model shown to be effective at increasing access to living-donor kidney transplantation for minority ethnic groups [42]. A focus on the potential benefits to family members from the education session (detection of undiagnosed kidney disease, how to optimise own health) could be emphasised. The use of "live donor champions" may also enable discussions to start: in this approach, a friend or family member is trained to undertake an advocate role, sharing information on the patient's behalf with the patient's wider social network [43]. Other approaches that may overcome "cultures of silence" include people with kidney disease, transplant recipients and donors sharing their experiences on an open web-platform such as healthtalk.org (http://healthtalk.org) and the living donation storytelling project (https://explorelivingdonation.org/) [44]. However, such approaches need to be formally evaluated for effectiveness.

Black, Asian and minority ethnic group respondents were more likely to report that potential donors were not the right blood group. Whether this represents true or perceived incompatibility requires further investigation. A single-centre study from the USA in 2002 found that more African-American donors than White donors were prevented from donating due to ABO incompatibility (9.7% vs. 5.6%, $p < 0.01$) [45]; however, to our knowledge this has not been examined in the UK. If found to be true, willingness to participate in the UK Living Kidney Sharing Scheme should be investigated, and participation encouraged.

This was a large, multicentre study utilising both quantitative and qualitative data. The questionnaire was evaluated in cognitive interviews prior to use and then piloted. The proportion of missing data was very small. However, the study has some limitations: (i) There is a risk of self-selection bias given our response rate, although this is comparable to other postal surveys in the UK [46,47] and the 47% response to a survey sent to Dutch and Swedish transplant recipients [48]. There is some evidence that Black, Asian and minority ethnic group individuals may have been under-represented but it is unclear whether the participants in the study would be different in respect to the reported reasons for non-donation. We suspect, if anything they would be more knowledgeable and engaged and so some of our results may underestimate the true associations. We did not have data on the ethnicity of non-responders and so we were unable to ascertain if there was a difference in response rate between the Black, Asian and minority ethnic group and White populations. (ii) Ethnicity can be described as a form of collective identity that draws on notions of ancestry, cultural commonality, geographical origins, and shared physical features. Ethnic identities are social constructs that are fluid across space and time [49]. In this study, ethnicity was coded using the UK's ONS 2011 census categories, but individuals may self-identify with several or none of the ethnic categories used in government statistics [49]. Any ethnic identify categorisation fails to respect the heterogeneity within a group due to differing cultures, religions, languages, HLA-types, whether a person was born in their place of residence or migrated to it, and for migrants, time resident. We analysed all Black, Asian and minority ethnic group respondents as one group as our sample size prevented analysis by more specific ethnic groups (e.g., Asian-Indian, Black British, Chinese). Study findings should be considered an indicator of a signal that requires further detailed investigation. (iii) The questionnaire was only available in English, as several survey tools had only been validated in English. Findings may therefore not be applicable to patients who do not read English, who may be from White or Black, Asian and minority ethnic group groups. (iv) Participants had all received a kidney transplant and findings may not be generalisable to transplant eligible people active on the transplant waiting list. Qualitative responses were limited to hand-written free-text entries and were all in English, which may have restricted participants for whom this was not a first language. In-depth interviews would allow for further investigation of the issues raised. This study describes patient-reported and patient-identified reasons potential donors were not considered suitable for kidney donation. Patients are gatekeepers to the process, making personal judgements as to suitability: both who to approach and whose offers to accept or decline. However, surveying non-donors about their reasons for non-donation would provide a different and important perspective, although such a study would be ethically and practically challenging [50].

5. Conclusions

We have identified multiple patient-identified barriers to living kidney donation in the UK Black, Asian and minority ethnic group population, which should be further investigated and addressed to reduce the ethnic inequity in living-donor kidney transplantation in the UK.

Supplementary Materials: The following are available online at http://www.mdpi.com/2077-0383/9/11/3751/s1, Supplementary Study sites, Supplementary Interactions, Table S1. Responders and non-responders, Table S2. Responders compared to national denominator population, Table S3. Missing data analysis, Table S4. Participant demographics—comparison of White and Black, Asian and minority ethnic group respondents, Table S5. Multivariable logistic regression analysis comparing reasons potential donor unsuitable between White and Black, Asian and minority ethnic group participants—missing explanatory variables imputed, Table S6. Characteristics of Black, Asian and minority ethnic group participants providing qualitative responses. Table S7. Themes and illustrative quotes from thematic analysis of White participant responses.

Author Contributions: Conceptualization, P.B., Y.B.-S., C.R.T.; methodology, P.B., Y.B.-S., S.M.; software, K.W., P.B.; formal analysis, K.W., P.B., S.M., A.O.-S.; investigation, K.W., P.B.; data curation, P.B.; writing—original draft preparation, K.W., P.B.; writing—review and editing, K.W., P.B., A.O.-S., S.M., F.J.D., Y.B.-S., C.R.T., F.C., D.I., S.B.; supervision, A.O.-S., Y.B.-S., C.R.T., F.C.; project administration, P.B.; funding acquisition, P.B. All authors have read and agreed to the published version of the manuscript.

Funding: This report is independent research arising from a Kidney Research UK Project Grant (Reference RP_028_20170302). Neither Kidney Research UK nor the University of Bristol had any role in study design, data collection, analysis, interpretation, manuscript preparation of the decision to submit the report for publication. K.W. is supported by the Elizabeth Blackwell Institute for Health Research, University of Bristol and the Wellcome Trust Institutional Strategic Support Fund. P.K.B. is funded by a Wellcome Trust Clinical Research Career Development Fellowship. Y.B.-S. is supported by the NIHR Applied Research Collaboration West (NIHR ARC West) as data science lead. The views expressed in this article are those of the author(s) and not necessarily those of the NIHR or the Department of Health and Social Care or any of the other funders.

Acknowledgments: The authors would like to thank all the study participants, the participating centre research nurses and coordinators (Hugh Murtagh, Nina Bleakley, Mary Dutton, Kulli Kuningas, Cecilio Bing Andujar, Ann-Marie O'Sullivan, Nicola Johnson, Kieron Clark, Thomas Walters, Mary Quashie-Akponeware, Jane Turner, Gillian Curry, Hannah Beer, Lynn.D Langhorne, Sarah Brand, Maria Weetman, Molly Campbell, Megan Bennett, Sharirose Abat, and Agyapong Kwame Ansu) and the local collaborators who facilitated the study (Sarah Heap, Mysore Phanish, Shafi Malik, Aisling Courtney, Adnan Sharif, Nicholas Torpey, Refik Gökmen, Michael Picton, Linda Bisset, Edward Sharples, and Simon Curran).

Conflicts of Interest: The authors declare no conflict of interest. The funders had no role in the design of the study; in the collection, analyses, or interpretation of data; in the writing of the manuscript, or in the decision to publish the results.

References

1. Cecka, J.M. Living donor transplants. *Clin. Transpl. Jan.* **1995**, 363–377. [PubMed]
2. Terasaki, P.I.; Cecka, J.M.; Gjertson, D.W.; Takemoto, S. High Survival Rates of Kidney Transplants from Spousal and Living Unrelated Donors. *N. Engl. J. Med.* **1995**, *333*, 333–336. [CrossRef] [PubMed]
3. Laupacis, A.; Keown, P.; Pus, N.; Krueger, H.; Ferguson, B.; Wong, C.; Muirhead, N. A study of the quality of life and cost-utility of renal transplantation. *Kidney Int.* **1996**, *50*, 235–242. [CrossRef] [PubMed]
4. Cecka, J.M. The OPTN/UNOS Renal Transplant Registry. *Clin Transpl.* **2005**, 1–16. [PubMed]
5. Roodnat, J.I.; Van Riemsdijk, I.C.; Mulder, P.G.H.; Doxiadis, I.; Claas, F.H.J.; Ijzermans, J.N.M.; Weimar, W. The superior results of living-donor renal transplantation are not completely caused by selection or short cold ischemia time: A single-center, multivariate analysis. *Transplantation* **2003**, *75*, 2014–2018. [CrossRef]
6. Annual Activity Report—ODT Clinical—NHS Blood and Transplant. Published 2019. Available online: https://www.odt.nhs.uk/statistics-and-reports/annual-activity-report/ (accessed on 19 February 2020).
7. Barnieh, L.; Manns, B.J.; Klarenbach, S.; McLaughlin, K.; Yilmaz, S.; Hemmelgarn, B.R. A description of the costs of living and standard criteria deceased donor kidney transplantation. *Am. J. Transpl.* **2011**, *11*, 478–488. [CrossRef]
8. Smith, C.R.; Woodward, R.S.; Cohen, D.S.; Singer, G.G.; Brennan, D.C.; Lowell, J.A.; Schnitzler, M.A. Cadaveric versus living donor kidney transplantation: A medicare payment analysis. *Transplantation* **2000**, *69*, 311–314. [CrossRef]

9. Maggiore, U.; Budde, K.; Heemann, U.; Hilbrands, L.; Oberbauer, R.; Oniscu, G.C.; Abramowicz, D. Long-term risks of kidney living donation: Review and position paper by the ERA-EDTA DESCARTES working group. *Nephrol. Dial. Transpl.* **2017**, *32*, 216–223. [CrossRef]
10. Muzaale, A.D.; Massie, A.B.; Wang, M.C.; Montgomery, R.A.; McBride, M.A.; Wainright, J.L.; Segev, D.L. Risk of end-stage renal disease following live kidney donation. *JAMA J. Am. Med. Assoc.* **2014**, *311*, 579–586. [CrossRef]
11. Massie, A.B.; Muzaale, A.D.; Luo, X.; Chow, E.K.; Locke, J.E.; Nguyen, A.Q.; Segev, D.L. Quantifying postdonation risk of ESRD in living kidney donors. *J. Am. Soc. Nephrol.* **2017**, *28*, 2749–2755. [CrossRef]
12. Segev, D.L.; Muzaale, A.D.; Caffo, B.S.; Mehta, S.H.; Singer, A.L.; Taranto, S.E.; Montgomery, R.A. Perioperative mortality and long-term survival following live kidney donation. *JAMA J. Am. Med. Assoc.* **2010**, *303*, 959–966. [CrossRef] [PubMed]
13. Lumsdaine, J.A.; Wray, A.; Power, M.J.; Jamieson, N.V.; Akyol, M.; Andrew Bradley, J.; Wigmore, S.J. Higher quality of life in living donor kidney transplantation: Prospective cohort study. *Transpl. Int.* **2005**, *18*, 975–980. [CrossRef] [PubMed]
14. Johnson, E.M.; Anderson, J.K.; Jacobs, C.; Suh, G.; Humar, A.; Suhr, B.D.; Matas, A.J. Long-term follow-up of living kidney donors: Quality of life after donation. *Transplantation* **1999**, *67*, 717–721. [CrossRef] [PubMed]
15. IRODaT—International Registry on Organ Donation and Transplantation. Available online: http://www.irodat.org/?p=database (accessed on 27 February 2020).
16. Udayaraj, U.; Ben-Shlomo, Y.; Roderick, P.; Casula, A.; Dudley, C.; Collett, D.; Caskey, F. Social deprivation, ethnicity, and uptake of living kidney donor transplantation in the United Kingdom. *Transplantation* **2012**, *93*, 610–616. [CrossRef]
17. Wu, D.A.; Robb, M.L.; Watson, C.J.E.; Forsythe, J.L.; Tomson, C.R.; Cairns, J.; Bradley, C. Barriers to living donor kidney transplantation in the United Kingdom: A national observational study. *Nephrol. Dial. Transpl.* **2017**, *32*, 890–900. [CrossRef]
18. Lentine, K.L.; Kasiske, B.L.; Levey, A.S.; Adams, P.L.; Alberú, J.; Bakr, M.A.; Segev, D.L. KDIGO Clinical Practice Guideline on the Evaluation and Care of Living Kidney Donors. *Transplantation* **2017**, *101*, S1–S109. [CrossRef]
19. Rodrigue, J.R.; Kazley, A.S.; Mandelbrot, D.A.; Hays, R.; Rudow, D.L.P.; Baliga, P. Living donor kidney transplantation: Overcoming disparities in live kidney donation in the US—Recommendations from a consensus conference. *Clin. J. Am. Soc. Nephrol.* **2015**, *10*, 1687–1695. [CrossRef]
20. Morgan, M.; Kenten, C.; Deedat, S.; on behalf of the Donation, Transplantation and Ethnicity (DonaTE) Programme Team. Attitudes to deceased organ donation and registration as a donor among minority ethnic groups in North America and the UK: A synthesis of quantitative and qualitative research. *Ethn. Health* **2013**, *18*, 367–390. [CrossRef]
21. Alnaes, A.H. Lost in translation: Cultural obstructions impede living kidney donation among minority ethnic patients. *Cambridge Q. Healthc. Ethics* **2012**, *21*, 505–516. [CrossRef]
22. Bailey, P.K.; Tomson, C.R.V.; MacNeill, S.; Marsden, A.; Cook, D.; Cooke, R.; Ben-Shlomo, Y. A multicenter cohort study of potential living kidney donors provides predictors of living kidney donation and non-donation. *Kidney Int.* **2017**, *92*, 1249–1260. [CrossRef]
23. Barbour, R.S. The case for combining qualitative and quantitative approaches in health services research. *J. Health Serv. Res. Policy* **1999**, *4*, 39–43. [CrossRef] [PubMed]
24. Bailey, P.K.; Tomson, C.R.V.; Ben-Shlomo, Y. What factors explain the association between socioeconomic deprivation and reduced likelihood of live-donor kidney transplantation? A questionnaire-based pilot case-control study. *BMJ Open* **2016**, *6*. [CrossRef]
25. Harris, P.A.; Taylor, R.; Thielke, R.; Payne, J.; Gonzalez, N.; Conde, J.G. Research electronic data capture (REDCap)-A metadata-driven methodology and workflow process for providing translational research informatics support. *J. Biomed. Inform.* **2009**, *42*, 377–381. [CrossRef] [PubMed]
26. Bailey, P.K.; Ben-Shlomo, Y.; Tomson, C.R.V.; Owen-Smith, A. Socioeconomic deprivation and barriers to live-donor kidney transplantation: A qualitative study of deceased-donor kidney transplant recipients. *BMJ Open* **2016**, *6*, e010605. [CrossRef]
27. 2011 Census Analysis: Ethnicity and Religion of the non-UK Born Population in England and Wales—Office for National Statistics. Available online: https://www.ons.gov.uk/peoplepopulationandcommunity/culturalidentity/ethnicity/articles/

2011censusanalysisethnicityandreligionofthenonukbornpopulationinenglandandwales/2015-06-18 (accessed on 19 February 2020).
28. StataCorp. *Stata Statistical Software: Release 15*; StataCorp LLC: College Station, TX, USA, 2017.
29. Miles, M.B.; Huberman, A.M.; Saldaña, J. *Qualitative Data Analysis A Methods Sourcebook*, 3rd ed.; SAGE Publications: Thousand Oaks, CA, USA, 2014.
30. Braun, V.; Clarke, V. Using thematic analysis in psychology. *Qual. Res. Psychol.* **2006**, *3*, 77–101. [CrossRef]
31. Von Elm, E.; Altman, D.G.; Egger, M.; Pocock, S.J.; Gøtzsche, P.C.; Vandenbroucke, J.P. Strengthening the reporting of observational studies in epidemiology (STROBE) statement: Guidelines for reporting observational studies. *BMJ* **2007**, *335*, 806–808. [CrossRef]
32. Tong, A.; Sainsbury, P.; Craig, J. Consolidated criteria for reporting qualitative research (COREQ): A 32-item checklist for interviews and focus groups. *Int. J. Qual. Health Care* **2007**, *19*, 349–357. [CrossRef]
33. NHS England. Commissioning Policy: Reimbursement of Expenses for Living Donors. Reference: NHS England A06/P/a June 2017. Available online: https://www.england.nhs.uk/publication/commissioning-policy-reimbursement-of-expenses-for-living-donors/ (accessed on 28 September 2020).
34. Bailey, P.K.; Caskey, F.J.; MacNeill, S.; Tomson, C.; Dor, F.J.M.F.; Ben-Shlomo, Y. Beliefs of UK Transplant Recipients about Living Kidney Donation and Transplantation: Findings from a Multicentre Questionnaire-Based Case–Control Study. *J. Clin. Med.* **2019**, *9*, 31. [CrossRef]
35. Zubair, M.; Jurisconsult, B. Organ Donation and Transplantation in Islam An Opinion. Available online: https://nhsbtdbe.blob.core.windows.net/umbraco-assets-corp/16300/organ-donation-fatwa.pdf (accessed on 20 November 2020).
36. Davis, L.A.; Grogan, T.M.; Cox, J.; Weng, F.L. Inter- and Intrapersonal Barriers to Living Donor Kidney Transplant among Black Recipients and Donors. *J. Racial Ethn. Health Disparities* **2017**, *4*, 671–679. [CrossRef]
37. Cerrato, A.; Avitable, M.; Hayman, L.L. The relationship between the sick role and functional ability: One center's experience. *Prog. Transpl.* **2008**, *18*, 192–198. [CrossRef]
38. Bailey, P.; Caskey, F.; MacNeill, S.; Tomson, C.; Dor, F.J.; Ben-Shlomo, Y. Mediators of socioeconomic inequity in living-donor kidney transplantation: Results from a UK multicenter case-control study. *Transpl. Direct.* **2020**, *6*, e540. [CrossRef] [PubMed]
39. Browne, T. The relationship between social networks and pathways to kidney transplant parity: Evidence from black Americans in Chicago. *Soc. Sci. Med.* **2011**, *73*, 663–667. [CrossRef] [PubMed]
40. Clark, C.R.; Hicks, L.S.; Keogh, J.H.; Epstein, A.M.; Ayanian, J.Z. Promoting access to renal transplantation: The role of social support networks in completing pre-transplant evaluations. *J. Gen. Intern. Med.* **2008**, *23*, 1187–1193. [CrossRef] [PubMed]
41. Lpez-Navas, A.; Ros, A.; Riquelme, A.; Martínez-Alarcón, L.; Pons, J.A.; Miras, M.; Parrilla, P. Psychological care: Social and family support for patients awaiting a liver transplant. *Transplant. Proc.* **2011**, *43*, 701–704. [CrossRef]
42. Ismail, S.Y.; Luchtenburg, A.E.; Timman, R.; Zuidema, W.C.; Boonstra, C.; Weimar, W.; Massey, E.K. Home-based family intervention increases knowledge, communication and living donation rates: A randomized controlled trial. *Am. J. Transpl.* **2014**, *14*, 1862–1869. [CrossRef]
43. Garonzik-Wang, J.M.; Berger, J.C.; Ros, R.L.; Kucirka, L.M.; Deshpande, N.A.; Boyarsky, B.J.; Segev, D.L. Live donor champion: Finding live kidney donors by separating the advocate from the patient. *Transplantation* **2012**, *93*, 1147–1150. [CrossRef]
44. Waterman, A.D.; Wood, E.H.; Ranasinghe, O.N.; Lipsey, A.F.; Anderson, C.; Balliet, W.; Salas, M.A.P. A Digital Library for Increasing Awareness About Living Donor Kidney Transplants: Formative Study. *JMIR Form. Res.* **2020**, *4*, e17441. [CrossRef]
45. Lunsford, S.L.; Simpson, K.S.; Chavin, K.D.; Menching, K.J.; Miles, L.G.; Shilling, L.M.; Baliga, P.K. Racial Disparities in Living Kidney Donation: Is There a Lack of Willing Donors or an Excess of Medically Unsuitable Candidates? *Transplantation* **2006**, *82*, 876–881. [CrossRef]
46. Robb, K.A.; Gatting, L.; Wardle, J. What impact do questionnaire length and monetary incentives have on mailed health psychology survey response? *Br. J. Health Psychol.* **2017**, *22*, 671–685. [CrossRef]
47. Harrison, S.; Henderson, J.; Alderdice, F.; Quigley, M.A. Methods to increase response rates to a population-based maternity survey: A comparison of two pilot studies. *BMC Med. Res. Methodol.* **2019**, *19*, 65. [CrossRef]

48. Slaats, D.; Lennerling, A.; Pronk, M.C.; van der Pant, K.A.; Dooper, I.M.; Wierdsma, J.M.; Zuidema, W.C. Donor and Recipient Perspectives on Anonymity in Kidney Donation From Live Donors: A Multicenter Survey Study. *Am. J. Kidney Dis.* **2018**, *71*, 52–64. [CrossRef] [PubMed]
49. Salway, S.; Holman, D.; Lee, C.; McGowan, V.; Ben-Shlomo, Y.; Saxena, S.; Nazroo, J. Transforming the health system for the UK's multiethnic population. *BMJ* **2020**, *368*, m268. [CrossRef] [PubMed]
50. Thiessen, C.; Kulkarni, S.; Reese, P.P.; Gordon, E.J. A Call for Research on Individuals Who Opt Out of Living Kidney Donation. *Transplantation* **2016**, *100*, 2527–2532. [CrossRef] [PubMed]

Publisher's Note: MDPI stays neutral with regard to jurisdictional claims in published maps and institutional affiliations.

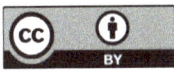

© 2020 by the authors. Licensee MDPI, Basel, Switzerland. This article is an open access article distributed under the terms and conditions of the Creative Commons Attribution (CC BY) license (http://creativecommons.org/licenses/by/4.0/).

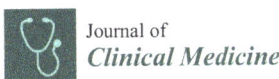 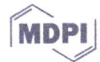

Article

Biopsy-Controlled Non-Invasive Quantification of Collagen Type VI in Kidney Transplant Recipients: A Post-Hoc Analysis of the MECANO Trial

Manuela Yepes-Calderón [1,†], Camilo G. Sotomayor [1,*,†], Daniel Guldager Kring Rasmussen [2], Ryanne S. Hijmans [1], Charlotte A. te Velde-Keyzer [1], Marco van Londen [1], Marja van Dijk [1], Arjan Diepstra [3], Stefan P. Berger [1], Morten Asser Karsdal [2], Frederike J. Bemelman [4], Johan W. de Fijter [5], Jesper Kers [6,7,8,9], Sandrine Florquin [6,7,8], Federica Genovese [2], Stephan J. L. Bakker [1], Jan-Stephan Sanders [1] and Jacob Van Den Born [1]

1. Division of Nephrology, Department of Internal Medicine, University Medical Center Groningen, University of Groningen, 9713 AV Groningen, The Netherlands; manueyepes@gmail.com (M.Y.-C.); r.s.hijmans@umcg.nl (R.S.H.); c.a.keyzer@umcg.nl (C.A.t.V.-K.); m.van.londen@umcg.nl (M.v.L.); m.van.dijk02@umcg.nl (M.v.D.); s.p.berger@umcg.nl (S.P.B.); s.j.l.bakker@umcg.nl (S.J.L.B.); j.sanders@umcg.nl (J.-S.S.); j.van.den.born@umcg.nl (J.V.D.B.)
2. Nordic Bioscience A/S, 2730 Herlev, Denmark; dgr@nordicbio.com (D.G.K.R.); MK@nordicbioscience.com (M.A.K.); fge@nordicbio.com (F.G.)
3. Department of Pathology and Medical Biology, University Medical Center Groningen, University of Groningen, 9713 AV Groningen, The Netherlands; a.diepstra@umcg.nl
4. Department of Nephrology, Amsterdam University Medical Center, University of Amsterdam, 1105 AZ Amsterdam, The Netherlands; f.j.bemelman@amsterdamumc.nl
5. Department of Nephrology, Leiden University Medical Center, University of Leiden, 2300 RC Leiden, The Netherlands; J.W.de_Fijter@lumc.nl
6. Amsterdam Institute for Infection and Immunity (AII), Amsterdam UMC, University of Amsterdam, 1098 XH Amsterdam, The Netherlands; j.kers@amsterdamumc.nl (J.K.); s.florquin@amsterdamumc.nl (S.F.)
7. Amsterdam Cardiovascular Sciences (ACS), Amsterdam UMC, University of Amsterdam, 1098 XH Amsterdam, The Netherlands
8. Leiden Transplant Center, Department of Pathology, Leiden University Medical Center, 2300 RC Leiden, The Netherlands
9. Van 't Hoff Institute for Molecular Sciences (HIMS), University of Amsterdam, 1098 XH Amsterdam, The Netherlands
* Correspondence: c.g.sotomayor.campos@umcg.nl; Tel.: +31-61-921-08-81
† These authors contributed equally to this work.

Received: 18 September 2020; Accepted: 2 October 2020; Published: 7 October 2020

Abstract: The PRO-C6 assay, a reflection of collagen type VI synthesis, has been proposed as a non-invasive early biomarker of kidney fibrosis. We aimed to investigate cross-sectional and longitudinal associations between plasma and urine PRO-C6 and proven histological changes after kidney transplantation. The current study is a post-hoc analysis of 94 participants of the MECANO trial, a 24-month prospective, multicenter, open-label, randomized, controlled trial aimed at comparing everolimus-based vs. cyclosporine-based immunosuppression. PRO-C6 was measured in plasma and urine samples collected 6 and 24 months post-transplantation. Fibrosis was evaluated in biopsies collected at the same time points by Banff interstitial fibrosis/tubular atrophy (IF/TA) scoring and collagen staining (Picro Sirius Red; PSR); inflammation was evaluated by the tubulo-interstitial inflammation score (ti-score). Linear regression analyses were performed. Six-month plasma PRO-C6 was cross-sectionally associated with IF/TA score (Std. β = 0.34), and prospectively with 24-month IF/TA score and ti-score (Std. β = 0.24 and 0.23, respectively) ($p < 0.05$ for all). No significant associations were found between urine PRO-C6 and any of the biopsy findings. Fibrotic changes and urine PRO-C6 behaved differentially over time according to immunosuppressive therapy. These results are a first step towards non-invasive fibrosis detection after kidney transplantation by means of collagen VI synthesis measurement, and further research is required.

Keywords: kidney transplantation; fibrosis; inflammation; extracellular matrix; collagen type VI

1. Introduction

Kidney transplantation is the best available treatment for patients with end-stage kidney disease [1,2]. In recent times, short-term graft survival has seen great improvement, which unfortunately has not been paralleled by equivalent improvement in long-term graft survival [3]. An important threat to long-term graft survival is progressive loss of kidney allograft function related to progressive fibrosis [4]. Despite its clinical importance, early identification of fibrosis appearance remains a challenge [5]. Currently, biopsy samples are the gold standard for the detection of established kidney fibrosis, but this has the evident drawback as a follow-up measurement of requiring an invasive procedure, which generates discomfort for the patients and can be complicated by bleeding. Other drawbacks are sampling variability and sampling errors [5,6]. Therefore, great interest exists in finding non-invasive biomarkers that can detect fibrosis formation, ideally at early stages [4].

Kidney allograft fibrosis reflects a pathological response to injury where the equilibrium between extracellular matrix formation and degradation is deregulated and progressive deposition of collagens, among other matrix constituents, takes place [7,8]. Assessment of active collagen formation may identify kidney transplant recipients (KTRs) at high risk of fibrosis progression and therefore development of chronic graft failure [9,10]. Among the different collagens, collagen type VI (COL VI) is found in the kidney and is constantly produced by fibroblasts at relative low levels in the interstitium, the intima and adventitia layers of the kidney vasculature, as well as in the glomeruli [11–13]. Under normal conditions, COL VI has an important physiological role in maintaining extracellular matrix (ECM) structure and function, controlling matrix and cell orientation [14]. However, under pathological conditions (e.g., chronic kidney disease), its active deposition in the kidneys is massively increased [9,12]. During production of COL VI, the C5 domain at the C-terminal of the $\alpha 3$ chain is released from the immediate pericellular matrix [15]. The PRO-C6 assay detects the C-terminal end of this domain and is proposed as a surrogate biomarker for COL VI active formation [9]. Moreover, the cleavage of part of this domain gives rise to a bioactive molecule, named endotrophin, which is also detected by the PRO-C6 assay [15,16]. Endotrophin has important biological effects, such as attracting macrophages, increasing transforming growth factor-β (TGFβ) signaling, promoting epithelial–mesenchymal transition, adipose tissue fibrosis, and metabolic dysfunction [17]. Increased plasma levels of PRO-C6 have previously been associated with the progression of chronic kidney disease and, specifically in the post-transplantation setting, with reduced graft function in KTR [4,9,18,19]. Whether associations between PRO-C6 and decreased graft function indeed correspond to increased fibrotic or inflammatory changes in the kidneys and whether it could be used as a non-invasive biomarker for fibrosis development in KTR remain unknown.

In the current study, we aimed to investigate the cross-sectional and longitudinal associations between PRO-C6 in plasma and urine, and proven histological changes in KTR of the minimization of maintenance immunosuppression early after kidney transplantation (MECANO) trial, which is a randomized, controlled, open-label, multicenter trial testing early cyclosporine A (CsA) elimination. Furthermore, since it is known that CsA nephrotoxicity includes pathological increased production and decreased degradation of extracellular matrix proteins, including collagen, and TGF-β up-regulation [20–22], we explored a potential differential role of PRO-C6 as a biomarker of fibrosis among patients under different immunosuppressive regimens.

2. Materials and Methods

2.1. Study Design and Population

Between November 2005 and June 2009, 361 de novo KTRs were recruited in three Dutch transplantation centers to participate in the MECANO trial (trial registration: NTR1615). The study was conducted according to the Good Clinical Practice guidelines, in accordance with the ethical principles of the Declaration of Helsinki, and was approved by the Dutch Medical Ethical Board for medical research (METC 04/154, 1 October 2004) [23,24]. All patients signed written informed consent forms. This study was a 24-month, prospective, multi-center, open-label, randomized, controlled trial, aiming at optimizing maintenance immunosuppression and reducing side effects. During the first six months after enrollment, all patients had a similar quadruple immunosuppressive regimen: induction with basiliximab, followed by CsA, mycophenolate sodium (MPS), and prednisolone [24]. At month six, a protocol biopsy was performed. When no histological signs of rejection were seen, patients were randomized to receive dual immunosuppressive therapy with CsA ($n = 89$), MPS, or everolimus (EVL) ($n = 96$), all in combination with prednisolone. In case of (borderline) rejection patients, were not randomized. The primary endpoint of the MECANO study was the development of interstitial fibrosis at the 24-months protocol biopsy.

After enrollment of 39 patients, the MPS-group was prematurely stopped by the Data Safety Monitoring Board because of an unacceptably high rejection percentage (21%). The trial continued as a two-group trial, comparing CsA and EVL. The results of the primary outcome of the study were published in 2016 [23].

2.2. Protocol Kidney Biopsies and Histological Analyses

Protocol biopsies were scheduled at 6 and 24 months after transplantation. At six months, biopsies were obtained in 99% and 98% of patients in the CsA group and the EVL group, respectively. Of the available biopsies, 78% and 81% in the CsA group and the EVL group were considered adequate, respectively. At 24 months, biopsies were obtained in 84% and 79% of patients in the CsA group and the EVL group, respectively. The prevalence of adequate samples was 81% and 73% in the CsA group and the EVL group, respectively ($p = 0.4$, two-tailed). The current study reports the results of the 94 patients (51 in the CsA group and 43 in the EVL group) whose 6-month biopsies met the minimal adequacy threshold of seven glomeruli and one artery.

Tissues were formalin-fixed and paraffin-embedded and stained with periodic-acid Schiff diastase, hematoxylin/eosin, and Jones' methenamine silver. Two independent kidney pathologists (Amsterdam University Medical Center (UMC) and Leiden UMC, The Netherlands), unaware of any clinical data, classified the biopsies according to the 2015 update of the Banff classification [25] and assigned a Banff interstitial fibrosis/tubular atrophy (IF/TA) score. Morphometric analysis of cortical interstitial fibrosis was centralized at the Amsterdam UMC. Adequate protocol biopsy sections were stained with Picro Sirius Red (PSR, Aldrich, Munich, Germany), which is used for the detection of collagen fibers. PSR-stained slides were digitalized using a slide virtual microscope system (Olympus, Tokyo, Japan) with a 20× magnification objective and saved in Tagged Image File Format (TIFF format). Image analyses were performed with the ImageJ software package (National Institutes of Health, Bethesda, MD, USA) where the PSR-stained area was automatically assessed by means of a macro. All input was verified manually. Inflammation was evaluated by the total percentage of inflamed cortical area (ti-score) as a continuous score [26].

2.3. PRO-C6 Detection

Plasma and urine PRO-C6 concentrations were measured using a competitive enzyme-linked immunosorbent assay (Nordic Bioscience, Herlev, Denmark) that specifically detects the last 10 amino acids of the alpha-3 chain of COL VI (3168'KPGVISVMGT3177') and is validated for both sample matrices [27]. The assay has a detection limit of 0.15 ng/mL and a 95% confidence interval for inter-

and intra-assay variability in plasma samples reported as 3.4%–12.4% and 1.1%–5.3%, respectively [19]. For urine samples, the detection limit was the same as plasma, and inter- and intra-assay variability are reported as 7.9% and 3.2%, respectively [9]. To account for variations in urine concentration, urinary PRO-C6 was divided by urinary creatinine, measured by the QuantiChrom™ Creatinine Assay Kit (BioAssay Systems, Hayward, CA, USA), and the PRO-C6/creatinine ratio was used in all analyses.

2.4. Statistical Analyses

Data analyses, computations, and graphs were performed with SPSS 25.0 software (IBM Corporation, Chicago, IL, USA). To test whether variables were normally distributed, a histogram was generated for each variable. For descriptive statistics data were presented as mean (standard deviation (SD)) for normally distributed data, and as median (interquartile range (IQR)) for variables with a non-normal distribution. Categorical data were expressed as number (percentage).

Differences in plasma and urine PRO-C6 and biopsy changes (IF/TA score, PSR, and ti-score) among subgroups of KTRs according to their treatment regimen and to their primary kidney disease were tested by one-way ANOVA for continuous variables with normal distribution, Mann–Whitney U test for continuous variables with skewed distribution, and X^2 test for categorical variables. Linear regression analyses were performed to study the association of plasma and urine PRO-C6 with biopsy changes at 6 and 24 months and the delta between the two visits. Furthermore, subgroup analyses were performed by dividing patients by the immunosuppressive regimen used. We also performed sensitivity analyses, in which patients who were grouped under "unknown cause" as primary kidney disease were recoded as if they have been suffering from glomerulonephritis as primary kidney disease. For all statistical analyses, a 2-sided $p < 0.05$ was considered significant.

3. Results

3.1. Baseline Characteristics

The characteristics at enrollment and at randomization of a total of 94 patients, 51 in the CsA group and 43 in the EVL group, are displayed in Tables 1 and 2. At enrollment, in the overall population, the mean (SD) age was 52 (13) years-old, and most patients were male and Caucasian. The main cause of end-stage kidney disease in this trial was polycystic kidney disease (24%), followed by glomerulonephritis (17%) and hypertension (16%). The mean donor age was 50 (13) years old, and the most frequent type of donors was living unrelated (31%), followed closely by deceased after brain death (30%). The median antigen mismatch was 3, and the median (IQR) of total time on kidney replacement therapy was 24 (5–46) months.

At randomization, 6 months after the beginning of the trial, patients had a mean graft function, as assessed by the estimated glomerular filtration rate (eGFR), of 49 (42–62) mL/min/1.73 m^2. Patients had a mean weight of 79 (14) kg and a mean systolic blood pressure of 144 (20) mmHg. Mean low-density lipoprotein (LDL) was 3.19 (2.39–3.75) mmol/L, and 59% of patients were statin users. Mean glycated hemoglobin was 6.08% (1.10), and only two patients had the diagnosis of diabetes mellitus. Fifteen patients (16%) were active smokers. Concerning subgroup differences, patients in the CsA group had an apparent higher weight (81 vs. 78 kg), a more frequent use of statins (63% vs. 54%), and a higher percentage were active smokers (20% vs. 12%) when compared to the EVL group. Also, the two diabetic patients were both in the EVL group. None of these differences was of statistical significance.

Table 1. Characteristics at enrollment of study population, overall kidney transplant recipients (KTRs), and randomization groups.

Characteristics at Enrollment	Overall	Randomized Group		p Value
		CsA	EVL	
Number of patients, n	94	51	43	
Age, years (SD)	52 (13)	51 (13)	54 (12)	0.30
Sex (male), n (%)	64 (68)	33 (65)	31 (72)	0.44
Race (Caucasian), n (%)	83 (88)	47 (92)	36 (84)	0.21
Primary kidney disease, n (%)				0.81
Polycystic kidney disease	24 (26)	13 (26)	11 (26)	
Glomerulonephritis	16 (17)	9 (18)	7 (16)	
Hypertension	15 (16)	7 (14)	8 (19)	
Urologic	8 (9)	3 (6)	5 (12)	
Vascular	5 (5)	2 (4)	3 (7)	
Focal segmental glomerulosclerosis	3 (3)	1 (2)	2 (5)	
Diabetes mellitus	3 (3)	2 (4)	1 (2)	
Unknown cause	16 (17)	11 (22)	5 (12)	
Donor type, n (%)				0.81
Living unrelated	29 (31)	15 (29)	14 (33)	
Deceased after brain death	28 (30)	15 (29)	13 (30)	
Living related	22 (23)	14 (28)	8 (19)	
Deceased after cardiac death	14 (15)	7 (14)	7 (16)	
Donor age, years (SD) [a]	50 (13)	51 (13)	49 (12)	0.55
Antigen mismatch, n (IQR)	3 (2–4)	3 (2–3)	3 (2–4)	0.52
TTKRT, months (IQR)	24 (5–46)	18 (6–46)	24 (5–48)	0.53

[a] Data available in 87 patients. CsA: cyclosporine A; EVL: everolimus; TTKRT: total time on kidney replacement therapy.

Table 2. Characteristics at randomization of study population, overall KTRs, and randomization groups.

Characteristics at Randomization	Overall	Randomized Group		p Value
		CsA	EVL	
eGFR, mL/min/1.73 m²	49 (42–62)	49 (43–57)	49 (40–67)	0.89
Weight, kg (SD) [a]	79 (14)	81 (15)	78 (13)	0.24
BMI, kg/m² (SD) [a]	26.7 (3.5)	26.0 (3.9)	25.4 (3.1)	0.44
SBP, mmHg (SD) [b]	144 (20)	144 (20)	145 (21)	0.82
DBP, mmHg (SD) [b]	84 (12)	84 (11)	83 (12)	0.68
LDL, mmol/L (SD) [b]	3.19 (2.39–3.75)	3.19 (2.37–3.95)	3.15 (2.40–3.70)	0.84
HDL, mmol/L (SD) [b]	1.39 (1.20–1.73)	1.30 (1.17–1.71)	1.49 (1.20–1.76)	0.49
Cholesterol, mmol/L (SD) [b]	5.13 (4.34–6.10)	5.16 (4.26–6.23)	5.08 (4.40–6.07)	0.92
Statins use, n (%)	55 (59)	32 (63)	23 (54)	0.36
Glucose, mmol/L [c]	5.10 (4.50–5.80)	5.10 (4.70–5.80)	4.90 (4.50–5.90)	0.35
HbA1c, % (SD) [c]	6.08 (1.10)	6.14 (1.25)	6.01 (0.88)	0.60
Diabetes mellitus, n (%)	2 (2)	0 (0)	2 (5)	0.12
Smoking current, n (%)	15 (16)	10 (20)	5 (12)	0.29

Data available in [a] 90, [b] 92, and [c] 88 patients. eGFR: estimated glomerular filtration rate; BMI: body mass index; SPB: systolic blood pressure; DBP: diastolic blood pressure; LDL: low-density lipoprotein; HDL: high-density lipoprotein; HbA1c: glycated hemoglobin.

3.2. PRO-C6 and Biopsy-Proven Histological Changes over Follow-Up

Mean (SD) plasma PRO-C6 at 6 and 24 months was 9.5 (3.4) and 9.4 (4.3) ng/mL, respectively, without significant differences between the two groups. As for urine, median (IQR) PRO-C6 at 6 and 24 months after correction by creatinine was 6.7 (4.8–12.4) and 5.9 (3.4–21.5) ng/mg, respectively. Plasma and urine PRO-C6 did not correlate at either 6 or 24 months (Spearman's ρ 0.226, $p = 0.09$; Spearman's ρ 0.311, $p = 0.11$; respectively). No difference in urine PRO-C6 between the two study groups was present at 6 months, but at 24 months mean urine PRO-C6 was significantly higher in the EVL group compared to the CsA group (7.5 vs. 4.5 ng/mg; $p = 0.02$). Delta plasma PRO-C6 was positive in both subgroups and was not significantly different. As for delta urine PRO-C6, it was positive in the EVL group and negative in the CsA group; this difference was statistically significant (0.9 vs. −1.4 ng/mg; $p = 0.01$). (Table 3).

Table 3. Biomarkers and histological characteristics during follow-up of overall KTRs and randomization groups.

Biomarkers and Histological Characteristics	Overall	Randomized Group		p
		CsA	EVL	
Biomarkers				
6 Months				
Plasma				
PRO-C6 (ng/mL) [a]	9.5 (3.4)	9.5 (3.1)	9.4 (3.9)	0.93
Creatinine, µmol/L (SD)	130 (33)	130 (31)	130 (35)	0.96
Urine				
PRO-C6 (ng/mg creat) [b]	6.7 (4.8–12.4)	6.6 (4.9–12.9)	6.8 (3.8–12.8)	0.70
24 Months				
Plasma				
PRO-C6 (ng/mL) [c]	9.4 (4.3)	9.6 (4.5)	9.1 (4.3)	0.72
Creatinine, µmol/L (SD)	143 (49)	149 (46)	136 (53)	0.22
Urine				
PRO-C6 (ng/mg creat) [b]	5.9 (3.4–21.5)	4.5 (3.2–10.2)	7.5 (4.6–40.7)	0.02
Delta$_{24-6}$				
Plasma				
PRO-C6 (ng/mL) [c]	0.3 (3.9)	0.6 (3.1)	0.01 (4.6)	0.67
Urine				
PRO-C6 (ng/mg creat) [b]	−0.5 (−2.6–4.8)	−1.4 (−3.6–−0.27)	0.9 (−2.2–23.9)	0.01
Histological analyses				
6 Months				
IF/TA-score	1 (0–1)	1 (0–1)	1 (1–2)	0.56
PSR, %	13.3 (6.0)	13.0 (6.1)	13.6 (6.0)	0.65
ti-score, %	10.0 (5.0–15.8)	10.0 (5.0–10.0)	10.0 (5.0–20.0)	0.38
24 Months				
IF/TA-score	1 (1–2)	1 (0–1)	1 (1–2)	0.36
PSR, %	17.3 (10.6)	19.7 (11.7)	14.5 (8.5)	0.02
ti-score, %	20.0 (10.0–41.3)	20.0 (10.0–50.0)	15.0 (10.0–30.0)	0.16
Delta$_{24-6}$				
IF/TA-score	0.5 (0–1)	1 (0–1)	0 (0–1)	0.23
PSR, %	4.0 (11.4)	6.7 (13.1)	0.9 (7.9)	0.01
ti-score, %	10 (0–30)	10 (0–45)	5 (0–20)	0.09

Data available in [a] 73, [b] 62, [c] 36 patients. CsA: cyclosporine group; EVL: everolimus group; PRO-C6: released pro-peptide of collagen type VI (endotrophin); IF/TA: interstitial fibrosis/tubular atrophy; PSR: Picro Sirius Red; ti-score: total inflammation score.

Histological analyses at 6 months showed a median IF/TA score of 1 (0–1) points and a mean PSR staining percentage of 13.3% (6.0), with no significant differences between patients in the CsA and EVL groups. Inflammation, as evaluated by the ti-score, was also not significantly different between the two groups. At 24 months, the overall population showed a higher IF/TA score, PSR percentage, and ti-score when compared to the previous biopsy. At this time point, the PSR staining percentage was higher in the CsA group compared to the EVL group (19.7% vs. 14.5%; $p = 0.02$); no significant difference was present in the other histological parameters (Table 3).

When patients were stratified by their primary kidney disease, no significant differences were found in the plasma and urine concentrations of PRO-C6 at any time point during follow-up. No significant difference was found either in fibrosis (IF/TA and PRO-C6) or inflammation (ti-score) at 6 and 24 months (Table S1). Also, no significant differences were found in sensitivity analyses in which all KTRs with unknown cause of primary kidney disease were considered as patients with glomerulonephritis as primary kidney disease (Table S2).

3.3. Association between PRO-C6 and Biopsy Changes

Plasma PRO-C6 at 6 months post transplantation was significantly associated with 6-month and 24-month IF/TA scores (Std. β = 0.34 and 0.24, respectively; both $p < 0.05$). A prospective association was also present for 6-month plasma PRO-C6 with 24-month biopsy proven inflammation (ti-score) and the delta inflammation between the two biopsies (Std. β = 0.23 and 0.22, respectively; both $p < 0.05$). No association was found between 6-month plasma PRO-C6 and 6- or 24-month PSR. Also, no cross-sectional association was found between 24-month plasma PRO-C6 and histological evidence of fibrosis or inflammation. Urine PRO-C6 at 6 months only showed a prospective and inverse association with 24-month PSR (Std. β = −0.30; $p < 0.05$), and there were no cross-sectional associations at 24 months. Delta plasma and urine PRO-C6 did not correlate with either histological evidence of fibrosis or inflammation (Table 4).

Table 4. Association of histological analyses with plasma and urine PRO-C6.

Histological Analyses	6-Months PRO-C6		24-Months PRO-C6		Delta$_{24-6}$ PRO-C6	
	Plasma, ng/mL	Urine, ng/mg	Plasma, ng/mL	Urine, ng/mg	Plasma, ng/mL	Urine, ng/mg
	Std. β	Std. β	Std. β	Std. β	Std. β	Std. β
6 Months						
IF/TA	0.34 **	0.20				
PSR	0.11	−0.18				
ti-score	0.04	0.08				
24 Months						
IF/TA	0.24 *	0.06	0.08	0.13	−0.04	0.02
PSR	0.01	−0.30 *	0.06	−0.24	−0.01	0.04
ti-score	0.23 *	0.23	0.16	0.09	0.05	−0.03
Delta$_{24-6}$						
IF/TA	−0.03	−0.08	−0.20	−0.07	−0.16	0.01
PSR	−0.06	−0.17	−0.009	−0.19	0.04	−0.04
ti-score	0.22 *	0.20	0.11	−0.02	0.01	−0.02

* p value < 0.05; ** p value < 0.01. Linear regression analyses were performed. Std. β coefficients represent the difference (in standard deviations) in each biomarker per 1 standard deviation increment in each individual biopsy score. PRO-C6: pro-peptide of collagen VI (endotrophin); Std. β: standardized beta coefficient; IF/TA: interstitial fibrosis/tubular atrophy; PSR: Picro Sirius Red; ti-score: total inflammation score.

When patients were divided by randomization group, no significant associations were found between 24-month plasma PRO-C6 and histological changes. Urine PRO-C6 was significantly and inversely associated with the delta of IF/TA score in patients among the CsA group, and no other significant association was found. Delta plasma and urine PRO-C6 were not significantly associated with any histological changes (Table 5).

Table 5. Association of histological analyses with plasma and urine PRO-C6 among CsA and EVL groups.

Histological Analyses	24 Months				Delta$_{24-6}$			
	Plasma PRO-C6, ng/mL		Urine PRO-C6, ng/mg		Plasma PRO-C6, ng/mL		Urine PRO-C6, ng/mg	
	CsA	EVL	CsA	EVL	CsA	EVL	CsA	EVL
	Std. β	Std. β	Std. β	Std. β	Std. β	Std. β	Std. β	Std. β
24 Months								
IF/TA	−0.11	0.32	−0.25	0.30	−0.31	0.16	0.13	−0.11
PSR	−0.07	0.18	−0.09	−0.31	−0.47	0.25	0.12	−0.11
ti-score	−0.07	0.40	0.18	0.14	−0.37	0.32	0.08	−0.07
Delta$_{24-6}$								
IF/TA	−0.30	−0.07	−0.43 *	0.07	−0.40	−0.01	0.12	−0.003
PSR	0.001	−0.06	−0.10	−0.27	−0.28	0.25	0.03	−0.18
ti-score	−0.08	0.33	0.07	0.05	−0.35	0.25	0.09	0.04

* p value < 0.05. Linear regression analyses were performed. Std. β coefficients represent the difference (in standard deviations) in each biomarker per 1 standard deviation increment in each individual biopsy score. PRO-C6: pro-peptide of collagen type VI (endotrophin); CsA: cyclosporine group; EVL: everolimus group; Std. β: standardized beta coefficient; IF/TA: interstitial fibrosis/tubular atrophy; PSR: Picro Sirius Red; ti-score: total inflammation score.

4. Discussion

This study shows, in a homogeneous well-characterized cohort of KTRs who were participants of the MECANO clinical trial, that 6-month post-transplant plasma concentration of PRO-C6 associates with graft biopsy-proven fibrotic and inflammatory changes, both cross-sectionally (IF/TA score) and longitudinally (IF/TA score and ti-score). Further, we show that these same associations are not found with 6-month urine PRO-C6, and that at 24 months, no cross-sectional association was present between fibrotic changes and either urine or plasma PRO-C6. Subgroup analyses comparing patients under CsA vs. EVL immunosuppressive therapy showed higher urinary concentration of PRO-C6 in the EVL group compared to the CsA groups during follow-up, despite lower fibrosis scorings.

The progression of kidney diseases is characterized by the appearance of progressive fibrosis, which reflects a pathological disequilibrium between the synthesis and degradation of ECM constituents, including collagens, within scarred kidneys [8,28]. COL VI is an ECM molecule distributed in the kidney interstitium, vasculature, and in the glomeruli, which is constantly produced by fibroblasts at relative low levels [12,13]. Under healthy conditions, it has an important physiological role in maintaining structure and function of the ECM by controlling organization and cell orientation [14]. However, its markedly increased synthesis and deposition has been reported under a wide spectrum of kidney pathologies [29,30].

COL VI biosynthesis and assembly involves a complex multi-step pathway [14,31]. During active deposition in the ECM, a pro-peptide in the α3 chain of COL VI is released; in turn, this gives rise to the bioactive molecule endotrophin [15,27], which is known to have a role in shaping a pro-inflammatory and pro-fibrotic microenvironment by, amongst other processes, triggering an increase in cytokines such as TGFβ [16]. The PRO-C6 assay measures both the release of endotrophin and of the pro-peptide, reflecting newly formed molecules of mature COL VI [9,27]. In the post-transplantation setting, the assessment of active collagen formation has been proposed as a way of early identifying KTRs that are at high risk of fibrosis progression [9,10], and since allograft function loss is closely related to the appearance and progression of interstitial fibrosis and tubular atrophy [10,32,33], it could identify also KTRs at future risk of developing chronic graft failure [9,10].

Clinically, increased deposition of COL VI has been reported in multiple scenarios of chronic kidney disease [28,31], and specifically in the post-transplantation setting, a strong association was found between increased plasma concentration of PRO-C6 and a decrease in graft function over time [4]. In agreement with this evidence, we found a positive prospective association between 6-month

PRO-C6 concentration and biopsy evidence of increased graft fibrosis (IF/TA). However, no associations were found with PSR staining. Following the evidence that patients receiving CsA are at risk of developing nephrotoxicity, which is also a condition with unregulated ECM deposition and TGF-β upregulation [20–22,34], we performed exploratory analysis by subgroups of immunosuppressive therapy. When dividing the population into subgroups, we found that patients in the CsA group had higher PSR% at 24 months, but urine PRO-C6 was higher in the EVL group.

This analysis shows that PRO-C6 measurement, as reflection of collagen VI synthesis, is associated with, but not identical to, quantification of fibrosis in transplanted kidneys, especially not under different treatment conditions. The next considerations should be taken into account: first, by measuring plasma or urine PRO-C6, the cells/tissues where the existing collagen VI synthesis takes place cannot be identified and might be (partially) different from the transplanted kidney. Second, PRO-C6, by definition, only measures a collagen split product of the alpha3 chain of collagen VI [15,27], whereas PSR staining is the resultant of all collagen deposits. As we know, there are >20 different types of collagens, all of which can be stained by PSR [35]. So, changes in PSR staining do not necessarily correspond with changes in COL VI synthesis. Third, the PRO-C6 assay measures a split product of collagen VI that is cleaved off after cellular synthesis and thus reflects synthesis of collagen VI. Collagen deposition in a tissue, however, is the resultant of collagen synthesis and collagen degradation (mainly by metalloproteinases). So, the PRO-C6 assay shows one side of the coin (synthesis), whereas the other side of the coin (degradation) is not measured. We anticipate that various treatment regimens might not only influence collagen VI synthesis but collagen VI degradation as well. Next, since we did not perform immunofluorescent studies, we cannot assure that there was recurrence or enhanced interstitial inflammation; however, when stratified analyses by primary kidney disease were performed, there was no significant difference in biomarkers or histological evidence of inflammation. Also, the possibility that incidence of glomerulonephritis was underestimated due to low use of immunofluorescence in the evaluation of biopsy materials in the regular clinical setting in which the current study was performed, and the possibility that such potential underestimation may have biased our results, is a limitation of our study. Although we performed sensitivity analyses in which we found no indication of the presence of such bias, it can, of course, not be excluded. Future studies are warranted to confirm our findings, and it would be relevant to apply immunofluorescence in such studies in order to maximize the accuracy of estimation of glomerulonephritis recurrence. It would also be interesting if future studies would compare the pre- and post-transplantation behavior of PRO-C6. Furthermore, patients receiving CsA had a more marked decline in eGFR compared to the EVL group, as was shown in the main outcomes of the MECANO publication [23]. This might have influenced both plasma and urine PRO-C6 values and differences between both treatment arms. Finally, we do not have information on eGFR at inclusion, therefore the eGFR changes before randomization could not be evaluated, and this prevents us from exploring the causes underlying early fibrotic lesions.

The present study has several strengths. Being a randomized clinical trial, we have a very homogenous population regarding time since transplantation and initial immunosuppressive regimen. Also, we studied PRO-C6 against the current gold standard for fibrosis detection, which is kidney biopsy [5,6], taken at the same time point as the biomarkers, allowing both cross-sectional and longitudinal analyses. Several limitations must also be considered. Most of our patients are from a European background, and care should be taken when extrapolating our findings to other ethnic groups. Also, especially at 24 months, we had a reduced number of available samples and a longer follow-up would have allowed us to further explore the prospective behavior of PRO-C6.

In conclusion, 6-month post-transplantation plasma concentration PRO-C6 has a good longitudinal association with graft biopsy-proven IFTA scores, which could make it potentially useful as a follow-up tool. On the other hand, urine PRO-C6 did not associate with fibrotic parameters measured at time of biopsy or in future protocol biopsies. Additionally, we showed a differential evolution of PRO-C6 during follow-up dependent on immunosuppressive regimen. For the first time, this study provides biopsy-controlled data of PRO-C6 as a potential non-invasive biomarker of graft fibrosis in KTRs.

This is a first step towards non-invasive detection by plasma PRO-C6 of pro-fibrotic ECM turnover early after transplantation. The potential utility of the implementation of PRO-C6 in clinical follow-up of KTRs requires further clinical studies.t The detection of causes underlying early kidney fibrosis was not the scope of the current study, yet we hold a plea for future studies aiming at evaluating whether primary kidney disease may influence he performance of PRO-C6 as a biomarker in KTRs. Furthermore, it would be interesting if future studies would also compare the pre- and post-transplantation behavior of PRO-C6.

Supplementary Materials: The following are available online at http://www.mdpi.com/2077-0383/9/10/3216/s1: Table S1. Biomarkers and histological characteristics during follow-up on KTRs by primary kidney disease. Table S2. Biomarkers and histological characteristics during follow-up on KTRs by primary kidney disease assuming all patients with unknown cause would have had glomerulonephritis as primary kidney disease.

Author Contributions: Conceptualization: C.G.S., D.G.K.R., and J.V.D.B.; Data curation: D.G.K.R., R.S.H., C.A.t.V.-K., M.v.L., M.v.D., and A.D.; Formal analysis: M.Y.-C., C.G.S., S.J.L.B., and J.V.D.B.; Investigation: D.G.K.R., R.S.H., C.A.t.V.-K., M.v.L., M.v.D., A.D., M.A.K., F.J.B., J.W.d.F., S.F., J.K., F.G., and S.J.L.B.; Methodology: S.P.B., M.A.K., F.J.B., J.W.d.F., S.F., J.K., and F.G.; Project administration: S.P.B., S.J.L.B., J.-S.S., and J.V.D.B.; Resources: D.G.K.R., M.A.K., and F.G.; Supervision: S.P.B., S.J.L.B, J.-S.S., and J.V.D.B.; Writing—original draft: M.Y.-C. and C.G.S.; Writing—review and editing: M.Y.-C., C.G.S., D.G.K.R., R.S.H, C.A.t.V.-K., M.v.L., M.v.D., A.D., S.P.B., M.A.K., F.J.B., J.W.d.F., S.F., J.K., F.G., S.J.L.B., J.-S.S., and J.V.D.B. All authors have read and agreed to the published version of the manuscript.

Funding: This work was supported by the Netherlands Organization For Health Research and Development (ZonMw; grant number 114021010, PO), the Danish Research Fund (Den Danske Forskningsfond), Novartis Pharma by means of an unrestricted grant, the Chilean National Commission of Scientific and Technological Investigation (CONICYT) (doctorate studies grant to Sotomayor [F 72190118]) and the Graduate School of Medical Sciences of the University Medical Center Groningen (MD/PhD grant to Hijmans).

Conflicts of Interest: D.G.K.R., M.A.K., and F.G. are full-time employees at Nordic Bioscience and M.A.K. and F.G. hold stocks. Nordic Bioscience is a privately-owned, small–medium-sized enterprise partly focused on the development of biomarkers and owns the patent for the ELISA used to measure PRO-C6 levels. None of the authors received fees, bonuses, or other benefits for the work described in the manuscript, and Nordic Biosicience did not have any role in the study design, data collection and analysis, decision to publish, or preparation of the manuscript. No other author declares conflict of interest.

References

1. Laupacis, A.; Keown, P.; Pus, N.; Krueger, H.; Ferguson, B.; Wong, C.; Muirhead, N. A study of the quality of life and cost-utility of renal transplantation. *Kidney Int.* **1996**, *50*, 235–242. [CrossRef] [PubMed]
2. Wolfe, R.A.; Ashby, V.B.; Milford, E.L.; Ojo, A.O.; Ettenger, R.E.; Agodoa, L.Y.C.; Held, P.J.; Port, F.K. Comparison of Mortality in All Patients on Dialysis, Patients on Dialysis Awaiting Transplantation, and Recipients of a First Cadaveric Transplant. *N. Engl. J. Med.* **1999**, *341*, 1725–1730. [CrossRef] [PubMed]
3. Meier-Kriesche, H.-U.; Schold, J.D.; Srinivas, T.R.; Kaplan, B. Lack of Improvement in Renal Allograft Survival Despite a Marked Decrease in Acute Rejection Rates Over the Most Recent Era. *Am. J. Transplant.* **2004**, *4*, 378–383. [CrossRef] [PubMed]
4. Stribos, E.G.D.; Nielsen, S.H.; Brix, S.; Karsdal, M.A.; Seelen, M.A.; van Goor, H.; Bakker, S.J.L.; Olinga, P.; Mutsaers, H.A.M.; Genovese, F. Non-invasive quantification of collagen turnover in renal transplant recipients. *PLoS ONE* **2017**, *12*, e0175898. [CrossRef]
5. Hijmans, R.S.; Rasmussen, D.G.K.; Yazdani, S.; Navis, G.; van Goor, H.; Karsdal, M.A.; Genovese, F.; van den Born, J. Urinary collagen degradation products as early markers of progressive renal fibrosis. *J. Transl. Med.* **2017**, *15*, 63. [CrossRef]
6. Farris, A.B.; Colvin, R.B. Renal interstitial fibrosis: Mechanisms and evaluation. *Curr. Opin. Nephrol. Hypertens.* **2012**, *21*, 289–300. [CrossRef]
7. Karsdal, M.A.; Nielsen, M.J.; Sand, J.M.; Henriksen, K.; Genovese, F.; Bay-Jensen, A.-C.; Smith, V.; Adamkewicz, J.I.; Christiansen, C.; Leeming, D.J. Extracellular matrix remodeling: The common denominator in connective tissue diseases. Possibilities for evaluation and current understanding of the matrix as more than a passive architecture, but a key player in tissue failure. *Assay Drug Dev. Technol.* **2013**, *11*, 70–92. [CrossRef]

8. Soylemezoglu, O.; Wild, G.; Dalley, A.J.; MacNeil, S.; Milford-Ward, A.; Brown, C.B.; el Nahas, A.M. Urinary and serum type III collagen: Markers of renal fibrosis. *Nephrol. Dial. Transplant.* **1997**, *12*, 1883–1889. [CrossRef]
9. Rasmussen, D.G.K.; Fenton, A.; Jesky, M.; Ferro, C.; Boor, P.; Tepel, M.; Karsdal, M.A.; Genovese, F.; Cockwell, P. Urinary endotrophin predicts disease progression in patients with chronic kidney disease. *Sci. Rep.* **2017**, *7*, 17328. [CrossRef]
10. Serón, D.; Moreso, F.; Ramón, J.M.; Hueso, M.; Condom, E.; Fulladosa, X.; Bover, J.; Gil-Vernet, S.; Castelao, A.M.; Alsina, J.; et al. Protocol renal allograft biopsies and the design of clinical trials aimed to prevent or treat chronic allograft nephropathy. *Transplantation* **2000**, *69*, 1849–1855. [CrossRef]
11. Magro, G.; Grasso, S.; Colombatti, A.; Lopes, M. Immunohistochemical distribution of type VI collagen in developing human kidney. *Histochem. J.* **1996**, *28*, 385–390. [CrossRef] [PubMed]
12. Groma, V. Demonstration of collagen type VI and alpha-smooth muscle actin in renal fibrotic injury in man. *Nephrol. Dial. Transplant.* **1998**, *13*, 305–312. [CrossRef] [PubMed]
13. Lennon, R.; Byron, A.; Humphries, J.D.; Randles, M.J.; Carisey, A.; Murphy, S.; Knight, D.; Brenchley, P.E.; Zent, R.; Humphries, M.J. Global analysis reveals the complexity of the human glomerular extracellular matrix. *J. Am. Soc. Nephrol.* **2014**, *25*, 939–951. [CrossRef]
14. Cescon, M.; Gattazzo, F.; Chen, P.; Bonaldo, P. Collagen VI at a glance. *J. Cell Sci.* **2015**, *128*, 3525–3531. [CrossRef] [PubMed]
15. Aigner, T.; Hambach, L.; Söder, S.; Schlötzer-Schrehardt, U.; Pöschl, E. The C5 domain of Col6A3 is cleaved off from the Col6 fibrils immediately after secretion. *Biochem. Biophys. Res. Commun.* **2002**, *290*, 743–748. [CrossRef] [PubMed]
16. Fenton, A.; Jesky, M.D.; Ferro, C.J.; Sørensen, J.; Karsdal, M.A.; Cockwell, P.; Genovese, F. Serum endotrophin, a type VI collagen cleavage product, is associated with increased mortality in chronic kidney disease. *PLoS ONE* **2017**, *12*, e0175200. [CrossRef]
17. Sun, K.; Park, J.; Gupta, O.T.; Holland, W.L.; Auerbach, P.; Zhang, N.; Goncalves Marangoni, R.; Nicoloro, S.M.; Czech, M.P.; Varga, J.; et al. Endotrophin triggers adipose tissue fibrosis and metabolic dysfunction. *Nat. Commun.* **2014**, *5*, 3485. [CrossRef]
18. Rasmussen, D.G.K.; Hansen, T.W.; von Scholten, B.J.; Nielsen, S.H.; Reinhard, H.; Parving, H.-H.; Tepel, M.; Karsdal, M.A.; Jacobsen, P.K.; Genovese, F.; et al. Higher Collagen VI Formation Is Associated with All-Cause Mortality in Patients with Type 2 Diabetes and Microalbuminuria. *Diabetes Care* **2018**, *41*, 1493–1500. [CrossRef]
19. Pilemann-Lyberg, S.; Rasmussen, D.G.K.; Hansen, T.W.; Tofte, N.; Winther, S.A.; Holm Nielsen, S.; Theilade, S.; Karsdal, M.A.; Genovese, F.; Rossing, P. Markers of Collagen Formation and Degradation Reflect Renal Function and Predict Adverse Outcomes in Patients with Type 1 Diabetes. *Diabetes Care* **2019**, *42*, 1760–1768. [CrossRef]
20. Gooch, J.L.; King, C.; Francis, C.E.; Garcia, P.S.; Bai, Y. Cyclosporine A alters expression of renal microRNAs: New insights into calcineurin inhibitor nephrotoxicity. *PLoS ONE* **2017**, *12*, e0175242. [CrossRef]
21. Sanchez-Pozos, K.; Lee-Montiel, F.; Perez-Villalva, R.; Uribe, N.; Gamba, G.; Bazan-Perkins, B.; Bobadilla, N.A. Polymerized type I collagen reduces chronic cyclosporine nephrotoxicity. *Nephrol. Dial. Transplant.* **2010**, *25*, 2150–2158. [CrossRef] [PubMed]
22. Slattery, C.; Campbell, E.; McMorrow, T.; Ryan, M.P. Cyclosporine A-Induced Renal Fibrosis. *Am. J. Pathol.* **2005**, *167*, 395–407. [CrossRef]
23. Bemelman, F.J.; de Fijter, J.W.; Kers, J.; Meyer, C.; Peters-Sengers, H.; de Maar, E.F.; van der Pant, K.A.M.I.; de Vries, A.P.J.; Sanders, J.-S.; Zwinderman, A.; et al. Early Conversion to Prednisolone/Everolimus as an Alternative Weaning Regimen Associates With Beneficial Renal Transplant Histology and Function: The Randomized-Controlled MECANO Trial. *Am. J. Transplant.* **2017**, *17*, 1020–1030. [CrossRef]
24. Bemelman, F.J.; de Maar, E.F.; Press, R.R.; van Kan, H.J.; ten Berge, I.J.; Homan van der Heide, J.J.; de Fijter, H.W. Minimization of Maintenance Immunosuppression Early After Renal Transplantation: An Interim Analysis. *Transplantation* **2009**, *88*, 421–428. [CrossRef]
25. Loupy, A.; Haas, M.; Solez, K.; Racusen, L.; Glotz, D.; Seron, D.; Nankivell, B.J.; Colvin, R.B.; Afrouzian, M.; Akalin, E.; et al. The Banff 2015 Kidney Meeting Report: Current Challenges in Rejection Classification and Prospects for Adopting Molecular Pathology. *Am. J. Transplant.* **2017**, *17*, 28–41. [CrossRef] [PubMed]

26. Mengel, M.; Reeve, J.; Bunnag, S.; Einecke, G.; Jhangri, G.S.; Sis, B.; Famulski, K.; Guembes-Hidalgo, L.; Halloran, P.F. Scoring Total Inflammation Is Superior to the Current Banff Inflammation Score in Predicting Outcome and the Degree of Molecular Disturbance in Renal Allografts. *Am. J. Transplant.* **2009**, *9*, 1859–1867. [CrossRef]
27. Sun, S.; Henriksen, K.; Karsdal, M.A.; Byrjalsen, I.; Rittweger, J.; Armbrecht, G.; Belavy, D.L.; Felsenberg, D.; Nedergaard, A.F. Collagen Type III and VI Turnover in Response to Long-Term Immobilization. *PLoS ONE* **2015**, *10*, e0144525. [CrossRef]
28. Bülow, R.D.; Boor, P. Extracellular Matrix in Kidney Fibrosis: More Than Just a Scaffold. *J. Histochem. Cytochem.* **2019**, *67*, 643–661. [CrossRef]
29. Nerlich, A.G.; Schleicher, E.D.; Wiest, I.; Specks, U.; Timpl, R. Immunohistochemical localization of collagen VI in diabetic glomeruli. *Kidney Int.* **1994**, *45*, 1648–1656. [CrossRef]
30. Wu, Q.; Jinde, K.; Nishina, M.; Tanabe, R.; Endoh, M.; Okada, Y.; Sakai, H.; Kurokawa, K. Analysis of prognostic predictors in idiopathic membranous nephropathy. *Am. J. Kidney Dis.* **2001**, *37*, 380–387. [CrossRef]
31. Knupp, C.; Pinali, C.; Munro, P.M.; Gruber, H.E.; Sherratt, M.J.; Baldock, C.; Squire, J.M. Structural correlation between collagen VI microfibrils and collagen VI banded aggregates. *J. Struct. Biol.* **2006**, *154*, 312–326. [CrossRef] [PubMed]
32. Boor, P.; Floege, J. Renal allograft fibrosis: Biology and therapeutic targets. *Am. J. Transplant.* **2015**, *15*, 863–886. [CrossRef] [PubMed]
33. Scian, M.J.; Maluf, D.G.; Archer, K.J.; Suh, J.L.; Massey, D.; Fassnacht, R.C.; Whitehill, B.; Sharma, A.; King, A.; Gehr, T.; et al. Gene expression changes are associated with loss of kidney graft function and interstitial fibrosis and tubular atrophy: Diagnosis versus prediction. *Transplantation* **2011**, *91*, 657–665. [CrossRef] [PubMed]
34. Busauschina, A.; Schnuelle, P.; van der Woude, F. Cyclosporine nephrotoxicity. *Transplant. Proc.* **2004**, *36*, S229–S233. [CrossRef] [PubMed]
35. Fitzgerald, J.; Holden, P.; Hansen, U. The expanded collagen VI family: New chains and new questions. *Connect. Tissue Res.* **2013**, *54*, 345–350. [CrossRef] [PubMed]

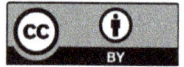

© 2020 by the authors. Licensee MDPI, Basel, Switzerland. This article is an open access article distributed under the terms and conditions of the Creative Commons Attribution (CC BY) license (http://creativecommons.org/licenses/by/4.0/).

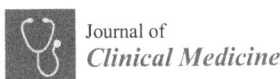 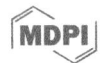

Article

Robot-Assisted versus Laparoscopic Donor Nephrectomy: A Comparison of 250 Cases

Philip Zeuschner [1], Linda Hennig [2], Robert Peters [2], Matthias Saar [1], Johannes Linxweiler [1], Stefan Siemer [1], Ahmed Magheli [3], Jürgen Kramer [3], Lutz Liefeldt [4], Klemens Budde [4], Thorsten Schlomm [2], Michael Stöckle [1,†] and Frank Friedersdorff [2,*,†]

1. Department of Urology and Pediatric Urology, Saarland University, Kirrberger Street 100, 66421 Homburg/Saar, Germany; philip.zeuschner@uks.eu (P.Z.); matthias.saar@uks.eu (M.S.); johannes.linxweiler@uks.eu (J.L.); stefan.siemer@uks.eu (S.S.); michael.stoeckle@uks.eu (M.S.)
2. Department of Urology, Charité-Universitätsmedizin Berlin, Corporate Member of Freie Universität Berlin, Humbold-Universität zu Berlin, and Berlin Institute of Health, Charitéplatz 1, 10117 Berlin, Germany; linda.hennig@charite.de (L.H.); robert.peters@charite.de (R.P.); thorsten.schlomm@charite.de (T.S.)
3. Department of Urology, Klinikum am Urban, 10967 Berlin, Germany; ahmed.magheli@vivantes.de (A.M.); juergen.kramer@vivantes.de (J.K.)
4. Department of Nephrology, Charité-Universitätsmedizin Berlin, Corporate Member of Freie Universität Berlin, Humbold-Universität zu Berlin, and Berlin Institute of Health, Charitéplatz 1, 10117 Berlin, Germany; lutz.liefeldt@charite.de (L.L.); klemens.budde@charite.de (K.B.)
* Correspondence: frank.friedersdorff@charite.de
† These authors contributed equally.

Received: 28 April 2020; Accepted: 22 May 2020; Published: 26 May 2020

Abstract: Living kidney donation is the best treatment for end-stage renal disease, however, the best surgical approach for minimally-invasive donor nephrectomy (DN) is still a matter of debate. This bi-centric study aimed to retrospectively compare perioperative outcomes and postoperative kidney function after 257 transperitoneal DNs including 52 robot-assisted (RDN) and 205 laparoscopic DNs (LDN). As primary outcomes, the intraoperative (operating time, warm ischemia time (WIT), major complications) and postoperative (length of stay, complications) results were compared. As secondary outcomes, postoperative kidney and graft function were analyzed including delayed graft function (DGF) rates, and the impact of the surgical approach was assessed. Overall, the type of minimally-invasive donor nephrectomy (RDN vs. LDN) did not affect primary outcomes, especially not operating time and WIT; and major complication and DGF rates were low in both groups. A history of smoking and preoperative kidney function, but not the surgical approach, were predictive for postoperative serum creatinine of the donor and recipient. To conclude, RDN and LDN have equivalent perioperative results in experienced centers. For this reason, not the surgical approach, but rather the graft- (preoperative kidney function) and patient-specific (history of smoking) aspects impacted postoperative kidney function.

Keywords: minimally-invasive donor nephrectomy; robot-assisted surgery; laparoscopic surgery; kidney transplantation; organ donation; living kidney donation

1. Introduction

Living kidney donation is the ultimate treatment for end-stage renal disease (ESRD) [1]. Since the first successful living kidney donation in 1955 was carried out by Murray et al., many advances in surgical techniques and immunosuppressive therapy have led to substantial improvements in life expectancy and quality of life, not only for kidney recipients, but also for kidney donors [2]. In particular, minimally-invasive approaches for donor nephrectomy (DN) have increased the incidence of living kidney donation since the first laparoscopic DN (LDN) in 1995 and the first robot-assisted DN (RDN) in 2000 [3–5]. Unfortunately, higher donation rates have not been able to compensate for higher demand, which has led to at least 120,000 patients worldwide waiting for a kidney transplant today.

Many variations of minimally-invasive DN techniques have been described so far. Apart from hand-assisted methods as a bridge to open surgery, DN has also been performed in a retroperitoneoscopic (hand-assisted) manner [6,7]. In line with shorter flank incisions for open DN ("minimally invasive" open DN), Gill et al. conducted the first LDN via a LESS approach (laparoendoscopic single site surgery) in 2008 and inserted all trocars through the umbilicus [8,9]. Others have even tried to perform DN as a NOTES (natural orifice transluminal endoscopic surgery), and Pietrabissa et al. were the first to report a transvaginal extraction of the kidney after RDN in 2010 [10]. Today, some high-volume centers have performed more than 100 RDNs or LESS single-port RDNs, and employ specialized robotic single-site platforms [11,12]. However, the robotic approach still accounts for less than 5% of all minimally-invasive DNs, with increasing incidence compared to conventional transperitoneal LDN at more than 50% [13].

Irrespective of this magnitude of variations, minimally-invasive approaches for donor nephrectomy represent the standard of care, and are recommended as "the preferential technique", according to the current guidelines for renal transplantation of the European Association of Urology (EAU) [14,15]. Multiple studies have shown that LDN is superior to open DN (ODN) in terms of hospital stay or postoperative pain, but the operating and warm ischemia time (WIT) are longer [16]. Importantly, LDN is not inferior in terms of complication rates, short- and long-term graft function. On the other hand, when comparing LDN with the robotic approach, RDN appears to have even less postoperative pain and less blood loss, but a longer WIT and operating time [17]. Nonetheless, analyses of cohorts with big sample sizes are still lacking, and the high variability of minimally-invasive DN renders it difficult to draw direct conclusions.

With this in mind, we conducted a retrospective bi-centric comparison of transperitoneal LDN with RDN and included more than 250 interventions. We aimed to compare perioperative outcomes as well as short- and mid-term kidney function of the donor and recipient up to four years after surgery. Alongside sub-analyses controlling for inherent learning, regression analyses to predict postoperative kidney and graft function were performed. All LDNs were conducted at the largest German kidney transplant program run by a urologic department that has been performing LDNs since 1999. All RDNs including the very first RDN in Germany in 2007, were performed at a urologic department highly specialized in robotic surgery [18].

2. Materials and Methods

In total, 257 DNs performed at two tertiary referral centers were retrospectively analyzed. All 205 LDNs were conducted by 11 surgeons with a median caseload of 11 (range 2–43) at a urologic department specialized in laparoscopic kidney surgery including LDNs. The 52 RDNs were performed at another urologic department, which is specialized in robotic surgery in general. All RDNs were conducted by five surgeons with a median caseload of 10 (range 2–29). The interventions were performed in a transperitoneal fashion between 2007–2020 (RDN) and 2011–2016 (LDN).

At the robotic department, the very first RDN in Germany was conducted [18]. Before 2007, all donor nephrectomies had been held in an open fashion, so none of the robotic surgeons had prior expertise in LDN, but in a large variety of other robotic interventions. Thereafter, DN was standardized to a robot-assisted approach. The other department in this study has been performing LDNs since 1999. Both departments always conducted DNs in a minimally-invasive fashion during the study period, unless the donor had a significant amount of prior abdominal surgeries and consequently high risk for conversion. The corresponding kidney transplantations were held in an open fashion, except for the last 18 (34.6%) cases at the robotic department. As a part of the EAU-RAKT working group (European Association of Urology working group for robotic kidney transplantation), the first RAKT in Germany was performed there in June 2016 [19,20]. From then, all RDNs were followed by RAKTs.

This entire analysis was conducted in adherence with the correct scientific research work terms of the Charité Medical University of Berlin and Saarland University including full anonymization of patient data. All the patients included in the analysis provided written informed consent.

2.1. Surgical Technique

All RDNs were performed using a transperitoneal approach, with either a DaVinci® Si or X system with four arms. The ports were placed pararectally. For the first RDNs, the graft was removed in a hand-assisted manner without a specimen bag via a Pfannenstiel incision, and later on via a periumbilically placed GelPOINT® trocar (Applied Medical, Los Angeles, CA, USA). For LDN, the approach was purely laparoscopic, without the hand-assisted technique, which has been described previously [21,22]. In brief, four ports were used, and the kidney was extracted through an enlarged lateral trocar incision measuring 5 to 6 cm.

2.2. Data Collection and Outcome Measures

For the donor characteristics, age, gender, body mass index (BMI, kg/m^2), pre-existing arterial hypertension, diabetes, and history of smoking were obtained. The graft's side, scintigraphic split-renal function (DTPA), and number of arteries and veins served as organ-specific factors. For the recipient characteristics, age, gender, BMI, implantation side, and individual number of prior kidney transplantations were obtained.

Intraoperative (operating time, WIT, complications) and postoperative (length of stay, major postoperative complications based on Clavien–Dindo grade ≥ 3 within 30 days after surgery) results were analyzed as *primary outcomes*. The comparison and prediction of postoperative kidney function of the donor and of the recipient up to four years after transplantation served as *secondary outcomes*. Delayed graft function (DGF), defined as dialysis within one week after transplantation or insufficient serum creatinine decline not below 2 mg/dL, was analyzed as a further kidney-related secondary outcome.

2.3. Statistical Analysis

Primary and secondary outcomes were compared between the LDN and RDN group. To assess whether perioperative outcome was affected by an inherent learning curve, both groups were split in half and the outcomes were compared within each group. The first 34 (65.4%) RDNs were followed by an open transplantation, but the last 18 (34.6%) were followed by a robot-assisted kidney transplantation. To ensure that RAKT did not affect the perioperative results of RDN, the last 18 RDNs were excluded in another sub-analysis. The impact of patient-, graft- or surgery-specific factors on postoperative kidney function of the donor at discharge was assessed by linear regression analysis. To predict kidney function of the recipient one week after surgery, donor and recipient characteristics, DN, and transplantation-specific aspects were included in another uni- and multivariate regression analysis.

Categorical variables were reported as frequencies and proportions, and continuous data as the median and range. Fisher's exact test and the Mann–Whitney U test were used to compare between groups. Covariates were included in the multiple regression analysis only if their respective effect was significant in the univariate analysis. The statistical analysis was performed by SPSS version 25 with Fix pack 2 installed (IBM, Armonk, NY, USA). All tests were two-sided, and p-values < 0.05 were considered significant.

3. Results

3.1. Overall Results: Primary Outcomes

In the RDN and LDN groups, most kidney donors were female (63–68%), 51–54 years old, and had a BMI of 25.4–25.9 (see Table 1). Donor characteristics only differed concerning the individual history of smoking, as there were more smokers in the LDN group (52.7 vs. 9.6%, $p < 0.001$). Donor organs were 20% right-sided and had a split-renal function of 50%. The number of organs with multiple arteries was no different between RDN and LDN (11.5% vs. 18.5%), but significantly more grafts in the LDN group had multiple veins (12.7% vs. none, $p < 0.01$). The groups did not differ regarding recipient characteristics. Most were male (67–70%), 42–45 years old, and had a BMI of 24.7–25.3. For more than 90% of recipients, it was their first kidney transplantation.

Table 1. Comparison of donor, graft, and recipient characteristics.

	RDN (n = 52)	LDN (n = 205)	p-Value
donor			
age (yr)	54 (20; 70)	51 (21; 78)	n.s.
male gender	16 (30.8%)	75 (36.6%)	n.s.
BMI (kg/m^2)	25.4 (17.6; 36.7)	25.9 (17.6; 36.1)	n.s.
pre-existing hypertension	15 (28.8%)	44 (21.5%)	n.s.
diabetes	1 (1.9%)	3 (1.5%)	n.s.
history of smoking	5 (9.6%)	108 (52.7%)	<0.001
graft			
right side	11 (21.2%)	45 (22%)	n.s.
multiple arteries	6 (11.5%)	38 (18.5%)	n.s.
multiple veins	0	26 (12.7%)	<0.01
scintigraphic function	50% (39; 57)	50% (38; 58)	n.s.
recipient			
age (yr)	42 (18; 66)	45 (6; 76)	n.s.
male gender	35 (67.3%)	144 (70.2%)	n.s.
BMI (kg/m^2)	25.1 (17.6; 37)	24.7 (16.8; 40.8)	n.s.
side left	8 (15.4%)	46 (22.4%)	n.s.
first transplantation	48 (92.3%)	187 (91.2%)	n.s.

Concerning primary outcomes, neither the median operating time (RDN 223.5 vs. LDN 213 min), WIT (3 vs. 2.45 min), nor intraoperative complication rate (5.7 vs. 2.9%) were significantly different between groups (see Table 2). One RDN had to be converted to open surgery because of massive obesity and multiple trocar dislocations. In two other cases, a malfunction of the stapler and a lumbal vein caused bleeding, which could be managed robotically without the need for blood transfusions. In the LDN group, in one case, bleeding from a dorsal branch of the renal vein could not be controlled laparoscopically, leading to a conversion to open surgery. In another LDN case, the renal vein was torn during kidney removal, but could be reconstructed. Once, the donor's spleen and the renal parenchyma were accidentally cut, and a small hole in the descending colon had to be sutured. A previously undetected obstructed ureteropelvic junction made one pyelovesicostomy necessary for a recipient in the LDN group.

The median length of stay of five days was no different between the LDN and RDN groups, nor was the postoperative major complication rate. In the RDN group, one patient had an ileus that dissolved after gastroscopy. In the LDN group, a bronchoscopy had to be performed because of dyspnea, and a retention of chylous ascites had to be punctured. In another case, continuous arterial bleeding from the abdominal internal oblique muscle made electrocoagulation necessary in the LDN group.

3.2. Learning Curve

When comparing the first half of the RDNs with the second half to analyze for inherent learning effects, the WIT, intra- and postoperative complication rate, and length of stay remained unchanged (see Table 3). Operating time significantly increased from 185 to 265 min in the RDN group ($p < 0.001$). This difference no longer remained significant when the last 18 RDN cases were excluded; in these cases, RDN was followed by robot-assisted kidney transplantation (185 vs. 226 min, n.s.). In the LDN group, the surgical results remained unchanged over time.

Table 2. Outcomes of 257 donor nephrectomies.

	RDN (n = 52)	LDN (n = 205)	p-Value
Intraoperative			
operating time (min)	223.5 (127; 363)	213 (120; 392)	n.s.
WIT (min)	3 (0.5; 1)	2.45 (0.4; 5.27)	n.s.
complications	3 (5.7%)	6 (2.9%)	n.s.
conversions	1 (1.9%)	1 (0.5%)	n.s.
postoperative			
length of stay (d)	5 (2; 12)	5 (3; 18)	n.s.
Clavien–Dindo			n.s.
grade 3	1 (1.9%)	1 (0.5%)	n.s.
grade 4	-	2 (1%)	n.s.
grade 5	-	-	n.s.
recipient			
DGF	6 (11.5%)	13 (6.3%)	n.s.

Table 3. Assessment for the inherent learning curves in RDN and LDN by comparing the first with the second half of cases within each group.

	RDN			LDN		
	1st half (n = 26)	2nd half (n = 26)	p	1st half (n = 102)	2nd half (n = 103)	p
Intraoperative						
operating time	185 (148; 284)	265 (127; 363)	<0.001 [1]	213 (135; 392)	216 (120; 363)	n.s.
WIT (min)	3 (0.5; 9)	2 (1; 10)	n.s.	2.4 (0.4; 5)	2.5 (0.5; 5.2)	n.s.
complications	2 (7.7%)	1 (3.8%)	n.s.	3 (2.9%)	3 (2.9%)	n.s.
conversions	1 (3.8%)	-	n.s.	-	1 (0.9%)	n.s.
postoperative						
length of stay (d)	5 (3–12)	5 (2–7)	n.s.	5 (3; 18)	5 (3; 11)	n.s.
Clavien–Dindo	0 (0; 2)	0 (0)	n.s.	0 (0; 4)	0 (0; 4)	n.s.
grade 3	1 (3.8%)	-	n.s.	1 (1%)	-	n.s.
grade 4	-	-	n.s.	1 (1%)	1 (1%)	n.s.
grade 5	-	-	n.s.	-	-	n.s.
recipient						
DGF	4 (15.4%)	2 (7.7%)	n.s.	6 (5.9%)	7 (6.8%)	n.s.

[1] When excluding the last 18 cases, where RDN was followed by robot-assisted kidney transplantation, the difference was no longer significant (185 vs. 226 min, n.s.).

3.3. Kidney Function of the Donor and Recipient: Secondary Outcomes

The type of surgical approach of DN did not impact the postoperative kidney function either of the donor or the recipient (see Figure 1). Among the donors, kidney function did not differ preoperatively or at discharge between groups. For recipients, kidney function significantly improved after transplantation, irrespective of the type of DN, and stayed stable thereafter.

DGF rates were 6.3 to 11.5% (LDN vs. RDN), and did not significantly differ between groups and did not change over time (see Tables 2 and 3). In the RDN group, DGF was caused by three (5.7%) suspected transplant renal artery stenoses, one (1.9%) perirenal hematoma due to double anticoagulation of the mechanic aortic valve and prolonged serum creatinine decline (no dialysis needed), one (1.9%) prolonged CIT (cold ischemia time) due to vascular complications during transplantation, and one (1.9%) insufficient serum creatinine decline without other cause. In the LDN group, DGF resulted from seven (3.4%) acute rejections, one (0.5%) lesion of the arterial anastomosis after the Fogarty maneuver, and one (0.5%) case of donor-related pre-existing vascular damage. One (0.5%) patient needed dialysis for depletion of potassium only, and in three (1.5%) other cases, the cause for DGF in the LDN group was unknown.

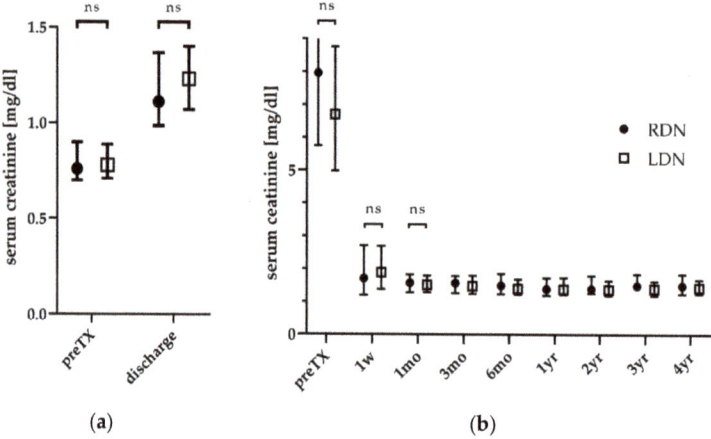

(a) (b)

Figure 1. Follow-up of kidney function of the donor (a) and graft (b). The kidney function did not differ between robot-assisted (RDN) and laparoscopic donor nephrectomy (LDN).

In the multivariate regression analysis, only patient-specific factors were found to have an impact on postoperative kidney function, but not surgical factors (see Table 4). Concerning the kidney function of the donor at discharge, male patient gender was predictive for worse kidney function (B-value 0.14, $p < 0.001$). Furthermore, worse preoperative kidney function was associated with worse postoperative function (B-value 1.0, $p < 0.001$). A history of smoking only had an impact on postoperative kidney function in the univariate analysis. No other (surgical) factors such as approach (LDN vs. RDN), operating time, intraoperative complications, WIT, kidney side, or number of arteries or veins, had an impact on the kidney function of the donor at discharge.

Table 4. Multivariable regression analysis to predict the serum creatinine (1) of the donor at discharge ("donor kidney function") or (2) of the recipient one week after transplantation ("graft function").

Variable	B-Value	p-Value
donor kidney function		
gender	0.14 (0.09; 0.19)	<0.001
preTX serum creatinine	1.00 (0.82; 1.18)	<0.001
surgical approach	-	n.s.
graft function		
smoking donor	0.63 (1.21; 0.05)	<0.05
preemptive Tx	-	n.s.
preTX serum creatinine	0.22 (0.12; 0.31)	<0.001
surgical approach	-	n.s.

A history of donor smoking also had a significant impact on the kidney function of the recipient in the multivariate regression analysis: a kidney donor with a history of smoking caused worse graft function one week after transplantation (B-value 0.63, $p < 0.05$, see Table 4). Again, the preoperative kidney function of the recipient was predictive for their postoperative graft function (B-value 0.22, $p < 0.001$). In the univariate, but not the multivariate analysis, a preemptive kidney transplantation predicted better graft function (B-value −0.72, $p < 0.05$). Again, no surgical factors, either the type of donor nephrectomy (LDN vs. RDN) or the type of transplantation (open vs. robot-assisted), had an impact on graft function one week after transplantation.

4. Discussion

In this bi-centric study, a comparison of 257 minimally-invasive donor nephrectomies with 205 laparoscopic and 52 robot-assisted DNs was conducted. Of note, this analysis included the very first RDN in Germany, and all LDNs were performed at a urologic department where LDNs have been conducted since 1999 [18].

Concerning the primary outcomes, operating time was no different between RDN and LDN (223.5 vs. 213 min, see Table 1). Most studies describe shorter operating times for LDNs, but report highly variable results [17]. Mean operating times for RDNs range from 144 to 306 min [23,24], and for LDNs between 178 and 270 min [25,26], even when only studies with cohorts larger than 100 patients are included. These differences could result from inherent learning curves: Horgan et al. and Janki et al. have shown that operating times in RDN shorten with growing expertise [27,28]. Interestingly, our data do not show an inherent learning effect, either in the RDN or in the LDN cohort. Outcomes remained unchanged over time (see Table 3). Conversely, operating time became significantly longer within the second half of the RDNs (185 vs. 265 min, $p < 0.001$).

This counterintuitive development resulted from the way transplantations were organized, as both institutions perform DNs and transplantations in different operating rooms simultaneously, but not sequentially. Two surgical teams work in parallel, but the graft is not removed unless the transplantation team is ready, to avoid long cold ischemia times. The RDN cohort not only comprised the first RDN, but also the first robot-assisted kidney transplantation in Germany (procedure #35) [18,20]. Operating times in the RDN cohort became longer from that point, as the learning curve for RAKTs had not yet been passed. Naturally, the RDN team started more than 30 min before the transplantation team, but RAKT proved to be much more challenging and time-consuming. When excluding the last 18 cases, when RDN was followed by RAKT, the operating times of the RDNs did not change over time. Thus, the obvious lack of a typical learning curve illustrates that for LDNs, the learning curve had already been passed and for RDNs, significant prior expertise in robotic surgery made it possible to reach stable results from the start [29].

As with the operating time, WIT was not different between RDNs and LDNs (3 vs. 2.45 min). In the RDNs, most grafts were extracted via a GelPOINT® trocar (Applied Medical, Los Angeles, CA, USA), which is an easy and fast, yet expensive method. Wang et al. illustrated significantly longer WIT for RDNs than LDNs in their meta-analysis, which is an often-stated argument against RDNs [17,30]. However, it is unlikely that differences of 30 or 60 s in WIT will harm the graft function in the long-, mid- or even short-term. It has clearly been shown that a WIT longer than 45 min impairs graft survival in living kidney donation [31]. Fortunately, neither our results nor those from other studies have documented WIT longer than 15 min for RDNs, keeping in mind that the consecutive CIT is again followed by another WIT during transplantation.

Intraoperative complication rates were low in both RDNs (5.7%) and LDNs (2.9%), and did not significantly differ. In line with others, most intraoperative complications were bleedings, whereof one in the LDN group made a conversion to open surgery necessary, but none in the RDN group [17]. In contrast, a patient with massive obesity had multiple trocar dislocations within the first minutes of surgery, so the RDN had to be converted to open surgery. Due to a technical defect of the stapler system for one patient in the RDN group, which made it cut but not staple, locking Hem-o-Lok clips were predominantly used later on, as described elsewhere [32]. During LDNs, Hem-o-Lok and titanium clips are used for the renal artery, a stapler for the right vein, and two Hem-o-Lok clips for the left vein. Not only intraoperative but also postoperative complication rates, according to Clavien–Dindo, were low and did not differ between LDN and RDN. Therefore, both surgical approaches had equivalent complication rates, while LDN has less costs, but RDN appears to be superior in complex situations such as bleedings.

The kidney donors were discharged five days after DN, irrespective of the type of surgery (see Table 2). Consequently, the median length of stay was longer than in most other works, ranging from 2–3 days for LDNs and RDNs [11,17,24]. This can be attributed to differences in national health care systems as (i) the German reimbursement system covers a longer hospital stay and (ii) most donors wanted to stay longer as inpatients for psychological reasons. In fact, only 15 (5.8%) patients were discharged two or three days after DN. Early discharge after RDN and LDN is possible from a surgical point of view, however, it has not been a crucial parameter for our perioperative approach, as long as neither patient satisfaction nor health care costs are affected.

As a secondary outcome, the impact of the surgical approach on postoperative kidney function was assessed. Kidney donors had a worse kidney function at discharge, which was comparable between groups and similar to results found in other studies (RDN 1.1 mg/dL vs. LDN 1.23 mg/dL; see Figure 1) [28,33]. Correspondingly, the preoperative kidney function, but not the type of surgical approach for DN, was predictive for the postoperative kidney function of the donor at discharge (see Table 4). Interestingly, patient gender also had a significant impact on postoperative kidney function. However, this should not be over-interpreted, as male kidney donors had a worse kidney function than women, with higher serum creatinine values preoperatively (0.9 vs. 0.72 mg/dL, $p < 0.001$) and postoperatively (1.42 vs. 1.1 mg/dL, $p < 0.001$) in this analysis. For this reason, (male) patient gender was predictive for (worse) postoperative kidney function; this may not be representative for other cohorts.

Similarly, Benoit et al. created a model to predict 1-year postoperative renal function of kidney donors after LDN, which has been externally validated [34,35]. The authors predicted postoperative eGFR by preoperative eGFR and patient age (postoperative eGFR = 31.71 + (0.5 × preoperative eGFR) − 0.314 × age at donation). In our model, patient age was not predictive for postoperative kidney function, potentially because we evaluated the short-term kidney function at discharge and not one year after DN.

Concerning recipients, the DGF rates of 6.3% (LDN) and 11.5% (RDN) did not significantly differ between groups. In general, there is a large variety of reported DGF rates in living kidney donation, ranging from 4 to 10% [36,37]. This not only results from center-specific differences, but also from inconsistent definitions: DGF can be defined by urine output per day, serum creatinine decline, or the need for dialysis after transplantation [36]. We applied a considerably broad definition for DGF (postoperative dialysis within one week after transplantation for any cause or insufficient creatinine decrease not below 2 mg/dL). DGF rates in the RDN group were 11.5% due to transplantation-related surgical, mainly vascular causes. One (1.9%) patient with a mechanic aortic valve developed a perirenal hematoma, causing prolonged creatinine decline without the need for dialysis. In the LDN group, DGF was mainly caused by acute rejections (3.4%), and also comprised one patient (0.5%) who required dialysis for potassium depletion only. Consequently, DGF did not result from the type of DN, but rather transplantation-specific causes.

Regardless, the kidney function of the recipients significantly improved after transplantation, and did not differ between groups during follow-up (see Figure 1). In the multiple regression analysis, not only the preoperative kidney function of the recipient, but also a history of donor smoking, had a significant impact on graft function one week after transplantation (see Table 4). Smoking is a well-known modifiable risk factor for the development of chronic and end-stage kidney disease [38,39]. A history of donor smoking has a negative impact not only on the survival of the donor, but also of the recipient [40]. In our cohort, a positive history of donor smoking increased serum creatinine one week after transplantation by 0.63 mg/dL. This highlights, again, the importance of informing not only transplant patients, but also potential kidney donors, about the risks of tobacco use, and the importance of helping patients to stop smoking.

This analysis is not devoid of limitations. As a bi-centric study, experienced but different surgeons and different teams conducted the RDNs and LDNs. Patient cohorts did not significantly differ in terms of characteristics, but were not equally balanced in terms of caseload. Although surgical results were not affected by inherent learning curves, at least the results in the RDN group were affected by simultaneous robot-assisted kidney transplantation. This procedural aspect highlights the complexity of comparing minimally-invasive donor nephrectomies: the surgical part itself is in high demand, but the high variability of the technical, procedural, and underlying ethical aspects also have to be taken into account [41].

5. Conclusions

Minimally-invasive surgical techniques have increased the acceptance of living kidney donation, but its high variability renders head-to-head comparisons of surgical approaches a complex task. In this bi-centric study, we compared more than 250 cases of 52 transperitoneal robotic DNs with 205 laparoscopic DNs. Operating time and length of stay were no different between groups, but slightly longer than elsewhere, as DNs and transplantations were conducted simultaneously to reduce CIT, and most other national health systems do not allow longer inpatient stays. Other perioperative results (complication rates, WIT) and mid-term kidney function including DGF rates were comparable with published data, and did not differ between RDN and LDN. This was possible because both centers already had prior expertise in either LDN itself or robotic surgery in general. For this reason, patient-specific factors (preoperative kidney function, history of donor smoking) were the more relevant impacts upon donor and graft function.

Author Contributions: P.Z., F.F., and M.S. (Michael Stöckle) designed the study; P.Z. analyzed the data and wrote the manuscript; L.H., R.P., M.S. (Matthias Saar), J.L., S.S., A.M., J.K., L.L., K.B., T.S., F.F., and M.S. (Michael Stöckle) drafted and revised the paper. All authors approved the final version of the manuscript.

Funding: This research received no external funding.

Acknowledgments: We would like to thank the working group for kidney transplantation ("Arbeitskreis Nierentransplantation", https://www.nieren-transplantation.com/) of the German Association of Urology for initiating this bi-centric work.

Conflicts of Interest: The authors declare no conflicts of interest.

References

1. Shapiro, R. End-stage renal disease in 2010: Innovative approaches to improve outcomes in transplantation. *Nat. Rev. Nephrol.* **2011**, *7*, 68–70. [CrossRef] [PubMed]
2. Murray, J.E.; Merrill, J.P.; Harrison, J.H. Renal homotransplantation in identical twins. *J. Am. Soc. Nephrol. JASN* **2001**, *12*, 201–204. [PubMed]
3. Schweitzer, E.J.; Wilson, J.; Jacobs, S.; Machan, C.H.; Philosophe, B.; Farney, A.; Colonna, J.; Jarrell, B.E.; Bartlett, S.T. Increased rates of donation with laparoscopic donor nephrectomy. *Ann. Surg.* **2000**, *232*, 392–400. [CrossRef] [PubMed]
4. Ratner, L.E.; Ciseck, L.J.; Moore, R.G.; Cigarroa, F.G.; Kaufman, H.S.; Kavoussi, L.R. Laparoscopic live donor nephrectomy. *Transplantation* **1995**, *60*, 1047–1049.
5. Pfaffl, M.W.; Horgan, G.W.; Dempfle, L. Relative expression software tool (REST) for group-wise comparison and statistical analysis of relative expression results in real-time PCR. *Nucleic Acids Res.* **2002**, *30*, e36. [CrossRef]
6. Wolf, J.S., Jr.; Tchetgen, M.B.; Merion, R.M. Hand-assisted laparoscopic live donor nephrectomy. *Urology* **1998**, *52*, 885–887. [CrossRef]
7. Wadstrom, J.; Lindstrom, P. Hand-assisted retroperitoneoscopic living-donor nephrectomy: Initial 10 cases. *Transplantation* **2002**, *73*, 1839–1840. [CrossRef]
8. Gill, I.S.; Canes, D.; Aron, M.; Haber, G.P.; Goldfarb, D.A.; Flechner, S.; Desai, M.R.; Kaouk, J.H.; Desai, M.M. Single port transumbilical (E-NOTES) donor nephrectomy. *J. Urol.* **2008**, *180*, 637–641, discussion 641. [CrossRef]

9. Janki, S.; Dor, F.J.; JN, I.J. Surgical aspects of live kidney donation: An updated review. *Front. Biosci.* **2015**, *7*, 346–365. [CrossRef]
10. Pietrabissa, A.; Abelli, M.; Spinillo, A.; Alessiani, M.; Zonta, S.; Ticozzelli, E.; Peri, A.; Dal Canton, A.; Dionigi, P. Robotic-assisted laparoscopic donor nephrectomy with transvaginal extraction of the kidney. *Am. J. Transplant.* **2010**, *10*, 2708–2711. [CrossRef]
11. LaMattina, J.C.; Alvarez-Casas, J.; Lu, I.; Powell, J.M.; Sultan, S.; Phelan, M.W.; Barth, R.N. Robotic-assisted single-port donor nephrectomy using the da Vinci single-site platform. *J. Surg. Res.* **2018**, *222*, 34–38. [CrossRef] [PubMed]
12. Tzvetanov, I.; Bejarano-Pineda, L.; Giulianotti, P.C.; Jeon, H.; Garcia-Roca, R.; Bianco, F.; Oberholzer, J.; Benedetti, E. State of the art of robotic surgery in organ transplantation. *World J. Surg.* **2013**, *37*, 2791–2799. [CrossRef] [PubMed]
13. Kortram, K.; Ijzermans, J.N.; Dor, F.J. Perioperative Events and Complications in Minimally Invasive Live Donor Nephrectomy: A Systematic Review and Meta-Analysis. *Transplantation* **2016**, *100*, 2264–2275. [CrossRef] [PubMed]
14. Abramowicz, D.; Cochat, P.; Claas, F.H.; Heemann, U.; Pascual, J.; Dudley, C.; Harden, P.; Hourmant, M.; Maggiore, U.; Salvadori, M.; et al. European Renal Best Practice Guideline on kidney donor and recipient evaluation and perioperative care. *Nephrol. Dial. Transplant.* **2015**, *30*, 1790–1797. [CrossRef]
15. Breda, A.; Budde, K.; Figueiredo, A.; Lledó García, E.; Olsburgh, J.; Regele, H.; Boissier, R.; Taylor, C.F.; Hevia, V.; Faba, O.R.; et al. *EAU Guidelines on Renal Transplantation*; EAU Guidelines Office: Arnhem, The Netherlands, 2020; ISBN 978-94-92671-07-3.
16. Wilson, C.H.; Sanni, A.; Rix, D.A.; Soomro, N.A. Laparoscopic versus open nephrectomy for live kidney donors. *Cochrane Database Syst. Rev.* **2011**, CD006124. [CrossRef] [PubMed]
17. Wang, H.; Chen, R.; Li, T.; Peng, L. Robot-assisted laparoscopic vs laparoscopic donor nephrectomy in renal transplantation: A meta-analysis. *Clin. Transplant.* **2019**, *33*, e13451. [CrossRef] [PubMed]
18. Janssen, M.S.U.; Kopper, B.; Gerber, M.; Ohlmann, C.-H.; Akcetin, Z.; Kamradt, D.; Siemer, S.; Stöckle, M. Lectures: 088 Robotic-assisted donor nephrectomy for living donor kidney transplantation—Results of the first series in Germany. *Transplant. Int.* **2011**, *24*, 3–24. [CrossRef]
19. Territo, A.; Gausa, L.; Alcaraz, A.; Musquera, M.; Doumerc, N.; Decaestecker, K.; Desender, L.; Stockle, M.; Janssen, M.; Fornara, P.; et al. European experience of robot-assisted kidney transplantation: Minimum of 1-year follow-up. *BJU Int.* **2018**, *122*, 255–262. [CrossRef] [PubMed]
20. Zeuschner, P.; Siemer, S.; Stockle, M. Robot-assisted kidney transplantation. *Urol. A* **2020**, *59*, 3–9. [CrossRef] [PubMed]
21. Turk, I.A.; Deger, S.; Davis, J.W.; Giesing, M.; Fabrizio, M.D.; Schonberger, B.; Jordan, G.H.; Loening, S.A. Laparoscopic live donor right nephrectomy: A new technique with preservation of vascular length. *J. Urol.* **2002**, *167*, 630–633. [CrossRef]
22. Giessing, M.; Deger, S.; Schonberger, B.; Turk, I.; Loening, S.A. Laparoscopic living donor nephrectomy: From alternative to standard procedure. *Transplant. Proc.* **2003**, *35*, 2093–2095. [CrossRef]
23. Cohen, A.J.; Williams, D.S.; Bohorquez, H.; Bruce, D.S.; Carmody, I.C.; Reichman, T.; Loss, G.E., Jr. Robotic-assisted laparoscopic donor nephrectomy: Decreasing length of stay. *Ochsner J.* **2015**, *15*, 19–24. [PubMed]
24. Serrano, O.K.; Kirchner, V.; Bangdiwala, A.; Vock, D.M.; Dunn, T.B.; Finger, E.B.; Payne, W.D.; Pruett, T.L.; Sutherland, D.E.; Najarian, J.S.; et al. Evolution of Living Donor Nephrectomy at a Single Center: Long-term Outcomes With 4 Different Techniques in Greater Than 4000 Donors Over 50 Years. *Transplantation* **2016**, *100*, 1299–1305. [CrossRef] [PubMed]
25. Basiri, A.; Simforoosh, N.; Heidari, M.; Moghaddam, S.M.; Otookesh, H. Laparoscopic v open donor nephrectomy for pediatric kidney recipients: Preliminary report of a randomized controlled trial. *J. Endourol.* **2007**, *21*, 1033–1036. [CrossRef] [PubMed]
26. Simforoosh, N.; Basiri, A.; Tabibi, A.; Shakhssalim, N.; Hosseini Moghaddam, S.M. Comparison of laparoscopic and open donor nephrectomy: A randomized controlled trial. *BJU Int.* **2005**, *95*, 851–855. [CrossRef] [PubMed]
27. Horgan, S.; Galvani, C.; Gorodner, M.V.; Jacobsen, G.R.; Moser, F.; Manzelli, A.; Oberholzer, J.; Fisichella, M.P.; Bogetti, D.; Testa, G.; et al. Effect of robotic assistance on the "learning curve" for laparoscopic hand-assisted donor nephrectomy. *Surg. Endosc.* **2007**, *21*, 1512–1517. [CrossRef] [PubMed]

28. Janki, S.; Klop, K.W.J.; Hagen, S.M.; Terkivatan, T.; Betjes, M.G.H.; Tran, T.C.K.; Ijzermans, J.N.M. Robotic surgery rapidly and successfully implemented in a high volume laparoscopic center on living kidney donation. *Int. J. Med. Robot.* **2017**, *13*. [CrossRef]
29. Friedersdorff, F.; Werthemann, P.; Cash, H.; Kempkensteffen, C.; Magheli, A.; Hinz, S.; Waiser, J.; Liefeldt, L.; Miller, K.; Deger, S.; et al. Outcomes after laparoscopic living donor nephrectomy: Comparison of two laparoscopic surgeons with different levels of expertise. *BJU Int.* **2013**, *111*, 95–100. [CrossRef]
30. Kawan, F.; Theil, G.; Fornara, P. Robotic Donor Nephrectomy: Against. *Eur. Urol. Focus* **2018**, *4*, 142–143. [CrossRef]
31. Hellegering, J.; Visser, J.; Kloke, H.J.; D'Ancona, F.C.; Hoitsma, A.J.; van der Vliet, J.A.; Warle, M.C. Deleterious influence of prolonged warm ischemia in living donor kidney transplantation. *Transplant. Proc.* **2012**, *44*, 1222–1226. [CrossRef]
32. Brunotte, M.; Rademacher, S.; Weber, J.; Sucher, E.; Lederer, A.; Hau, H.-M.; Stolzenburg, J.-U.; Seehofer, D.; Sucher, R. Robotic assisted nephrectomy for living kidney donation (RANLD) with use of multiple locking clips or ligatures for renal vascular closure. *Ann. Transl. Med.* **2020**, *8*, 305. [CrossRef] [PubMed]
33. Luke, P.P.; Aquil, S.; Alharbi, B.; Sharma, H.; Sener, A. First Canadian experience with robotic laparoendoscopic single-site vs. standard laparoscopic living-donor nephrectomy: A prospective comparative study. *Can. Urol. Assoc. J.* **2018**, *12*, E440–E446. [CrossRef] [PubMed]
34. Benoit, T.; Game, X.; Roumiguie, M.; Sallusto, F.; Doumerc, N.; Beauval, J.B.; Rischmann, P.; Kamar, N.; Soulie, M.; Malavaud, B. Predictive model of 1-year postoperative renal function after living donor nephrectomy. *Int. Urol. Nephrol.* **2017**, *49*, 793–801. [CrossRef] [PubMed]
35. Kulik, U.; Gwiasda, J.; Oldhafer, F.; Kaltenborn, A.; Arelin, V.; Gueler, F.; Richter, N.; Klempnauer, J.; Schrem, H. External validation of a proposed prognostic model for the prediction of 1-year postoperative eGFR after living donor nephrectomy. *Int. Urol. Nephrol.* **2017**, *49*, 1937–1940. [CrossRef]
36. Perico, N.; Cattaneo, D.; Sayegh, M.H.; Remuzzi, G. Delayed graft function in kidney transplantation. *Lancet* **2004**, *364*, 1814–1827. [CrossRef]
37. Narayanan, R.; Cardella, C.J.; Cattran, D.C.; Cole, E.H.; Tinckam, K.J.; Schiff, J.; Kim, S.J. Delayed graft function and the risk of death with graft function in living donor kidney transplant recipients. *Am. J. Kidney Dis.* **2010**, *56*, 961–970. [CrossRef]
38. Xia, J.; Wang, L.; Ma, Z.; Zhong, L.; Wang, Y.; Gao, Y.; He, L.; Su, X. Cigarette smoking and chronic kidney disease in the general population: A systematic review and meta-analysis of prospective cohort studies. *Nephrol. Dial. Transplant.* **2017**, *32*, 475–487. [CrossRef]
39. Orth, S.R.; Hallan, S.I. Smoking: A risk factor for progression of chronic kidney disease and for cardiovascular morbidity and mortality in renal patients–absence of evidence or evidence of absence? *Clin. J. Am. Soc. Nephrol.* **2008**, *3*, 226–236. [CrossRef]
40. Aref, A.; Sharma, A.; Halawa, A. Smoking in Renal Transplantation; Facts beyond Myth. *World J. Transplant.* **2017**, *7*, 129–133. [CrossRef]
41. Ahlawat, R.K.; Jindal, T. Robotic Donor Nephrectomy: The Right Way Forward. *Eur. Urol. Focus* **2018**, *4*, 140–141. [CrossRef]

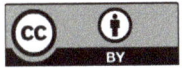

© 2020 by the authors. Licensee MDPI, Basel, Switzerland. This article is an open access article distributed under the terms and conditions of the Creative Commons Attribution (CC BY) license (http://creativecommons.org/licenses/by/4.0/).

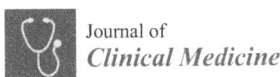

Article

Should We Perform Old-For-Old Kidney Transplantation during the COVID-19 Pandemic? The Risk for Post-Operative Intensive Stay

Philip Zeuschner [1], Urban Sester [2], Michael Stöckle [1], Matthias Saar [1], Ilias Zompolas [3], Nasrin El-Bandar [3], Lutz Liefeldt [4], Klemens Budde [4], Robert Öllinger [5], Paul Ritschl [5], Thorsten Schlomm [3], Janine Mihm [2,†] and Frank Friedersdorff [3,*,†]

1. Department of Urology and Pediatric Urology, Saarland University, Kirrberger Street 100, 66421 Homburg/Saar, Germany; philip.zeuschner@uks.eu (P.Z.); michael.stoeckle@uks.eu (M.S.); matthias.saar@uks.eu (M.S.)
2. Department of Nephrology and Hypertension, Internal Medicine IV, Saarland University, Kirrberger Street 100, 66421 Homburg/Saar, Germany; urban.sester@uks.eu (U.S.); janine.mihm@uks.eu (J.M.)
3. Department of Urology, Charité-Universitätsmedizin Berlin, Corporate Member of Freie Universität Berlin, Humbold-Universität zu Berlin, and Berlin Institute of Health, Charitéplatz 1, 10117 Berlin, Germany; ilias.zompolas@charite.de (I.Z.); nasrin.el-bandar@charite.de (N.E.-B.); thorsten.schlomm@charite.de (T.S.)
4. Department of Nephrology, Charité-Universitätsmedizin Berlin, Corporate Member of Freie Universität Berlin, Humbold-Universität zu Berlin, and Berlin Institute of Health, Charitéplatz 1, 10117 Berlin, Germany; lutz.liefeldt@charite.de (L.L.); klemens.budde@charite.de (K.B.)
5. Department of Surgery, Campus Charité Mitte/Campus Virchow-Klinikum CCM/CVK, Charité-Universitätsmedizin Berlin, Corporate Member of Freie Universität Berlin, Humbold-Universität zu Berlin, and Berlin Institute of Health, Charitéplatz 1, 10117 Berlin, Germany; robert.oellinger@charite.de (R.Ö.); paul.ritschl@charite.de (P.R.)

* Correspondence: frank.friedersdorff@charite.de
† Both authors contributed equally.

Received: 29 May 2020; Accepted: 10 June 2020; Published: 12 June 2020

Abstract: Health care systems worldwide have been facing major challenges since the outbreak of the SARS-CoV-2 pandemic. Kidney transplantation (KT) has been tremendously affected due to limited personal protective equipment (PPE) and intensive care unit (ICU) capacities. To provide valid information on risk factors for ICU admission in a high-risk cohort of old kidney recipients from old donors in the Eurotransplant Senior Program (ESP), we retrospectively conducted a bi-centric analysis. Overall, 17 (16.2%) patients out of 105 KTs were admitted to the ICU. They had a lower BMI, and both coronary artery disease (CAD) and hypertensive nephropathy were more frequent. A risk model combining BMI, CAD and hypertensive nephropathy gained a sensitivity of 94.1% and a negative predictive value of 97.8%, rendering it a valuable search test, but with low specificity (51.1%). ICU admission also proved to be an excellent parameter identifying patients at risk for short patient and graft survivals. Patients admitted to the ICU had shorter patient (1-year 57% vs. 90%) and graft (5-year 49% vs. 77%) survival. To conclude, potential kidney recipients with a low BMI, CAD and hypertensive nephropathy should only be transplanted in the ESP in times of SARS-CoV-2 pandemic if the local health situation can provide sufficient ICU capacities.

Keywords: kidney transplantation; organ donation; deceased donor; Eurotransplant Senior Program; risk stratification; intensive care

1. Introduction

Health care systems all over the world have been facing major and unprecedented challenges since the outbreak of Coronavirus Disease 2019 (COVID-19). Extensive restrictions and nation-wide lockdowns were implemented to contain the spread of the novel coronavirus SARS-CoV-2. Its special features contributed to its fast and widespread transmission, including (1) being highly contagious, (2) the possible transmission from asymptomatic individuals and (3) causing mild symptoms in most of the infected patients [1,2]. Some countries were unexpectedly overwhelmed by a considerable increase in patients admitted to hospitals in need of intensive care [3]. Meanwhile, a worldwide shortage of personal protective equipment (PPE) in conjunction with limited bed capacities at intensive care units (ICU) resulted in suspension of elective surgeries. PPE and ICU beds were urgently needed as scarce medical resources for the management of COVID-19 cases and for the protection of the medical staff [4,5]. Another reason for postponing elective surgeries was the fear that patients admitted to hospital for elective surgery would become vectors for the transmission of a nosocomial infection with SARS-CoV-2 [3,4].

The outbreak of the pandemic also resulted in restrictions and cancellations in terms of kidney transplantation (KT) [6–9]. In Italy, a notable decrease in solid organ transplantation and procurement has already been observed in the first four weeks of the pandemic [10]. Currently, decisions on prioritizing certain procedures—including KT—are based on expert opinions rather than on evidence, contributing to different spread-dependent restrictions between regions [7]. In addition, it is unclear which immunosuppressive induction regimen can be administered safely. Especially, the administration of thymoglobulins causing long-lasting lymphopenia has been discussed critically, as a low lymphocyte count has been negatively associated with the disease severity of SARS-CoV-2 infection [1,11,12]. Even planned immunosuppression in living donation has been questioned [1]. The American Society of Transplantation and the European Association of Urology currently recommend to defer non-urgent KTs with living donors, but to perform urgent KTs—depending on the local situation [13,14]. However, the main aim should be rationing scarce medical resources, especially PPE, ventilators and ICU beds, while providing the best possible medical care to our patients [4].

The costs and benefits of a kidney transplantation during a pandemic should be counterbalanced [2]. We know that KT is the best treatment option for patients suffering from end-stage kidney disease (ESKD), with an improved survival rate and quality of life [15]. On the other hand, we lack information about the risk for admission to ICU after KT. In the context of scarce ICU resources, knowing about risk factors for ICU admission is crucial. Especially, older patients with comorbidities could have a higher risk for admission to ICU. The Eurotransplant Senior Program (ESP) is a special kidney transplant program which was initiated in 1999 to reduce waiting times by allocating kidneys from deceased donors aged ≥65 years to old recipients aged ≥65 years. Before that date, only 3% of patients aged 65 years or older actually received a KT offer within the Eurotransplant region, because younger patients with more favorable outcomes were prioritized [16]. In ESP, organ allocation is not based on immunological compatibility, but on local, regional or national allocation and AB0-compatibility, in order to reduce cold ischemia time (CIT). For this reason, risk assessment scores such as the Kidney Donor Risk Index (KDRI) are not integrated into the standard allocation protocols [17]. Double kidney allocation is not allowed at the beginning of the allocation procedure. Within the regular Eurotransplant Kidney Allocation System (ETKAS), kidneys can be allocated for donation after brain death (DCB) and, if allowed by national law, donation after cardiocirculatory death (DCD). Within the first 10 years, ESP has significantly increased the number of old kidney recipients. Local allocation resulted in shorter CITs and lower delayed graft function (DGF) rates compared to old kidney recipients in the regular Eurotransplant Kidney Allocation System (ETKAS) [18,19].

We lately had to decide whether or not to accept an allocated kidney from a 66 year old donor with a negative SARS-CoV-2 test result, allocated within ESP. The recipient was a 70 year old male with a solitary kidney who had an underlying hypertensive nephropathy. He had been on dialysis for 36 months and additionally suffered from coronary artery disease (CAD). This was the first organ offer within the ESP program at our department since the beginning of the SARS-CoV-2 pandemic. To provide valid information and thereby help decision-making in times of SARS-CoV-2, we conducted the first risk assessment for post-operative ICU stay among patients in the ESP so far. Additionally, the impact of an ICU admission on further outcome was assessed in this bi-center study.

2. Materials and Methods

In total, 105 KTs in the ESP performed at two tertiary referral centers were retrospectively analyzed. From 2010 to 2020, 40 (38.1%) and 65 (61.9%) kidneys were locally allocated to two transplant centers. In accordance with local law, all donors were brain-dead. No double kidney transplantations were included. All KTs were conducted in an open fashion by experienced transplant surgeons. After KT, the patients were admitted to an intermediate care unit by default. Only in the case of severe complications which could not be treated in an intermediate care unit, patients were admitted to the ICU. All kidney recipients received basiliximab as an induction treatment in combination with tacrolimus, mycophenolate mofetil and (methyl)prednisolone as the standard immunosuppressive regimen in both transplant centers.

This entire analysis was conducted in adherence with the correct scientific research work terms of the Charité Medical University of Berlin and Saarland University. Patients provided written informed consent and patient data was fully anonymized.

2.1. Data Collection and Outcome Measures

For the recipient characteristics, age, gender, BMI (kg/m^2) and relevant health-conditions (arterial hypertension, CAD, diabetes mellitus, history of smoking) were obtained. The underlying cause for ESKD, duration and type of dialysis, and number of prior kidney transplantations characterized recipient's nephrological history. For the graft characteristics, donor age, number of HLA-mismatches and cold ischemia time (CIT) were obtained. Regarding KT, operating time, warm ischemia time (WIT) and intraoperative complications served as surgical outcomes. Admission to ICU, length of ICU stay, complications based on Clavien Dindo within 30 days after surgery (major complications defined as ≥grade 3a) and length of hospital stay characterized the recipient's postoperative course. The graft function was assessed by DGF rates, defined as the need for dialysis within 7 days after transplantation, and serum creatinine during follow-up. Over 10 years, graft and patient survival were compared.

As the primary outcome, risk factors for ICU admission after KT in ESP were identified. Therefore, patients with ICU admission were compared with patients without an ICU stay. To assess the influence of recipient and donor age on ICU admission, age-dependent comparisons were conducted, considering very old donors ≥75 years (very old-for-old vs. old-for-old) and very old recipients ≥70 years (old-for-very old vs. old-for-old). A multivariate binary logistic regression analysis identified significant risk predictors for ICU stay, which were used to create a risk model.

As the secondary outcome, the impact of ICU admission on further outcome was assessed. For this objective, survival and regression analyses identifying factors impacting graft and overall survival were calculated. Graft survival was always censored for death with functioning graft (DWFG).

2.2. Statistical Analysis

Categorical variables were reported as frequencies and proportions, and continuous data as the median and range. Fisher's exact test and Mann-Whitney U test were conducted to compare between the groups. Kaplan Meier analyses compared graft and patient survival between groups by log-rank test. For binary logistic and cox regression analyses, covariates were included in multivariate regression analysis only if the respective effect was significant in the univariate analysis. For multivariate regression analyses, forward Wald selection was applied. The best cut-off for predicted probability of ICU stay in the multivariate risk model was estimated via ROC-analysis and Youden index. Statistical analyses were performed by SPSS version 25 with Fix pack 2 installed (IBM, Armonk, NY, USA). All tests were two-sided, and p-values < 0.05 were considered significant.

3. Results

3.1. Overall Results Regarding ICU Admission

Overall, 17 (16.2%) patients were admitted to the ICU for a median length of 2 days (range 1–27). The main reason for ICU admission was significant hypotension requiring catecholamines in the absence of acute bleeding in five (29.4%) patients. Three (17.6%) patients were admitted for respiratory insufficiency, three (17.6%) for sepsis with multiple organ failure, and two (11.7%) for cardiac infarction. One (5.9%) patient had hyperkalemia, another a compartment syndrome due to occlusion of iliac arteries. One (5.9%) patient had a significant bleeding requiring surgical re-exploration, another had his graft surgically removed because of arterial stenosis and consecutive graft necrosis, and required intensive care thereafter. The median time between KT and ICU admission was 0 days, as 10 (58.8%) patients were admitted to the ICU immediately after KT. In total, 4 (23.5%) patients were admitted on postoperative day (POD) 2 to 4, and 2 (11.7%) patients on POD 8 and 9. One (5.9%) patient was admitted to the ICU on POD 36; he suffered from a late-onset sepsis. The admission rate to the ICU did not differ between the two transplant centers.

Patients admitted to the ICU were insignificantly older than patients without an ICU stay (71 vs. 69 years, n.s.) (see Table 1). They had a lower BMI (24.2 vs. 26.7, $p < 0.05$) and CAD twice as often (64.7% vs. 35.2%, $p < 0.05$). Regarding the underlying renal disease, hypertensive nephropathy was more common in patients admitted to the ICU (35.3% vs. 10.2%, $p < 0.05$). In both groups, the median number of HLA-mismatches was four (range 1–6, n.s.). There was a tendency towards longer CIT for patients admitted to the ICU (667.8 vs. 552.3 min), but it was not significant.

Table 1. Comparison of patient characteristics with or without ICU stay after kidney transplantation in the ESP program.

	Σ (n = 105)	ICU Yes (n = 17)	ICU No (n = 88)	p
Recipient				
age (year)	69 (65; 82)	71 (65; 80)	69 (65; 82)	n.s.
male gender	68 (64.8%)	10 (58.8%)	58 (65.9%)	n.s.
BMI (kg/m^2)	26.3 (19.2; 37.9)	24.2 (19.3; 31)	26.7 (19.2; 37.9)	0.014
Pre-transplant				
hypertension	101 (96.2%)	17 (100%)	84 (95.5%)	n.s.
CAD	42 (40%)	11 (64.7%)	31 (35.2%)	0.031
diabetes	41 (39%)	6 (35.3%)	35 (39.8%)	n.s.
history of smoking	18 (17.1%)	2 (11.8%)	16 (18.2%)	n.s.
Cause for ESKD				
chronic GN	23 (18.9%)	1 (5.9%)	22 (25%)	n.s.
diabetic NP	17 (13.9%)	2 (11.8%)	15 (17%)	n.s.
hypertensive NP	15 (12.3%)	6 (35.3%)	9 (10.2%)	0.015
other *	50 (47.6%)	9 (52.9%)	46 (52.2%)	n.s.
time on dialysis (d)	918.5 (2; 3830)	1384 (484; 3830)	855.5 (12; 3302)	n.s.
hemodialysis	84 (80%)	16 (94.1%)	68 (77.3%)	n.s.
first Tx	101 (96.2%)	17 (100%)	84 (95.5%)	n.s.
Graft				
donor age (year)	71 (65; 85)	71 (66; 82)	71 (65; 85)	n.s.
HLA-mismatches	4 (1; 6)	4 (1; 6)	4 (1; 6)	n.s.
CIT (min)	571.8 (181.2; 1236)	667.8 (228; 1166.4)	552.3 (181.2; 1236)	0.053

* see Appendix A Table A3 for further information.

Regarding KTs, patients admitted to the ICU had slightly longer operating times (212 vs. 180 min, $p = 0.053$), and neither WIT nor intraoperative complication rates differed (see Table 2). During the postoperative course, patients with an ICU stay suffered from more frequent and higher complications based on Clavien Dindo, although this was not significant. Although there were fewer minor complications, 9 (52.9%) patients admitted to the ICU had more complications at grade 5 (17.6% vs. 0, $p < 0.01$). Patients with an ICU stay were discharged insignificantly later (21.5 vs. 18 days, n.s.).

Table 2. Perioperative outcome.

	Σ (n = 105)	ICU Yes (n = 17)	ICU No (n = 88)	p-Value
Transplantation				
operating time (min)	184 (116; 436)	212 (129; 268)	180 (116; 436)	n.s.
WIT (min)	46.5 (21; 126)	47 (35; 70)	46 (21; 126)	n.s.
complications	12 (11.4%)	2 (11.8%)	10 (11.4%)	n.s.
Postoperative				
complications				n.s.
none	42 (40%)	5 (29.4%)	37 (42%)	n.s.
minor	28 (26.7%)	3 (17.6%)	25 (28.4%)	n.s.
major	35 (33.3%)	9 (52.9%)	26 (29.5%)	n.s.
length of stay	19 (8–66)	21.5 (12–66)	18 (8–62)	n.s.
Graft Function				
DGF rate	42 (40%)	9 (52.9%)	33 (37.5%)	n.s.

DGF rates were higher for patients admitted to the ICU (52.9% vs. 37.5%, n.s.) (see Table 2). Serum creatinine significantly declined after KT ($p < 0.05$) and did not differ between patients with or without ICU stay (see Figure 1).

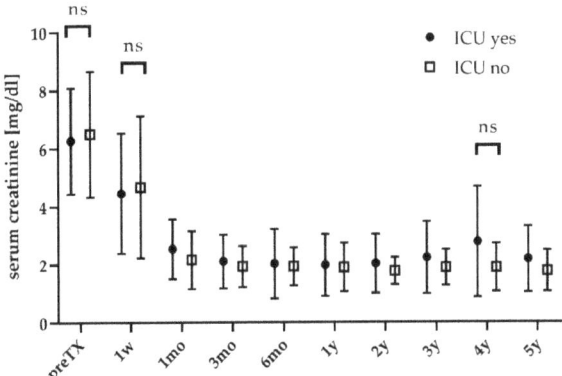

Figure 1. Graft function during follow-up. w: week; mo: month; y: year.

3.2. Donor- and Recipient-Age-Dependent Comparison

In total, 28 (26.7%) patients received a graft from very old donors ≥75 years, compared to 77 (73.3%) old donors ('old-for-old') (see Table 3). When stratifying for donor age (very old-for-old vs. old-for-old), neither recipient nor graft characteristics differed. Grafts from very old donors had a tendency towards a longer CIT, which was not significant (677.1 vs. 540.6 min). Kidney recipients of very old donors had a tendency to be admitted to the ICU more frequently (21.4% vs. 14.3%, n.s.), but were discharged significantly earlier (16 vs. 20 days, $p < 0.05$). Neither DGF rates nor the kidney function differed during follow-up.

When stratifying for recipient age (old-for-very old vs. old-for-old), 47 (44.7%) recipients were ≥70 years old, and thereby were considered as very old (see Table 3). Regarding recipient characteristics, only the history of smoking differed, as fewer very old recipients had a history of smoking (8.5% vs. 24.1%, $p < 0.05$). Neither graft nor transplantation-specific factors were different. Very old recipients were admitted to the ICU insignificantly more often (21.3% vs. 12.1%). Graft function one week after KT was the only parameter that differed when comparing very old to old recipients, as very old recipients had a lower serum creatinine than old recipients (3.35 vs. 5.36, $p < 0.01$). During follow-up, the kidney function became equivalent.

Table 3. Age-dependent comparison stratifying for donor age (very old donors ≥75 years vs. old donors) or recipient age (very old recipients ≥70 years vs. old recipients).

	Donors: Very Old-For-Old vs. Old-For-Old			Recipients: Old-For-Very Old vs. Old-For-Old		
	Very Old (n = 28)	Old (n = 77)	p	Very Old (n = 47)	Old (n = 58)	p
Transplantation						
operating time	180 (120; 281)	188 (116; 436)	n.s.	190 (128; 268)	181 (116; 436)	n.s.
WIT (min)	46 (21; 126)	49.5 (32; 85)	n.s.	48 (32; 104)	46 (21; 126)	n.s.
complications	4 (14.3%)	8 (10.4%)	n.s.	6 (12.8%)	6 (10.3%)	n.s.
Postoperative						
ICU admission	6 (21.4%)	11 (14.3%)	n.s.	10 (21.3%)	7 (12.1%)	n.s.
Clavien–Dindo			n.s.			n.s.
none	13 (46.4%)	29 (37.7%)		16 (34%)	26 (44.8%)	
minor	10 (35.7%)	18 (23.4%)		13 (27.7%)	15 (25.9%)	
major	5 (17.9%)	30 (39%)		18 (38.3%)	17 (29.3%)	
length of stay	16 (12; 46)	20 (8; 66)	0.028	20 (10; 66)	18.5 (8; 65)	
Graft Function						
DGF	14 (50%)	28 (36.4%)	n.s.	19 (40.4%)	23 (39.7%)	n.s.

3.3. Risk Model for ICU Stay

Among recipient and graft characteristics as well as transplantation-specific outcomes, the BMI of the recipient, an underlying hypertensive nephropathy and CAD were the only significant predictors for ICU admission in univariate and multivariate analysis (see Table 4). A higher BMI lowered the OR for ICU admission (OR 0.8, $p < 0.01$), but a hypertensive nephropathy (OR 4.0, $p < 0.05$) and CAD (OR 4.46, $p < 0.05$) significantly increased the OR for ICU admission during the hospital stay. Donor or recipient age did not impact the risk for ICU admission.

Table 4. Multivariate regression analysis to predict an ICU admission during the hospital stay.

Variable	OR (95% CI)	p-Value
BMI	0.80 (0.68; 0.94)	0.008
hypertensive nephropathy	4 (1.02; 15.67)	0.046
coronary artery disease	4.46 (1.32; 15.07)	0.016

When combining these three factors in a risk model to estimate the probability for ICU admission, the c-index reached 0.789 ($p < 0.001$) (see Figure A1). When setting the cut-off for the predicted probability of ICU admission to 0.08, which had highest Youden-index, the risk model reached a sensitivity of 94.1%, specificity of 51.1%, false positive rate (FPR) of 48.9%, false negative rate (FNR) of 5.9%, positive predictive value (PPV) of 27.1% and negative predictive value (NPV) of 97.8% (see Table A1).

3.4. Survival Analysis

For all 105 patients, the median length of follow-up was 49.5 months. The overall graft survival at 1, 5 and 9 years was 84%, 73% and 42%, respectively, with a median death-censored graft survival of 113.9 months. Median patient survival was 108.2 months, with a 1-, 5- and 9-year survival of 85%, 62% and 38%, respectively.

When stratifying for ICU admission, patients admitted to the ICU had a significantly shorter graft survival (59.1 vs. 115.7 months, $p = 0.049$) (see Figure 2a). Their 1- and 5-year graft survivals were 75% and 49%, and thereby worse compared to patients without an ICU stay (86% and 77%). Over the whole study period, the death-rate for patients with an ICU stay was almost three times higher compared to patients without an ICU stay (70.6% vs. 26.1%, $p < 0.001$). Consequently, the median patient survival for patients admitted to the ICU was significantly shorter (ICU 36.9 vs. 114.9 months, $p < 0.001$) (see Figure 2b). 1- and 5-year patient survival for patients admitted to an ICU was 57% and 0% and for patients without an ICU stay 90% (1 year), 72% (5 years) and 44% after 9 years, respectively. In total, 17 (48.6%) patients died with a functioning graft, and the DWFG rate did not differ between groups (ICU 50% vs. 47.8%, n.s.). Neither the age of the donor nor the recipient affected graft or patient survival (see Table A2).

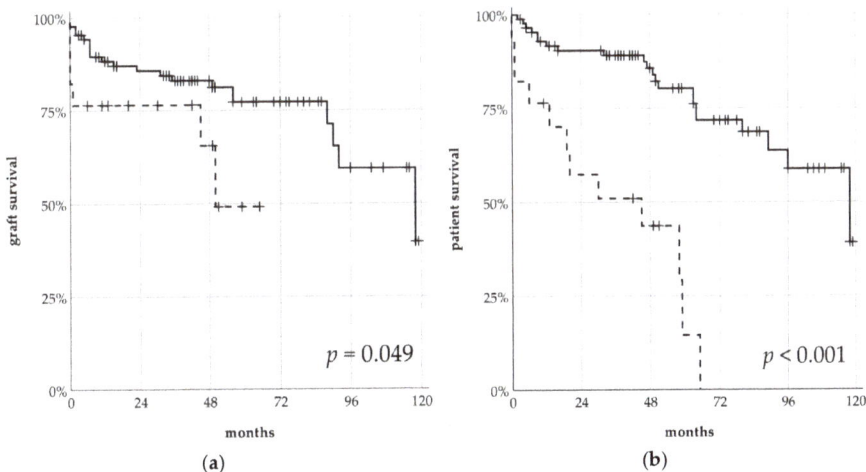

Figure 2. Death-censored graft survival (**a**) and patient survival (**b**) comparing patients admitted to the ICU (**dashed line**) vs. patients not admitted to the ICU (**solid line**) after kidney transplantation in the ESP program.

In a multivariate cox regression, higher numbers of prior KTs and HLA-mismatches significantly shortened graft survival (hazard ratio (HR) for graft loss 9.66, $p = 0.001$; HR 1.53, $p < 0.05$) (see Table 5). Additionally, higher serum creatinine 1 month after KT was associated with worse graft survival (HR 1.37, $p < 0.05$). ICU admission during the hospital stay after KT did not affect graft survival. Regarding patient survival, a pre-transplant diabetes mellitus and an ICU admission during the hospital stay were significant predictors for worse outcomes in the multivariate analysis (HR for patient death 2.22, $p < 0.05$, HR 4.7, $p < 0.001$). Major complications during the hospital stay and the serum creatinine 1 month after KT were only associated with patient survival in univariate analysis.

Table 5. Significant impact factors on graft loss and patient death in multivariate cox regression.

Variable	HR (95% CI)	p-Value
Graft Loss		
number of Tx	9.66 (2.48; 37.69)	0.001
HLA-mismatches	1.53 (1.03; 2.27)	0.033
serum creatinine 1 mo	1.37 (1.01; 1.87)	0.04
Patient Death		
pre-transplant diabetes	2.22 (1.02; 4.86)	0.046
ICU admission	4.72 (2.02; 11.03)	<0.001

4. Discussion

In this bi-centric study, an analysis of 105 kidney transplantations of deceased donors, allocated within the Eurotransplant Senior Program, was conducted. We aimed to identify risk factors for ICU admission after KT during a hospital stay in times of shortened PPE and ICU capacities because of the SARS-CoV-2 pandemic.

Overall, recipient and graft characteristics were comparable with other cohorts [19–22]. CIT was lower, lasting on average 9.5 h, while most other ESP programs have CITs averaging 10 to 12 h [19,20]. ESP aims to reduce CIT by prioritizing local organ allocation, as longer CITs have been clearly linked with higher DGF rates. Nonetheless, our DGF rate of 40% is higher than that of one of the largest ESP cohorts so far, with 1406 KTs, by Frei et al. They reported a median DGF rate of 29.7% [19]. In contrast, other groups have comparable DGF rates ranging between 34.7 to 41.1% in their ESP cohorts [22,23]. Chavalitdhamrong et al. even stated a DGF rate of 60.4% for 601 KTs, but for organs allocated by ECD (extended criteria donors) for donors aged 50–69 years, and 63.9% for donors aged ≥70 years [24].

In a high-risk cohort like ESP recipients, complications are common. There were 11.4% intraoperative complications, and 26.7% minor and 33.3% major complications occurred postoperatively, according to Clavien–Dindo. Reports on complication rates state highly variable results, mainly due to inconsistent definitions. Bentas et al. have "surgical complications" in 47% of cases in their ESP program, whereas Bahde et al. reported 15.7% intraoperative and 22.5% post-operative surgical complications among their recipients [23,25]. Only Gallinat et al. defined postoperative complications according to Clavien–Dindo. In their comparison of very old donors in the ECD program, the rate for major complications was 48%, defined as ≥grade 3b [26].

During follow-up, death-censored graft survival (1- and 5-year: 84% and 73%) and patient survival (1- and 5-year: 85% and 62%) were superior to Frei et al. and comparable with Quast et al., who retrospectively analyzed 217 ESP transplantations at their department from 1998 to 2014, considering donor age [19,20] (see Table 6). In accordance with Boesmueller and Giessing et al., the main reason for graft loss was death with functioning graft [18,22]. Our analysis comprises one of the longest follow-ups in ESP so far. Overall, graft-survival after 9 years was 42%, and patient survival was 38%. Quast et al. reported a 10-year patient survival of 40% for old donors, and 35% for very old donors, whereas graft survival was 30% and 10%, respectively.

Table 6. Comparison of death-censored graft and patient survival in ESP programs.

	Frei [19] n = 1406	Quast [20] n = 217	Bahde [23] n = 89	Jacobi [21] n = 89	Our Results n = 105
Graft Survival					
1-year	75%	76.4% [1]	n.a.	87%	84%
5-year	47%	57.3% [1]	77%	63%	73%
Patient Survival					
1-year	86%	88.2% [1]	n.a.	87%	85%
5-year	60%	71.8% [1]	69.8%	63%	62%

[1] Only considering old, but not very old, donors.

Based on this data, we have identified risk factors for ICU admission during a hospital stay in the ESP. In times of the SARS-CoV-2 pandemic with a shortage of ICU capacities, risk stratification is crucial to identify patients at high risk for ICU admission (after KT). This aspect has rarely been addressed so far. To the best of our knowledge, only three working groups have stratified their data for ICU admission [27–29]. Two working groups focused on ICU admission at any time after KT, even years after KT, which clearly does not help when trying to decide whether or not to perform a KT during the present SARS-CoV-2 pandemic. Abrol et al. retrospectively analyzed 1527 kidney transplantations between 2007 and 2016 and found higher age, increasing BMI, pre-transplant dialysis and deceased donor transplantation to be associated with ICU admission in their multivariate analysis. Living donor KT and preemptive KT were associated with a lower risk [27]. Nonetheless, 82.8% of the included KTs were living kidney transplantations. As such, we are the first to report on the risk for ICU admission immediately after kidney transplantation in the ESP.

17 (16.2%) patients in our cohort were admitted to the ICU for a mean time of 2 days. More than 80% of patients were admitted directly postoperatively or within four days after KT. The main cause for ICU admission was significant hypotension requiring catecholamines. Overall, patients admitted to the ICU had a lower BMI, and CAD as well as hypertensive nephropathy were more common. Graft characteristics and surgical outcomes during transplantation did not differ. The DGF rate of patients admitted to the ICU was high, with 52.9%, but did not significantly differ from patients without an ICU stay (37.5%).

As stated elsewhere, neither the donor nor the recipient's age had an impact on the postoperative course [18,20]. Therefore, age did not affect ICU admission rates in the regression analysis. We assume that within this (very) old patient cohort, age differences were not as important as in younger patient cohorts due to preselection during the workup for listing. As patients admitted to the ICU had a lower BMI, an increasing BMI lowered the risk for ICU admission (OR 0.8, see Table 4). This is an interesting finding, referring to the 'obesity paradox', which describes the association of obesity with higher mortality in the general population on the one hand, but with a survival advantage among obese patients with several diseases on the other hand. In this regard, meta-analyses have shown that patients with a higher BMI might have (i) a reduced risk of ICU admission or death when suffering from pneumonia, (ii) a reduced adjusted mortality when admitted to the ICU with sepsis, severe sepsis or shock, and (iii) a lower mortality on mechanical ventilation in an ICU [30–32]. Although the concept of the obesity paradox has been questioned, there is also convincing evidence for underlying molecular mechanisms, i.e., that a lower energy reservoir in underweight patients cannot equally counteract the adverse influence of increased catabolic stress [33,34].

As further variables, hypertensive nephropathy and CAD increased the OR for ICU admission by 4 and 4.5, respectively. Most patients were admitted to the ICU because of hypotension as a major symptom for cardiac insufficiency, which is more likely in patients with CAD. In addition, hypertensive nephropathy has been linked with a higher risk for cardiovascular events and death [35]. When combining these three independent risk factors in a risk model, it gained a c-index of 0.789 with a sensitivity of 94.1%, a FNR of 5.9% and a NPV of 97.8% (see Table A1). For this reason, our risk model is highly valuable for the identification of patients at high risk for ICU admission. When applied to our cohort, the risk model was false negative in only one case. We are aware that it has a rather low specificity and PPV, whereas the FPR is high. Furthermore, the confidence intervals for the corresponding odds ratios are large, because only 17 (16.2%) patients were admitted to the ICU and not all of them suffered from hypertensive nephropathy or CAD (see Table 1). However, the high sensitivity and NPV of more than 94% render our risk model an ideal search test.

Our patient who had an organ offer in ESP during the SARS-CoV-2 pandemic had a probability of 92.8% to be admitted to the ICU according to our risk model, with a hypertensive nephropathy, CAD and BMI of 29.4 kg/m^2 (see A1 for further explanation). Of note, this patient was not included within the analyzed cohort. Indeed, after transplantation, he had to be admitted to the ICU on postoperative day seven due to urosepsis and suspected cardiac infarction. Infectious complications are common among old kidney recipients and have been shown to be their second most frequent cause for DWFG [16]. In our cohort, 3 out of 17 (17.6%) patients had to be admitted to the ICU because of sepsis. Especially in the context of the ongoing SARS-CoV-2 pandemic, the question of how to manage immunosuppression for KT recipients is still a matter of debate [11,12].

As standard, all patients were administered tacrolimus, mycophenolate mofetil, (methyl)prednisolone and basiliximab for induction therapy. Consequently, the regimen did not affect ICU admission rates. Since lymphopenia has been associated both with a higher risk for SARS-CoV-2 infection and for severe forms of Covid-19, the questions (i) whether or not to perform the transplantation at all and (ii) whether the induction therapy should be reduced were intensively discussed at the transplant center which had an organ offer in ESP during the SARS-CoV-2 pandemic [11]. Finally, the patient was transplanted and received an induction therapy with basiliximab, and unfortunately suffered from sepsis and neutropenia. For this reason, mycophenolate mofetil was stopped and the dose of prednisolone reduced. Of note, SARS-CoV-2 had been ruled out prior to transplantation and after the onset of sepsis again; as we have not experienced a major shortage of ICU capacities, we could guarantee maximum care for this patient at all times. However, we might decide differently if we receive another organ offer in the ESP program during the ongoing SARS-CoV-2 pandemic again.

Interestingly, ICU admission also proved to be an excellent indicator for the identification of patients at risk for short graft and patient survival. In Kaplan–Meier analysis, patients admitted to the ICU had a significantly shorter graft survival of 59.1 months; all of them died within five years (see Figure 2). Consequently, ICU admission impacted patient survival with a HR of 4.72, but did not impact graft survival in Cox regression (see Table 5). Diabetes mellitus was the only other covariate impacting patient survival. Other studies were inconclusive about the effect of pre-transplant diabetes mellitus or new-onset diabetes mellitus (NODAT) on patient survival. Some studies have found associations with NODAT, but not pre-transplant diabetes, with mortality and graft failure, and others the inverse [36–38]. By contrast, ICU admission did not impact death-censored graft survival in Cox regression. The individual number of kidney transplantations per patient (HR 9.66), number of HLA-mismatches (HR 1.53) and the serum creatinine one month after transplantation (HR 1.37) were significant. The negative impact of increasing HLA-mismatches on graft survival was reported more than two decades ago [39]. To shorten waiting times for old recipients, ESP does not integrate HLA-matching in the allocation algorithm.

This analysis is not devoid of limitation. To exclude center-specific factors and enlarge cohort size, we performed a bicentric analysis and included 105 patients. This is a rather low sample size, but big sample sizes in ESP programs are rare. Due to its retrospective nature, we could not test our new risk model for ICU admission in a prospective, independent manner. Before extrapolating our results to other centers, an external validation of our risk model will be needed. For this reason, we encourage other transplantation centers to test our risk model to further enhance its validity. With a bigger cohort size, the confidence intervals for the risk factors BMI, CAD and hypertensive nephropathy will potentially be reduced. Currently, our risk model is an excellent search test, but has a rather low PPV and therefore cannot replace individual and local risk assessment in times of reduced ICU capacities during the SARS-CoV-2 pandemic.

5. Conclusions

The SARS-CoV-2 pandemic has impacted health care systems tremendously worldwide, making the deferral of elective and non-urgent surgical interventions necessary due to limited PPE and ICU capacities. To provide a valid risk assessment tool concerning the risk of ICU admission for old patients in the Eurotransplant Senior Program, we have identified a low BMI, coronary artery disease and hypertensive nephropathy as significant predictors for ICU admission. For this reason, each transplant center should always carefully discuss whether local ICU capacities allow high-risk KT or not.

Author Contributions: Conceptualization, P.Z., J.M., F.F.; methodology, P.Z.; software, P.Z.; validation, P.Z., J.M., F.F.; formal analysis, P.Z.; investigation, P.Z. and F.F.; data curation, P.Z., J.M., F.F.; writing—original draft preparation, P.Z.; writing—review and editing, all authors, P.Z., U.S., M.S. (Michael Stöckle), M.S. (Matthias Saar), I.Z., N.E.-B., L.L., K.B., R.Ö., P.R., T.S., J.M. and F.F.; visualization, P.Z.; supervision, F.F., All authors have read and agreed to the published version of the manuscript.

Funding: This research received no external funding.

Conflicts of Interest: The authors declare no conflict of interest.

Appendix A

Appendix A.1. Risk Model for ICU Admission

In a multivariate binary logistic regression analysis, BMI, hypertensive nephropathy and coronary artery disease had significant impact on ICU admission. The prediction probability (P) of an ICU stay for each individual patient was calculated with the equation

$$P = \frac{1}{1 + e^{-z}}$$

in which the logit z is

$$z = 3.557 + 4.004 \times HN + 1.495 \times CAD - 0.221 \times BMI$$

- HN: presence of hypertensive nephropathy (binary: no = 0, yes = 1)
- CAD: presence of coronary artery disease (binary: no = 0, yes = 1)
- BMI: body-mass-index in kg/m^2 (continuous)

The optimal cut-off for the predicted probability of ICU admission was calculated via ROC analysis by using a Youden index (see Figure A1). By setting the cut-off to 0.08, this risk model gained a sensitivity of 94.1%, specificity of 51.1%, false positive rate of 48.9%, false negative rate of 5.9%, positive predictive value of 27.1% and negative predictive value of 97.8% (see Table A1).

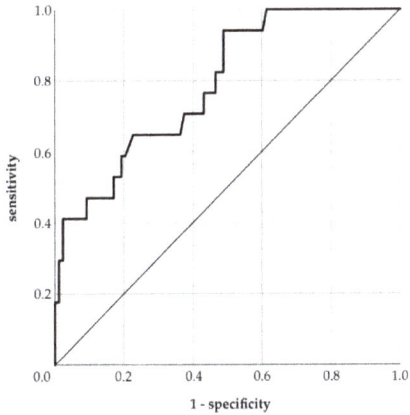

Figure A1. ROC analysis examining the relationship between the predicted probability of ICU stay and actual ICU admission.

Table A1. Crosstabulation illustrating case assignment in our cohort by risk model.

	ICU Yes	ICU No	Σ
risk model: ICU yes	16	43	59
risk model: ICU no	1	45	46
Σ	17	88	105

Appendix A.2. Graft and Patient Survival Stratified for Donor and Recipient Age

Table A2. Mortality table with age-dependent comparison stratified for donor age (very old donors ≥75 vs. old donors) or recipient age (very old recipients ≥70 years vs. old recipients).

	Donors: Very Old-For-Old vs. Old-For-Old			Recipients: Old-For-Very Old vs. Old-For-Old		
	Very Old ($n = 28$)	Old ($n = 77$)	p	Very Old ($n = 47$)	Old ($n = 58$)	p
Graft Survival			n.s.			n.s.
1 year	22 (78%)	61 (86%)		37 (87%)	46 (82%)	
5 years	11 (78%)	25 (72%)		18 (73%)	18 (75%)	
9 years	2 (58%)	6 (41%)		108 (60%)	4 (35%)	
Patient Survival			n.s.			n.s.
1 year	25 (78%)	63 (90%)		39 (82%)	49 (87%)	
5 years	12 (74%)	28 (59%)		21 (60%)	19 (63%)	
9 years	1 (36%)	6 (54%)		2 (55%)	5 (33%)	

Appendix A.3. Underlying Renal Diseases

Table A3. Underlying renal diseases for patients with or without ICU stay after KT.

	Σ ($n = 105$)	ICU Yes ($n = 17$)	ICU No ($n = 88$)	p-Value
ADPKD	11 (10.5%)	2 (11.8%)	9 (10.2%)	n.s.
amyloidosis	3 (2.9%)	-	3 (3.4%)	n.s.
analgesic nephropathy	3 (2.9%)	1 (5.9%)	2 (2.3%)	n.s.
chronic glomerulonephritis	23 (21.9%)	1 (5.9%)	22 (25%)	n.s.
cardiac cirrhosis	1 (1%)	-	1 (1.1%)	n.s.
diabetic nephropathy	17 (16.2%)	2 (11.8%)	15 (17%)	n.s.
FSGS	2 (1.9%)	-	2 (2.3%)	n.s.
goodpasture syndrome	2 (1.9%)	-	2 (2.3%)	n.s.
hypertensive nephropathy	15 (14.3%)	6 (35.3%)	9 (10.2%)	<0.05
IgA nephropathy	3 (2.9%)	-	3 (3.4%)	n.s.
kidney cirrhosis	8 (7.6%)	2 (11.8%)	6 (6.8%)	n.s.
nephrosclerosis	7 (6.7%)	2 (11.8%)	5 (5.7%)	n.s.
other cystic disease	3 (2.9%)	1 (5.9%)	2 (2.2%)	n.s.
renal cell carcinoma	2 (1.9%)	1 (5.9%)	1 (1.1%)	n.s.
vascular nephropathy	7 (6.7%)	3 (17.6%)	4 (4.5%)	n.s.
vasculitis	2 (1.9%)	1 (5.9%)	1 (1.1%)	n.s.
not known	13 (12.5%)	-	13 (14.8%)	n.s.

References

1. Kumar, D.; Manuel, O.; Natori, Y.; Egawa, H.; Grossi, P.; Han, S.-H.; Fernández-Ruiz, M.; Humar, A. COVID-19: A global transplant perspective on successfully navigating a pandemic. *Arab. Archaeol. Epigr.* **2020**. [CrossRef]
2. Gori, A.; Dondossola, D.; Antonelli, B.; Mangioni, D.; Alagna, L.; Reggiani, P.; Bandera, A.; Rossi, G. Coronavirus disease 2019 and transplantation: A view from the inside. *Am. J. Transplant. Off. J. Am. Soc. Transplant. Am. Soc. Transpl. Surg.* **2020**. [CrossRef]
3. Nacoti, M.; Ciocca, A.; Giupponi, A.; Brambillasca, P.; Lussana, F.; Pisano, M.; Goisis, G.; Bonacina, D.; Fazzi, F.; Naspro, R.; et al. *At the Epicenter of the Covid-19 Pandemic and Humanitarian Crises in Italy: Changing Perspectives on Preparation and Mitigation*; NEJM Catalyst: Waltham, MA, USA, 2020.
4. Stahel, P.F. How to risk-stratify elective surgery during the COVID-19 pandemic? *Patient Saf. Surg.* **2020**, *14*, 1–4. [CrossRef] [PubMed]

5. Phua, J.; Weng, L.; Ling, L.; Egi, M.; Lim, C.-M.; Divatia, J.V.; Shrestha, B.R.; Arabi, Y.M.; Ng, J.; Gomersall, C.D.; et al. Intensive care management of coronavirus disease 2019 (COVID-19): Challenges and recommendations. *Lancet Respir. Med.* **2020**, *8*, 506–517. [CrossRef]
6. Stensland, K.D.; Morgan, T.M.; Moinzadeh, A.; Lee, C.T.; Briganti, A.; Catto, J.W.; Canes, D. Considerations in the Triage of Urologic Surgeries During the COVID-19 Pandemic. *Eur. Urol.* **2020**, *77*, 663–666. [CrossRef]
7. Boyarsky, B.J.; Chiang, T.P.-Y.; Werbel, W.A.; Durand, C.M.; Avery, R.; Getsin, S.N.; Jackson, K.R.; Kernodle, A.B.; Rasmussen, S.E.V.P.; Massie, A.B.; et al. Early impact of COVID-19 on transplant center practices and policies in the United States. *Arab. Archaeol. Epigr.* **2020**. [CrossRef] [PubMed]
8. Akalin, E.; Azzi, Y.; Bartash, R.; Seethamraju, H.; Parides, M.; Hemmige, V.; Ross, M.; Forest, S.; Goldstein, Y.D.; Ajaimy, M.; et al. Covid-19 and Kidney Transplantation. *N. Engl. J. Med.* **2020**. [CrossRef] [PubMed]
9. Ritschl, P.; Nevermann, N.; Wiering, L.; Wu, H.H.; Morodor, P.; Brandl, A.; Hillebrandt, K.; Tacke, F.; Friedersdorff, F.; Schlomm, T.; et al. Solid organ transplantation programs facing lack of empiric evidence in the COVID-19 pandemic: A By-proxy Society Recommendation Consensus approach. *Arab. Archaeol. Epigr.* **2020**. [CrossRef]
10. Angelico, R.; Trapani, S.; Manzia, T.M.; Lombardini, L.; Tisone, G.; Cardillo, M. The COVID-19 outbreak in Italy: Initial implications for organ transplantation programs. *Arab. Archaeol. Epigr.* **2020**. [CrossRef]
11. Kronbichler, A.; Gauckler, P.; Windpessl, M.; Shin, J.I.; Jha, V.; Rovin, B.H.; Oberbauer, R. COVID-19: implications for immunosuppression in kidney disease and transplantation. *Nat. Rev. Nephrol.* **2020**, 1–3. [CrossRef]
12. Maggiore, U.; Abramowicz, D.; Crespo, M.; Mariat, C.; Mjoen, G.; Peruzzi, L.; Sever, M.S.; Oniscu, G.C.; Hilbrands, L.; Watschinger, B. How should I manage immunosuppression in a kidney transplant patient with COVID-19? An Era-Edta Descartes expert opinion. *Nephrol. Dial. Transplant. Off. Publ. Eur. Dial. Transpl. Assoc. Eur. Ren. Assoc.* **2020**. [CrossRef] [PubMed]
13. American Society of, T. FAQs for Organ Transplantation. Available online: https://www.myast.org/sites/default/files/internal/COVID19%20FAQ%20Tx%20Centers%2005.11.2020.pdf (accessed on 18 May 2020).
14. Ribal, M.J.; Cornford, P.; Briganti, A.; Knoll, T.; Gravas, S.; Babjuk, M.; Harding, C.; Breda, A.; Bex, A.; Rassweiler, J.J.; et al. European Association of Urology Guidelines Office Rapid Reaction Group: An Organisation-wide Collaborative Effort to Adapt the European Association of Urology Guidelines Recommendations to the Coronavirus Disease 2019 Era. *Eur. Urol.* **2020**. [CrossRef] [PubMed]
15. Garcia, G.G.; World Kidney Day Steering Committee 2012; Harden, P.; Chapman, J. The global role of kidney transplantation. *J. Nephrol.* **2012**, *25*, 1–6. [CrossRef] [PubMed]
16. Dreyer, G.J.; De Fijter, J.W. Transplanting the Elderly: Mandatory Age- and Minimal Histocompatibility Matching. *Front. Immunol.* **2020**, *11*, 359. [CrossRef]
17. Lehner, L.J.; Kleinsteuber, A.; Halleck, F.; Khadzhynov, D.; Schrezenmeier, E.; Duerr, M.; Eckardt, K.-U.; Budde, K.; Staeck, O. Assessment of the Kidney Donor Profile Index in a European cohort. *Nephrol. Dial. Transplant.* **2018**, *33*, 1465–1472. [CrossRef]
18. Giessing, M.; Fuller, T.F.; Friedersdorff, F.; Deger, S.; Wille, A.; Neumayer, H.-H.; Schmidt, D.; Budde, K.; Liefeldt, L. Outcomes of transplanting deceased-donor kidneys between elderly donors and recipients. *J. Am. Soc. Nephrol.* **2008**, *20*, 37–40. [CrossRef] [PubMed]
19. Frei, U.; Noeldeke, J.; Machold-Fabrizii, V.; Arbogast, H.; Margreiter, R.; Fricke, L.; Voiculescu, A.; Kliem, V.; Ebel, H.; Albert, U.; et al. Prospective Age-Matching in Elderly Kidney Transplant Recipients—A 5-Year Analysis of the Eurotransplant Senior Program. *Arab. Archaeol. Epigr.* **2007**, *8*, 50. [CrossRef]
20. Quast, L.S.; Grzella, S.; Lengenfeld, T.; Pillokeit, N.; Hummels, M.; Zgoura, P.; Westhoff, T.H.; Viebahn, R.; Schenker, P. Outcome of Kidney Transplantation Using Organs From Brain-dead Donors Older Than 75 Years. *Transplant. Proc.* **2020**, *52*, 119–126. [CrossRef]
21. Jacobi, J.; Beckmann, S.; Heller, K.; Hilgers, K.F.; Apel, H.; Spriewald, B.; Eckardt, K.-U.; Amann, K.U. Deceased Donor Kidney Transplantation in the Eurotransplant Senior Program (ESP): A Single-Center Experience from 2008 to 2013. *Ann. Transplant.* **2016**, *21*, 94–104. [CrossRef]
22. Boesmueller, C.; Biebl, M.; Scheidl, S.; Öllinger, R.; Margreiter, C.; Pratschke, J.; Margreiter, R.; Schneeberger, S. Long-Term Outcome in Kidney Transplant Recipients Over 70 Years in the Eurotransplant Senior Kidney Transplant Program: A Single Center Experience. *Transplantation* **2011**, *92*, 210–216. [CrossRef]

23. Wolters, H.; Bahde, R.; Vowinkel, T.; Unser, J.; Anthoni, C.; Hölzen, J.P.; Suwelack, B.; Senninger, N. Prognostic factors for kidney allograft survival in the Eurotransplant Senior Program. *Ann. Transplant.* **2014**, *19*, 201–209. [CrossRef]
24. Chavalitdhamrong, D.; Gill, J.; Takemoto, S.; Madhira, B.R.; Cho, Y.W.; Shah, T.; Bunnapradist, S. Patient and Graft Outcomes from Deceased Kidney Donors Age 70 Years and Older: An Analysis of the Organ Procurement Transplant Network/United Network of Organ Sharing Database. *Transplantation* **2008**, *85*, 1573–1579. [CrossRef]
25. Bentas, W.; Jones, J.; Karaoguz, A.; Tilp, U.; Probst, M.; Scheuermann, E.; Hauser, I.A.; Jonas, D.; Gossmann, J. Renal transplantation in the elderly: surgical complications and outcome with special emphasis on the Eurotransplant Senior Programme. *Nephrol. Dial. Transplant.* **2008**, *23*, 2043–2051. [CrossRef] [PubMed]
26. Gallinat, A.; Feldkamp, T.; Schaffer, R.; Radunz, S.; Treckmann, J.W.; Minor, T.; Witzke, O.; Paul, A.; Sotiropoulos, G.C. Single-Center Experience With Kidney Transplantation Using Deceased Donors Older Than 75 Years. *Transplantation* **2011**, *92*, 76–81. [CrossRef] [PubMed]
27. Abrol, N.; Kashyap, R.; Frank, R.D.; Iyer, V.N.; Dean, P.G.; Stegall, M.D.; Prieto, M.; Kashani, K.B.; Taner, T. Preoperative Factors Predicting Admission to the Intensive Care Unit After Kidney Transplantation. *Mayo Clin. Proc. Innov. Qual. Outcomes* **2019**, *3*, 285–293. [CrossRef] [PubMed]
28. De Freitas, F.G.R.; Lombardi, F.; Pacheco, E.S.; De Sandes-Freitas, T.V.; Viana, L.A.; Junior, H.T.-S.; Medina-Pestana, J.O.; Bafi, A.T.; Machado, F.R. Clinical Features of Kidney Transplant Recipients Admitted to the Intensive Care Unit. *Prog. Transplant.* **2017**, *28*, 56–62. [CrossRef]
29. Marques, I.; Caires, R.A.; Machado, D.; Goldenstein, P.; Rodrigues, C.; Pegas, J.; De Paula, F.; David-Neto, E.; Costa, M. Outcomes and Mortality in Renal Transplant Recipients Admitted to the Intensive Care Unit. *Transplant. Proc.* **2015**, *47*, 2694–2699. [CrossRef]
30. Cai, F.; Wang, M.; Wu, X.D.; Xu, X.M.; Su, X.; Shi, Y. Body mass index is associated with the risk of ICU admission and death among patients with pneumonia: A systematic review and meta-analysis. *Int. J. Clin. Exp. Med.* **2016**, *9*, 5269–5278.
31. Pepper, D.J.; Sun, J.; Welsh, J.; Cui, X.; Suffredini, A.F.; Eichacker, P.Q. Increased body mass index and adjusted mortality in ICU patients with sepsis or septic shock: A systematic review and meta-analysis. *Crit. Care* **2016**, *20*, 181. [CrossRef]
32. Zhao, Y.; Li, Z.; Yang, T.; Wang, M.; Xi, X. Is body mass index associated with outcomes of mechanically ventilated adult patients in intensive critical units? A systematic review and meta-analysis. *PLoS ONE* **2018**, *13*, e0198669. [CrossRef]
33. Banack, H.R.; Stokes, A. The 'obesity paradox' may not be a paradox at all. *Int. J. Obes.* **2017**, *41*, 1162–1163. [CrossRef] [PubMed]
34. Antonopoulos, A.S.; Tousoulis, D. The molecular mechanisms of obesity paradox. *Cardiovasc. Res.* **2017**, *113*, 1074–1086. [CrossRef] [PubMed]
35. Nakayama, M.; Sato, T.; Miyazaki, M.; Matsushima, M.; Sato, H.; Taguma, Y.; Ito, S. Increased risk of cardiovascular events and mortality among non-diabetic chronic kidney disease patients with hypertensive nephropathy: The Gonryo study. *Hypertens. Res.* **2011**, *34*, 1106–1110. [CrossRef] [PubMed]
36. Kasiske, B.L.; Snyder, J.J.; Gilbertson, D.; Matas, A.J. Diabetes mellitus after kidney transplantation in the United States. *Arab. Archaeol. Epigr.* **2003**, *3*, 178–185. [CrossRef]
37. Cosio, F.G.; Pesavento, T.E.; Kim, S.; Osei, K.; Henry, M.; Ferguson, R.M. Patient survival after renal transplantation: IV. Impact of post-transplant diabetes. *Kidney Int.* **2002**, *62*, 1440–1446. [CrossRef]
38. Kuo, H.-T.; Sampaio, M.S.; Vincenti, F.; Bunnapradist, S. Associations of Pretransplant Diabetes Mellitus, New-Onset Diabetes After Transplant, and Acute Rejection With Transplant Outcomes: An Analysis of the Organ Procurement and Transplant Network/United Network for Organ Sharing (OPTN/UNOS) Database. *Am. J. Kidney Dis.* **2010**, *56*, 1127–1139. [CrossRef]
39. Held, P.J.; Kahan, B.D.; Hunsicker, L.G.; Liska, D.; Wolfe, R.A.; Port, F.K.; Gaylin, D.S.; García, J.R.; Agodoa, L.; Krakauer, H. The Impact of HLA Mismatches on the Survival of First Cadaveric Kidney Transplants. *N. Engl. J. Med.* **1994**, *331*, 765–770. [CrossRef]

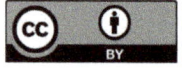

© 2020 by the authors. Licensee MDPI, Basel, Switzerland. This article is an open access article distributed under the terms and conditions of the Creative Commons Attribution (CC BY) license (http://creativecommons.org/licenses/by/4.0/).

MDPI
St. Alban-Anlage 66
4052 Basel
Switzerland
Tel. +41 61 683 77 34
Fax +41 61 302 89 18
www.mdpi.com

Journal of Clinical Medicine Editorial Office
E-mail: jcm@mdpi.com
www.mdpi.com/journal/jcm